Ions in the Brain

Ions in the Brain

Normal Function, Seizures, and Stroke

GEORGE G. SOMJEN
Department of Cell Biology and Neurobiology
Duke University Medical Center

OXFORD
UNIVERSITY PRESS
2004

OXFORD

UNIVERSITY PRESS

Oxford   New York
Auckland   Bangkok   Buenos Aires   Cape Town   Chennai
Dar es Salaam   Delhi   Hong Kong   Istanbul   Karachi   Kolkata
Kuala Lumpur   Madrid   Melbourne   Mexico City   Mumbai   Nairobi
São Paulo   Shanghai   Taipei   Tokyo   Toronto

Published by Oxford University Press, Inc.,
198 Madison Avenue, New York, New York 10016

www.oup.com

Oxford is a registered trademark of Oxford University Press

Library of Congress Cataloging-in-Publication Data
Somjen, George G.
Ions in the brain : normal function, seizures, and stroke /
George G. Somjen.
p. ; cm.   Includes bibliographical references and index.
ISBN 0-19-515171-2 (cloth)
1. Brain—Pathophysiology.   2. Epilepsy—Pathophysiology.
3. Cerebrovascular disease—Pathophysiology.
4. Ion channels.   5. Neurochemistry.
6. Neurotransmission.
I. Title.
[DNLM: 1. Brain—physiopathology.   2. Brain Diseases—physiopathology.
3. Ions—metabolism.
WL 348 S696i 2004]   RC386.2.S66 2004   616.8'047—dc21   2003049867

9 8 7 6 5 4 3 2 1

Printed in the United States of America
on acid-free paper

Illustrations were used in this book from the following sources with permission from their respective publishers and authors:

Figure 1–4: Modified from Schielke and Betz (1992) in *Physiology and Pharmacology of the Blood–Brain Barrier*, p. 23, by permission of Springer Verlag.

Figure 2–2: Modified from Hallows and Knauf (1994) by permission of CRC Press.

Figure 2–9: Modified from Conners et al. (1979), in *Neuroscience Letters*, 13, p. 149, by permission of Elsevier Science.

Figure 2–10: Modified from Joyner and Somjen (1973), *Progress in Neurobiology*, pp. 222–237, by permission of Elsevier Science.

Figure 2–11B: Modified from Cordingley and Somjen (1978), in *Brain Research*, 151, p. 294, by permission of Elsevier Science.

Figure 2–12: Modified from Lothman et al. (1975), in *Brain Research*, 88, p. 21 and 26, by permission of Elsevier Science.

Figure 3–1A: Modified from Hallows and Knauf (1994) by permission of CRC Press.

Figure 4–2: Modified from Balestrino et al. (1986) in *Brain Research*, 377, p. 233, by permission of Elsevier Science.

Figure 4–3: Modified from Somjen and Müller (2000) in *Brain Research*, 885, p. 109, by permission of Elsevier Science.

Figure 4–4: Modified from Dingledine and Somjen (1981) in *Brain Research*, 207, p. 220, by permission of Elsevier Science.

Figure 4–5: Modified from Balestrino et al. (1986) in *Brain Research*, 377, p. 235, by permission of Elsevier Science.

Figure 4–6: Modified from Chebabo et al. (1995) in *Brain Research*, 695, p. 205, by permission of Elsevier Science.

Figure 4–8: Modified from Somjen (1999) in *Brain Research*, 852, p. 194, by permission of Elsevier Science.

Figure 4–9: Modified from Somjen (1999) in *Brain Research*, 852, p. 195, by permission of Elsevier Science.

Figure 4–14: Modifed from Drouin and The (1969) in *Pflügers Archiv*, 313, p. 85, by permission of Springer Verlag.

Figure 5–1A: Reproduced from Engel et al. (1975) in *Brain*, 98, p. 138, by permission of Oxford University Press.

Figure 5–1B: Modified from Avoli and Gloor (1987) in *Encyclopedia of Neuroscience*, p. 401, by permission of Springer Verlag.

Figure 5–1C: Reproduced from Walton (1985) in *Brain's Diseases of the Nervous System*, p. 618, by permission of Oxford University Press.

Figure 5–2: Reproduced from Gastaut and Broughton (1972) in *Epileptic Seizures*, p. 39, courtesy of Charles C. Thomas, Publisher Ltd.

Figure 6–3: Modified from Bliss and Collingridge (1993), by permission of Nature Publishing Group.

Figure 6–4: Modified from Racine (1972) in *Electroencephalography and Clinical Neurophysiology*, 32, pp. 281–294, by permission of Elsevier Science.

Figure 7–1: Modified from Ward (1969) in *Basic Mechanisms of the Epilepsies*, by permission of Lippincott, Williams and Wilkins.

Figure 7–2: Modified from Connors and Gutnick (1990) in *Trends in Neurosciences*, 13, p. 100 and p. 102, by permission of Elsevier Science.

Figure 7–4: Modified from Kostopoulos (2000), in *Clinical Neurophysiology*, 111 (Suppl. 2), S27–S38, by permission of Elsevier Science.

Figure 7–5: Reproduced from Steriade et al. (1990), *Thalamic Oscillations and Signaling*, p. 36, by permission of Wiley and Sons, Inc.

Figure 7–6: Modified from Coulter (1998) in *Epilepsy, a Comprehensive Textbook*, p. 343, by permission of Lippincott, Williams and Wilkins.

Figure 7–7: Modified from Coulter (1998) in *Epilepsy, a Comprehensive Textbook*, p. 347, by permission of Lippincott, Williams and Wilkins.

Figure 7–10: Modified from Wadman et al. (1992) in *Brain Research*, 570, p. 89, by permission of Elsevier Science.

Figure 9–8B: Redrawn after Fertziger and Ranck (1970) in Experimental Neurology, 26, pp. 571–585, by permission of Elsevier Science.

Figure 8–4: Modified from Lothman et al. (1975), in *Brain Research*, 88, p. 29, by permission of Elsevier Science.

Figure 12–2: Modified from Herreras and Somjen, (1993a) in *Brain Research*, 610, p. 284, by permission of Elsevier Science.

Figure 12–4: Modified from Herreras and Somjen, (1993a) in *Brain Research*, 610, p. 287, by permission of Elsevier Science.

Figure 13–6: Modified from Somjen, (1984) in *Brain Research*, 311, p. 187, by permission of Elsevier Science.

Figure 13–7: Modified from Lothman et al. (1975), in *Brain Research*, 88, p. 30, by permission of Elsevier Science.

Figure 14–1: Modified from Czéh et al. (1993) in *Brain Research*, 632, p. 197, by permission of Elsevier Science.

Figure 17–2B: Modified from Brierley and Graham (1984) by permission of Edward Arnold Publisher.

Figure 17–3: Modified from Sick et al. (1987) in *Brain Research*, 418, p. 229, by permission of Elsevier Science.

Figure 17–4: Modified from Balestrino et al. (1989) in *Brain Research*, 497, p. 104, by permission of Elsevier Science.

Figure 18–3: Modified from Young and Somjen (1992) in *Brain Research*, 573, p. 73, by permission of Elsevier Science.

Figure 18–4: Modified from Czéh and Somjen (1990) in *Brain Research*, 527, p. 230, by permission of Elsevier Science.

Figure 19–1: Modified from Czéh et al. (1993) in *Brain Research*, 632, p. 198, by permission of Elsevier Science.

Figure 19–3: Modified from Young et al. (1991) in *Brain Research*, 548, p. 344, by permission of Elsevier Science.

Figure 19–4: Modified from Jing et al. (1991) in *Brain Research*, 557, p. 180, by permission of Elsevier Science.

Figure 19–7: Modified from Mitani et al. (1992), in *Neuroscience*, 48, pp. 307–313, by permission of Elsevier Science.

Figure 19–8: Modified from Mitani et al. (1994), by permission of Blackwell Publishers.

Figure 19–9: Modified from Siesjö et al. (1999) in *Journal of Cerebral Blood Flow and Metabolism*, 19, pp. 19–26, by permission of Lippincott, Williams and Wilkins.

*I dedicate this volume to the young, whose work will reveal
all that still is obscure.*

*And to Amalia
wife, companion, best friend
whose valiant and victorious struggle against
the aftermath of brain surgery brought parts of this text
all too close to home.*

Preface

Neuroscience research has come to a paradoxical stage. During the past century and a half, we have learned a great deal about the elementary processes that govern the functioning of individual neurons and glial cells and of the junctions that connect them. Yet, we must admit that we have no solid theory, not even a conceptual framework, of the workings of the system as a whole. The paradox lies in the fact that, in spite of our bafflement and frustrating inability to understand its normal operation, we have gained considerable insight into the ways in which cerebral function can go wrong. This, the mechanisms of some of the most severe afflictions that can befall the brain, is a main topic of this volume.

In this matter, the pathophysiology of the brain, we might say that a major chapter has just been completed, at least in outline, while the next one is just beginning to be written. We have a good understanding of the way in which cells and groups of cells behave when seized by epileptic fits and of what happens, on a microscopic scale, when brain cells are deprived of oxygen. We have been able to observe the tides of ions flowing into and out of cells, and we have learned how ion fluxes feed back on the ion channels through which they pass. This is the part that is more or less complete, save some missing details, and it is the main topic of this book. The next chapter, dealing with molecular and submolecular processes, which is still in an incipient stage, is touched on but not reviewed in detail.

My goals are twofold. One is to explain to clinicians the errant biophysical mechanisms causing the brain diseases with which they deal in practice. The other is to introduce research scientists who are not medically trained to the problems faced by their clinical colleagues. This is, emphatically, not a clinical manual but an attempt to bridge the gap between research and practice.

There are four parts to this book. Part I reviews the regulation of brain ion levels and describes the influence that altered ion levels can have on the functioning of brain cells. Parts II, III, and IV deal with the pathological conditions in which ion channels and ion fluxes have a decisive role. The data suggest that ion maldistributions created by faulty membrane transport underlie many pathological responses and cause injury to energy-deprived cells. Computer simulations based on data from live tissues support these notions.

The emphasis in the book is on advances made in the past few decades, without neglecting the road by which we have arrived at the present stage of knowledge. A true historical survey cannot be accommodated in this small volume, but each major topic is introduced by highlighting the historical background, casting a backward glance at the origins and the evolution of current ideas. Each chapter concludes with a selection of the major theses developed on the preceding pages. As the reference section attests, the literature is enormous. My list of references is far from complete, and I apologize to all whose contributions are not fully represented. Still, I did attempt to present a comprehensive review of the available data. Where interpretations by experts diverge, I tried to give a balanced summary of contrasting opinions, not concealing my own view, yet allowing the reader to draw informed conclusions that may in some cases differ from my own.

Although this is not an introductory book, there are scattered "notes" intended as summaries of some basic concepts. Other similar notes concern technical matters. Chapter 5 is mainly for readers who are not medically trained. All these materials can be safely skipped by those who already know their content.

Acknowledgments

I am grateful for many suggestions to Michael Müller, who read an early version of the manuscript, and to Joseph LaManna, Steven Schiff, Tom Sick, Dennis Turner, and Wytse Wadman, who read parts.

I would also like to thank copyright holders and authors for permission to use previously published figures.

And, of course, to the staff of Oxford University Press for all their help and expert guidance.

Contents

PART II   CEREBRAL SEIZURES

PART III   SPREADING DEPRESSION OF LEÃO

Illustrations

Abbreviations

ACh	acetylcholine
AChR	acetylcholine receptor. nAChR: nicotinic acetylcholine receptor. mAChR: muscarinic acetylcholine receptor
ACSF	Artificial cerebrospinal fluid
ADP	afterdepolarization, same as DAP: depolarizing afterpotential
AED	antiepileptic drug
AHP	afterhyperpolarization, same as HAP: hyperpolarizing afterpotential
AIF	apoptosis inducing factor
AMPA	α-amino-3-hydroxy-5-methyl-4-isoxalepropionic acid. A selective agonist of one of the three ionotropic glutamate receptors.
4-AP	4-aminopyridine.
ATP	adenosine triphosphate
ATPase	adenosine triphosphatase
AVD	apoptotic volume decrease
BAPTA	1,2-*bis*(o-aminophenosy)ethane-N,N,N',N'-tetraacetic acid. A calcium chelating agent.
BBB	blood–brain barrier

BDNF	brain-derived neurotrophic factor
CBF	cerebral blood flow
CICR	calcium-induced calcium release. The release of Ca^{2+} from sequestration in endoplasmic (or sarcoplasmic) reticulum by way of ryanodine receptor channels into the cytosol under the influence of Ca^{2+} entering through membrane channels from the extracellular medium.
CNS	central nervous system
CSD	Current source density. CSD analysis is the computation of the second spatial derivative of voltage, ideally in three dimensions; in practice it is usually one-dimensional, based on recordings of extracellular voltage by a row of closely spaced microelectrodes.
CSF	cerebrospinal fluid
CsNSC	calcium sensing non-selective cation channel
DAP	depolarizing afterpotential. Same as ADP: afterdepolarization
DG	dentate gyrus. *Gyrus dentatus* according to the international *Nomina Anatomica*. Also known as *fascia dentata* (FD)
DIDS	4,4'-diisothiocyanatostilbene-2,2'-disulfonic acid. An inhibitor of the Cl^-/HCO_3^- exchange transport
DRG	dorsal root ganglion
ECF	extracellular fluid
ECG	electrocardiogram
ECoG	electrocorticogram, an extracellular electrical recording from the neocortex
ECT	electroconvulsive therapy; electroconvulsive shock applied to psychiatric patients
EEG	electroencephalogram; electroencephalography
EPSP	excitatory postsynaptic potential
fEPSP	focally recorded (extracellular, or field) EPSP
EPSC	excitatory postsynaptic current
ER	endoplasmic reticulum
FAD	(oxidized) flavin adenine dinucleotide
FGPE	feline generalized penicillin epilepsy; a model of absence seizures
GABA	γ-aminobutyric acid. $GABA_A$: GABA-A receptor, controlling fast Cl^- (and HCO_3^-)-permeable anion channels; $GABA_B$: GABA-B receptor, controlling slow, second messenger–operated K^+ selective channels

GABAR	GABA receptor
GAERS	genetic absence epilepsy rat from Strasbourg
GDNF	glia-derived nerve growth factor
GEFS+	generalized epilepsy with febrile seizures
GEPR	genetically epilepsy prone rat
GHK	Goldman-Hodgkin-Katz equation
GluR	glutamate receptor
GTCS	generalized tonic-clonic seizures
HAP	hyperpolarizing afterpotential. Same as AHP: afterhyperpolarization
HIF	hypoxia-inducible factor
HSD	hypoxic spreading depression–like depolarization; also known as *anoxic depolarization* (AD)
HVA or I_{HVA}	high-voltage activated current; usually referring collectively to L, N, P, and Q type Ca^{2+} currents
I	current
I_{Na}	Na^+ current
$I_{Na,T}$	transient Na^+ current or "Hodgkin-Huxley-style" Na^+ current
$I_{Na,P}$	persistent (slowly inactivating) Na^+ current
I_K	K^+ currents in general, but sometimes also used for the delayed rectifier type K-current
$I_{K,DR}$	delayed rectifier, persistent K^+ current
$I_{K,A}$ or I_A	A current, transient K^+ current
$I_{Ca,T}$ or I_T	T-current, low voltage activated or transient Ca^{2+} current
$I_{Ca,L}$ or I_L	L-current, lasting or persistent high voltage activated Ca^{2+} current
$I_{Ca,N}$ or I_N	N-type calcium current
$I_{P/Q}$	P-Q type calcium current
iEEG	intracranial EEG
IOS	intrinsic optical signals
IP_3 or $InsP_3$	inositol-1,4,5- trisphosphate
IPSP	inhibitory postsynaptic potential
ISF	interstitial fluid
ISM	ion-selective microelectrode
ISVF	interstitial volume fraction
KA	kainic acid
LTD	long-term depression

LTP	long-term potentiation
LVA or I_{LVA}	Low-voltage activated Ca^{2+} current; synonym for transient or T-current, $I_{Ca,T}$.
MGluR	metabotropic glutamate receptor
MK-801	dizocilpine maleate; A noncompetitive NMDA antagonist drug (in high concentration it is not absolutely selective)
MPT	mitochondrial permeability transition
mPTP	mitochondrial permeability transition pore
MTLE	mesial temporal lobe epilepsy; See also TLE (almost but not quite a synonym)
NAD^+	oxidized nicotinamide adenine dinucleotide
NADH	reduced NAD
NGF	nerve growth factor
NMDA	N-methyl-D-aspartate
NO	nitric oxide
NRT	nucleus reticularis thalami
OGD	oxygen-glucose deprivation; sometimes called *in vitro ischemia*
OVLT	organum vasculosum of the lamina terminals
PDS	paroxysmal depolarizing shift; synonym: depolarizing shift (DS)
PID	peri-infarct depolarization; same as peri-infarct spreading depression wave
Po_2, (P_{CO2})	partial pressure of oxygen (carbon dioxide)
PS	population spike; compound action potential recorded by extracellular electrodes in gray matter
PTP	posttetanic potentiation
PTX	picrotoxin
PTZ	pentylenetetrazol; synonym: pentamethylenetetrazol, metrazol
REM	rapid eye movement, typical of a sleep stage
ROS	reactive oxygen species
RVD	regulatory volume decrease
RVI	regulatory volume increase
SD	spreading depression (also known as *cortical spreading depression, CSD*)
SE	standard error
S.E.M.	standard error of the mean
SERCA	sarcoplasmic/endoplasmic reticulum ATP-fueled calcium pump
SR	sarcoplasmic reticulum

SW	spike-and-wave
SWD	spike-wave discharge
SW	also: slow wave
TCA	tricarboxylic acid
TEA	tetraethylammonium
TEA^+	the TEA cation
TLE	temporal lobe epilepsy; see also MTLE
TMA	tetramethyl-ammonium
TMA^+	the TMA cation
TTX	tetrodotoxin, a highly selective blocker of voltage-gated sodium channels
TUNEL	terminal deoxynucleotidyltransferase-mediated nick-end labeling; A marker of apoptosis
VDAC	voltage-dependent anion channel
VGCC	voltage-gated calcium channel. Synonyms: Voltage-operated calcium channel (VOCC), voltage-controlled
V_m	(trans-) membrane potential
V_o	extracellular voltage
V_I	intracellular voltage, measured against a distant ground potential. $V_m = V_i - V_o$. (V_o may be neglected only if it remains close to zero (= ground) potential). ΔV: shift of voltage

I

IONS AND WATER
IN THE BRAIN

1

The Blood–Brain Barrier

Certain substances injected into the blood stream appear only in trace amounts in the brain and spinal cord, yet others pass unhindered from capillaries into the cerebral tissue. The selective filtering at the interface between blood and central nervous tissue could be thought of as a protective device, except that some of the compounds that are freely admitted into the brain are more harmful than some of those that are excluded. Rather than being a filter, the blood–brain barrier acts as an active regulator of the internal environment of brain cells. For clinicians, the barrier is sometimes a hindrance that must be overcome in order to deliver drugs to their targets in central nervous tissues.

This chapter discusses the nature of the barrier that separates the nervous system from the rest of the organism.

The discovery of the blood–brain barrier

Well before the end of the nineteenth century, Paul Ehrlich and others noticed that certain dyes injected into live animals, a procedure known as *intravital staining* (*Vitalfärbung*), colored all organs except the brain, eyes, peripheral nerves, and testes. Ehrlich also noted the absence of bilirubin in brain tissue in cases of generalized jaundice. He attributed the failure of intravital staining in certain organs to lack of affinity or *attraction* (*Anziehung*) for the dye by the protoplasm of

3

the cells in the spared tissues (Ehrlich, 1885). The idea of a blood–brain barrier (BBB) came later.

Edwin E. Goldmann (1913) is usually credited with the discovery of the BBB, but he acknowledged the precedence of several others, among them Bouffard (1906) and Lewandowsky. Lewandowsky (1900) wrote that "the walls of cerebral capillaries hinder the transit of certain compounds and not that of others." He believed this, because he saw that quite small amounts of sodium ferrocyanide injected into the subarachnoid space of a dog's spinal cord caused violent convulsions, yet much larger amounts injected systemically were well tolerated. This contrasted with the action of strychnine, which caused lethal cramps when administered either way. Lewandowsky was probably the first to postulate a selective barrier to diffusion into the central nervous system (CNS) and certainly the first to attribute a barrier function to a unique specialization of CNS capillaries.

As may be guessed, Lewandovsky's suggestion aroused much skepticism. Ehrlich, among others, forcefully resisted the notion that capillaries in the unstained tissues would differ in some mysterious way from all other capillaries in the body. This lapse of insight need not detract from the overall image of Ehrlich, who, without doubt, was a great figure in the history of experimental biology.

In the end, it was Goldmann who provided convincing proof of a barrier between blood and brain. In his first major work, he gives a detailed account of the distribution of staining in animals that had repeatedly been injected with trypan blue (Goldmann, 1909). Most tissues became vividly blue, with the expected sparing of the central and peripheral nervous systems, the eyes, and the gonads. There is an engaging picture of a live mouse with bright blue ears and tail in this paper. At this time, Goldmann still shared Ehrlich's opinion that the selective staining was due to variations in tissue affinity to the dye. A few years later, however, Goldmann put the idea of selective tissue *affinity* to a critical test. In what has subsequently become known as *Goldmann's second experiment*, he injected the same dye, trypan blue, into the subarachnoid space. Administered in this manner, it stained CNS tissue vividly, proving that, given a chance, brain cells can attract trypan blue as well as all other cells (Goldmann, 1913).

Yet the concept remained controversial for some time, and even in 1962 Tschirgi asked whether the BBB was "fact or fancy" (Tschirgi, 1962). Doubt about a real barrier was revived when early electron micrographs showed little or no space between cellular elements of cortical tissue. This suggested that indicator substances could be excluded from the CNS simply because there was no room for them (Horstmann and Meves, 1959). Later it turned out that the absence of interstitial space was an artifact caused by the swelling of cells during tissue preparation. Van Harreveld found ample space between cell membranes when he fixed the tissue by freeze-substitution after rapidly freezing the cortex (Van Harreveld et al., 1965). Besides, extracellular markers such as inulin, administered by ventriculo-cisternal perfusion, also indicated the existence of a sizable extracellular space (Katzman and Pappius, 1973; Rall et al., 1962). More recent estimates based on the dilution of iontophoretically administered marker ions show an interstitial volume fraction close to 20% of the total volume in most gray matter areas, with extremes of 13% and 30% in some regions (McBain et al., 1990; Nicholson and Syková, 1998). The morphological substrate of the BBB remained uncertain for several decades even to those who accepted its existence. The two chief contenders were the capillary wall and the pericapillary glial tissue. By the end of the nineteenth century, it was well known that the small vessels in brain tissue are surrounded by the endfeet of astrocyte processes. Golgi believed that the glial processes transported nutritional materials from the blood to the nerve cells (for historic references, see Somjen, 1988). Ramón y Cajal (1913), quoting Achúcarro, called the layer of glial endfeet around capillaries and venules *aparatos chupadores*, meaning "suction devices" or "absorption apparatus." To Goldmann (1913) this *gliöse Grenzmembran* (glial limiting membrane) formed by the astrocyte endfeet seemed to be the likely selective filter that could keep certain compounds out of the brain, and several authors concurred (Tschirgi, 1962). The notion of the glial barrier became untenable when it turned out that large molecule tracer substances such as horseradish peroxidase pass unhindered through gaps between the perivascular glial endfeet but are reliably stopped by the layer of endothelium forming the capillary wall (Brightman, 1992; Brightman and Reese, 1969). As we shall see later, even though the astrocyte processes do not form the BBB, they probably do participate in important ways in the regulation of brain ion levels (Abbott, 2002).

Figure 1–1 is a diagram of fluid spaces in and around the brain, and Figure 1–2 is a schematic representation of the BBB and other fluid interfaces.

The blood–brain barrier is not just a hindrance to free diffusion, but an active tissue

Detailed reviews of the BBB and the cerebrospinal fluid (CSF) may be found in several major works (Bradbury, 1979; Davson and Segal, 1996). A brief summary will have to suffice here.

By the 1970s, it was well accepted that in most vertebrates, with the exception of elasmobranch fish, the BBB is formed by the capillary endothelium (Abbott, 1992; Bradbury, 1979). The *tight* endothelial wall of cerebral capillaries differs from the capillaries of most other organs that are either *leaky* or *fenestrated*. The tightness is due to the presence of continuous seams of *tight junctions* between adjacent endothelial cells (Brightman and Reese, 1969; Huber et al., 2001) (Fig. 1–2). Cerebral capillaries are transformed from leaky to tight under the influence of glial cells during embryonic development, and the transformation can be replicated by coculturing astrocytes with endothelial cells (Abbott, 2002; Brightman, 1992;

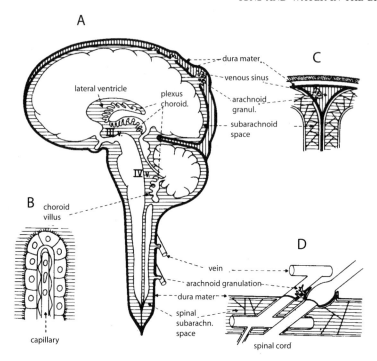

FIGURE 1–1. Schematic representation of fluid spaces in and around the brain (not to scale). A: Overview of cerebrospinal fluid. Cerebrospinal fluid is formed by the choroid villi (B) of the choroid plexuses. It flows from the lateral ventricles into the third ventricle (III.v) and then into the fourth (IV.v.), from where it makes its way through one median and two lateral openings (foramina of Magendie and Luschka, not illustrated) into the subarachnoid spaces around the brain, cerebellum, and spinal cord. It is absorbed from the subarachnoid space into venous blood through the arachnoid granulations (C, D). (Modified from Somjen, 1983.)

Cancilla et al., 1993; Janzer and Raff, 1987). The influence appears to be mutual, for there is also recent evidence that endothelial cells induce differentiation in astrocytes (Mi et al., 2001).

The situation is different at the boundary between blood and CSF in the *choroid plexus*. Here even large molecules can move from the capillary lumen into the tissue of the plexus, but not through the ***ependyma*** that secretes the CSF (Fig. 1–2). Goldmann (1909) remarked on the contrast between the pale brain and the bright blue choroid plexus of his vitally stained mice. Thus the blood–CSF barrier is formed by the choroid ependyma, which has the properties of a secreting epithelium.

Cerebrospinal fluid is continuously secreted in the ***choroid plexuses*** of the four cerebral ventricles (Fig. 1–1). In addition, fluid is moved from the blood into the interstitial space of CNS tissue through the BBB, that is, through the capillary walls.

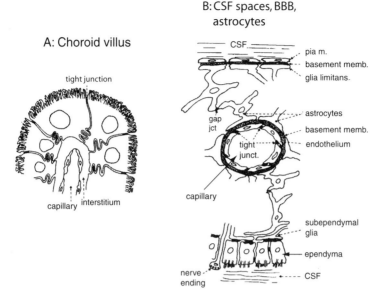

A: Choroid villus

tight junction

capillary interstitium

B: CSF spaces, BBB, astrocytes

CSF

pia m.
basement memb.
glia limitans.

gap jct
astrocytes
basement memb.
tight junct.
endothelium

capillary

subependymal glia
ependyma
nerve ending
CSF

FIGURE 1–2. Schematic representation of the blood–cerebrospinal fluid (CSF) barrier and blood–brain barrier (BBB). A: The capillaries in the core of a choroid villus are lined with leaky endothelium. The secretory cells that line the villus are modified ependymal cells, joined by seams of tight junctions, which seal the blood–CSF barrier. B: In brain tissue, capillaries are lined by a tight endothelium, the endothelial cells being joined by tight junctions. The capillaries are surrounded by endfeet of astrocytes, but the gaps between the glial processes permit free diffusion of solutes. (Not shown are *pericytes* or perivascular cells.) Gap junctions connect astrocytes. The ependymal lining of the cerebral ventricles and the pia mater and basement membrane at the brain surface are permeable to water and to solutes. (Modified from Somjen, 1983.)

Excess interstitial fluid finds its way into the cerebral ventricles seeping through the ependyma lining the ventricular walls, and also along connective tissue in the walls of cerebral vessels into the lymphatic system of the head (Bradbury et al. 1981; Cserr and Patlak, 1992). But while in most of the body interstitial fluid is formed by ultrafiltration, in the CNS it is produced by ***active transport.*** As Betz (1985) and others have emphasized, even though the walls of cerebral capillaries look like endothelia, they behave as secreting epithelia (Fig. 1–4). The product of endothelial secretion is the interstitial fluid of the CNS.

Solute traffic through the BBB is two-way, with ions, nutrients, hormones, and metabolic waste each going their own way. Various compounds can permeate the BBB to varying degrees. Generally speaking, lipid-soluble substances encounter little hindrance, because they can diffuse through the lipid bilayer that forms much of the plasma membrane of the endothelial cells—hence the ease with which many anesthetics such as diethyl ether and chloroform penetrate, and also that favorite of many, ethanol. Water-soluble substances are largely excluded from the lipid bilayer, but some can gain slow access through the tight junctions (Anderson and Van Itallie, 1995). As a general rule, ions are less permeant than nonionized molecules, but none is completely excluded (Fig. 1–3). To supply the brain with what it needs, to rid it of metabolic waste, and to regulate its ion levels, the plasma membrane of the cerebral capillary endothelial cells is endowed with numerous specialized transporters (Fig. 1–4), and it also has unusually large numbers of mitochondria to generate the energy required for active transport (Betz, 1985; Oldendorf et al., 1977; Schielke and Betz, 1992).

Once the controversy about barriers between blood and CSF and between blood and brain had been settled, there was discussion of a barrier between CSF and cerebral interstitium. It turns out that the ependymal lining of the cerebral ventricles permits the diffusion of even large molecules, so that the ventricular CSF communicates freely with the interstitial fluid of the CNS (Cserr, 1974). Thus, in mature mammals, the impenetrable ependyma of the choroid plexus differs markedly from the penetrable lining of the ventricles, even if they share the same name and embryological derivation. Similarly to the ventricular ependyma, the pia mater

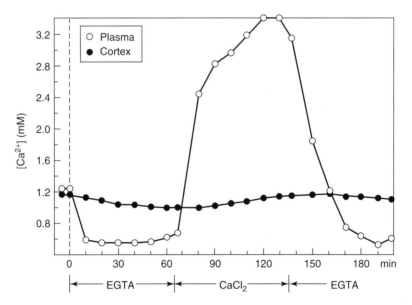

FIGURE 1–3. The blood–brain barrier limits the exchange of ions between blood and cerebral interstitial fluid. Experiment on an anesthetized cat. The arterial plasma Ca^{2+} concentration was measured by a calcium-selective electrode in an extracorporeal loop inserted into one carotid artery. $[Ca^{2+}]_o$ in brain was measured with a calcium-selective microelectrode in the neocortex of the same side. The free calcium level in circulating blood was lowered by the intravenous infusion of ethylene glycol tetraacetic acid (EGTA), and it was raised by the infusion of $CaCl_2$. (From Somjen et al., 1987a.)

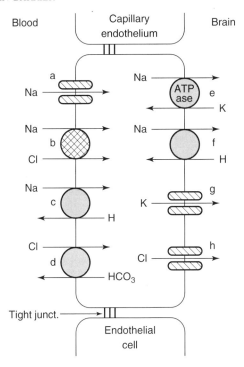

Figure 1–4. Ion transporters in brain capillary endothelial cells. a: Na⁺ channel. b: Na-Cl cotransporter (symport). c: Na/H exchanger (antiport). d: Cl/HCO₃ exchanger. e: 3Na/2K ATPase ion pump. f: Na/H exchanger. g: K⁺ channel. h: Cl⁻ channel. Note that, except for the Na/H exchanger, the transporters on the blood side differ from those on the brain side. Not shown are numerous other transporters, for example for glucose, amino acids, and others, several of which involve coupled movement of Na⁺. (Modified from Schielke and Betz, 1992.)

of the cerebral convexity permits the diffusional exchange of solutes between CSF and interstitial fluid (Bradbury, 1979; Davson and Segal, 1996; Katzman and Pappius, 1973).

Parenteral magnesium therapy: Is the effect central or peripheral?

Magnesium ions scarcely penetrate the BBB (Hilmy and Somjen, 1968; Kemény et al., 1961), yet magnesium sulfate ($MgSO_4$) is used to treat *eclampsia*, a serious complication of pregnancy that can cause epileptiform seizures (Möhnle and Goetz, 2001; Pritchard, 1979). The forerunners of eclampsia are *toxemia* of pregnancy and *preeclampsia*, characterized by hypertension due to renal malfunction. More recently, Mg^{2+} salts have also been recommended for the treatment of stroke (Ames et al., 1995; Muir, 1998). The logic is impeccable, because elevated $[Mg^{2+}]_o$ reduces neuronal excitability by screening surface charges, limits the output of synaptic transmitters by competing with Ca^{2+} at presynaptic terminals, and blocks N-methyl-D-aspartate (NMDA) receptor-mediated ion currents (see Chapter 4, "Calcium and magnesium"). All three effects tend to soothe hyperexcitable brain tissue, counteract the tendency toward seizures, and limit excitotoxic neuron injury, at least in vitro (Kass et al., 1988; Marcoux et al., 1990; Traynelis and Dingledine, 1989; Young et al., 1991). In the past, magnesium salt was also used in laboratories to (supposedly) anesthetize experimental animals, especially rabbits, and at least one report appeared of surgery on three human patients under magnesium anesthesia (Peck and Meltzer, 1916). The question is this: how can the parenteral systemic administration of magnesium salts be effective if ions cannot penetrate the BBB?

Years ago, while investigating the mode of action of various anesthetic agents, I tested the supposedly central effect of intravenous administration of Mg^{2+} salts. At the time, the BBB was still a controversial concept. Disappointingly, intravenous magnesium chloride ($MgCl_2$), while paralyzing neuromuscular junctions, had no effect on spinal reflexes, nor on the electroencephalographic (EEG) activity of the cerebral cortex of cats and rabbits (Somjen, 1967). There appeared to be only one way to determine whether Mg^{2+} salts in fact act as general anesthetics. To settle the issue, we persuaded the chief anesthesiologist at our university hospital to infuse a solution of $MgCl_2$, first into my vein and later into that of my student, Dr. Mehdi Hilmy. As expected, we became partially paralyzed but, not as expected, we remained conscious, if somewhat dazed (Somjen et al., 1966). The total dose each of us received was 1.32 mmol/kg and 1.53 mmol/kg body weight over 44 and 57 minutes, respectively, raising the total plasma magnesium concentration (free + bound) to 12.6 and 12.3 mM, respectively (well above the toxic levels listed by Möhnle and Goetz (2001) and above the intravenous dose recommended for emergencies (Fawcett et al., 1999; Möhnle and Goetz, 2001). We also measured the accumulation of Mg^{2+} in various organs after administering large loads of Mg^{2+} salts to rabbits. The increase in cerebral tissue Mg^{2+} content was quite small compared to that in skeletal muscle or liver tissue (Hilmy and Somjen, 1968). These data on tissue uptake agreed with an earlier report by Kemény, Boldizsár and Pethes (1961), who found that large intravenous infusions of a variety of ions, including Mg^{2+}, raised CSF concentrations only slightly. In recent clinical trials in which plasma levels of Mg^{2+} had doubled after therapeutic doses were administered, the CSF concentration rose only by 20%–25% (Muir, 1998). It is doubtful that elevating cerebral $[Mg^{2+}]_o$ from about 1.0–1.2 mM to 1.2–1.5 mM would profoundly influence neuronal function; indeed, Link et al. (1991) were not able to control metrazol-induced seizures in rats with parenterally administered Mg^{2+}.

To repeat the question: if Mg^{2+} crosses the BBB only sparingly, how does $MgSO_4$ suppress eclampsic convulsions or mitigate neuron injury caused by stroke? There are two possible answers, which are not mutually exclusive. First,

BBB permeability is affected by disease states, and the BBB may be more than normally permeable in the eclampsic state and after stroke (Huber et al., 2001; Tomkins et al., 2001). Second, the therapeutic effect may depend on the peripheral actions of Mg^{2+}. An elevated plasma concentration of this ion relaxes smooth muscle and therefore dilates blood vessels (Viveros and Somjen, 1968), including those in the brain that tend to be in spasm during eclampsia. By its action on vascular smooth muscle, high Mg^{2+} lowers blood pressure, mitigating toxemic hypertension (Pritchard, 1979), and it is also an effective diuretic. These actions are beneficial in controlling eclampsia. A high Mg^{2+} concentration also reduces the tendency toward intravascular blood clotting by competing with Ca^{2+}. Together with cerebral vasodilatation, this can improve blood perfusion in the penumbral area surrounding the ischemic focus in thrombotic or embolic cerebral stroke (see Chapter 19: "The ischemic penumbra . . .") (Saris et al., 2000).

Breaching the barrier

There are small regions in the brain, close to the ventricles, where the capillary endothelium is normally leaky. These are known as ***circumventricular organs*** and include the *area postrema* in the floor of the fourth ventricle, and the *organum vasculosum of the lamina terminalis (OVLT)*. The absence of an effective BBB at these sites is related to the specialized function of the resident neurons. For example, neurons in the OVLT sense the osmolarity of the blood.

The BBB can be breached artificially. Raising the pressure in cerebral capillaries and injecting very strongly hyperosmotic solutions into a cerebral artery can do this. The BBB can also become defective in pathological conditions (Davson and Segal, 1996; Huber et al., 2001)—for example, in very severe, prolonged seizures (status epilepticus) and in prolonged cerebral ischemia. In ischemia, the leakiness is not immediate but takes time to develop (Suzuki et al., 1983a). A leaky BBB is one of the causes of cerebral edema (see Chapter 3, "Three kinds of cerebral edema").

Key points

A diffusion barrier between blood and CNS tissue exists not only in the brain but in all parts of the CNS, including the brain stem and spinal cord, except for a few specialized regions such as the area postrema and the circumventricular organs.

In all mammals and most other vertebrates, the BBB is formed by the capillary endothelium. Brain endothelial cells are welded together by continuous seams of tight junctions that are not present in the capillary linings in most other organs.

The CSF is secreted by the specialized ependymal cell layer in the choroid plexuses. This ependyma is the barrier between blood and CSF. Cerebrospinal fluid is drained in bulk by one-way valve action through arachnoid granulations into venous sinuses.

The ependymal lining of the cerebral ventricles and the pia mater of the CNS surface are permeable to the solutes in CSF.

Lipid-soluble substances diffuse unhindered through the BBB. Water-soluble ions and molecules require specialized transport molecules in the plasma membrane of endothelial cells. Cerebral capillary endothelium resembles secreting epithelial cells in richness of mitochondria and the ability to actively transport key ions. These features, and the tight junctions, set cerebral capillaries apart from capillaries elsewhere. Cerebral capillary endothelium acquires its special properties during embryonal development, induced by pericapillary glial cells.

Magnesium therapy of eclampsia and stroke probably works mainly by causing vasodilatation, lowering blood pressure, inhibiting blood clotting, and increasing diuresis while influencing brain function only slightly, if at all.

Astrocyte endfeet surround cerebral capillaries and have important functions in the exchange of substances between CNS interstitial fluid and capillary blood.

The permeability of the BBB can be artificially increased by raising intracapillary pressure and elevating the osmolarity of the blood. Under certain pathological conditions the BBB breaks down.

2

The Regulation of Brain Ions

The blood–brain barrier stabilizes ion levels in the central nervous system in the face of fluctuations in circulating blood, but even when all is quiet, the composition of the extracellular fluids in the brain differs from that in the rest of the body. The differences may seem small at first sight, but they are functionally important.

This chapter presents an overview of the mechanisms that control ions inside and around brain cells, and the brain-body ion differences.

Ion concentrations and ion activities

Some definitions

It may be useful to define here the terms ***concentration***, ***free ion concentration***, and ***ion activity***. The differences among these terms are best illustrated in the example of calcium (Fig. 2–1). The largest fractions of the univalent ions in physiological fluids are free and active, but this is not the case for Ca^{2+}. Of the total concentration of calcium in blood plasma, much is bound to proteins, while a smaller but still important fraction is bound (chelated) by bicarbonate and even less by phosphate and citrate. The calcium atoms that are so bound are not ionized, because their electric charge is neutralized by the negative charge of the molecules to which they are attached. Less easily grasped is the fact that not all the ions that are *free* are also *active*. The fraction that is free but not active is *screened* electrically by ions of opposite charge without being chemically bound by them. The ratio of active to free ion levels is expressed as the ***activity coefficient***. In physiological fluids the activity coefficient for Na^+ and K^+ is close to unity, but this is not so for Ca^{2+}. Activity is conventionally denoted as a_{ion} — for example, for calcium as a_{Ca} — whereas (total) concentration is c_{Ca} and free ion concentration is usually shown as $[Ca^{2+}]$. The symbol for extracellular concentration is either $[Ca^{2+}]_o$ or $[Ca^{2+}]_e$, and for intracellular cytosolic concentration it is $[Ca^{2+}]_i$ or sometimes $[Ca^{2+}]_c$. Even though only the active fraction exerts biophysical effects, in this book free ion concentrations are almost always given because these are usually measured and reported most often in the literature. This is justified because activity coefficients do not usually change as long as total ion concentration (ionic strength) remains constant; therefore, whenever concentrations change, activities change in equal proportions. In the normal traffic of ions across cell membranes, (total)

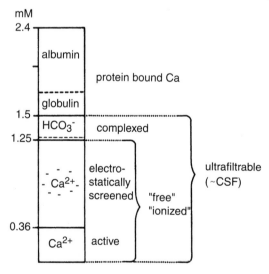

FIGURE 2–1. Calcium fractions in blood plasma. Of the approximately 2.4 mM calcium in plasma, only about half is ionized and even less is active. The complexed and ionized fractions are ultrafiltrable (and dialyzable). (Modified after Siggaard-Andersen et al., 1980, and Somjen et al., 1987a.)

ionic strength remains constant both inside and outside cells. Pathological exceptions occur during salt loss, water poisoning, salt retention, and water deprivation.

The calcium that is bound, chelated, or screened in blood plasma (Fig. 2–1) is in reversible equilibrium with the active fraction. This means that the inactive calcium acts as a ready reserve, available to be released in active form whenever the active fraction declines. Changes in pH, however, do alter the binding of calcium to protein as well as its chelation by small anions, and therefore influence the ratio of the active/bound amount even if there is no change in total calcium concentration. This will be discussed in some detail later (see Chapter 4: "Alkalotic tetany . . ."). Severe protein deficiency also changes the ratio of the free/bound calcium fractions.

Zinc is somewhat similar to calcium in that most of it is bound and little of it is free. Its concentration, however, is some two orders of magnitude lower than that of calcium. It is also different in that some of it is tightly bound to globulin, that is, it is not exchangeable; only the fraction attached to albumin and chelated by small molecules is reversibly bound. The active fraction in plasma is very low, much lower even that that of protons (Takeda, 2001). (For more about Zn^{2+}, see Chapter 19: "*Zinc*, the guardian of neurons or the new villian?".)

Mechanisms of the regulation of ion content and ion concentrations in and around cells

Table 2–1 shows average values of extracellular and intracellular concentrations of the most important ions.

Extracellular Ion Concentrations and Body Content Are Regulated By Coordinated Actions of Internal and External Secreting Organs

Before we consider brain ions, a few remarks concerning the general physiology of ion regulation are in order. Ion concentrations in the circulating blood plasma are kept within physiological limits by the coordinated functions of the gut, kidneys, adrenal and parathyroid glands, and, to lesser degrees, the sweat and salivary glands. The lungs and kidneys are the main regulators of the concentration of protons (i.e., pH). The control mechanisms of the body content and plasma concentrations of sodium, potassium, calcium, chloride, phosphate, and bicarbonate, as well as total osmolarity, are in broad outline well known, yet frequently missing is an insight into the method by which the body measures some of the variables it controls so well. The sensors for blood glucose, oxygen, pH, osmolarity, and perhaps calcium have been identified and the mechanism of their me-

TABLE 2–1. Ion Concentrations in Body Fluids, in Millimoles, and Equilibrium Potentials E_{eq} in Millivolts

	ARTERIAL PLASMA		CSF		CNS NEURON	ASTROCYTE	E_{EQ}, NEURON
	HUMAN	RAT	HUMAN	RAT			
Na^+	150	148	147	152	10	55	72
K^+	4.6	5.3	2.9	3.4	125	80	–100
Ca, total	2.4	3.1	1.14	1.1	0.75		
Ca^{2+}, free	1.4	1.5	1.0	1.0	0.00006		131
pCa					7.22		
Mg, total	0.86	0.8	1.15	1.3	8		
Mg^{2+}, free	0.47	0.44	0.7	0.88	0.5		4.5
H^+	0.000039	0.000032	0.000047	0.00005	0.000057	0.000079	–5.5
pH	7.41	7.5	7.3	7.3	7.24	7.1	
Cl^-	99		119		6.6	30[a]	–77
HCO_3^-	26.8	31	23.3	28	18	11	–6.9

[a]Reported levels range from 6 to 40 mM (see "pH is regulated both inside and outside cells" later in this chapter). CNS, central nervous system; CSF, cerebrospinal fluid.

Sources: Ballanyi, 1995; Bevensee and Boron, 1998; Davson and Segal, 1996; Deitmer, 1995; Forsythe and Redman, 1988; Kaila, 1994; Katzman and Pappius, 1973; Kimelberg, 1990; Rose and Ransom, 1998; Walz, 1995.

tering is generally understood, but we know less about the sensors for the overall average levels of K^+ and Na^+. For ions in general and for Na^+ and Cl^- especially, not only the *concentration* in various body fluids but also the *total content* in the body is relevant and appears to be physiologically regulated. Chronically patho-logical conditions, in which the intake of Na^+ (and Cl^-) exceeds its elimination, cause generalized edema, because the kidneys retain water as they keep osmolar-ity within physiological limits. Conversely, if Na^+ is lost from the system, total extracellular fluid (ECF) volume tends to decrease, threatening circulatory shock. The mechanisms that regulate the total body content of NaCl, and with it the amount of body water, are topics of intensive research, which has not yet yielded clear or simple answers.

Capillaries in most tissues are freely permeable to ions and water, and there-fore local deviations from the normal concentrations in tissues are restored within physiological limits by diffusional exchange between capillary blood and tissue interstitium. By guarding the ionic composition of blood plasma, the systemic regulating mechanisms automatically take care of the interstitial fluid. Equilibra-tion between tissues and capillaries does take time, however, and ion levels can fluctuate transiently and locally as ions move into and out of cells. Such short-lived ion shifts play a part in normal function, but they become especially impor-tant in pathophysiology. For example, abnormal level of $[K^+]_o$ in heart muscle can cause certain cardiac arrhythmias (Carmeliet, 1999).

Intracellular Concentration and Cell Content of Ions Depend on a Balance of Intake and Output

We know less about the mechanisms regulating intracellular ion levels than about those governing extracellular ions. It is quite clear that cytosolic ions are normally also kept within well-defined narrow limits; the question is how the cell "knows" what it contains and how it keeps track of intake and output. Typical values for the most important extra- and intracellular ions are shown in Table 2–1. The ion concentrations inside and outside cells are very different, indicating independent regulation of the two phases. The independence cannot be absolute, of course, for cells depend on the supply of ions and of nutrients on the extracellular milieu. Severe deficiencies or excesses in blood cannot be compensated for and are re-flected in deviations in the ion household of cells. For example, depletion of in-tracellular K^+ is an important factor in chronic hypokalemic syndromes.

At the dawn of biophysics, all ion exchange across cell membranes was thought to happen by diffusion, "downhill" along energetic gradients and driven by elec-trochemical force. With the development of radioactive tracers, it became clear that there is a steady, incessant trickle of Na^+ ions into and K^+ ions out of cells. In order to explain the constancy of ion concentration gradients across cell mem-branes, it became necessary to postulate metabolically fueled *active* transport systems, dubbed *ion pumps*, that move ions "uphill," at a rate equal to but in the direction opposite to the downhill diffusion. This notion was soon confirmed to be correct when it turned out that depriving cells of metabolic energy stops active transport and causes the rundown of transmembrane ion gradients. All cell membranes have a low but finite permeability for all ions, even when at rest. When ion channels are activated, larger ion flows occur. The standing gradients are maintained by active transport, ultimately fueled by the splitting of high-energy phosphate bonds, principally of adenosine triphosphate (ATP). There is thus no truly resting state for a live cell, because work must go on to maintain a steady state. In what we nevertheless call *rest*, that is, the absence of excitation, influx and outflux of each ion must be equal and constant. When excited into activity, the ion content of excitable, contractile, and secretory cells is transiently perturbed, and it must be subsequently restored (see "Keeping ions in their place . . ." below). A small army of researchers has investigated the numerous and varied active and passive transport processes of cell membranes (Fig. 2–2). Yet while the membrane machinery that moves ions has gradually become clear, we are at a loss to explain

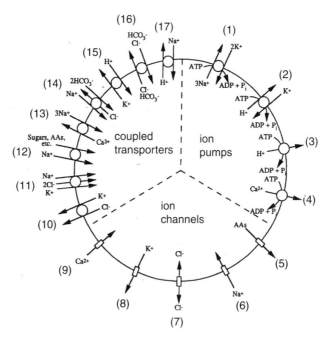

FIGURE 2–2. Summary of the better-known ion transporters. Note that most ion pumps and ion channels transport unequal charges and are therefore electrogenic. Of the coupled transporters, some are electrically neutral (e.g., 10, 11) but others are electrogenic (e.g., 13). Number 12 represents a class of secondary active cotransporters coupling Na^+ to glucose or amino acids (AAs), which, in most cases, are also electrogenic. ADP: adenosine diphosphate. ATP: adenosine triphosphate. (Modified from Hallows and Knauf, 1994.)

how the cell knows how many ions it has, let alone how many it needs for normal function. (For historical reviews, see Eccles, 1953; Katz, 1966.)

Channels, pumps and transporters

Ions move across membranes through ion ***channels***, ***ion pumps***, and ***transporters*** (Fig. 2–2). Channels are large, integral membrane proteins constructed of several subunits, with a central water-filled pore through which the ions can move (Hille, 2001). The channel can flicker between the open and closed states, controlled either by the transmembrane voltage (***voltage-gated*** or *voltage-operated* channels, VOCCs) or by chemical agents or *ligands* (from the Latin *ligare*, meaning "to bind") (***ligand-gated*** or *ligand-operated* channels). Most channels have a selectivity filter that allows easy passage of one or a few ion species and keeps out others. ***Transporters*** are transmembrane molecules that bind the transported ion or another particle on one side of the membrane, move it across, and release it on the other side. Some transporters enable the movement of one ion and are called ***uniporters***. In others, two or more ions move in the same direction; these are called ***symporters*** or *coupled* or *cotransporters*. Still others enable the exchange of one or more ions going one way against (an)other ion(s) moving in the opposite direction; these are ***antiporters***, ***exchangers***, or *countertransporters*. If equal charges are exchanged or if equal charges of opposite sign move in the same direction, the transport is ***electrically neutral***. If the flux of charges is not balanced, the transport creates a current and it is then called ***electrogenic*** or *rheogenic*. Transporters have no pore. They have a limited binding capacity; therefore, they are ***saturable***. Transporters are either *passive*, which means that the flux is energetically downhill, enabled by the electrochemical gradient of the transported particle, or *active* if the transporter has its own power supply. Only active transport can move ions against a gradient; without it, standing gradients cannot be maintained (except for the trivial case of impermeable barriers). ***Primary active transport*** is fueled by ***ATP*** and, in all well-characterized examples, a component of the transporter molecular complex itself functions as an ATPase. Like an internal combustion engine and unlike a steam engine, such ***ion pumps*** produce the power and the motion (work) within the same structure, because as they split ATP, they provide the energy required to move ions uphill against an electrochemical gradient (see below: "The 3Na/2K triphosphatase . . ." and "Intracellular calcium ion activity . . ."). By contrast, ***secondary active transport*** relies on energy stored in standing ion gradients, most often that of Na^+. As Na^+ moves downhill into a cell, it can drag with it another ion or compound in cotransport . Glucose and amino acids are taken into cells this way. Alternatively, the inflow of Na^+ can energize the extrusion of another ion of molecule in *countertransport*. For example,

Ca^{2+} and H^+ are in many cases moved across barriers by secondary active countertransport (see below). One can visualize this mechanism as a waterwheel, the downhill flow of Na^+ being the river that moves the wheel, which raises the Ca^{2+} or H^+ up the hill. The waterwheel of the exchange transporters is kept moving only as long as the Na^+ gradient across the plasma membrane is kept up, and this requires the continuous work of primary active ion pumps, mainly the *3Na/2K ATPase* pump. When oxygen or oxidizable substrate is in short supply, the ATP-dependent ion pumps slow or stop, and soon, so do the Na-dependent *secondary active* transporters and exchangers.

Total Solute Content Determines Cell Volume

As we have seen, besides the *concentration* of individual ions, the total ion *content* of cells is also important because ions represent the bulk of the osmotically active particles in cells. Two general physiological rules are valid, with only few exceptions: *First*, in the tissues of mammals, the osmolarity of intracellular fluid is at equilibrium with that of extracellular fluid. *Second*, the majority of the osmotically active particles are ions. The ion content of the cell is therefore the most important determinant of cell volume, because changes in ion content cause osmotically driven water flow.

A number of amendments modify these general concepts. In certain conditions, nonionized compounds become osmotically important, for example in *diabetes mellitus* (elevated glucose and ketone bodies) or in *renal failure* (blood urea nitrogen). Also, osmotic equilibration is not instantaneous, because water cannot flow through membranes at infinite speed. Water permeability—known in the specialized literature as *hydraulic conductivity*—of plasma membranes varies among cells. Synthetic pure lipid bilayers have low conductivity, and most of the water moving across living cell membranes flows through channels built of protein. Specialized water channel proteins are known as *aquaporins*, and the cells that secrete or absorb large quantities of water are well endowed with them. For our narrative, it is worthwhile to mention that astrocytes and ependymal cells are rich in aquaporins, while neurons are apparently deficient (Nagelhus et al., 1996; Nielsen et al., 1997). Water also seeps through ion channels, but the magnitude of water flow through this route is a matter for debate. Osmotic effects will be discussed in greater detail later (Chapter 3).

The 3Na/2K Adenosine Triphosphatase Exchange Pump Does Most of
the Active Work of Ion Transport Across Cell Membranes

A major breakthrough in biophysics occurred when Skou (1975) demonstrated the existence of a membrane constituent macromolecule that splits ATP into adenine diphosphate (ADP) plus inorganic phosphate and uses the energy so obtained to transport sodium out of and potassium into the cell. Known variously as membrane *Na/K ATPase* or the *Na/K pump*, it is present in all cell plasma membranes. The molecular structure is now known. It is a constituent membrane protein composed of four subunits, and it exists in a number of related variants (Läuger, 1991).

Skou (1975) determined that the Na/K adenosine triphosphatase (ATPase) moves 3 Na^+ ions outward against 2 K^+ ions inward across the cell membrane. Moving unequal charges creates a voltage, and therefore the 3Na/2K pump is *electrogenic* (or *rheogenic*, meaning current-generating). As it removes three positive charges from the cell while admitting just two, this pump makes the cell's interior more negative than the outside. The voltage generated by the ion pump is added to the larger fraction of the membrane potential, which is created by the unequal distribution and unequal rate of diffusion of ions. The main fraction of the membrane potential is defined by the well-known **Goldman-Hodgkin-Katz (GHK)** equation (Eq. 4–1) (Hille, 2001). It is the ATP-fueled pump that maintains the unequal distribution. Even though the pump voltage is a small fraction of the total membrane potential, it is important because it makes the cytoplasm *more negative* than it would be under purely passive conditions. The 3Na/2K ion pump is stimulated to greater effort whenever $[Na^+]_i$ and (or) $[K^+]_o$ increase. Following the firing of an action potential, and especially after a burst of several impulses, the pump works harder to restore resting ion levels. The electrogenic voltage of the pump contributes to the ***afterhyperpolarization***, merging its voltage into that generated by the current through K^+ channels.

Charge balance in the face of unequal membrane transport

This should be well remembered: Think of an imaginary demon straddling the membrane of a resting neuron, counting all the Na^+ and K^+ ions crossing. This demon would find that exactly the same number of each ion moves in and out per unit time as needed in order to maintain a steady state. This is true even though the 3Na/2K ATPase ion pump moves more Na^+ out than it moves K^+ in, and the K^+ conductance of the resting membrane is greater than its Na^+ conductance. Unequal membrane transports are counterbalanced by opposite, unequal driving forces. The extra voltage generated by the 3Na/2K pump heightens the force pulling K^+ into the cell and lessens the force pushing Na^+ out, so that in the steady state of rest the passive and active fluxes balance exactly. If this were not so, there would be no rest.

A different theoretical question concerns the balance of the charges within the bulk solutions. As a practical matter, the sum of all positive charges and the sum of all negative charges within the cytosol are taken to be equal, even though there is a standing voltage across the plasma membrane. Strictly speaking, this cannot be true; the transmembrane voltage implies some inequality of positive and negative charges. The discrepancy (excess of negatively charged ions over positive ones inside cells) is, however, so small as to be negligible. Of course, this applies only to a resting cell; excitation sends momentarily unbalanced ion surges across membranes.

Keeping K^+ inside and Na^+ out is not the only accomplishment of the 3Na/2K ATPase pump. The transmembrane gradient of Na^+ established by the pump represents stored potential energy that is utilized by a number of transport processes to move materials uphill against a chemical gradient (see "Channels, pumps, and transporters" above). It is estimated that half of all the energy turnover in brain tissue is spent fueling the 3Na/2K ATPase pump (Ames, 2000).

Intracellular Calcium Ion Activity Is Kept Low by Several Coordinated Buffer and Transport Mechanisms

As shown in Table 2–1, the gradient of free Ca^{2+} concentrations across cell membranes is huge, amounting to four orders of magnitude. Add to this the negative intracellular potential, and it is clear that a tremendous force is pulling Ca^{2+} into cells. The resting permeability of the plasma membranes of most neurons for Ca^{2+} is quite low, so that in spite of the powerful driving force, few calcium ions manage to slip through it. Central neurons are equipped with highly selective voltage- and ligand-gated Ca^{2+} channels that open only when adequately stimulated and then permit accurately dosed, short-lived but intensive inward surges. There are exceptions among neurons that have calcium channels with a sizable *window* region near the resting potential (see Chapter 7: "The roles of thalamic relay nuclei") (Williams et al., 1997). This specialization endows these cells with unusual responses (Hughes et al., 1999).

Most of the calcium inside cells is either bound to specialized *calcium-binding proteins* or sequestered inside organelles, most notably the *endoplasmic reticulum (ER)* (*sarcoplasmic reticulum [SR]* in muscle), as well as the *Golgi apparatus* and *mitochondria* (Meech and Thomas, 1980; Rizzuto, 2001, Kann et al., 2003), leaving only a small fraction in free solution (Fig. 2–3). The total concentration of intracellular calcium, defined as all of the calcium in the cell divided by the cell volume, is several orders of magnitude higher than the free ionized concentration (Table 2–1). The proteins and the organelles together act as a buffer system, preventing excessive increase of $[Ca^{2+}]_i$. Calcium-binding proteins are, however, not mere passive buffers of $[Ca^{2+}]_i$. Three of these—*calmodulin, calbindin*, and *calcineurin*—interact with each other, as well as with regulatory and structural proteins, and are active participants in cell function. When calmodulin-binding sites are occupied by calcium, they react with calmodulin-binding-proteins, which then catalyze further reactions or activate early genes in the nucleus (Shibasaki et al., 2002; Solà et al., 2001).

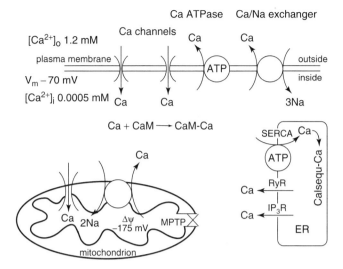

FIGURE 2–3. Schematic representation of the regulation of calcium in cells. CaM: calmodulin. $\Delta\Psi$: mitochondrial membrane potential (relative to cytoplasm). mPTP: mitochondrial permeability transition port, normally closed. ER: endoplasmic reticulum. SERCA: sarcoplasmic/endoplasmic reticulum adenosine triphosphate (ATP)–fueled calcium pump. Calsequ: calsequestrin, one of the calcium-binding proteins in ER. RyR: ryanodine receptor–controlled calcium channel. IP$_3$R: inositol-1,4,5- trisphosphate–controlled calcium channel. For further description see the section "Intracellular calcium activity is kept low . . ."

The membranes of mitochondria and of ER have channels and pumps moving Ca^{2+} both into and out of the organelles (Babcock and Hille, 1998; Duchen, 1999; Gunter et al., 1994; Rose and Konnerth, 2001b) (Fig. 2–3). Calcium itself is a signal for a variety of cell functions, and the ER membrane contains receptors that respond to second messenger signals that induce the release of Ca^{2+} from storage into the cytosol, as required (Blaustein and Golovina, 2001; Rose and Konnerth, 2001b). Calmodulin also interacts with other intracellular components, depending on its saturation with calcium. Changes in calcium-binding proteins appear to be involved in epileptogenesis and other pathological conditions (Freund et al., 1990a; Maglóczky et al., 1997; Mattson et al., 1991; Morris et al., 1995; Picone et al., 1989; Shibasaki et al., 2002; Sloviter, 1989; Solá et al., 2001).

When calcium channels in the plasma membrane open, they let in a measured quantity of Ca^{2+}, which, once it performs its job, is rapidly removed from cytosol by binding to buffer proteins and uptake into organelles. Yet, however good the buffers, excess Ca^{2+} that found its way into cells must eventually be extruded into the external milieu. Among a number of known calcium transporters, two are present in the plasma membrane of most cells and seem to do most of the work of keeping $[Ca^{2+}]_i$ low. ***Calcium-activated ATPase*** pumps Ca^{2+} outward using energy provided by the splitting of ATP. This is a uniporter; it carries no ion other than Ca^{2+}, and therefore it generates an outward current, aiding membrane polarization (negative inside). However, the magnitude of the current is small, as it involves few ions compared to the 3Na/2K ATPase ion pump.

Another mechanism moving Ca^{2+} across the membrane is the ***3Na/Ca exchanger***, the properties of which have been reviewed by Blaustein and Lederer (1999). This is an *antiporter*. It moves Na^+ ions inward against Ca^{2+} outward and is therefore an example of secondary active transport, because it uses the energy stored in the standing transmembrane gradient of Na^+ ions to power the uphill transport of Ca^{2+} (like the mill powered by a waterwheel, described above; see "Channels, pumps, and transporters"). Neuronal 3Na/Ca exchangers are preferentially located in the plasma membrane near junctional ER elements, in presynaptic terminals and dendritic spines, sites where membrane traffic of Ca^{2+} is functionally most important. Even though ATP does not supply the energy for the work, its presence is obligatory because it activates the exchanger by phosphorylating a critical site. The proportions of the transported ions apparently vary in different membranes, but in central neurons 3 Na^+ ions are exchanged against one Ca^{2+}. Since Ca^{2+} carries two charges compared to the one on Na^+, the turnover represents a three to two excess in the direction in which Na^+ is moving. This makes the transport electrogenic (or rheogenic, similarly to the 3Na/2K ion pump) (Fig. 2–4). Under normal conditions, the exchanger moves Ca^{2+} out of the cell at the expense of allowing Na^+ to flow in, creating a net inward electric current, but if either the membrane potential or the ion gradients shift by much, the "wheel" can also turn in reverse. The direction of the transport is determined by the difference between the prevailing membrane potential and the equilibrium potential of the exchanger (Fig. 2–4). Blaustein and Lederer (1999) define this equilibrium as follows:

$$E_{Na/Ca} = 3E_{Na} - 2E_{Ca} \qquad (2-1)$$

where $E_{Na/Ca}$ is the equilibrium potential of the 3Na/2Ca exchanger and E_{Na} and E_{Ca} are the equilibrium potentials of the ions, Na^+ and Ca^{2+}.

In healthy resting neurons, where E_{Na} is about +72 mV and E_{Ca} is between +116 and +134 mV (see Table 2–1), $E_{Na/Ca}$ is between –50 and –19 mV. Figure 2–4 illustrates the operation of the exchanger for the situation in which $E_{Na/Ca}$, is near –50 mV. As long as the membrane potential, V_m, is more negative than $E_{Na/Ca}$, Na^+ is flowing inward and Ca^{2+} is being driven outward, and the exchanger is said to operate in the *Ca^{2+} exit mode*. When V_m levels become more positive than –50 mV, the fluxes reverse and the exchanger works in the *Ca^{2+} entry mode*. At rest with V_m at around –70 mV, the exchanger works in the Ca^{2+} exit mode, but if the cell depolarizes, the exchanger becomes an avenue for Ca^{2+} uptake. This happens briefly with each action potential. Besides V_m, the direction of the exchange also depends on the distribution of both Na^+ and Ca^{2+}, because these values set

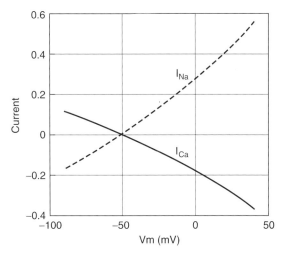

FIGURE 2–4. The voltage dependence of the Na^+ and Ca^{2+} currents of the 3Na/Ca exchanger. Computation based on $E_{Na/Ca}$ near –50 mV. When V_m is more negative than $E_{Na/Ca}$, Na^+ flows into and Ca^{2+} is driven out of the cell: Ca exit mode. When V_m is more positive than $E_{Na/Ca}$, the exchanger reverses to the Ca entry mode. See also the section "Intracellular calcium activity is kept low . . ." and Figures 2–3 and 16–4B. (Computation by H. Kager, unpublished.)

the equilibrium levels. Whenever the cell takes up extra Na^+, reducing the $[Na^+]_o/[Na^+]_i$ ratio, the curves of Figure 2–4 shift in the negative direction, limiting the driving force of Ca^{2+} and enhancing that of Na^+. On the other hand, intake of Ca^{2+}, which reduces $[Ca^{2+}]_o/[Ca^{2+}]_i$, shifts the current-voltage curves in the positive direction, boosting Ca^{2+} extrusion (or limiting its influx if the exchanger has already worked in the calcium-entry mode). When both ratios decrease, as happens during seizures, spreading depression (SD), and hypoxia, there is a tug of war. Using values likely to occur during such pathophysiological processes, one can calculate the outcome. During seizures $E_{Na/Ca}$ probably shifts to a slightly more positive level, aiding Ca^{2+} extrusion, but during hypoxic SD-like depolarization the reverse happens (see Fig. 16–4). The combined effect of V_m depolarizing (becoming more positive) and $E_{Na/Ca}$ becoming more negative at first hinders the outward transport of Ca^{2+}; then the exchanger turns in the "wrong" direction. The pump and the also activated Ca^{2+} channels then let a great deal of Ca^{2+} accumulate in the cell, aggravating the deleterious effect of hypoxia and stroke (Chapter 19). Reversal of the Na/Ca exchanger has been blamed for the accumulation of Ca^{2+} not only in neurons but also in hypoxic glial cells and optic nerve axons (Stys et al., 1992b).

To complicate matters, in many cells, including some neurons, there are other transporters next to the Na/Ca exchanger. These include a ***Ca/H antiporter***, which transports Ca^{2+} out and H^+ in, or the reverse, depending on prevailing conditions, influencing not only $[Ca^{2+}]_i$ but also cell pH (Trapp et al., 1996).

Ca²⁺ Acts as a Second Messenger for Numerous Cell Functions

Acting as a signal, $[Ca^{2+}]_i$ can momentarily increase from its resting level of 0.05–0.1 μM to several micromoles. The source is either calcium entering from the outside through its channels in the plasma membrane or calcium released from sequestration in intracellular stores into the cytosol. For the latter purpose, the ER membrane contains two classes of channels, both controlled by intracellular messenger compounds. One is opened by *inositol triphosphate* (*IP₃* or InsP₃); the other is sensitive to *ryanodine* and is opened by Ca^{2+} itself, mediating *calcium-induced calcium release* (*CICR*) (Rizzuto, 2001) (Fig. 2–3). Since calcium is supposed to be the signal for a multitude of different functions, how can the cell know which task it is supposed to perform? This matter is addressed in recent reviews by Blaustein and Golovina (2001) and Bootman et al. (2001). The answer lies in the concept of *microdomains* or, some say, nanodomains. Physiological elevation of $[Ca^{2+}]_i$ is not uniform, but is limited to the parts of the cell where it is needed. Nonuniform distribution is achieved because the release of calcium from the ER, as well as its admission through membrane channels from the outside, are limited in time as well as in space. Diffusion of calcium inside cells is (relatively) slow, and on their way from one microregion to another, Ca^{2+} ions can be intercepted by calcium-binding proteins and by uptake into the ER/SR or mitochondria. As a result, for a short time, there can be steep concentration gradients within the cell, the concentration being much higher in strategic locations where it is needed than the average in the cell as a whole. High-resolution imaging has in fact revealed such gradients (Tank et al., 1988). In microdomains or nanodomains, Ca^{2+} concentrations can momentarily reach tens or even hundreds of micromoles (Augustine, 2001). The gates in the surface membrane of the ER that open to let the Ca^{2+} enter are usually close to and linked to the target organelle or macromolecular complex whose function the Ca^{2+} is called on to stimulate.

When $[Ca^{2+}]_i$ remains high for an extended period throughout the cell, it can activate processes that damage the cell (Schanne et al., 1979; reviewed by Duchen, 2000; see also Figs. 19–3, 19–4, and 19–9, and Chapter 19). The calcium-binding proteins that are supposed to buffer $[Ca^{2+}]_i$ should exert a protective effect against calcium-induced cell injury. Diligent attempts to demonstrate such protection have so far been disappointing (Bouilleret et al., 2000; Freund et al., 1990a; Sloviter, 1989). Endoplasmic reticulum and, to a lesser degree, mitochondria do, however, have undisputed roles in protecting neurons against excessive rise of $[Ca^{2+}]_i$ (Duchen, 1999).

A simplified diagram of the main transport pathways for calcium is presented in Figure 2–3. In reality, the ER forms an extensive, continuous intracellular network with a large, folded, continuous membrane surface suitable for the rapid, localized transfer of Ca^{2+} between cytosol and the interior of the ER (Berridge, 1998). The intrareticular calcium-binding proteins *calsequestrin* and *calreticulin* enable the storage of (relatively) large amounts of calcium (in the millimolar range) without raising the free concentration inside the ER excessively (Fill and Copello, 2002; Rizzuto, 2001). Uptake into and release from the ER can occur in very restricted regions, preventing excessive fluctuation of the overall average cytosol concentration. There are sites where the ER forms functional complexes with the plasma membrane, where the two membranes come into close proximity, called *plasmERosomes* by Blaustein and Golovina (2001). The ***IP₃*** receptor-operated channel is controlled by the intracellular messenger ***inositol triphosphate***, which is formed at the plasma membrane in a complex mechanism, stimulated among others by ***metabotropic glutamate receptors (mGluR)***. The IP_3 receptor is also modulated by the prevailing cytosolic Ca^{2+} level (Blaustein and Golovina, 2001). Unlike IP_3, ***ryanodine*** is not a physiological stimulus of the channel; it is a plant poison originally intended for use as an insecticide. The natural stimulus for the ryanodine receptor channel is cytosolic calcium. (There may be others, not yet disclosed.) Its opening underlies calcium-induced calcium release. In skeletal muscle it serves *excitation-contraction coupling* (Fill and Copello, 2002). In astrocytes it is the probable mediator of ***calcium waves*** (Finkbeiner, 1992) (see Chapter 14: "In spreading depression neurons lead and glial cells follow").

Not all is clear concerning calcium traffic across the mitochondrial membrane (Duchen, 2000). Mitochondria are enveloped in a double membrane. Most of the relevant transporters are in the inner membrane. The high ***mitochondrial membrane potential*** ($\Delta\psi_{mit}$), some 150–200 mV negative relative to the cytosol, drives the uptake of Ca^{2+} through a channel-like pathway. Ca^{2+} is removed from mitochondria by complex systems involving exchanges with Na^+ and H^+, which can be either electrogenic or electrically neutral. Under normal conditions, the intramitochondrial calcium concentration ($[Ca]_{mit}$) is in the micromolar range, which is very high compared to cytosol but lower than expected from electrochemical equilibrium and much lower than in ER (Duchen, 2000; Rutter et al., 1998). The ***mitochondrial permeability transition pore (mPTP)*** is a normally closed pathway, which is not selective and which opens (or is being assembled from scattered subunits) on depolarization of the mitochondrial membrane. When the mitochondrial membrane potential collapses, for example in anoxic conditions, Ca^{2+} can flood the cytosol through the open mPTP. If this condition persists, it heralds the demise of the cell. Conversely, excessive accumulation of Ca^{2+} in cytosol can open the mPTP and drive an overload of Ca^{2+} into the mitochondria, which can impair mitochondrial function and cause failure of energy metabolism and eventual cell death (Duchen, 2000; Zoratti and Szabó, 1995; see also Figs. 19–8 and 19–9).

Not shown in Figure 2–3 is the phenomenon of ***store-dependent*** or ***capacitative calcium entry***. When intracellular calcium stores are empty, the uptake into cells is stimulated. The significance of this for neuronal function is uncertain.

*Can Calmodulin and Mitochondria Regulate Calcium and
at the Same Time Be Regulated by It?*

Here is a problem. If calmodulin and mitochondria act as buffers of excess calcium, then they are obligated to bind and store an excess, regardless of their other functions. On the other hand, experimental data indicate that Ca^{2+} stimulates the functions of calmodulin and mitochondria (Shibasaki et al., 2002; Kann et al., 2003). The two statements are compatible only if there is an unalterable and obligatory link between the amount of Ca^{2+} stored and its signaling function. For instance, consider the case of Ca^{2+} uptake due to excitation. The facts are these: with each action potential a certain amount of Ca^{2+} enters the neuron. Some of the Ca^{2+} is taken into mitochondria, which are then stimulated to make more ATP. Extra ATP is indeed needed to fuel the ion pumps that restore ion balance in the wake of each nerve impulse. If this were the purpose of mitochondrial Ca^{2+}, then, to dose the Ca^{2+} signal properly, the rising ATP level would have to inhibit Ca^{2+} intake into mitochondria. Such inhibition would act as negative feedback regulation. In this scenario, storage would be incidental and subordinate to the role of Ca^{2+} as a signal.

The exact relationship between Ca^{2+} storage and the role of Ca^{2+} as an intracellular signal is not explicitly addressed in recent reviews (that I have found). Given the large amount of work devoted to intracellular calcium, clear answers should be forthcoming soon.

Meanwhile, at least the role of the ER is not ambiguous. It appears to be a bona fide storage organ, keeping large amounts of calcium safe and dispensing measured amounts to the cytosol as needed.

Intracellular Ionized Magnesium Is Maintained Below Equilibrium Level

Magnesium has been called the body's *orphan ion* because there seems to be no specific endocrine mechanism regulating its plasma concentration (reviews by Fawcett et al., 1999; Saris et al., 2000). It is also a bit of an orphan in cell biology research, for less is known about its cellular regulation than about the other major ions. In part this is so because measuring its intracellular concentration is more difficult than measuring that of calcium. It is well known that about 90% of the magnesium contained in cells is in bound form. The concentration of free, active ionized Mg^{2+} in cytosol is not very different from that in the extracellular fluids of the CNS (see Table 2–1). Nevertheless, because of the negative-inside V_m, the intracellular concentration is far from equilibrium. The main outward transport that keeps $[Mg^{2+}]_i$ low is believed to be either an electrogenic 3Na/Mg exchange transport, similar to the 3Na/Ca exchanger (Flatman, 1991), or an electrically neutral 2Na/Mg antiport (Saris et al., 2000). The existence of an ATP-dependent active magnesium pump is not definitely established.

pH is regulated both inside and outside cells

Introductory textbooks usually state that the pH of body fluids is tightly regulated and normally does not vary by more than 0.1 up or down. This statement is true, but it is also a bit misleading. Small changes in pH mean relatively large changes in proton concentration, [H+], as is emphasized in Figure 2–5, which illustrates the two ways of expressing the same variable. The normal range of arterial pH_o is 7.36–7.44 (Katzman and Pappius, 1973), which corresponds to a proton concentration of approximately 36.3–43.7 nM. Reckoned as a fraction of the average, the concentration of $[H^+]_o$ is in fact more variable than that of $[Na^+]_o$, the limits of which are stated in textbooks to be 136–145 mM.

The regulation of blood plasma pH is the task of the kidneys and the lungs working in concert. For a detailed treatment of pH regulation the reader is referred to standard physiology texts. Here the main points will be reviewed briefly. The kidneys can set the blood plasma pH by varying the excretion of H+ ions and of bicarbonate. To compensate for acidosis, excretion of the former increases while excretion of the latter decreases. In alkalosis the compensatory adjustments are reversed. Respiration can influence blood pH by varying the amount of CO_2 released from the body. Carbon dioxide itself is not an acid but carbonic acid is, and CO_2 reacts with water to form H_2CO_3, which in turn dissociates in large part into H+ and HCO_3^- according to the **Henderson-Hasselbalch** equation:

$$CO_2 + H_2O \leftrightarrows H_2CO_3 \leftrightarrows H^+ + HCO_3^- \tag{2–2}$$

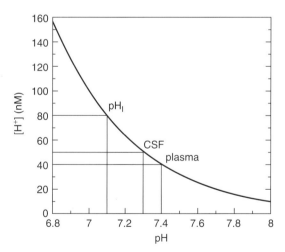

FIGURE 2–5. Interpreting the pH scale: proton concentration versus pH. The indicated levels for arterial blood plasma, cerebrospinal fluid (CSF), and neuron cytosol pH_i are approximate average values. See also Table 2–1.

The reactions are reversible, so that changes in $[CO_2]$ automatically change $[H^+]$ as well. *Carbonic anhydrase* speeds the dissociation of carbonic acid in either direction. Carbon dioxide is often referred to as a *volatile acid*, which is an incorrect but easy shorthand way to describe its behavior in water. Acidosis stimulates alveolar respiration, causing breathing to become both deeper and faster, a pattern known as *Kussmaul's* breathing. The concentration of H^+ in the blood is being sensed by two sets of receptors that influence breathing: the *arterial chemoreceptors* of the carotid and aortic bodies and the *brain stem respiratory region* within the CNS itself. Neurons in the respiratory areas respond to H^+ in ways that differs from those of other neurons (see Chapter 4: "Acidosis generally lowers and alkalosis boosts excitability"). Increased alveolar ventilation reduces $[CO_2]$ in blood and drives the reaction in the alkaline direction. Thus, against an acid load, hyperventilation is the first line of defense. Conversely, when the lungs are diseased, failing respiration causes the buildup of CO_2, resulting in the condition known as *respiratory acidosis*. Up to certain limits, healthy kidneys can compensate for respiratory acidosis and alkalosis. Removal of H^+ and retention of HCO_3^- by the kidneys is slower than the reflexive stimulation of respiration but, in the long run, renal compensation is more effective in restoring physiological conditions.

Besides respiratory acidosis, clinicians recognize so-called *metabolic acidosis*. This term refers not only to metabolic pathology such as severe diabetes or liver failure, but also to any acid load that is not due to impaired respiration. The important distinction is this: In respiratory acidosis, CO_2 and therefore the HCO_3^- concentration in blood is *increased*. In metabolic acidosis, respiration is stimulated and both CO_2 and HCO_3^- are *decreased*. Brain pH is influenced by CO_2, and the importance of this difference will become clear as we proceed to discuss the effect of pH on brain function (see below: "The sometimes paradoxical behavior of brain pH", and Chapter 4: "Acidosis generally lowers and alkalosis boosts excitability").

Cells regulate their internal pH by transport mechanisms built into the plasma membrane (Fig. 2–6) (Bevensee and Boron, 1998; Bonnet et al., 2000; Chesler, 1990). The main task of these membrane transporters is to get rid of excess acid or to accumulate base. There are at least three reasons for the ever-present need to remove acid from cells. First, at rest in healthy brain cells, $[H^+]_i$ is lower (i.e., pH is higher) than would be expected for passive distribution. The equilibrium potential of H^+ is about -5.5 mV in neurons, much positive relative to the resting membrane potential (Table 2–1). Therefore, the membrane potential continually attracts H^+ ions into the cell, so that the steady state can be maintained only by matching the inward leakage by constant active or uphill regulatory outward transport. By contrast, the problem with the distribution of bicarbonate is the opposite: there is more HCO_3^- inside cells than there would be at equilibrium. If the resulting tendency of bicarbonate to move outward proceeded unchecked, it too would increase acidity. The

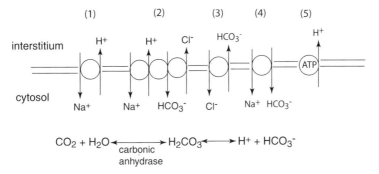

FIGURE 2–6. Schematic representation of transporters mediating pH regulation in neurons and glial cells. (1) Na/H exchanger. (2) Na/H/HCO₃/Cl exchanger. (3) Cl/HCO₃ exchanger. (4) Na-HCO₃⁻ cotransport. (5) Proton adenosine triphosphatase (ATPase) pump. Much of the carbonic anhydrase in brain is bound to membranes and myelin and, of the soluble fraction, glial cells contain more than do neurons.

final reason mandating regulatory outward transport of acid (or inward transport of alkali) is that CO_2 and organic acid residues are generated all the time by metabolism, creating new H^+ ions. Less commonly, under certain pathological conditions, cells must defend themselves against an overload of alkali.

A variety of membrane channels, transporters, and pumps that keep pH_i within limits have been identified. Different cell types contain different sets of these. Brief descriptions of those that are most important in brain cells follow. Figure 2–6 is a diagram of the chief regulators of pH. The numbers in parentheses over the figure refer to the following numbered paragraphs:

1. The **Na/H exchanger** moves Na^+ into and H^+ out of cells. The energy for this exchange is derived from the inwardly directed electrochemical gradient of Na^+. The gradient of H^+ is also inward and would, if it could, move the transport in the opposite direction, but the driving force acting on H^+ is weaker than that on Na^+, and Na^+ wins the tug of war.

2. A sodium-dependent **bicarbonate/chloride exchanger** couples the inflow of Na^+ plus HCO_3^- to the outward transport of H^+ plus Cl^-. The net effect is an increase in pH. Like the Na/H exchanger, the Na/HCO₃/Cl/H exchanger is driven by the transmembrane Na^+ gradient.

3. A sodium-independent **Cl/HCO₃ exchanger** exists in many but not all brain cells. Unlike the former two, this transporter increases acidity (decreases pH) as it moves Cl^- into and HCO_3^- out of cells. The main driving force is the outwardly directed electrochemical gradient of HCO_3^-. There is almost as much bicarbonate inside as outside cells (Table 2–1), and therefore the negative intracellular potential exerts an outward drive on this negatively charged ion. The electrochemical position of the counter-ion, Cl^-, varies among cells.

The level for glial cells varies from a $[Cl^-]_i$ of more than 35 mM in astrocytes, according to Walz (2002), to only 6 mM, according to Ballanyi et al. (1987). In oligodendrocytes Cl^- is passively distributed, and Walz (2002) suggests that perhaps the cells recorded by Ballanyi et al. (1987) were in fact oligocytes, not astrocytes. Astrocytes have γ-aminobutyric acid-A (GABA$_A$) and glycine-sensitive channels and respond with depolarization when these channels are opened. In contrast to glial cells, in most brain and spinal cord neurons an outwardly transporting Cl pump reduces $[Cl^-]_i$ below the level expected for passive distribution. This sets the equilibrium potential for Cl^- at a more negative level than the resting potential, and it enables the inward flow of Cl^- that is mainly responsible for the hyperpolarizing inhibitory postsynaptic potentials (IPSPs) of inhibitory synapses operated by GABA$_A$ and glycine receptors. In dorsal root ganglion cells, and during the first few days of life of rodents, in all brain neurons there is, however, more Cl^- than is required for equilibrium, and activation of GABA$_A$ receptor–operated channels depolarizes these membranes (Ben-Ari et al., 1997).

4. In glial cells but not in neurons there is also coupled ***Na-HCO$_3$ cotransport***, moving both ions inward and alkalinizing the cytosol. The two ions do not, however, move in tandem. In different cells, either two or three bicarbonate ions move with each sodium ion and the transport is therefore electrogenic. Moreover, the transporter is activated by depolarization, and it appears to be responsible for the *depolarization-induced alkalinization* of glial cells (Deitmer, 1995).

5. Finally, the existence of an *ATP-fueled **H$^+$ pump*** has been suggested by some data on certain cells. This is a vacuolar transport mechanism resembling exocytosis.

These five pH-regulating membrane transports are shown schematically in Figure 2–6. For reviews, see Bevensee and Boron (1998), Bonnet et al. (2000), and Chesler (1990).

The independent regulation of the ion levels in the central nervous system

Ion concentrations in the extracellular fluids (ECF) of the brain and the spinal cord differ in small but functionally important ways from those in most of the body. In the CNS, ECF include both the cerebrospinal fluid (CSF) and the interstitial fluids (ISF). By and large, the two are similar, although the composition of CSF changes slightly as it flows from its sources in the choroid plexuses through the lateral ventricles and the third and fourth ventricles and into the arachnoid spaces of the brain and spinal cord (Davson and Segal, 1996). Also, as in heart and skeletal muscles, locally and transiently ISF can be modified by the activity of neurons.

The overall similarity of cerebral ISF and CSF is maintained by the relatively free exchange between them. Unlike the "tight" endothelial lining of capillaries separating blood from cerebral ISF, the ependyma and the pia mater that form the boundary layers between ISF and CSF are permeable to the solutes in these fluids.

As Table 2–1 shows, there is less K^+ but more protons and Mg^{2+} in brain ECF than in blood plasma or systemic ISF. The 1 to 1.5 mM difference in $[K^+]_o$ between brain and blood may seem unimpressive, but in relative terms this amounts to 30%–50%. Similarly, the typical plasma pH of 7.4 seems very close to the 7.3 typically measured in CSF, but when pH is converted to proton concentration, the $[H^+]_o$ of 40 nM (blood) versus 60 nM (brain) represents a functionally significant gradient across the BBB. The lower $[K^+]_o$ and the higher $[H^+]_o$ and $[Mg^{2+}]_o$ modulate the excitability of central neurons (Chapter 4). Calcium has a special position. It is often stated that CSF has much less calcium than does blood plasma. This, however, refers mainly to total calcium. The difference in concentration of free ionized calcium is smaller on the two sides of the BBB. The difference in total Ca is due mainly to the presence of calcium bound to albumin in plasma (Fig. 2–1); in CSF and in brain ISF there are normally only trace amounts of protein.

Rapidly raising or lowering ion levels in the blood of experimental animals has only a slight effect on CSF or brain ISF concentrations (Fig. 1–3; Hilmy and Somjen, 1968; Kemény et al., 1961). This cannot be said of the clinically more relevant conditions lasting for days, weeks, or months. Low-calcium tetany, that is, the excessive irritability resulting from severe rickets or hypoparathyroidism, has both peripheral and central components. Similarly, in chronic hypo- or hyperkalemia, the brain suffers along with the rest of the body, although the deviation in CSF and cerebral ISF usually remains less severe even in long-lasting disease. It must be said, then, that while the BBB protects the brain well against sudden, short-lived fluctuations in blood ion composition, this protection is not absolute, and it becomes less effective the longer the disturbance lasts.

Like cell membranes, the BBB is not completely impervious to ions. Radioactive tracer measurements have long shown that ions such as Na^+ and K^+ do cross the barrier, even if much more slowly than through capillary walls elsewhere in the body. Some of the leaking of small molecules, ions, and water itself into and out of the brain probably occurs through the tight junctions between endothelial cells rather than through the cells (Gloor et al., 2001; Huber et al., 2001). This is true even though tight junctions form continuous and complete seams that seal the gaps among the endothelial cells in CNS capillaries. Few rules in biology are absolute, and so it is with the tightness of the BBB. Moreover, there is evidence that the permeability of the tight junctions can vary with conditions, such as elevated capillary pressure, and it may be under humoral control (Huber et al., 2001).

Unlike leaks, most of the regulated traffic is through the endothelial cells rather than through the tight junctions between them. In addition to the transporters shown in Figure 1–4, endothelial cells are endowed with *aquaporin water channels* (Nielsen et al., 1995; Nico et al., 2001). The diffusion of water through the BBB is influenced, among other things, by *catecholamines* and *vasopressin* (Hartmann et al., 1980; Raichle, 1980). Besides the membrane transporters, water and solutes may also be carried through endothelial cells by the traffic of vesicles, a process called *transcytosis*.

Realization that ions can and do diffuse across the BBB has led to the inevitable conclusion that ion levels in brain ECF must be maintained by active transport. For each ion slipping across the barrier by diffusion, another one of the same species is transported in the opposite direction. At first, this idea was difficult to accept because under the light microscope cerebral endothelial cells do not seem different from those in capillaries elsewhere. It seemed strange that these thin cells could behave like the secreting epithelia in kidneys and glands. As it turned out, the endothelial cells of CNS capillaries are well endowed with mitochondria that can supply the energy for the work of transporting ions against electrochemical gradients (Oldendorf et al., 1977).

It is generally accepted that the endothelium of cerebral and spinal capillaries is functionally equivalent to secreting epithelia. In common with secretory cells, the plasma membranes of the cerebral endothelial cells contain a rich variety of ion channels, pumps, and other transport proteins (Fig. 1–4). There is a different collection of these transporters at the two faces of the capillary wall, the side of the blood and the side of the brain. This too is similar to the situation of secreting epithelial cells, which typically contain different sets of channels and transporters at their basolateral and apical membranes. Such polarization is necessary for the well-controlled and directed transcellular traffic of solutes (Schielke and Betz, 1992).

The special case of the blood–brain pH gradient

The pH of CSF is more acid than that of arterial blood plasma by about 0.1 pH, [H^+] being higher and [HCO_3^-] lower (Table 2–1). The pH of CSF is, however, closer to that of venous than to that of arterial blood pH (Katzman and Pappius, 1973). The blood–CSF difference has been attributed to the presence of the barriers at the choroid plexus and at the cerebral capillary endothelium (Davson and Segal, 1996; Held et al., 1964). It seems fair to conclude that the extracellular environment of the brain is regulated to contain more H^+ than the ECF of other tissues. This is functionally significant, for as we shall see shortly (Chapter 4: "Acidosis generally lowers and alkalosis boosts excitability"), a slightly acidic pH has a calming effect on neurons and synapses.

Regulation of cerebral pH_o at the BBB is believed to be the work of the endo-thelial cells and of the ependymal cells of the choroid plexuses that secrete the CSF. Whether the transport is active or passive has been a matter of controversy (Fencl, 1971; Messeter and Siesjö, 1971). It is now clear that, as with other ions, the maintenance of an H^+ concentration gradient is achieved by the coordinated action of pumps and transporters in the membranes of the cells that form the BBB and the blood–CSF barriers, which do contain transporters for H^+, HCO_3^-, and Cl^- (Fig. 1–4). There is an electrical potential difference of a few millivolts be-tween blood and CSF and a similar voltage difference between blood and cere-bral ISF. The *positive voltage in CSF* relative to blood accentuates the acid–base disequilibrium, since the electrical force tends to drive cerebral $[H^+]_o$ lower and $[HCO_3^-]_o$ higher, the opposite of what we find. The standing electrical potential is altered when the pH of the blood changes (Fig. 4–11). It has been suggested that the voltage shift is generated by electrogenic ion transport associated with the regulation of pH across the BBB (Held et al., 1964). Confusing the issue is the fact that in rats, rabbits, dogs, and goats, blood acidosis causes a positive shift of the brain potential relative to its normal level (Fig. 4–11), but in cats and mon-keys the shift is negative (Balestrino and Somjen, 1988; Besson et al., 1971; Car-penter et al., 1974; Held et al., 1964; Speckmann and Caspers, 1969). To solve the mystery, Besson et al. (1971) suggested that the positive voltage shift is gen-erated by ion transport across the BBB but the negative shift is a streaming arti-fact due to increased cerebral blood flow. In some species the former and in others the latter effect would dominate. Whatever their origin, the slow voltage shifts as-sociated with pH changes must be reckoned with in clinical electrophysiology. This is not a factor in routine EEG, for standard EEG machines do not register DC volt-ages, but they do in DC-coupled recordings of slow potentials, sometimes favored in psychophysiological and specialized clinical studies (Voipio et al., 2003).

The acidity of the CSF and the cerebral ISF compared to the pH of blood plasma is, according to Messeter and Siesjö (1971), the consequence of metabolic acid production. In brain slices in vitro, the pH_o of the interstitial fluid is more acid by about 0.1 pH than the standard bath fluid (Schiff and Somjen, 1987). There is, of course, no specialized barrier to diffusion at the cut surface of such tissue slices, and this raises the question whether in the brain there is also a pH gradient be-tween ISF and CSF. This need not be the case. Tissue slices are at a disadvantage because they lack capillary circulation, and the distance for diffusional exchange between the depth of the slice and the bath in vitro is greater than that between interstitium and capillary in situ. Besides, the standard bathing fluids do not con-tain carbonic anhydrase. Both of these differences favor accumulation of CO_2 in the slice, and this may be the cause of the relative acidosis. Measurements of in-terstitial pH_o in intact brains reveal values around 7.3, which is similar to the av-erage pH of CSF in mammals, suggesting near-equilibrium conditions between ISF and CSF.

The Sometimes Paradoxical Behavior of Brain pH

During respiratory acidosis and alkalosis, the pH of blood and of brain CSF and ISF change in the same sense, if not necessarily to the same degree. This is expected, since CO_2 is lipid soluble and penetrates the BBB without hindrance. The CO_2 concentration in CNS changes in the same direction as it does in blood when respiration is either insufficient or exaggerated. An excess of CO_2 combines with water according to the Henderson-Hasselbalch reaction (Eq. 2–2), so it creates excess H^+ ions. In contrast to respiratory changes, during metabolic pH disturbances the pH in brain can shift in the opposite direction than the rest of the body, at least initially (Sørensen, 1971). In metabolic acidosis the CSF (and the cerebral ISF) can become alkaline, and in metabolic alkalosis they can become acid. The explanation for this paradox is as follows. The primary "metabolic" pH disturbance is, by definition, an altered strong ion difference in the blood, and lipid-insoluble strong acids and bases do not penetrate the BBB. The first line of defense against metabolic acidosis is hyperventilation, stimulated by the arterial chemoreceptors. Hyperventilation drives CO_2 out of the system and lowers the P_{CO_2} level in blood. Since CO_2 does diffuse freely through the cerebral capillary walls, the low blood P_{CO_2} level also forces the cerebral CO_2 concentration down and makes the brain paradoxically alkalotic. The reverse occurs during acute metabolic alkalosis, because alveolar ventilation is reduced, CO_2 accumulates in the system, and the excess CO_2 makes the brain more acidic. For a similar reason, caution is recommended in treating diabetic acidosis by rapid infusion of an alkaline solution, lest it inhibits respiration, causing accumulation of CO_2 and paradoxical central acidosis with worsening coma (Posner and Plum, 1967).

In spite of the free passage of CO_2 through the BBB, sudden respiratory pH changes are milder in ISF of the cerebral cortex than in blood. The direction of the change is the same, but the magnitude is not. It appears that ion regulation can partially counteract the effect of CO_2 on the pH in the brain. This is probably achieved by transferring some of the excess protons generated by the excess CO_2 from the brain into the capillary blood and by transporting base in the reverse direction. The paradoxical shifts occur only during rapid metabolic pH changes; in chronic conditions, brain tissue compensates more effectively for metabolic pH deviations than does the rest of the body (Fencl, 1971). The situation is different when the primary metabolic malfunction is within the brain itself, for example during cerebral hypoxia, in which case cerebral tissue acidosis can be marked (Fig. 19–10).

In the specialized region of the medulla oblongata that controls respiration, neurons respond acutely to arterial CO_2-dependent pH changes. It is the pH of the ISF and not molecular CO_2 that stimulates respiratory neurons (Fencl et al. 1966). Excitation by acid is an intrinsic property of these respiratory neurons; it requires no synaptic input (Dean et al., 1990). In this respect, respiratory neurons differ from most other neurons, which are typically depressed by low pH.

Glial cells regulate ion levels in several ways

As we have seen, overall ion levels in the CSF and brain ISF are set by active transport across the blood–CSF barrier and the BBB. The ependyma of the choroid plexus and the endothelium of cerebral capillaries are the active participants in this regulation. These regulatory mechanisms maintain the global ion composition of cerebral fluids, but they cannot completely prevent localized ion concentration changes in the narrow interstitial spaces. Neuronal activity requires ions to move across neuron membranes, and such flux perturbs the composition of the extracellular environment of the very cells that are active.

Neuroglia and the Regulation of Potassium

The fate of potassium in the CNS demands special attention. K^+ ions are discharged from excited neurons with each action potential, each excitatory postsynaptic potential (EPSP), and each $GABA_B$ receptor–controlled IPSP. Loss of K^+ to the extracellular medium raises the $[K^+]_o/[K^+]_i$ ratio, and this can profoundly influence neuron function. Since $[K^+]_o$ in brain is between 2.9 and 3.4 mM, while $[K^+]_i$ is about 125 mM, and since the fractional volume of neurons is several times greater than that of the interstitial space, it is easy to see that neuronal activity will raise $[K^+]_o$ more than it lowers $[K^+]_i$. The likely magnitude of the fluctuations of $[K^+]_o$ during normal and pathological events, and their significance for cerebral function, will be reviewed below in the section "Neuronal activity alters ion distributions" below and in Chapter 4. Here we consider the mechanisms that guard against undue increases in $[K^+]_o$ that could, if unrestrained, impair cerebral function.

Excess $[K^+]_o$ can be restored to normal by the cooperation of several mechanisms (Fig. 2–7).

1. The K^+ that is lost must, of course, be *recaptured by the neurons* that lost them; this is the job of the ATP-fueled membrane 3Na/2K pump. During low-frequency firing, which is the most common normal mode of operation of neurons, the pump can almost keep up with outflow. Following each spike, all or most of the K^+ that has been released is returned to the neuron. $[K^+]_o$ is raised only slightly and transiently (Fig. 2–9).

2. During high-frequency firing, other processes must intervene. If the high level of excitation is confined to a small focal area, then the excess K^+ that is not immediately recaptured can *diffuse* into the quieter region surrounding the active focus. This can dissipate the excess if and only if a sufficiently steep gradient of the K^+ concentration has been created; it will not work if $[K^+]_o$ is elevated in a large volume of tissue. Once the high rate of firing has abated, as the stimulated 3Na/2K ATPase pumps K^+ back into the previously excited neurons, a local low-$[K^+]_o$ region (sink) is created, described as the *postexcitation undershoot* (Heinemann and Lux, 1975). Into this sink the

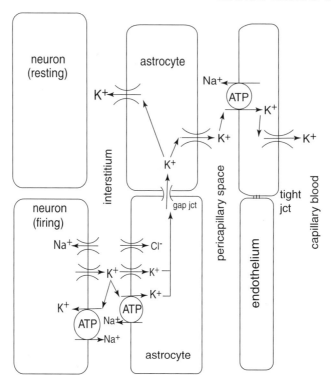

FIGURE 2–7. Diagram of the fate of K⁺ released from neurons. K⁺ is released through voltage-gated channels with action potentials and synaptic potentials. Normally, most of it is recaptured by the 3Na/2K ATPase ion pump. If retrieval does not keep pace with release, much of the excess is mopped up by glial cells, in part by the glial 3Na/2K adenosine triphosphatase (ATPase), and in part driven by an electrochemical gradient through K⁺ channels. Cl⁻ is forced into the astrocyte with K⁺ to maintain charge balance (see also Fig. 2–8). Excess K⁺ can move from one glial cell into its neighbors through gap junctions, causing K⁺ release through K⁺ channels at some distance into the interstitial (spatial buffering) or pericapillary spaces (siphoning). From the pericapillary space endothelial cells can take it up by the 3Na/2K ATPase ion pump and then discharge it into the capillary (see also Fig. 1–4).

dispersed K⁺ ions can return, and both $[K^+]_o$ and $[K^+]_i$ recover to baseline levels.

3. When neuronal reuptake and extracellular diffusion fail to keep $[K^+]_o$ within safe limits, glial cells, mainly *astrocytes*, probably in cooperation with capillary endothelium, are believed to play an important part in the regulation of $[K^+]_o$ (Fig. 2–7). More than one biophysical process cooperates in the glial regulation of $[K^+]_o$. *Net uptake* of K⁺ from ISF into glial cells can occur, either (a) *passively*, in combination with anions, chiefly Cl⁻, or (b) by active uptake in exchange against Na⁺ by the *glial Na/K pump*, stimulated by elevated

$[K^+]_o$. The net uptake of K^+ raises the glial intracellular K^+ concentration (Fig. 2–8). (c) *Spatial buffering* through the network of glial cells coupled by gap junctions achieves dispersion and dilution of K^+ ions more efficiently than diffusion through the interstitial spaces. A special case of spatial dispersion is the *siphoning* of K^+ ions, a goal-directed transport from perineuronal interstitium to the pericapillary spaces, from which it can be dumped into the bloodstream. We shall consider each of these glial mechanisms in turn, but first we must discuss the basic biophysical properties of glial cells. Simplified diagrams are presented in Figures 2–7 and 2–10.

As shown by Ransom et al. (1995), excess $[K^+]_o$ in the optic nerve is cleared by a combination of temperature-sensitive and temperature-insensitive processes. The former are presumably active, that is, energy-demanding, while the latter are passive, energy-dissipating mechanisms. Adenosine triphosphate–fueled active uptake by both glial and axonal membrane ion pumps appears to play a part (Ransom et al., 2000).

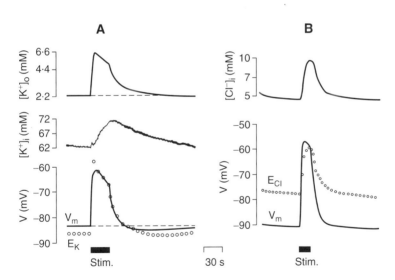

FIGURE 2–8. Uptake of K^+ and Cl^- in glial cells. Recordings from glial cells in guinea pig hippocampal tissue slices. Responses are evoked by repetitive afferent stimulation (Stim.). **A:** Extracellular and intracellular K^+ concentrations ($[K^+]_o$ and $[K^+]_i$ recorded with ion-selective microelectrodes, membrane potential (V_m), and calculated equilibrium potential of K^+ (E_K, open circles) during repetitive afferent stimulation. E_K is slightly more negative than V_m during rest , briefly overshoots V_m at the height of the depolarization, and coincides closely with V_m during repolarization. **B:** Rise of glial intracellular Cl^- concentration in another glial cell. The calculated large difference between E_{Cl} and V_m in the resting state is probably overestimated. (Modified from Ballanyi et al., 1987.)

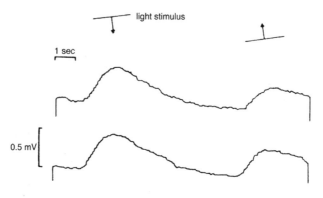

FIGURE 2–9. Responses of $[K^+]_o$ in visual cortex to visual stimulation. Recording with an ion-selective microelectrode from area 17 in the cerebral cortex of an anesthetized cat. Stimulation is produced by moving a slit of light, projected on a screen in front of the animal, first down and then up through the receptive field of the recorded cortical cell column. The calibration bar of 0.5 mV represents a change of slightly less than 0.5 mM from the resting $[K^+]_o$, which was between 3.0 and 3.5 mM. (Modified from Connors et al., 1979.)

The Plasma Membrane of Astrocytes

In a series of experiments by now considered classics, Kuffler and associates defined for the first time the most striking biophysical properties of glial cells as they found them in the nervous system of leeches and mudpuppies (Kuffler, 1967; Kuffler and Nicholls, 1966). Glial plasma membranes are highly selectively permeable to K^+ and for this reason behave as *good potassium electrodes*. This means that the glial membrane potential very nearly equals the equilibrium potential for K^+ ions, and when $[K^+]_o$, changes, the glial membrane potential follows, as predicted by the Nernst equation (Eq. 4–2). The other ions have very little influence. In this respect glial cells differ from neurons, the membrane potential of which is significantly influenced by Na^+ (Fig. 4–1). Glial cells do not generate action potentials or other active electrical signals. Also, glial cells are linked one to another by low-resistance pathways formed by *gap junctions*, so that a population of glial cells acts as a *functional and electrical syncytium*. In true syncytia the cytoplasm of adjacent cells is continuous, without intervening membranes. Myocardium and astrocyte networks behave electrically as if they were syncytia, but since their cells are bounded by complete membranes, they are only quasi-syncytia.

The original studies were done on glial tissue in invertebrates and amphibia, but their salient properties have been confirmed in glial cells in mammalian CNS in situ (reviewed by Somjen, 1975, 1995). Like those of invertebrates, the mem-

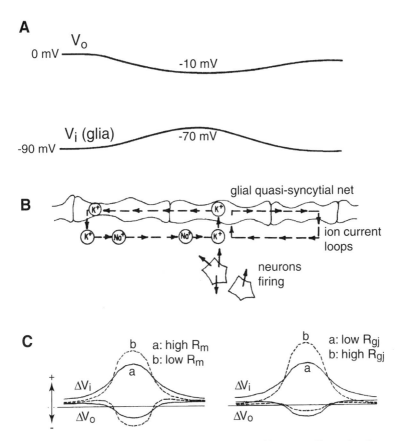

Figure 2–10. Simplified model of the voltages generated by a one-dimensional array of glial cells, acting as a spatial buffer of K$^+$. **A:** Schematic (conceptual) representation of spatial profiles of voltage shifts outside (V$_o$), and inside glial cells (V$_i$), referred to a fixed ground potential. **B:** A row of model glial cells that could generate a voltage shifts similar to those shown in **A**. The glial cells are joined by gap junctions that are permeable to K$^+$. At the center of the row, K$^+$ has been released from neurons. Excess K$^+$ taken into the central glial cell initiates a current through gap junctions into its neighbors, causing the discharge of K$^+$ into the extracellular medium at some distance. The current loop is completed by Na$^+$ flowing in the extracellular medium from the "resting" toward the "excited" region. **C:** Computed voltage shifts inside and outside (ΔV$_i$ and ΔV$_o$) generated by a row of connected model cells. High membrane resistance (R$_m$) and low gap junction resistance (R$_{gj}$) make the ΔV shifts to spread farther. (Computation by R. Joyner. Modified from Joyner and Somjen, 1973.)

branes of mammalian glial cells appeared to be inexcitable and behaved passively. *Inexcitable* means that no action potentials could be triggered, and *passivity* implies that the membrane resistance was *ohmic*, that is, it remained constant or changed only very slightly over a wide range of membrane voltages, not only under a *current clamp* (Ransom and Goldring, 1973b; Somjen, 1970) but also under a whole-cell voltage clamp (Czéh et al., 1992; Somjen, 1995) (Fig. 14–2). It is true that, at first, it seemed that, unlike those in leech ganglia, mammalian astrocytes were less than perfect K^+ electrodes. The plot of glial intracellular potential against $[K^+]_o$ was linear, but the slope of the function was less steep then expected from the Nernst equation (Ransom and Goldring, 1973a). As pointed out by the authors, however, in these trials the K^+-induced depolarization may have been underestimated for technical reasons. Indeed, when the true membrane potential was measured by referring intracellular voltage to the extracellular voltage measured in the vicinity of the cell instead of a distant, constant ground reference potential, the $\Delta V_m/\log[K^+]_o$ slope did follow the Nernst relationship (Lothman and Somjen, 1975), as it also did in glial cells in tissue slices from both human and guinea pig brains (Picker et al., 1981). The similarity of the trajectories of glial depolarization and the rise of $[K^+]_o$ evoked by afferent nerve stimulation is illustrated in Figure 2–11A. The membrane of cultured *oligodendrocytes* also behaved as a "good potassium electrode," provided that the rise of both $[K^+]_i$ and $[K^+]_o$, was taken into account (Kettenmann et al., 1983).

Like glia in leech and frog, the glial cells of the mammalian brain were found coupled to one another through gap junctions (Gutnick et al., 1981). The coupling could be demonstrated electrically and also by the spread of an indicator dye that, when injected into one cell, also stained its neighbors (termed *dye coupling*). The electrical continuity enables the generation of extracellular current loops over long distances, which could underlie slow extracellular potential shifts (Figs. 2–10, 2–11A). Indeed, there is a three-way linear correlation among sustained potential shifts, glial depolarization, and the increase of $[K^+]_o$, all three recorded simultaneously and evoked by prolonged stimulation of synaptically transmitted responses in mammalian spinal cord or neocortex (Lothman and Somjen, 1975; Lothman et al., 1975). This strongly suggests that at least a major component of these voltages is generated by glial tissue (Cordingley and Somjen, 1978; Dietzel et al., 1989; Ransom, 1974; Somjen, 1973, 1993) (Figs. 2–10, 2–11).

Channels in Glial Membranes

In these early studies, the glial membrane was considered to behave passively and the highly selective K^+ conductance was assumed to be, as it were, an ion leak. It was a major surprise when reports began to appear of the existence of voltage-gated K^+, Na^+, and Ca^{2+} currents in glial cells (Barres et al., 1990; Kimelberg et al., 1993; MacVicar, 1984; Sontheimer and Ritchie, 1995). In the words of Duffy and

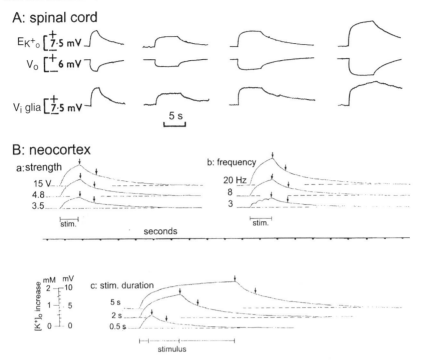

FIGURE 2–11. Extracellular K^+ concentration, voltage shifts, and glial intracellular potentials during repetitive electrical stimulation of afferent fibers. **A:** Recording in spinal gray matter. Simultaneous recordings of the ion-selective electrode ($E_{K,o}$) and extracellular potential (V_o) with a double-barreled ion-selective electrode and glial intracellular potential (V_i) with an attached intracellular electrode. Each triplet of traces was recorded during stimulation at varying stimulus strengths and durations. Intracellular penetration was lost at the end of the last V_i recording. **B:** Recording from the neocortex of an anesthetized cat. Trains of surface stimulations were at varied strength (a), frequency (b), and train duration (c). (**A:** modfied from Lothman and Somjen, 1975; **B:** modified from Cordingley and Somjen, 1978.)

MacVicar (1993), "the variety of ion channels observed is difficult to reconcile with the passive electrical responses of astroglia recorded *in situ*." There is a difference between the behavior of glial cells in culture and in tissue slices (Walz and MacVicar, 1988), and the expression of Na^+ and Ca^{2+} channels decreases with age (Chvátal et al., 1995; Ransom and Sontheimer, 1992). Still, some feeble voltage-dependent and tetrodotoxin (TTX)-sensitive Na^+ currents have also been recorded from astrocytes in tissue slices and in astrocytes freshly isolated from young mature rats (Sontheimer and Ritchie, 1995; Zhou and Kimelberg, 2000). Yet none of the glial cells found in mature mammalian CNS generate action potentials under ordinary conditions, when stimulated in ways that reliably excite neurons. For now, the function of Na^+ and Ca^{2+} channels of glial cells is a matter of speculation. Ritchie proposed that Schwann cells and astrocytes could donate and transfer the Na^+ channels they manufacture to axonal nodes of Ranvier and neurons in order to supplement those made by the neurons themselves. This is a plausible guess, but so far just a guess (see the review by Sontheimer and Ritchie, 1995).

Voltage-Gated Channels, but Voltage-Independent Membrane Resistance?

The topic of greatest importance is the nature of the K^+ conductance of glial membranes. Deviating from the earlier assumption of a purely passive ohmic glial membrane, recent reports emphasize the presence of several types of K^+ channels in astrocyte plasma membranes, some of which are wide open at rest and some of which are voltage dependent and strongly rectifying, either inward or outward (Duffy et al., 1995; Zhou and Kimelberg, 2000). Nonetheless, typical astrocytes in mature rat and frog spinal cords, tested by Syková and collaborators with voltage clamp-controlled potential steps, responded with currents that were symmetrical, that is, that were identical in amplitude for hyperpolarizing and depolarizing steps and did not decay with time (Chvátal et al., 1995, 2001). Also, in hippocampal tissue slices, Czéh et al. (1992) recorded linear current current-voltage functions from glial elements in a whole-cell patch-clamp configuration (Fig. 14–2). Oligodendrocytes generated more complex currents, and glial precursor cells displayed a rich array of voltage-dependent currents. Nevertheless, they also behave almost as ideal potassium electrodes, at least in cell culture (Kettenmann et al., 1983).

Two points must be borne in mind if one is to reconcile the seemingly passive or ohmic behavior regularly and reliably observed when recordings were made from glial cells in situ in brain and spinal cord with the equally convincing demonstration of voltage-gated nonlinear currents generated by similar cells in culture and in isolation, especially when examined under voltage clamp. The input resistance (R_{in}) of glial cells in situ is orders of magnitude lower than that of similar cells in isolation. The low R_{in} arises from the electrical continuity among populations of glial cells in situ. Current injected into one cell passes through extensive gap junctional connections to the cell's neighbors. The shunting not only lowers the effective input resistance but can also mask active responses and create the appearance of passive behavior. This, however, cannot be the complete explanation, because the glial membrane potential also behaves as though it were a passive potassium-selective electrode when $[K^+]_o$ is raised in the tissue (Lothman and Somjen, 1975; Ransom and Goldring, 1973a). When all glial cells in the vicinity are exposed to the same rising $[K^+]_o$, they must depolarize equally, and shunting through gap junctions cannot take place. An alternative explanation for the seemingly ohmic behavior was offered by Barres (1991): Both inwardly and outwardly rectifying K^+ channels present in the same membrane could complement one another in such a way that the current-voltage function (I-V curve) becomes nearly linear over a wide range of voltages. This indeed has been observed, for example by Zhou and Kimelberg (2000) in many but not all the astrocytes freshly isolated from rat hippocampus.

There is mounting evidence of at least two and perhaps more distinct types of astrocytes, some having *linear* membrane electrophysiology and no detectable voltage-dependent conductances (like the ones reported by Syková and coworkers; see Chvátal et al., 1995) and others endowed with a variety of voltage-gated, rectifying K^+ channels (D'Ambrosio et al., 1998; Steinhäuser et al., 1993). The existence of passive glial cells has, however, been challenged on technical grounds (Bordey and Sontheimer, 1998). To resolve the controversy, Walz (2000a) suggested that astrocytes can undergo rapid changes, depending on environmental conditions, and the heterogeneity of membrane properties reflects functional plasticity rather than the existence of permanent subtypes. Potassium currents in both types of astrocytes described by Zhou and Kimelberg (2000, 2001) were voltage dependent, but one of these populations had only outwardly rectifying channels, whereas the other had *variably rectifying* currents that combined to produce near-linear I-V functions. Judged by input resistance and input capacitance, the variably rectifying cells were probably much larger in size than the purely outwardly rectifying cells. It is likely that, as one searches blindly for glial cells with microelectrodes in intact CNS tissue, successful recordings are almost always established with the largest cells. Thus it is possible that all the glial cells we have studied behaved as if they were true potassium electrodes with invariant membrane resistance (Lothman and Somjen, 1975; Somjen, 1970, 1995) and presented linear whole-cell I-V function upon patch clamping (Czéh et al., 1992; Somjen, 1995) because of bias in sampling.

In conclusion

Some astrocytes probably have genuinely passive membranes, meaning that their ion channels are of the ohmic, leaky-current type. How common these cells are, and whether they increase in relative numbers with age, remains to be determined (see also the discussion in Zhou et al., 2000). It is also likely that, under certain recording conditions, the I-V functions of glial cells with variably rectifying K^+ channels could mistakenly be taken to be linear.

The Spatial Buffer Concept

Based on the properties of leech and mudpuppy glial cells, Orkand et al. (1966) first suggested the possibility that the quasi-syncytial network of gap junction–coupled glial cells could act as a *spatial buffer* for the K^+ ions that spilled out of neurons. It is expected that near a focus of excited neurons, locally elevated $[K^+]_o$ would drive K^+ into nearby glial cells through open K^+ channels. The driving force for uptake would arise from the raised $[K^+]_o/[K^+]_i$ ratio that moves the K^+ equilibrium potential away from the glial resting potential. The accumulated intraglial excess K^+ would then initiate a current through intercellular gap junctions from cell to cell; finally, K^+ would be released from glia at some distant location where neurons have been quiet and therefore $[K^+]_o$ has remained low (Figs. 2–7 and 2–10). The spatial buffer does not neutralize K^+ in the manner of a pH buffer, but disperses and therefore dilutes the excess. (For a detailed discussion, see Chen and Nicholson, 2000; Dietzel et al., 1989; Somjen, 1973, 1995.)

It is important to understand that the K^+ taken into one glial cell is not the same ion as the one released by another cell at a distance. The dispersion is not by diffusion but by ion current. To understand the difference, think of a row of marbles in a groove: add one at one end, and another will fall off at the other end. The important point is this: while diffusion over a distance is slow, current conduction is extremely fast.

As already emphasized by Kuffler (1967), spatial buffering works well if clusters of excited neurons are surrounded by quiescent cells but not when many neurons in a wide area are active. Besides, for such a spatial buffer to be effective, glial membranes must be highly permeable to K^+. Kuffler (1967) estimated the specific membrane resistance of glial cells in the leech nervous system to be high, and therefore judged the importance of the glial syncytium in the regulation of $[K^+]_o$ to be minor. In mammals the resting membrane resistance of glial cells is, however, probably much lower than that of neurons (Trachtenberg and Pollen, 1970). In line with the spatial buffer concept, Gardner-Medwin and Nicholson (1983) found that K^+ propelled by electrochemical force flows not just in the interstitial spaces but also through cells. While their method did not distinguish flux through glia from flux through neurons, the higher resting K^+ conductance of glial cells and the greater abundance of gap junctions among them should favor the flow through the glial net.

Voltage-Gated Channels in the Service of the Spatial Buffer

When the potassium buffer hypothesis was presented, glial cell membranes were considered to be purely passive. Has the discovery of voltage-gated ion channels modified this concept? The presence of small numbers of Na^+ and Ca^{2+} channels is probably irrelevant, not only because of their scarcity but also because they inactivate rapidly and therefore do not conduct during sustained elevation of $[K^+]_o$. But how about rectifying voltage-gated K^+ channels? Zhou and Kimelberg (2000) reported that only variably rectifying astrocytes generate vigorous inward current when exposed to elevated $[K^+]_o$, while the outwardly rectifying cells do not. They therefore proposed the following: in a net of connected astrocytes, the variably rectifying cells take K^+ in and forward the load to the outwardly rectifying members of the net, which then discharge the excess at some distance, where $[K^+]_o$ is low.

Can Spatial Buffering Have Unintended Consequences?

According to the spatial buffer concept, for each K^+ absorbed into a glial cell near excited neurons, another K^+ ion will be extruded at some distance and deposited in the vicinity of a quiescent neuron (Figs. 2–7, 2–10) (Dietzel et al., 1980; Orkand et al., 1966; Somjen, 1973). This causes a dispersal of excess K^+, which could be a factor in the spread of seizures and of SD (Amzica et al., 2002; Heinemann et al., 1991, 1995; Lux et al., 1986). If so, one might expect that interdicting cell-to-cell communication would inhibit or retard SD. In fact, however, selectively poisoning glial cells (Largo et al., 1996, 1997b) or disconnecting them by genetically deleting the glia-specific connexin building block of gap junctions (Theis et al., 2003) has the opposite effect: it facilitates SD and hypoxic SD-like depolarization. Therefore, it seems that SD propagation is not facilitated by glial dispersal of K^+, and spatial buffering inhibits rather than promotes SD (Chapter 14: "In SD neurons lead, glial cells follow"). No similar data are available on the spread of seizures.

Siphoning

The spatial buffer concept acquired a new aspect when Newman reported that K^+ channels are not evenly distributed over the surface of glial cells, but are found at highest density at the exposed extremities of cell processes (Brew et al., 1986; Newman, 1984, 1986, 1995). In the Müller cells of the retina, high K conductivity is located so as to channel K^+ from the region where neurons discharge it toward the vitreous substance, where it can do no harm. In brain tissue, K^+ conductance is maximal in the *astrocyte endfeet*. This location suggests that the pericapillary endfeet act as floodgates for K^+, discharging the overload to the endothelial cells, which can then transport it into the blood. Newman coined the term *siphoning* to describe the process.

   Chen and Nicholson (2000) analyzed the movements of excess K^+ in a computer model incorporating extracellular diffusion, passive uptake in glia, and spatial buffering/siphoning. They defined the theoretically optimal conditions for the most efficient glial buffer function. How well the properties of glial cells in live brain tissue conform to this model remains to be discovered. Values for geometry and electrical parameters in several representative cytoarchitectonic regions are needed to resolve this issue.

Net uptake of K^+

Besides moving K^+ from regions of high to regions of low concentration, glial tissue may relieve K^+ flooding by taking up and temporarily storing the excess (Henn et al., 1972; Hertz, 1978; Kimelberg et al., 1993; Walz, 2000b). Such net uptake of K^+ could occur in exchange against Na^+, or K^+ could be accompanied by an anion, Cl^- and/or HCO_3^-. In brain tissue slices, Ballanyi et al. (1987) found that $[K^+]_i$ and $[Cl^-]_i$ increased in glial cytoplasm (Fig. 2–8) but also that $[Na^+]_i$ decreased during neuronal activity, indicating that both methods were employed. Releasing Na^+ while taking in K^+ provides dual benefits, for it not only reduces accumulation of extracellular K^+ but also partially replenishes a deficit of Na^+. Because the aggregate volume of astrocytes is larger than the interstitial space, a comparatively small increase in glial $[K^+]_i$ can buffer a much larger increase in $[K^+]_o$. Alternatively or additionally, K^+ ions can be taken up together with anions, principally Cl^- and HCO_3^-. Uptake of KCl must lead to osmotic cell swelling, as argued by Boyle and Conway (1941) in a now classical paper. Cultured astrocytes exposed to high $[K^+]_o$ do indeed swell, as expected (e.g., Kimelberg et al., 1992; Walz, 1987). In brain in situ cell swelling is limited due to constraints of space.

In each of the alternative mechanisms, whether glial tissue functions as a spatial buffer, a siphon, a temporary storage space, or all of these, the K^+ lost from neurons must eventually be returned to them by a reversal of the flow pattern, from glial cells into interstitium and from there back into neurons.

Astrocytes and pH$_o$

Glial cells may also play a part in modulating brain pH, but their role here is not clear. Both astrocytes and oligodendrocytes contain more carbonic anhydrase than do neurons. The astrocyte membrane has several transporters for H^+ and HCO_3^-, and Deitmer (1995) emphasized that, using these transporters, glial cells could serve as "H^+ caretakers similarly as has been postulated for K^+." The true role of neuroglia may, however, be more complicated. The rise of $[K^+]_o$ caused by intense neuronal excitation is accompanied by transient extracellular alkalinization followed by slow acidification (Deitmer, 1995; Kraig et al., 1983; Urbanics et al., 1978). Glial cells depolarize when $[K^+]_o$ is increased and glial depolarization stimulates uptake of $NaHCO_3$, resulting in alkalinization of the glial cytoplasm, while the ISF undergoes an acidic shift in pH (Chesler, 1990). This mechanism could mitigate the initial excitation-induced extracellular alkalinization, but it would add to the subsequent acidification (Fig. 13–6).

Astrocytes and Calcium

Among the channels of glial cells there are some that are selectively or unselectively permeable to calcium (Barres et al., 1990; MacVicar, 1984; Verkhratsky and Kettenmann, 1996). The problem with much of the published data is that many of the experiments were done on cultures of cells originally harvested from immature brains. As the brain matures, the properties of glial cells change and the expression of ion channels in glia changes drastically in the course of postnatal development. It is an open question whether cells in culture undergo the same transformation as they do in intact brain. Moreover, the culture medium and the cell population represented in the culture might deviate from the natural environment and could influence the cells in ways that are different from in situ conditions. Reviewing the evidence, Verkhratsky and Kettenmann (1996) emphasize that different populations of glial cells express very different sets of channels and that even within the same population there are variations. Insofar as they possess voltage-gated and glutamate-dependent channels, glial cells could take up Ca^{2+} whenever they are depolarized by high $[K^+]_o$ or by glutamate released by excited neurons. And since some of the calcium transporters operate in either direction, depending on the driving force (Fig. 2–4), glial cells could also release Ca^{2+} when their milieu is depleted due to uptake by neurons, glia could buffer external $[Ca^{2+}]_o$ fluctuations in either direction. This matter has not been explored and deserves attention by laboratory workers and computer modelers alike.

Neuronal activity alters ion distributions

The transmembrane exchange of ions inherent in normal excitation can feed back and influence the very cell whose activity caused the movement of ions in the first place. This was first demonstrated by Frankenhaeuser and Hodgkin (1956). Their indirect and ingenious method consisted of measuring the hyperpolarizations that followed each spike during repetitive stimulation of a squid axon. The successive hyperpolarizing afterpotentials gradually decreased in amplitude, producing a positive shift of the envelope of the repeating waves. From earlier work, it was known that the hyperpolarizing afterpotential is generated by K^+ current. Frankenhaeuser and Hodgkin concluded that K^+ ions released with the spikes accumulated in the restricted periaxonal space, and their buildup reduced the outward K^+ current and therefore repressed the hyperpolarization. The narrow gap between the axolemma of the squid giant axon and its Schwann cell sheath is often referred to as the *Frankenhaeuser-Hodgkin space*.

Extracellular Potassium Responses in Mammalian Brain Tissue

The interstitial volume fraction (ISVF) in the CNS amounts to 13%–30% of the total tissue volume in different regions and is generally close to 20% (McBain et al., 1990; Nicholson and Syková, 1998). It may be expected that, similarly to the squid periaxonal space, ion concentrations would be altered in the cerebral interstitium by ion flow during neuron activation. The first indication that this is so was reported as a side issue by Kelly and Van Essen (1974), who studied neuron responses in the visual receiving area of cat cortex but also happened to record the intracellular potential of a few glial cells. Adequate optical stimuli caused transient depolarization of the glial cells. Since the membrane potential of a few glial cells was assumed to be dominated by K^+ (Kuffler, 1967), their depolarization was taken to indicate an increase an in cortical $[K^+]_o$.

More precise measurement with ion-selective microelectrodes showed transient $[K^+]_o$ responses in cat visual cortex, amounting maximally to 0.5 mM or less (Connors et al., 1979; Singer and Lux, 1975) (Fig. 2–9). Intermittent photic stimulation evoked similar $[K^+]_o$ responses in the neocortex of baboons (Heinemann et al., 1986). Other recordings of $[K^+]_o$ during physiological stimulation in central sensory receiving areas also showed responses that were moderate in magnitude (Somjen, 1978, 1979; Somjen et al., 1976; Syková et al., 1974). Because of technical difficulties, there are few data on ion levels in the CNS of freely moving, unanesthetized animals (Korytová, 1977). Spontaneous fluctuations of $[K^+]_o$ in the various regions of the CNS related to sleep spindles or burst firing were in the range of 0.2–0.5 mM measured with ion-selective electrodes in barbiturate anesthesia (Somjen, 1979) and up to 1.5 mM as estimated from glial depolarization waves during slow-wave sleep (Amzica and Neckelmann, 1999). In isolated eyecup-retina preparations, stimulation by light evoked $[K^+]_o$ increases of 0.5 mM or less (Karwoski and Proenza, 1978; Karwoski et al., 1985). Larger responses were sometimes seen in the spinal cord, where touching the skin raised $[K^+]_o$ by only 0.4 mM, but rhythmic flexion-extension of the knee joint caused it to increase by 1.7 mM (Heinemann et al., 1990a), and prolonged noxious cutaneous stimulation raised it on average by 1.6 mM and in the extreme case by 3 mM (Svoboda et al., 1988).

Much more drastic changes were recorded when afferent pathways to brain or spinal cord were stimulated by repetitive electrical pulses and during epileptiform seizures, which can drive $[K^+]_o$ to several times its normal level. During prolonged maximal stimulation, $[K^+]_o$ rises to a more or less steady *ceiling* level between 6 and 12 mM, depending on the CNS region and the stimulated pathway (Heinemann and Lux, 1977; Moody et al., 1974). The ceiling is higher in immature than in mature animals (Hablitz and Heinemann, 1989).

How Much Excess Extracellular K^+ Is Cleared Through Each
Route Shown in Figure 2–7?

We do not have a reliable answer to this basic question, so we must rely on educated guesswork. It is evident that if the neurons are healthy and the metabolic energy supply is adequate, eventually all the K^+ lost from neurons will be pumped back by the membrane 3Na/2K ATPase. As long as neurons fire sporadically and not in synchrony, it may be expected that, after each action potential, the pump can reclaim all the K^+ that had exited before the next spike is fired. As Figure 2–9 shows, when a cell column in the visual cortex is stimulated by a physiologically adequate stimulus, there is a small but reproducible increase in $[K^+]_o$. We know from many studies that during such stimulation many neurons within the functional column fire repeatedly. Even if individual spikes are not exactly synchronized, their combined output of K^+ ions adds up, causing the brief increase in $[K^+]_o$. For estimating diffusion in the tissue, it is worth noting that the so-called cortical columns are not cylindrical but are shaped more like thin slabs. At the boundaries of the stimulated column, some of the K^+ is expected to diffuse from the excited into the resting region, but this type of loss is probably minimal because the concentration gradient is shallow. For the same reason, glial uptake is probably also small. It seems likely that most of the excess K^+ represented by the small waves of $[K^+]_o$ increase seen in Figure 2–9 remains near the active cells, and at the end of stimulation it returns to the neurons without having been dispersed. The absence of poststimulus undershooting of $[K^+]_o$ supports this contention; if much K^+ had been dispersed, then in the wake of stimulation, $[K^+]_o$ should have dropped below its resting baseline (Heinemann and Lux, 1975).

The situation is very different during prolonged, artificial, massive electrical stimulation and during seizures. When most or all of the neurons in a region are forced to fire for an extended period of time, $[K^+]_o$ increases until it comes to a high but steady level somewhere between 8 and 12 mM (Moody et al., 1974) dubbed the *ceiling* by Heinemann and Lux (1977) (Figs. 2–11, 8–2, 8–3D, 9–5A). The ceiling is reached when the K^+ clearing mechanisms (Fig. 2–7) are sufficiently turned on to balance the release. In the wake of such maximal discharge, $[K^+]_o$ undershoots its resting baseline (Heinemann and Lux, 1975), indicating that much of the previously released K^+ has been removed from the vicinity of the previously excited neurons. Dietzel, Heinemann, and Lux (1989) analyzed ion movements in neocortex during and after intense stimulation and paroxysmal afterdischarge, using a computer model and experimental data. They had to make a number of assumptions, and more recent data indicate that some of these assumptions may not be accurate. Nonetheless, the main conclusions appear to be sound. The main actor setting the limit to the $[K^+]_o$ increase, as represented by the ceiling level, is the glial system. The Dietzel et al. model suggests that dispersal by the spatial buffer current and uptake by the glial 3Na/2K ATPase exchange pump remove about equal amounts of K^+, while the coupled K-Cl cotransport contributes a smaller amount.

Dietzel et al. (1989) considered washout of excess of K^+ by the circulating blood to be negligible. This conclusion was based on data from Mutsuga et al. (1976), who measured the K^+ concentration in the venous blood leaving the cortex, as well as $[K^+]_o$ in the cortex during electrical stimulation and seizure. They estimated the amount carried away by the blood as less than 10% of the K^+ that is released during a seizure, but in a later study they did show that ischemia retarded the clearing of excess $[K^+]_o$ (Vern et al., 1979). Bradbury and Stulcova (1970) measured the fraction cleared by blood during ventriculo-cisternal perfusion of a high-K^+ solution and estimated it to amount to 37%. The truth may lay in between.

K^+ administered through the ventricular system is not really representative of K^+ released from neurons within the gray matter. On the other hand, Mutsuga et al.'s numbers may be in error for two reasons. The rate of local blood flow may have been underestimated. Also, Mutsuga et al. were using single-barrel electrodes in the cerebral veins. Referring the electrode potential against a distant ground instead of a reference barrel in the bloodstream could have biased the recording. Spurious potentials (streaming potential, transendothelial voltage, etc.) may have interfered with the measurement.

In conclusion

We do not know how much excess K^+ is washed out by blood during a seizure, but some undoubtedly is. The 3Na/2K ATPase in the endothelial membrane (Fig 1–4) does have some work to do.

Responses of Extracellular Sodium and Chloride

Electrical stimulation of afferent pathways and seizure discharges cause $[Na^+]_o$ to decrease, while $[Cl^-]_o$ tends to increase slightly (Dietzel et al., 1982; Heinemann et al., 1978; Lehmenkühler et al., 1982a; Nicholson et al., 1978; Pumain and Heinemann, 1985). The decrease in $[Na^+]_o$ reflects influx into cells, while the increase in $[Cl^-]_o$ is ascribed to the shrinkage of the interstitial space caused by cell swelling (see Chapter 8: "Na^+, Cl^-, and cell volume changes . . ."). There are no data on changes in these ions during normal physiological activity.

As ions move across neuron membranes, extracellular concentration changes must be accompanied by reciprocal changes in intracellular levels. Since, however, the volume of neurons is larger than that of the surrounding interstitial space, intracellular concentrations are expected to change less than extracellular levels.

During SD and hypoxic spreading depression-like depolarization, both $[Na^+]_o$ and $[Cl^-]_o$ drop markedly (Chapter 13).

Extracellular Calcium Responses

$[Ca^{2+}]_o$ levels do not always show measurable changes during mild stimulation of the kind that does evoke $[K^+]_o$ responses (Somjen, 1980). Small changes in $[Ca^{2+}]_o$ have been recorded in normal brain and spinal cord tissue during slow-wave sleep as well as during EEG spindle activity induced by general anesthesia (Massimini and Amzica, 2001; Somjen, 1980). Larger responses were evoked by strong trains of electrical stimulation (Heinemann et al., 1978; Nicholson et al., 1978; Somjen, 1980). Usually $[Ca^{2+}]_o$ decreased when large numbers of neurons were simultaneously activated for an extended period of time, but small, slow increases were also seen. The extracellular calcium level is reduced because Ca^{2+} ions leave the interstitial space, entering cells through voltage-gated and NMDA receptor–

operated Ca^{2+} channels (Bollmann et al., 1998; Helmchen et al., 1999; Regehr et al., 1989).

The mechanism of the occasional increase in $[Ca^{2+}]_o$ is less obvious. Ca^{2+} can be pumped out of cells by one or other transporter, for example the Na/Ca exchanger or the Ca-ATPase ion pump (Fig. 2–3), but extrusion is unlikely to exceed uptake and therefore is unlikely to raise $[Ca^{2+}]_o$. More probably, the main reason for the concentration increase is the movement of water from the interstitial space into cells due to osmotic flow, which shrinks the interstitial space and concentrates its solutes. Only when more calcium than water leaves the interstitial space can $[Ca^{2+}]_o$ start to decline.

During seizures the decrease in $[Ca^{2+}]_o$ is much more marked than during the stimulation of normal tissue, because more cells are excited and depolarization and firing rates are higher and perhaps glutamate is overflowing in the interstitium, activating NMDA receptor-controlled channels (Amzica et al., 2002; Heinemann et al., 1977; Somjen, 1980; Somjen and Giacchino, 1985) (see also Fig. 8–3B).

Calcium Changes May Be Drastic in the Restricted Volume of Synaptic Clefts

Ion-selective electrodes are made from double-barreled glass capillaries, and even when pulled to the finest possible combined tip, they produce a small cavity in the tissue that is large compared to the interstitial spaces. The concentration that is measured is a local average that does not resolve short-distance gradients.

Synapses are usually surrounded by a glial envelope that is both a barrier to diffusion and an active system coordinating the removal and replenishment of transmitter substances (Kimelberg et al., 1993; Rusakov et al., 1999). Inasmuch as this perisynaptic sheath hinders diffusion into and out of the subsynaptic cleft, ion changes within the cleft may be much greater than those measured by ion-selective electrodes. This concerns especially Ca^{2+}, because voltage-gated and transmitter-operated calcium channels are known to be concentrated in both the pre- and postsynaptic membranes.

Excitatory or inhibitory postsynaptic potentials evoked in rapid succession tend to decrease with repetition. This has been attributed in part to desensitization of postsynaptic receptors and in part to exhaustion of readily available transmitter. A third factor is now taken into consideration, namely, the depletion of Ca^{2+} within the synaptic cleft. Theoretical computations suggested that the subsynaptic space can be almost completely emptied of Ca^{2+} if the synapse is activated several times in rapid succession (Dittman and Regehr, 1998; King et al., 2001; Rusakov, 2001). These calculations did not take into account the possible buffering of calcium by the astrocytes that form the perisynaptic envelope; Ca^{2+} transport mechanisms are bidirectional and could be reversed during extracellular dearth. Nonetheless, with the view of the dependence of synaptic transmission on available extracellular calcium, a plausible case can be made for a role of $[Ca^{2+}]_o$ in regulating $_{\smile}$ .apses and even more so for shaping the mechanism of seizure discharges (Chapter 8: "Calcium, magnesium and seizures").

Do Stimulus-Induced Ion Changes Matter?

Do stimulus-induced ion changes alter the functioning of the neurons that caused the ion shifts? In other words, do they represent feedback? As far as the healthy brain is concerned, this is debatable, because the ion shifts are small. It should be remembered that electrical pulses as used in experimentation, forcing large numbers of nerve fibers or cells into synchronous firing, evoke a pattern that is very different from normal neuronal activity. From the sparse available data, it seems fair to conclude that in the course of normal activity in healthy forebrains, fluctuations of $[K^+]_o$ amount to no more than 0.5 mM, except perhaps during slow-wave sleep, when waves of 1.5 mM may occur in neocortex (see above). Responses in spinal cord could be greater. For $[Ca^{2+}]_o$ the normal fluctuations may be especially small. Yet, as we shall see in Chapter 4, relatively small changes in ion levels can have small but significant effects on synaptic transmission. It is at least possible that "mental fatigue" and other subtle normal psychological states are contingent on small changes in CSF and ISF ion levels. A guess that is worthy of exploration.

During pathological events, especially seizures, SD, and hypoxia, the normal limits are breached. There can be no doubt that these major pathological ion shifts profoundly affect brain function. We shall address some of these questions in Chapters 3, 4, 8, and 9.

Keeping ions in their place (or putting them back where they belong) is hard work

Primary active transport is fueled by the splitting of a phosphate from ATP, converting it into ADP. An increase in the ADP concentration is the primary stimulus for increased cellular energy metabolism. Of the several ion pumps, the 3Na/2K ATPase ion exchanger uses the largest amount of energy, estimated to amount to about 50% of all the energy used by brain cells (Ames, 2000). Elevation of $[K^+]_o$ and/or $[Na^+]_i$ stimulates the 3Na/2K pump, which, while doing its work, produces ADP, which then stimulates cellular energy metabolism, which then restores ATP by rephosphorylating ADP.

Intramitochondrial Respiratory Enzymes Are Oxidized During Excitation in Intact Brain with Normal Blood Circulation

One of the main coenzymes in energy metabolism is *nicotinamide adenine dinucleotide*, which exists in reduced and oxidized forms as ***NADH*** and ***NAD+***, respectively. It is a major participant in cytoplasmic glycolysis, the tricarboxylic acid (TCA) cycle, and mitochondrial oxidative phosphorylation. Several decades ago, Chance and Jöbsis worked out a fluorometric method to measure the changes in the level of NADH in intact cells (Chance et al., 1962; see also the review by Jöbsis, 1964). Since *NADH fluoresces* but NAD^+ does not, the fluorescence signal of the correct wavelength provides a measure of the reduced form, NADH. As long as the total amount of the dinucleotide (NADH + NAD^+) remains constant, changes in NADH level indicate changes in the *redox* level of the enzyme, that is, the ratio of NADH to NAD^+.

This method was later adapted for use with intact brain by Jöbsis et al. (1971; O'Connor et al., 1972; Rosenthal and Jöbsis, 1971). To avoid artifacts, changes in cortical NADH autofluorescence were corrected for changes in the light scattered from the surface of the brain. Excitation by electrical stimulation or by epileptiform seizures of neocortex or hippocampal formation was invariably associated with a decrease in the corrected NADH fluorescence, indicating oxidation, as long as blood flow and oxygen delivery were normal. If, however, the preparation was made hypoxic by slowing or stopping artificial respiration, or if the circulation was impeded, the baseline fluorescence level rose. Also, under hypoxic conditions, neuron excitation also induced transient fluorescence increases instead of the usual decreases. In a tightly reasoned, cogent discussion based on the data and on previous work of several laboratories, Jöbsis and coworkers concluded that the corrected fluorescence signal represented NADH contained mainly in mitochondria and mainly in neurons. Previous data indicated that the NADH in mitochondria fluoresces 10–20 times more intensely than the NADH in cytosol. Furthermore, neurons contain far more mitochondria than do glial cells (Jöbsis et al., 1971). Diminished NADH fluorescence was therefore taken to mean oxidation of intramitochondrial NADH to NAD^+. In prior experiments on isolated mitochondria, this occurred whenever ATP production by oxidative phosphorylation was stimulated. Also, as expected, when oxygen was in short supply, NAD^+ was reduced to NADH, as shown by increased fluorescence. (For discussions of cellular respiration, see the reviews both old [Jöbsis, 1964] and new [Beattie, 2002]).

These basic observations were confirmed by Mayevski and Chance (1975) and by Lewis and colleagues (Lewis and Schuette, 1975; Lewis et al., 1974). In a joint project with the Jöbsis laboratory, we then related the oxidation of NADH to extracellular voltage shifts and the responses of $[K^+]_o$, during electrical stimulation, seizures, and SD (Lothman et al., 1975; Rosenthal and Somjen, 1973). During electrical stimulation at various intensities, the increase in $[K^+]_o$ was linearly correlated with the response of the corrected NADH fluorescence (Fig. 2–12). During seizures, however, the oxidation of NADH increased disproportionately more than did the $[K^+]_o$, which hovered around a steady ceiling (Fig. 8–4) (Lothman et al., 1975). We concluded that seizures demanded the expenditure of extra energy for processes other than those spent on ion regulation. In retrospect, it could be argued that the ion pumps had to go into overdrive in order to guard against

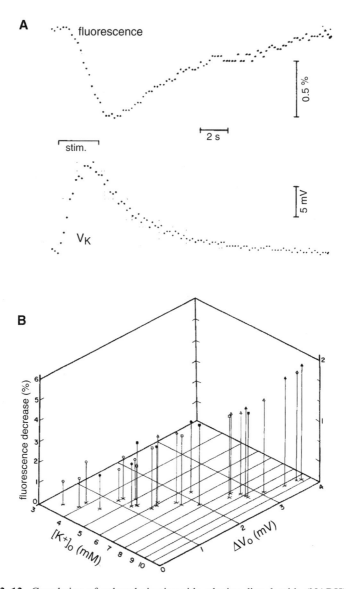

Figure 2–12. Correlation of reduced nicotinamide adenine dinucleotide (NADH) oxidation, extracellular potassium, and sustained extracellular potential responses in cat neocortex in situ. **A:** Corrected NADH autofluorescence and potassium-selective microelectrode responses evoked by a train of stimuli applied to a nearby cortical surface (20 Hz). Decreasing fluorescence indicates NADH oxidation. The traces are the averages of eight trials. **B:** The three-way correlation of NADH oxidation (fluorescence decrease), peak level of $[K^+]_o$ (scaled logarithmically), and negative potential shift (ΔV_o) recorded simultaneously, in one session from the same cortical site. Responses evoked by stimulus trains of varying intensity and duration. (Modifed from (Lothman et al., 1975.)

the breaching of the $[K^+]_o$ ceiling in the face of massive outflow of K^+ from seized neurons. In part, the extra expenditure of energy could have been due to pumping by the glial 3Na/2K ATPase, which may have been recruited into action only at dangerously high $[K^+]_o$ levels. It is, of course, also possible that, as we originally suggested, other demands for metabolic energy, such as the disposal of excess transmitter substances, created the disproportionate demand for NADH oxidation. Be that as it may, in seizures the ceiling for $[K^+]_o$ was respected, and when the ceiling was breached, SD ensued (see Chapter 13).

Later, Jöbsis et al. (1977) used differential reflectance spectrophotometry to assay the redox state of cytochromes a and a_3 in cerebral cortex (the method did not distinguish a from a_3). Electrical stimulation of the cortex evoked slight oxidation of these cytochromes, and during SD much more marked oxidation occurred. Depriving the brain of blood flow or of oxygen caused the expected reduction of cytochromes a and a_3. Seizure discharges were also usually accompanied by oxidation of cytochromes a and a_3, but when seizures recurred at frequent intervals, the oxidation responses were eventually replaced by reductions, and at this time each seizure was accompanied by lowering of the partial pressure of oxygen in the tissue (Kreisman et al., 1983a). The cytochrome signal was corrected for changes in intracortical blood volume, using the simultaneously recorded hemoglobin signal. Blood volume decreased during ischemia and increased during hypoxia, so that the hemoglobin signal changed in opposite directions in the two conditions, but the corrected cytochrome signal indicated reduction during both hypoxia and ischemia, confirming the appropriateness of the correction.

In Isolated Neurons and Brain Tissue Slice Preparations, Excitation Is Accompanied by Brief Initial Oxidation Followed by Long-Lasting Reduction of Reduced/Oxidized Nictotinamide Adenine Dinucleotide and Reduced/Oxidized Flavin Adenine Dinucleotide

A consistent picture emerged from the works just mentioned, and the many related publications cited therein (Jöbsis et al., 1971, 1977; Kreisman et al., 1981, 1983a; Lothman et al., 1975; O'Connor et al., 1972; Rosenthal and Jöbsis, 1971; Rosenthal et al., 1976). They demonstrated that increased activity of central neurons in healthy brain tissue stimulates a regulated increase of cerebral blood flow (CBF), oxygen delivery, and oxidation of the enzymes of mitochondrial respiration. Surprisingly, isolated neurons, organotypic cultures, and brain tissue slices in vitro behave differently. In such isolated CNS preparations, increased excitation is accompanied by an initial decrease followed by a prolonged increase of reduced nicotinamide adenine dinucleotide (NADH) fluorescence, indicating initial transient oxidation of NADH followed by prolonged and more intense reduction of NAD^+ to NADH (Fig. 2–13) (Duchen, 1992; Fayuk et al., 2000; Heinemann et al., 2002b; Kann et al., 2003; Kovács et al., 2001; Schuchmann et al., 2001;

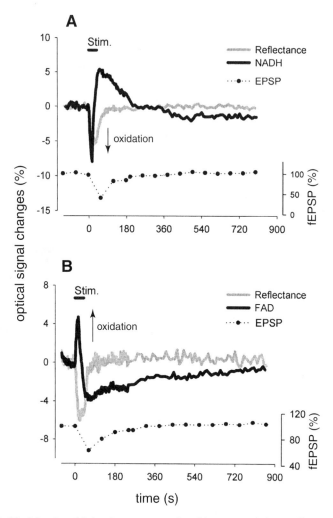

Figure 2–13. Mitochondrial redox responses in a hippocampal tissue slice. A: Reduced nicotinamide adenine dinucleotide (NADH) autofluorescence, reflected light intensity (intrinsic optical signal) and extracellular excitatory postsynaptic potential (EPSP)—focally recorded EPSP (fEPSP) amplitude in stratum radiatum of CA1 in a rat hippocampal tissue slice. Beginning at zero time, 10 Hz stimulation for 40 seconds. Focally recorded EPSPs were evoked by single shocks. Following the train, the fEPSP was depressed. Diminished NADH fluorescence indicates oxidation, followed by increased fluorescence indicating reduction. Diminished reflectance indicates diminished light scattering due to (mild) cell swelling. B: Similar to A, but in the case of flavin adenine dinucleotide (FAD), increased fluorescence indicates oxidation. A and B from different slices. (Unpublished figure by D. Fayuk and D.A. Turner; see also Turner and Fayuk, 2002.)

D. Fayuk and D.A. Turner, personal communication). The reduction outlasts the neuron excitation, whereas in the previous experiments on brains in situ, oxidation was maintained throughout excitation and gradually subsided thereafter. Duchen (1992b) and Fayuk and Turner (personal communication) recorded the fluorescence of flavin adenine dinucleotide (FAD) in addition to that of NADH. Whereas NADH is present in cytoplasm as well as in mitochondria, FAD (as also cytochromes) is purely mitochondrial. Like NADH, FAD underwent brief oxidation followed by more prolonged reduction during stimulation, but the time courses of the NADH and FAD changes were different. When 2-deoxyglucose was substituted for glucose and pyruvate was added as a metabolic substrate, the reduction responses of both NAD^+ and FAD were depressed but the oxidation responses were still evoked, suggesting that the reduction was mainly an expression of cytoplasmic glycolysis, while the oxidation related to the stimulation of mitochondrial oxidative metabolism ((Fayuk et al., 2000; Turner and Fayuk, 2002 and personal communication). Duchen (1992, 1999) and Kovács et al. (2001) interpreted this differently: they related the reduction of NAD^+ to its role in the TCA cycle. The two views do not, of course, contradict one another. Indeed, there are steps in both the glycolytic pathway and the TCA cycle where NAD^+ is reduced to NADH, but at the "entrance" to the electron transport chain NADH is oxidized when cellular respiration is stimulated by ADP, provided that oxygen is available at the other end of the chain (reviewed in Beattie, 2002; Harris, 2002; Jöbsis, 1964). Reactive oxygen species (ROS) can also oxidize the respiratory enzymes (Schuchmann et al., 2001), but under normal conditions this is probably a minor and evanescent event.

Why Is There a Difference Between Brain In Situ and Brain Tissue In Vitro?

It is remarkable that the data obtained in experiments on intact brains by several laboratories were quite consistent, as were the more recently reported results of trials in various brain cell and tissue preparations in vitro. Is there a way to reconcile the two data sets? The following is a tentative attempt to explain the divergent findings.

Low oxygen availability favors reduction of NAD^+ and FAD over their oxidation, because it slows oxidative metabolism and relaxes the brake on glycolysis (diminished Pasteur effect). Glial cells are relatively poor in mitochondria (see O'Connor et al., 1972, and references therein) but rich in glycogen and in glycolytic enzymes (Hamprecht and Dringen, 1995). The fluorescence signal is derived from all the NADH in the tissue, and the question is, which fraction dominates under which conditions? There are differences in oxygen availability in intact brain compared to CNS tissue in vitro. In normal brain with intact circulation, neurons are never far from capillaries. In the unstimulated, anesthetized, resting brain tissue the partial pressure of oxygen is, however, considerably lower than in arterial blood (Feng et al., 1988), keeping respiratory enzymes partially reduced (LaManna et al., 1987; O'Connor et al., 1972). Nonetheless, the supply of molecular oxygen is abundant because, as it is consumed, it is readily replenished by the large amount carried by hemoglobin. During stimulation and during seizures, the supply of oxygen through dilated vessels increases even more than the demand, so that tissue P_{o2} actually rises in the face of increased oxygen consumption, except when the cerebral circulation fails (Kreisman et al., 1981, 1983b; Leniger-Follert, 1984). Compared to their relatively reduced resting state, NADH and the cytochromes become oxidized as the tissue is oversupplied with oxygen. Exuberant local blood flow is ensured by vasodilatation mediated perhaps by nitric oxide or K^+ or CO_2 or H^+ and lactic acid or acetylcholine or most probably by a combination of several factors. Compared to brain tissue in situ, the partial pressure of oxygen at the surface of brain tissue slices in vitro is very high, but at the center of the slice it is much lower than at the surface (Sick and Somjen, 1998). Around isolated neurons and organotypic slice cultures, P_{O_2} is usually higher than in blood-perfused CNS. However, in preparations in vitro, the oxygen supply does not increase with demand. More importantly, since the solubility and diffusibility of oxygen in water are low, the supply of molecular oxygen is limited where it is needed, at the inner membrane of mitochondria. The availability of oxygen to mitochondria may therefore fall short on the long run during prolonged activity, even though the P_{O_2} pressure in the bath is constant. The initial oxidation response of $NADH/NAD^+$ and $FADH_2/FAD$ then turns into reduction, as it does in hypoxic intact brain.

In conclusion

In brains with normal circulation, the redox status of energy metabolic enzymes follows tissue oxygen tension, which depends on capillary blood flow. In brain cells in vitro, the tissue oxygen tension (and therefore the redox status) falls and rises with oxygen consumption.

The discussion in the preceding paragraphs perhaps simplifies a complex issue. (It is, after all, an electrophysiologist's view of biochemistry.) Be that as it may, the measured changes in redox level of the enzymes of energy metabolism probably are valid indices of the rate of energy turnover, regardless of the direction in which they move, and therefore they can be useful in investigations of energy sufficiency. For example, Schuchmann et al. (1999) found that during recurrent low Mg^{2+}-induced seizures in vitro, the NAD^+ reduction responses became smaller and smaller after a certain number of repetitions, and they never recovered. The authors interpreted the fading of the fluorescence responses as caused by irreversible energy failure (see also Heinemann et al., 2002b).

Key points

The total amount of solute inside cells determines their volume, because cell osmolarity is regulated to keep it equal to the osmolarity of the extracellular milieu. Ions make up the bulk of osmotically active particles inside and outside cells.

The concentration of each ion inside cells is regulated. The channels, exchangers, and pumps mediating membrane transport have been studied in great detail, but understanding of the mechanisms that sense intracellular molecular content and ion concentrations, and of the biophysical method of determining set points, is sketchy.

Ion pumps serving primary active transport are built of membrane-spanning giant molecular subunits. The same structure performs the transport and derives the necessary energy from splitting the high-energy phosphate bond of ATP. These structures are therefore also called ATPases. In central neurons the 3Na/2K ATPase is by far the largest consumer of ATP. Additional ATPase pumps include one transporting Ca^{2+} out of cells and probably also one for H^+. Primary active ion transport is electrogenic (rheogenic).

The ADP produced from ATP is the chief normal stimulus regulating energy metabolism. In neurons, most of the ATP is produced in mitochondria by oxidative phosphorylation by the electron transport chain.

Secondary active transport derives its energy from energetically downhill flow of one ion, enabling the uphill transport of another ion. Influx of Na^+ into cells is the driver of many such transporters. In some cases, driver and driven ions move together in the same direction (cotransport or symport); in others, one is exchanged against another (countertransport or antiport). Transporters can be electrogenic or electrically neutral, depending on the balance of charges.

Ion channels consist of membrane-spanning subunits with a water-filled pore. They are equipped with selectivity filters and usually also with molecular gates operated either by membrane voltage or by ligand molecules. An important difference between transporters and ion channels is that transporters require reversible bonding of the transported ion to limited binding sites, and transport is therefore saturable.

Neuron membrane transport influences both intra- and extracellular ion concentrations. The composition of interstitial fluid is additionally regulated by glial cells and by exchange with blood through transport across the capillary endothelium.

Astrocytes regulate the interstitial K^+ level ($[K^+]_o$) by net uptake through both active transport and passive flux through ion channels. Spatial buffering and siphoning disperse excess K^+ and help its discharge into circulating blood.

The cytosolic free Ca^{2+} concentration is very low; pCa is similar to pH. Total cellular calcium concentration is much higher, but most of the intracellular calcium is either bound to protein or sequestered in the ER, mitochondria, and Golgi apparatus. Transient, strictly localized $[Ca^{2+}]_i$ increases serve as signals regulating cellular functions, including the activities of calmodulin and mitochondrial function. Probably only the ER serves as a true storehouse for calcium.

Astrocytes contain more carbonic anhydrase than do neurons and probably aid in maintaining pH. They also take up excess glutamate and probably have a role in maintaining other ion levels within physiological limits.

Intensive neuronal activity can cause spatially limited local fluctuations in interstitial ion levels. $[K^+]_o$ can increase and $[Na^+]_o$ can decrease somewhat, and very small changes in $[Ca^{2+}]_o$ and $[Cl^-]_o$ may occur, but under normal conditions, neuronal and glial regulation keeps these changes within physiological limits. During seizures, hypoxia, brain trauma, and probably also other pathologies, ion levels can drastically change and influence neuronal function for the worse.

3

Osmotic Stress and the Brain

When thinking of biophysical and biochemical processes, we are used to consider the concentrations (or activities) of the ions and other active ingredients dissolved in the water of the cytosol and of the extracellular fluids. Yet water itself has a concentration (and activity), which is in a reciprocal relationship to the sum of the concentrations of all the solutes for which it is the solvent. Osmolarity expresses the activity of water, and it is a key parameter in vital processes.

Chapter 3 reviews the regulation of osmolarity in brain cells and in the brain as a whole, and the reasons for its failures. Biophysical effects of deviant osmolarity will be considered later, in Chapter 4.

Osmotic pressure in biological systems

Some definitions as reminders

Osmotic concentration refers to the sum total of dissolved particles in a solution. It is determined by adding up the molar concentrations of nonelectrolytes and ion concentrations of dissociated compounds. The osmotic concentration of 1 M sucrose is 1 osmol, abbreviated 1 Osm, but for 1 M NaCl it is 2 Osm.

Osmolarity refers to ***osmotic activity***. It is usually not equal to osmotic concentration, yet it too is measured in osmols. Concentration is related to activity by the ***osmotic coefficient***. Different solutes have different osmotic coefficients and, to make matters more complicated, the coefficients usually vary with the concentration. For salts the osmotic coefficient is usually less than 1; for some sugars it is very slightly more than 1. Osmolarity determines not only the osmotic pressure but also other ***colligative*** properties, such as *freezing* and *boiling points* and *vapor pressure*. Most laboratory osmometers measure either freezing point or vapor pressure, not osmotic pressure, and report the result in (milli)osmols.

Tonicity refers to ***osmotic pressure***. In comparing two solutions, one can be called hypo- or hyperosmolar relative to the other. It is common to speak of *isotonic, hypotonic,* and *hypertonic* solutions but, strictly speaking, this is not correct. *Osmotic pressure is exerted across a semipermeable membrane* that separates two solutions of different osmolarity, but a solution in a glass beaker does not exert an osmotic pressure. Thus blood plasma is correctly described as being isotonic to the cytosol of erythrocytes. In everyday jargon and in clinical parlance, *isotonic saline* is used as a synonym for *normal saline*, meaning osmolarity equal to that of normal blood plasma, even though the solution itself, in a glass vessel, exerts no pressure. The distinction may seem petty, and indeed it may be safely ignored as long as it is not completely forgotten, for it speaks to the essence of the concept.

Osmotic Pressure Depends on Kinetic Energy of Water Molecules

The following equation sums up the relationship:

$$\pi = RT\phi ic \tag{3-1}$$

where π is the *osmotic pressure*, R is the *gas constant*, T is the *absolute temperature*, ϕ is the *osmotic coefficient*, i is the number of ions into which the compound dissociates (unity for nonelectrolytes), and c is the molar concentration of the solute.

Yet remember this: even though osmolarity is expressed in terms of the *solute* concentration, the actual pressure is generated by the *kinetic energy of water molecules*, not by the dissolved particles. Where there is less solute, there is more water, and therefore *water will tend to move from the hypotonic into the hypertonic solution*. As a result, pressure will build up on the hypertonic side. In a closed vessel containing two solutions separated by a *semipermeable membrane*, the hydraulic pressure measured on the hypertonic side of the membrane is the force that resists the flow of water across the membrane in the face of the energy difference between the two solutions on the two sides of the membrane.

Another point is sometimes overlooked and yet is important for understanding physiological osmotic effects: Equation 3–1 calculates the osmotic pressure that is obtained once ***equilibrium*** has been attained. If osmolarity is suddenly changed in an ideal system with perfectly rigid walls and an unyielding membrane, equilibrium will rapidly be reached because only a very small amount of water must pass through the membrane to build the pressure that will stop further flow. In living systems, however, membranes are somewhat yielding, and they will be stretched when water flows into a cell. The water is propelled by its kinetic energy, manifested as the osmotic force. Pressure will build gradually, and equilibrium will be reached only after the membrane has been stretched to its limit. The rate of water flow is set by both the permeability of the membrane for water and the elastic yield of the membrane and (in the case of living cells) of its supporting cytoskeleton. Water permeability is expressed technically as **hydraulic conductivity**. *If hydraulic conductivity is zero, then there will be no osmotic pressure, no matter how large the difference in the osmolarities of the two solutions.*

All the previous considerations apply only to ideally semipermeable membranes, which let solvent pass without hindrance and solutes not at all. Few real membranes behave ideally, and certainly none of the physiological membranes do. Deviation from ideality are expressed by the **reflection coefficient** of solutes. It is determined by the properties of both the dissolved particle and the membrane.

$$V_w = \sigma L \Delta \pi \qquad\qquad (3\text{–}2)$$

where V_w is the volume flow of water, σ is the reflection coefficient, L is the hydraulic conductivity of the membrane, and $\Delta \pi$ is the difference in osmolarity between the two sides of the membrane. Note that the closer σ is to unity, the more nearly ideal is the system. Note also the simplification: there is no account in Eq. 3–2 of the elasticity of the membrane.

Here are a few more points to keep in mind in the next few pages:

1. While most of the time most cells of mammals live in an isotonic *milieu interieur* and therefore experience no osmotic force across the plasma membrane, this is not always the case, either in health or in disease (think of kidneys).
2. More importantly, the isotonicity of cells is not the result of equilibrium, but of the hard work of pumps and other transport systems in the plasma membrane, which ensure osmolar balance between cytosol and interstitial fluid. If the pumps stop, cells swell (see "Volume regulation . . . " below).
3. Biological membranes are not truly semipermeable. The various solutes in body fluids have widely ranging reflection coefficients.
4. Hydraulic conductivity (water permeability) of the plasma membrane varies among cell types. In some cells it can be controlled by physiological mechanisms, such as the insertion of aquaporin channels in response to specific signals.
5. Plasma membranes can be stretched to some degree, variably among cells. As a result, cells can swell or shrink under the influence of osmotic changes.

Cell swelling is restrained by the cytoskeleton that is anchored in the plasma membrane. It is constrained by the presence of neighboring cells and connective tissue fibers; and the assembly of cells is constrained by the architecture of the organ as a whole, which may be encased in a stiff capsule or, in the case of the brain, the rigid skull.

Water poisoning and other causes of cerebral edema

Miners' and Stokers' Cramps Are Prevented by Common Salt

In a hot, humid environment, sweat glands are the main guardians protecting the body from overheating. Losing heat through evaporation from the skin surface becomes especially important when performing heavy labor in a tropical climate. When we perspire, we lose salt and water. Compared to body fluids, sweat contains more water than salt. As excess water is lost, the osmolarity of body fluids rises. If water loss is severe, the volume of circulating blood plasma shrinks, and not only the osmolarity but also the viscosity of the blood rises. An individual so suffering is very thirsty and, given a chance, will drink water copiously. Replacing sweat that contains salt, with water, which does not, reverses the hyperosmolarity previously caused by the sweating and dilutes the blood.

The primary dangers of prolonged heavy physical exertion in a tropical environment are, first, overheating and then collapse of the circulation. Drinking a large volume of water after heavy perspiration can lead to seizures and delirium, a condition formerly known as *miners'* or *stokers' cramps*. These convulsions are caused by the hypotonicity of blood, and their mechanism will be the topic of the next two sections and Chapter 4: "Sodium, chloride and osmotic effects in the central nervous system." The cramps can be prevented by taking common salt together with the water. Adding other electrolytes, especially potassium in smaller amounts, to the water may have some added benefit, but the main ingredient should be NaCl.

Stokers' cramp is a form of water poisoning. Ordinarily, it is hard to drink enough water so fast that the kidneys can't keep up with the excess. After heavy perspiration, the motivation for excessive water intake is excessive thirst stimulated by both the raised osmolarity and the reduced volume of circulating blood. Without thirst, healthy persons are not inclined to ingest more water than they need, except for some chronic schizophrenic patients, who seem to have an inappropriate urge for excessive water intake.

How water is transported across biological membranes

There is no biological reverse osmosis. No biological water pumps exist that can transport free water against an osmotic gradient across biological membranes. This was a matter for debate in the past, but the argument was settled in the negative, apparently for good (Robinson, 1960). Nonetheless, glands and kidneys can secrete fluids of a tonicity very different from that of extracellular fluid (ECF), even though ECF provides the raw material for such secretion. The question then is, how can a secreted fluid be diluted, if not by pumping water? To move water across membranes, solutes must always primarily be transported, and water is dragged secondarily, driven by the osmotic force generated by the transported solutes. Then how is hypotonicity achieved? Secreting organs solve the problem by proceeding in two or more stages. At first an isotonic fluid is produced, as salt and other solutes are either secreted or filtered together with water in iso-osmolar proportion. From this iso-osmolar solution, solute is removed in the next stage, leaving a hypotonic solution behind. Dilution is achieved while the primary isotonic fluid is led along a duct or tubule, the wall of which is (nearly) impermeable to water but is endowed with active transporters for one or more solutes, such as salts and sugars. Selected dissolved ingredients are removed from the lumen of the duct and reabsorbed into the blood, while water is not, and the fluid retained in the duct becomes hypo-osmolar relative to plasma.

The Brain Is Subject to Osmotic Swelling and Shrinkage

The ECF of the brain, comprising the CSF and ISF, is normally isotonic with blood plasma. Problems arise when the osmolarity either of circulating blood or of the fluids in the brain changes rapidly. The hydraulic conductivity of the BBB is lower than that of peripheral capillaries, but its permeability to water is still much higher than the passive permeability to electrolytes or glucose. Because of this difference, the brain is said to behave as an *osmometer*; that is, it tends to swell when plasma osmolarity decreases and to shrink when the plasma becomes hypertonic. The former condition is edema, the latter is dehydration, and both conditions affect CNS function adversely. Both hypo- and hyperosmolarity powerfully affect synaptic transmission and neuronal excitability, as will be outlined in Chapter 4 ("Sodium, chloride, and osmotic effects . . .").

A Potential Vicious Circle Occurs in Brain Swelling

Besides affecting CNS excitability, cerebral edema has a mechanical effect that can be life-threatening. *Edema* means waterlogging of tissues, which is undesirable in any organ. Cerebral edema can be catastrophic, because the skull is rigid and does not accommodate large changes in the size of the brain. If the brain swells, intracranial pressure rises and blood vessels are compressed. Compression of the vessels increases the resistance to blood flow, impairing cerebral circulation. Even more dangerously, elevated intracranial pressure can wedge the base of the brain into the foramen magnum and so impede the drainage of CSF from the cerebral ventricles. If CSF continues to be secreted but cannot be drained, the result is a vicious circle of rising intracranial pressure, which worsens the outflow blockage, which further elevates pressure. To save the patient in this condition, plasma osmolarity must be raised to draw water from the swollen brain. In practice, this requires the administration of a solution that is hyperosmolar relative to plasma. For this purpose, a compound must be selected that does not penetrate the BBB (has a high reflection coefficient), is not toxic, is not metabolized or taken up by cells but is excreted slowly by the kidneys, and has a low molecular weight so that an osmotically significant amount can rapidly be administered intravenously. Clinicians prefer mannitol to prevent or to reverse cerebral edema in short-term settings in the face of normal plasma sodium levels, which may occur during surgical procedures.

Three Kinds of Cerebral Edema

As we have just seen, cerebral edema can be caused by the ***lowering of systemic osmolarity***, as in water poisoning or salt loss, but it can also be the result of cerebral pathology, without disturbance of the overall salt and water balance of body fluids. Pathologists distinguish between ***vasogenic*** and ***cytotoxic*** cerebral edema. In vasogenic edema the capillary endothelium is injured, and it becomes permeable to various solutes including plasma proteins. It is essentially a breakdown of the BBB (Davson and Segal, 1996). Normally, the protein concentration in brain ISF is very low. The extravasation of albumin after BBB breakdown raises ***colloid osmotic*** (synonym: *oncotic*) ***pressure*** in the interstitial fluid, drawing water from the capillaries and causing vasogenic edema. In cytotoxic edema, the primary cause is an accumulation of excess metabolites that raise osmotic pressure in cell cytoplasm, drawing water into the cells. This can occur if membrane transport fails, for example due to lack of oxygen, and *Gibbs-Donnan* forces take over (see "Volume regulation . . ." below); or it can be due to faulty metabolism. Tissue acidosis, elevated $[K^+]_o$, and the extracellular accumulation of glutamate cause cell swelling, especially of astrocytes, less so of neuron dendrites, and least of all of neuron somas (Kimelberg, 2000). During hypoxia all three metabolic factors operate, in addition to the depressed outward transport of Na^+ caused by reduced ATP.

Edema has two aspects: the accumulation of excess water in interstitial spaces and the uptake of water by cells. Vasogenic edema is also called ***extracellular edema***, and a synonym for cytotoxic edema is ***intracellular edema*** (Kempski, 2001). It is important to realize that, even though in the case of vasogenic edema water is accumulating at first in the interstitium and only secondarily inside cells, while in cytotoxic edema cell swelling is the primary problem, in the end there is excess water in both extra- and intracellular compartments in both types, and only the *relative distributions* differ. In cases of water poisoning, water accumulates primarily in the interstitium, driven by the osmotic force across the BBB. Then, as soon as the interstitial fluid is diluted, water also moves into brain cells. By contrast, in vasogenic edema, much of the fluid remains extracellular, because the extravasated albumin is not taken up by cells since it cannot pass plasma membranes. Cytotoxic (metabolic) edema is primarily intracellular, for it occurs inside cells where excess osmotic particles are being produced. Once the excess metabolic products are released from cells, however, water will be drawn from circulating blood into the interstitial fluid as well. The topic of cell swelling will be picked up again in the discussion of the effects of cerebral ischemia (Chapter 19: "Two mechanisms cause the acute swelling . . .").

Most of the traffic in water, electrolytes, and other bioactive compounds goes through endothelial cells, which are well equipped with aquaporin water channels (Nico et al., 2001). Genetically altered mice deficient in aquaporin expression are apparently protected against the cerebral edema that results from BBB damage after intense seizures (Binder et al., 2001b). This is a rare example of a genetic defect that confers some advantage, although, one suspects, at the expense of other functions.

Volume regulation of cells and of the brain

Cellular Volume Regulation Requires Active Transport

Cells that are deprived of metabolic energy swell. Osmolarity of the cytosol is kept equal to that of the extracellular milieu by active membrane transport, and in the absence of such transport, cells acquire excess osmols, with water following. The reason is the presence of impermeant anions inside the cell, and of more permeant anions on the outside than in the cytosol. The forces that drive ion and water movement in these cases have been defined by Gibbs and Donnan (Kutchai, 1993). Since there are more permeant anions outside, they are driven by a chemical gradient into the cells; as they penetrate, they drag permeant cations with them, building an osmotic gradient and forcing water to flow into the cell. In an inanimate system, a twofold equilibrium sets in when the inward flow of water is balanced by hydrostatic *pressure* (osmotic pressure) and ion movement is stopped by *voltage* (the equilibrium potential) across the membrane. In live animals the cell membranes cannot sustain a large hydrostatic pressure. Instead, in healthy cells, the influx of ions driven by **Gibbs-Donnan forces** is countered by outward transport by ion pumps, chiefly the 3Na/2K ATPase pump, maintaining osmotic balance at the expense of steady work. How the pumping is precisely regulated to maintain cell volume and satisfy the electrical as well as the osmotic steady state is not clear. If the pump stops, cells swell and eventually the membrane becomes incontinent and its contents leak, including all normally impermeant ingredients (*lysis*). This presumably is an irreversible terminal condition heralding cell death. We shall return to hypoxic cell swelling in Chapter 19 (see "Two mechanisms cause the acute swelling . . .").

Osmotic Volume Changes and Volume Regulation

During introductory physiology courses, many readers will have put a drop of their blood in hypotonic salt solution and under the microscope saw erythrocytes swell, followed by *hemolysis*. Similar cells in hypertonic solution shrank and became crenellated. Rarely mentioned at the introductory level is the fact that most cells left in a moderately hypo- or hypertonic environment for more than a very short time tend to have their volume restored, at least partially (unless they undergo lysis, of course). In a hypotonic bath, cells swell at first, but then they shrink partway back toward their normal volume. The partial compensatory restoration of size in the face of hypotonic treatment is called *hypotonic regulatory volume decrease* (*RVD*) (Fig. 3–1). Conversely, in moderately hypertonic solution, cells first shrink and then undergo *hypertonic regulatory volume increase* (*RVI*) (Hallows and Knauf, 1994).

Regulatory volume changes are achieved by solute transport across the plasma membrane. Usually K^+ and Cl^- are released from the cytosol during the first phase of RVD, followed later by the efflux of K^+ coupled with organic anions, notably taurine and other amino acids (Kimelberg et al., 1990; Walz, 2002). Among the amino acids there may be excitatory compounds such as glutamate and aspartate, with profound consequences, as we shall see later (Chapter 15). For the sake of RVI, electrolytes are taken up from the ECF. When normal bath osmolarity is being restored following an osmotic challenge, cells that have previously undergone RVD or RVI will transiently under- or overshoot their original size before returning to normal. This is because a cell that has given up some of its intracellular osmotic particles during RVD will experience normal extracellular osmolarity as if it was hypertonicity, and therefore it will shrink when bath osmolarity is restored. Before the cell can finally return to its usual size, it has to retrieve the solutes it had lost during RVD. Conversely, a cell that has undergone RVI during hypertonic challenge will transiently swell before recovering.

Among brain cells, astrocytes show marked volume changes under osmotic challenge, as well as vigorous regulatory volume changes if the challenge continues for more than a few minutes (Fig. 3–1B) (Kempski et al., 1991; Kimelberg, 2000; Kimelberg and Goderie, 1988; Walz, 2002). The plasma membrane of astrocytes has been shown to be richly endowed with aquaporin water channels (Nielsen et al., 1997), as well as Cl^-, K^+, and organic anion transporters. For volume regulation, the most important channels are stretch-sensitive (or volume-operated) membrane channels that open when the cell swells and allow the unloading of solutes (Walz, 2002).

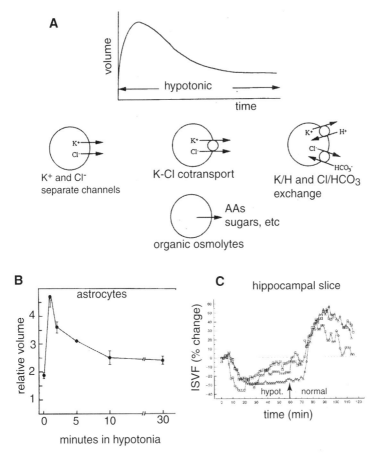

Figure 3-1. Regulatory volume decrease (RVD). **A:** Illustration of the RVD concept. The graph is an idealized representation of initial cell swelling followed by RVD during hypotonic exposure. The four diagrams below the graph show various mechanisms by which cells lose osmotic particles as they achieve RVD. Potassium chloride is removed first. The combined action of K/H and Cl/ HCO$_3$ exchangers results in the exit of KCl and uptake of protons and bicarbonate; H$^+$ + HCO$_3^-$ then combine into water and CO$_2$ under the influence of carbonic anhydrase. The CO$_2$ diffuses out of the cell and the water dilutes the cytosol, aiding equilibration with the hypotonic extracellular medium. AAs: amino acids. **B:** Regulatory volume decrease in a culture of astrocytes. **C:** The slow RVD of three hippocampal tissue slices during 60 min of hypotonic exposure and its aftermath. The interstitial volume fraction (ISVF) was measured by recording the extracellular concentration of TMA$^+$ (Chapter 2: "Osmotic volume changes . . ."). Shrinkage of ISVF indicates cell swelling. Note that one of the three slices showed no overt RVD during hypotonia, but all three slices underwent major cell shrinkage when normal osmolarity was restored (after 60 min), indicating loss of solutes from the cells during the preceding hypotonia. (**A:** modified from Hallows and Knauf, 1994; **B:** modified from Kimelberg and Frangakis, 1986; **C:** from Chebabo et al., 1995b.)

For neurons the evidence is uncertain. There is evidence of RVD in hippo-campal tissue slices (Fig. 3–1) (Chebabo et al., 1995b). Cell volume changes were ascertained from the reciprocal changes in ***interstitial volume fraction (ISVF)*** according to the method of Nicholson et al. (1979), Nicholson and Rice (1988), and Dietzel et al. (1980). The ISVF was assayed from the concentration of marker ions, tetramethyl ammonium (TMA^+) or tetraethyl ammonium (TEA^+), delivered by ionophoretic pulses from microelectrodes into the tissue and mea-sured with a nearby ion-selective microelectrode (see the example in Fig. 13–2). During hypotonic exposure ISVF became much smaller, as expected for cell swelling; then in most slices it slowly but steadily began to recover, demonstrat-ing RVD. Returning the bath to normal osmolarity caused a large overshooting of ISVF in all slices, indicating cell shrinkage even in those slices that did not show RVD during hypotonia (Fig. 3–1C). The posthypotonic cell shrinkage suggests that even in these slices there was "latent RVD" that presumably pre-vented even greater cell swelling. Tissue resistance measurements (R_T) con-firmed hypotonic cell swelling, RVD, and posthypotonic cell shrinkage in hippocampal slices (Chebabo et al., 1995b). Osmotic volume regulation of ce-rebral tissue slices in vitro has been disputed (Andrew et al., 1997), yet it clearly does occur, albeit slowly (Fig. 3–1C). The problem is that these data do not distinguish glial tissue from neurons.

Swelling of neuron dendrites is a prominent feature in electron micrographs of brain tissue prepared from pathological specimens (Van Harreveld and Schadé, 1960). On the other hand, freshly harvested isolated neurons change their size only very sluggishly when exposed to anisosmotic bathing solutions and, once they swell or shrink, do not show RVD or RVI (Aitken et al., 1998a). The reluctant osmotic response suggests low hydraulic conductivity of neuronal plasma membranes that limits or at least slows neuron swelling. Freshly disso-ciated neurons lose their dendritic tree in the process of preparation, and what is left is the soma with a stump of the shaft of the apical dendrite and short pieces of the basal dendrites. Another experimental approach is the recording of light scattering by live brain tissue slices in vitro. Light scattering is a time-honored means to measuring cell volume changes (Aitken et al., 1999) (see Chapter 13: "Spreading depression–related intrinsic optical signals"). When hippocampal tissue slices are placed in hypo-osmotic artificial cerebrospinal fluid (ACSF), light scattering decreases markedly in the layers that contain neuron dendrites and glial cells (neuropil) but much less so in cell body layers that contain few glial processes (Fayuk et al., 2002). This suggests that neuron somata swell only slightly, while glial processes and perhaps also neuron dendrites respond much more strongly. Concordant with slow swelling of neurons, aquaporins have not (yet) been found in or on neurons but are abundant on glial membranes (Nielsen et al., 1997).

Volume Regulation of the Brain

There is also evidence that the brain as a whole undergoes regulatory volume changes in the face of changing osmolarity of the blood (Gullans and Verbalis, 1993; Lundbaek et al., 1990). This acts as a defense, albeit an imperfect defense, against cerebral edema. During systemic hypotonia (water poisoning) of rats, cerebral interstitial volume remained relatively constant while brain cellular volume increased, but not as much as would be expected in the absence of regulatory compensation (Lundbaek et al., 1990; Sager et al., 1996). By contrast, during severe systemic hypertonia of anesthetized rats, cerebral interstitial fluid was depleted, with relatively little change in average brain cell volume (Cserr et al., 1991). The mechanism of cerebral volume regulation is not completely clear, but it must involve solute transport across the BBB, presumably through the astrocyte-endothelial system.

Key points

Osmotic pressure is exerted by the kinetic energy of water molecules. The pressure can develop only through a membrane that is more permeable to water than to (some of the) solutes.

The BBB is more permeable to water than to solutes; therefore, if the osmolarity of blood plasma changes, the brain can swell or shrink. Because the brain is enclosed in the skull, once the arachnoid space is filled, further swelling can have catastrophic consequences.

Osmolarity inside the cells of animals is normally kept equal to the milieu by active transport of solutes. Energy-deprived cells swell.

When exposed to a hypotonic environment, the swelling of cells is, to some degree, counteracted by RVD; osmotic cell shrinkage is limited by RVI. RVD is achieved, first, by release of KCl and later by the release of organic osmolytes. RVI requires uptake of ions from the ECF.

Among brain cells, glial cells swell more, but also have more effective osmotic volume regulation, than do neurons.

4

The Influence of Ion Concentrations
on Neuron Functions

As we have seen, the brain—similarly to the eye and the testicles—has a privileged position, protected by the BBB against undue fluctuations of ion levels and other unwanted intrusions. In the pages that follow, we will see why this is important. We will explore how deviations from the normal range of ion levels can disrupt neuron function. Later, we will also ask, under what conditions do ion levels in brain move outside their normal range?

Ringer's fluid

Rarely does a technical mistake lead to a major discovery, and such serendipity comes only to an exceptional mind. An example is seen in a landmark paper, beginning with this admission by Sidney Ringer: "After publication of [an earlier] paper in the Journal of Physiology, . . . I discovered, that the saline solution which I had used had not been prepared with distilled water, but with pipe water supplied by the New River Water Company" (Ringer, 1883). The actual events were as follows. Ringer had been experimenting with excised frog hearts perfused with a solution of NaCl. Thus treated, hearts usually continued to beat, perhaps for 20 minutes. On this lucky day, however, the heart never stopped until the hour when Dr. Ringer was "obliged to leave." Because on subsequent days he could not repeat this observation, Ringer began to interrogate his assistant about the solution he had prepared on that earlier occasion, when all went exceptionally well. As he now admitted, the assistant had run out of distilled water and used tap water instead. Next, Ringer obtained a chemical analysis of the water supplied by the New River Water Company, and then he began to determine systematically which of the ingredients "present in minute quantities" was responsible for preserving the heart for so many hours. Thus *Ringer's fluid* was born. The recipe contained, besides the usual NaCl, KCl, $CaCl_2$ and $NaHCO_3$, the last intended to "neutralize the acid produced by the beating heart."

Frog Ringer had to be modified for use with mammals, first because the osmolarity had to be higher. Ringer ignored magnesium; this was the only important mistake. After Mg^{2+}, sulfate and phosphate, sometimes lactate, and frequently glucose were added in later formulations. The physiological pH of 7.4 can be achieved if the solution contains 24 mM $NaHCO_3$ and is saturated with gas containing 5% CO_2, but the pH can also be stabilized by sodium-lactate/lactic acid, phosphate, or HEPES buffer. Brain tissue slices are bathed in *artificial CSF* (*ACSF*), with ion levels slightly different from those of other standard solutions such as Tyrode's and Krebs' solutions.

A brief review of elementary membrane physiology

The resting membrane potential (***resting V_m***) of mammalian neurons is usually between –60 and –75 mV. (As we have seen, rest does not mean metabolic inaction.) Since the dawn of membrane biophysics more than 100 year ago, it has been clear that this voltage is generated by a selective permeability of cell membranes for K^+ ions. A general expression of the relationship of V_m to ion concentrations and ion permeabilities was formulated in the mid-twentieth century and is known as the ***Goldman-Hodgkin-Katz (GHK)*** equation (Hille, 2001):

$$V_m = \frac{RT}{F} \ln \frac{P_k[K+]_o + P_{Na}[Na+]_o + P_{Cl}[Cl-]_i}{P_k[K+]_i + P_{Na}[Na+]_i + P_{Cl}[Cl]_o} \qquad (4\text{--}1)$$

where R is the gas constant, T is the absolute temperature, F is Faraday's number, P_k is the permeability of K^+, and $[K^+]_o$, and so on, have the usual meaning of ion concentrations outside or inside the cell.

Equation 4–1 is the original GHK equation intended for axon membrane potentials, but other ions, especially Ca^{2+}, H^+, and HCO_3^-, also contribute to the membrane potential of central neurons and should be included to better approximate reality. Divalent ions contribute only half of the voltage provided by univalent ions, so for calcium the expression would be $(P_{Ca}/2)[Ca^{2+}]$. The GHK equation is based on a number of assumptions (Hille, 2001), one of them being a constant field across the membrane, and this concept has been challenged. Nonetheless, this simple formula proved to be an adequate approximation of experimental observations, and it is widely used in theoretical treatment of data and in computer simulations. The equation states that the contribution of each ion to the membrane potential is determined by the ion's distribution between the inside and outside of the cell, as well as by its permeability through the membrane. The permeability, P, is assumed to be symmetrical, that is, the same for crossing the membrane in either direction.

Since $[K^+]_o < [K^+]_i$, the gradient tends to drive K^+ outward and therefore to make the inside of cells electrically negative. For Na^+ the gradient is inwardly directed but, since in neurons at rest $P_K \gg P_{Na}$, the resting V_m is close to but not equal to the **equilibrium potential** of K^+, E_K. E_K is expressed as follows:

$$E_K = \frac{RT}{F} \ln \frac{[K+]_o}{[K+]_i} \tag{4-2}$$

Equation 4–2 is known as the **Nernst equation** for potassium. (At room temperature, the Nernst equation predicts that E_K changes by $= 58$ mV $* \log_{10}([K^+]_o/[K^+]_i.)$ At the physiological temperature of 37°C the magic number is 61.5 mV for each decade of $([K^+]_o/[K^+]_i.)$ change. E_K is negative because $[K^+]_o < [K^+]_i$. This, of course, is a matter of convention. The ratio in the Nernst equation could have been inverted to read $[K^+]_i/[K^+]_o$ but it is customary to consider the average outside potential to be zero and to refer the voltage inside cells to the outside. During the firing of action potentials $P_{Na} \gg P_K$ and, since $[Na^+]_o > [Na^+]_i$, the membrane potential becomes positive for a brief moment.

The unequal distribution of ions between the inside and outside of cells is maintained by active transport driven by metabolic energy. The most important ion pump moves 2 K^+ into cells against 3 Na^+ ions moving out, and it is fueled by ATP. The enzyme splitting the ATP is built into the same integral membrane protein complex that is moving the ions, and the assembly is referred to as *Na/K ATPase*. Because more positive charges are pumped out than in, the transport is electrogenic: it adds a negative voltage to the membrane potential that is summed with the one defined by the GHK equation. The pump voltage is small compared to the GHK voltage, but it becomes important in certain situations, as we shall see later (see also Chapter 2: "Mechanisms of the regulation of ion content . . .")

For anions the electrical gradient is the opposite of the chemical gradient. This again is a matter of convention, since we regard electric current as the movement of positive charge. Therefore the Nernst equation for Cl^- is:

$$E_{Cl} = RT/F \ln [Cl^-]_i/[Cl^-]_o \tag{4-3}$$

exactly as for K^+, except that the inside concentration is divided by the outside concentration.

The resting P_{Cl} of neurons is usually low. If Cl^- ions are not actively transported, the inside-negative resting potential, keeps $[Cl^-]_i < [Cl]_o$. In fact, in skeletal muscle, where resting P_{Cl} is higher, E_{Cl} is nearly equal to V_m, and Cl^- is said to be passively distributed. This is not the case in most central neurons, where active transport keeps $[Cl^-]_i$ even lower than it would be if it remained at equilibrium, so that E_{Cl} is more negative than the resting potential

The importance of reference potential

Here a technical note is in order. In electrophysiological practice (and in clinical electrocardiography [EKG] and EEG), it is customary to connect the body of an experimental animal or the organ bath of isolated tissues to **ground** (**earth** in the United Kingdom), which could be a metal rod sunk into the earth or the third pole of an electric plug or simply the plumbing of the building. Intracellular voltages are then measured against ground, which is taken to be constant and equal to the potential outside the cell. This is as it should be as long as the voltage in the interstitial spaces indeed remains more or less constant. A problem arises, however, when the extracellular voltage changes significantly, as it does, for example, during epileptiform discharges or SD (Figs. 7–8, 12–2). In these cases, recording the *intracellular voltage* (V_i) against ground does not yield the true transmembrane voltage, because the recorded change of voltage is the sum of the extracellular and intracellular potential shifts. To obtain the true (trans)membrane potential (V_m), the intracellular voltage must be referred to the voltage outside the cell, which can be obtained if, in addition to the intracellular electrode, an extracellular microelectrode is inserted close to the cell ($\Delta V_m = \Delta V_I - \Delta V_o$) (Figs. 13–1 and 19–1 have been produced this way). This precaution is occasionally neglected even by seasoned neuroscientists.

Changing potassium levels influence excitability, synaptic transmission, and Na⁺ channel function

Potassium Effects on Membrane Potential

From the preceding section, it follows that raising $[K^+]_o$ (to be more precise, *increasing* $[K^+]_o/[K^+]_i$) *depolarizes* neuron membranes (diminishes the inside negative membrane potential). As we have seen, however, potassium is not the only ion governing the resting potential. Because P_{Na} is not zero, V_m is not a linear function of $\ln([K^+]_o/[K^+]_i)$. Especially within the normal range, where $[K^+]_o$ is low and $[Na]_o$ is high, the depolarization induced by a given increment of $[K^+]_o$ is milder than expected from the Nernst equation (Eq. 4–2), but as $[K^+]_o$ rises higher and higher, V_m more and more approaches the value predicted by the Nernst equation (Fig. 4–1) (Forsythe and Redman, 1988; Kuffler, 1967; Somjen et al., 1981). This has important consequences. In the milieu of central neurons $[K^+]_o$ is normally between 2.7 and 3.5 mM, which is even lower than in the ECF of the rest of the

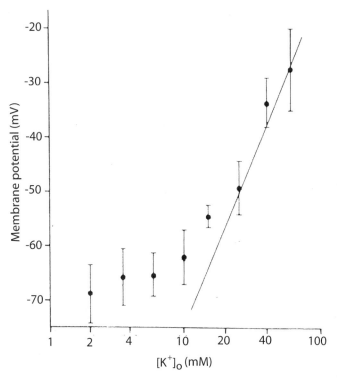

FIGURE 4–1. The dependence of neuronal membrane potential on extracellular potassium concentration. Each point on the mean V_m ($\pm$SD) of four to six cells in rat dorsal root ganglia in vitro. Note the logarithmic abscissal scale. The straight line is the Nernst function (Eq. I–6). Note the deviation from the Nernst function at $[K^+]_o$ less than 10 mM. (From Connors, 1979, and modified from Somjen et al., 1981.)

body (4.5 mM; Table 2–1). It seems that keeping $[K^+]_o$ low protects central neurons from undue influence by fluctuating $[K^+]_o$ levels. While $[K^+]_o$ is not absolutely constant, the small fluctuations during normal activity (Fig. 2–9) keep it within the range of *relative indifference*. The indifference is relative, and even moderate changes in $[K^+]_o$ slightly influence synaptic function (Fig. 4-2). But only under pathological conditions does $[K^+]_o$ increase so much that it can seriously perturb neuron function.

As V_m moves closer to or further from the threshold of firing, excitability becomes greater or smaller. Since the membrane potential governs voltage-controlled membrane ion channels, when $[K^+]_o$ is raised, neurons not only depolarize, but the membrane resistance decreases (Pan and Stringer, 1997) because opening probabilities of voltage-gated ion channels start to increase. As a general rule, under acute pathological conditions $[K^+]_o$ changes to a greater degree than does $[K^+]_i$, but the reverse is true in chronic hypo- or hyperkalemia. Of course, during experiments on brain tissue and on isolated cells or cell cultures, only $[K^+]_o$ can easily be controlled by the experimenter.

Synaptic transmission is affected in complex ways. The efficiency of excitatory synaptic transmission depends on both the readiness of postsynaptic cells to respond—that is, their excitability—and the amount of transmitter released from presynaptic terminals with each afferent impulse. The function of both sides of the synapse is affected by membrane potential and therefore by $[K^+]_o/[K^+]_i$. Hyperpolarization moves V_m away from threshold voltage and therefore depresses excitability, while mild depolarization increases excitability. More severe depolarization, however, has an opposite effect because it inactivates some voltage-gated ion channels, raising the threshold of firing and eventually rendering neurons inexcitable (known as **depolarization block** or, in the earlier literature, as *cathodal block*). As $[K^+]_o$ or, more precisely, $[K^+]_o/[K^+]_i$ moves from very low to very high, excitability first increases and then decreases (Hablitz and Lundervold, 1981; Matsuura, 1969).

Variation of $[K^+]_o$ influences the membrane potential of presynaptic terminals as well. Therefore, it also modulates synaptic transmission.

The outcome of the various competing effects of abnormal levels of $[K^+]_o$ on pre- and postsynaptic functions cannot be predicted theoretically. For one thing, different types of synapses are not uniformly sensitive to its effects. When tested, the results varied not only among different synapses, but in some cases even in similar preparations in the hands of different experimenters. The results may have been influenced by the age and breed of the experimental animals or by other experimental conditions.

Input-output functions in the analysis of synaptic efficacy

Overall efficiency of excitatory synaptic transmission may be expressed as an input-output function by plotting postsynaptic population spike amplitude (output) as a function of presynaptic spike amplitude (input) (Figs. 4–2, 4–4, 4–5). Successive elements in the transmission chain can be decomposed. The excitability of afferent axons can be gauged from the size of the presynaptic volley evoked by varying electrical stimulus pulses. This function has a threshold: the stimulus that is just sufficient to fire one afferent fiber. In the lowest range, the afferent fiber volley (number of afferent axons firing) grows almost linearly with stimulus intensity, but the slope soon decreases as the function approaches the absolute maximum, when all axons are excited. Next, one can plot the amplitude of the extracellularly recorded EPSP (fEPSP) as a function of the presynaptic volley. This is a gauge of presynaptic transmitter output. In an ideal synapse its origin is at the zero intercept because even a single incoming afferent impulse will evoke a small EPSP. This function is also nearly linear at first but approaches an absolute maximum in the higher range. Plotting the postsynaptic population spike amplitude as a function of fEPSP measures postsynaptic neuron excitabil-

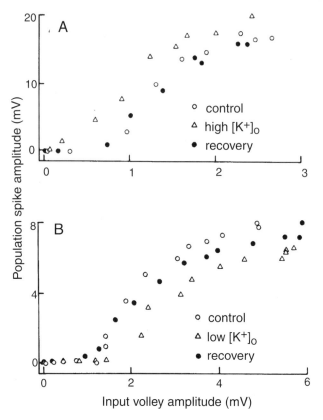

FIGURE 4–2. The influence of extracellular K^+ concentration on synaptic transmission. Input-output curves from two hippocampal tissue slices. Variable stimulus pulses applied to the Schaffer collateral-commissural bundle; responses recorded in CA1. Input volley: compound action potential of afferent fibers recorded in stratum (st.) radiatum. Population spike recorded in st. pyramidale. Normal $[K^+]_o$ was 3.5 mM. A: high $[K^+]_o$ = 5 mM. B: low $[K^+]_o$ = 2 mM. (Modified from Balestrino et al., 1986.)

ity. This function has a threshold: the smallest-population EPSP that fires at least one postsynaptic target neuron; beyond that the function is sigmoid, again with an absolute maximal value (Balestrino and Somjen, 1988; Balestrino et al., 1986). This must be remembered: the amplitude of population spikes (synonym, *compound action potentials*) is a function of the number of unit elements firing a spike. The amplitude of the action potentials fired by individual axons or cell bodies is usually more or less constant (all-or-none), except in severely pathological conditions, but different cells contribute different unit spikes to the aggregate (depending on the distance from the recording electrode, cell geometry, etc.). This is not so for the extracellularly recorded (focal or field) fEPSP. The contribution of each postsynaptic target neuron to the fEPSP can vary greatly because each receives input from many afferent fibers. The magnitude of the EPSP generated by each postsynaptic neuron therefore varies with the number of afferent impulses it receives.

Potassium Effects on Synaptic Transmission

Release of transmitter from synaptic terminals is governed by influx of Ca^{2+} through voltage-gated channels and therefore, in turn, by presynaptic impulse amplitude (Katz, 1966). Depolarization of presynaptic axon endings has long been considered a mechanism of presynaptic inhibition (Eccles, 1964). Presynaptic depolarization inactivates Na^+ and Ca^{2+} channels, reducing action potential amplitude and calcium uptake and thus transmitter output. Moderately elevated $[K^+]_o$ may be expected to cause a tug of war between pre- and postsynaptic effects, because postsynaptic neurons become more excitable, while transmitter output may be depressed. Beyond a certain level of raised $[K^+]_o$, all excitability is abolished due to depolarization-induced inactivation of voltage-gated Na^+ current. With inhibitory synapses, the picture changes. A reduced output of inhibitory transmitter substances (***disinhibition***) combined with enhanced excitability of the postsynaptic targets renders inhibition less effective than it normally is. Since very high $[K^+]_o$ inactivates all nerve cells, it renders both inhibitory and excitatory synapses irrelevant. In view of these multiple effects, the influence of varying the K^+ concentration cannot be predicted, and actual testing yields a variable outcome.

In the isolated mouse spinal cord, reflex transmission from the dorsal to the ventral root was barely changed by varying tissue $[K^+]_o$ between 2.0 and 5.5. mM, but it was depressed at both lower and higher concentrations (Czéh et al., 1988). In brain slices, mild elevation of $[K^+]_o$ enhanced synaptic transmission, whereas a more drastic increase depressed it. In rat hippocampal tissue slices, when $[K^+]_o$ was raised from the normal 3.5 mM to 5.0 mM, the population spike evoked by a given presynaptic volley increased by almost 50%, while fEPSP was unchanged, indicating increased postsynaptic excitability of pyramidal neurons with no change in transmitter release (Balestrino et al., 1986; Rausche et al., 1990) (Fig. 4-2). Further raising $[K^+]_o$ to 6.25 or 9.25 mM actually enhanced the fEPSP amplitude, indicating enhanced synaptic release (Hablitz and Lundervold, 1981). According to Poolos and Kocsis (1990), at 7.5 mM $[K^+]_o$ EPSPs acquired an NMDA receptor–mediated component. Only at 12.25 mM was there indication of reduced synaptic efficacy. In another study, at 6.25 mM, both fEPSP and the postsynaptic population spike were increased, indicating enhanced transmitter release plus enhanced postsynaptic excitability (Hablitz and Lundervold, 1981). A further increase to 9.25 mM still enhanced transmission, according to Hablitz and Lundervold (1981), but even 8 mM caused depression, according to another report (Rausche et al., 1990).

The $[K^+]_o$ levels applied to the various preparations listed in the previous paragraph should be seen in the context of the $\Delta[K^+]_o$ responses seen in CNS tissues. As we have seen (Chapter 2: "Extracellular potassium responses . . ."), 5 mM is probably never reached in healthy forebrain, but possibly it does occur in spinal dorsal horn. During seizures, however, 8–12 mM can easily be reached.

Potassium on Persistent Na^+ Current

Besides setting the membrane potential and influencing synaptic transmission, elevated $[K^+]_o$ potentiates persistent (slowly inactivating) Na^+ current ($I_{Na,P}$) of neurons (Somjen and Müller, 2000) (Fig. 4–3). This usually small voltage-gated current is probably generated by a rarer variant of the more common, rapidly inactivating Na^+ channel, although it is also possible that an entirely different channel is responsible (Crill, 1996). Its significance will become clear when we consider the generation of seizure discharges (Chapters 7 and 9).

Potassium Effects in Intact Central Nervous System

Perennial doubt lingers about the validity of results from tissues excised from brains and kept in dishes under artificial conditions. Unfortunately, it is very difficult to alter the ionic environment within intact brains in a well-controlled manner. Superfusing the exposed hippocampus of anesthetized rats with fluid of increasing K^+ concentration resulted in an increase in synaptically evoked responses (Izquierdo et al., 1970). Many years earlier, Feldberg and Sherwood (1957) injected KCl solution through permanently implanted cannulae into the lateral ventricle of alert rabbits. Raising $[K^+]_o$ in this rather crude manner caused epileptiform convulsions. Other investigators have exposed hippocampus or neocortex in anesthetized animals and applied a solution containing a high concentration of K^+ to the surface of the brain, which caused EEG discharges similar to seizures (Zuckermann and Glaser, 1968). The CA3 region of hippocampal tissue in vitro became spontaneously active when $[K^+]_o$ was increased above 6.5 or 7 mM, generating discharges resembling interictal epileptic activity, and at about 8.5 mM, electrographic ictal-like seizures erupted in the CA1 region as well (Chamberlin and Dingledine, 1988; Jensen and Yaari, 1997; Korn et al., 1987; Pan and Stringer, 1997). At even higher levels, $[K^+]_o$ can induce SD. Later, we will consider the likely role of K^+ in the generation of seizures and of SD in detail (Chapter 8: "Potassium and seizures," and Chapters 9 and 15).

We have attempted to raise $[K^+]_o$ in the brains in situ of anesthetized rats in a more controlled manner by first opening the BBB and then administering KCl through the internal carotid artery (Somjen et al., 1991). In spite of the apparently successful breach of the barrier, nothing much changed at first. $[K^+]_o$ in neocor-

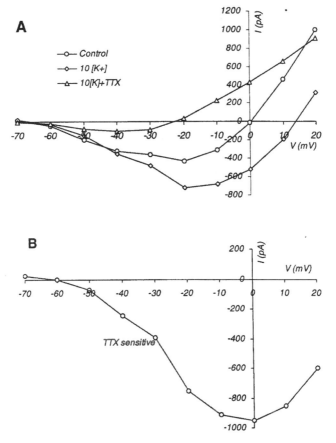

FIGURE 4–3. Elevated extracellular K$^+$ concentration potentiates persistent Na$^+$ current. Whole-cell current-voltage (I-V) curves of patch-clamped CA1 pyramidal cells in hippocampal tissue slices. Average data from four cells in four slices. The current was measured near the end of a 600 ms test voltage step (V_h = –65 mV; pre-pulse before test step: to –90 mV) . A: Current-voltage curves in normal artificial cerebiospinal fluid (3.5 mM [K$^+$]) during exposure to 10 mM [K$^+$] and exposure to 10 mM [K$^+$] with 1.0 µM tetrodotoxin (TTX) added. B: Subtracting the data obtained under 10 mM [K$^+$] + TTX from those obtained in 10 mM [K$^+$] yields the TTX-sensitive (Na$^+$-dependent) fraction of the potentiated persistent current. (From Somjen and Müller, 2000.)

tex and in hippocampus remained constant for a considerable time; then, instead of the well-controlled, gradual increase we hoped to achieve, SD erupted. The conclusion: active regulation can defend the internal environment of the brain even when the BBB is defective, up to a point. And this defense is essential, because once it is overwhelmed, SD immediately arrests normal brain function.

Calcium and magnesium

Ca²⁺–Mg²⁺ Synergism: Surface Charge Screening

Ringer credits Biederman with first noticing that excised skeletal muscle left in an isotonic NaCl solution starts to twitch spontaneously. Ringer then showed that adding a small amount of calcium to the bath quiets the muscle (Ringer, 1886). The need for calcium for brain function was emphasized by Sabbatani (1901), who reported experiments by his assistant, P. Regoli. Small amounts of citrate or oxalate solution applied to the exposed cerebral cortex increased the excitability of the brain, culminating in epileptiform seizures. Sabbatani correctly reasoned that the excitation was caused by the binding of calcium, and not by the citrate or oxalate itself. A very small amount of a calcium salt administered in the same manner had a calming effect. Sabbatani concluded that the "minute amounts of calcium normally present in the cortex have a moderating effect" on cortical excitability. This conclusion stood the test of time, and we shall devote much attention to the complex roles of calcium and, as it turns out, magnesium in normal and abnormal neuron function.

Huge amounts of calcium are present in bone, but its concentration in free, ionized form is only about 1.0–1.5 mM in all ECF (Table 2–1). There is a fair amount of calcium inside cells, but most of it is either bound to specific proteins or sequestered in organelles, principally the ER (or, in muscle cells, the SR) and mitochondria, as well as in Golgi apparatus (Fig. 2–3) (Chapter 2: "Intracellular calcium ion activity . . .").

Extracellular Mg^{2+} levels are about the same as free Ca^{2+} levels, but inside cells the cytosol concentration of free Mg^{2+} is much higher than that of Ca^{2+}. The precise adjustment of the levels of Ca^{2+} and Mg^{2+} both inside and outside cells is crucial for the functioning of excitable tissues. It is useful to discuss these two main divalent cations together, because they interact in interesting ways. In some respects they act synergistically, while in others they antagonize each other's effects.

Divalent cations have long been considered to be ***membrane stabilizers*** because raising their extracellular concentrations reduces excitability and increases membrane resistance, while lowering them makes tissues more irritable (Gordon and Sauerheber, 1982; Shanes, 1958). Today embrane stabilization is defined more precisely as ***surface charge screening*** (Hille et al., 1975; Madeja, 2000). At the outer surface of cell membranes, and especially around the entrance to ion channels, there are negatively charged residues. These fixed negative charges on the outer surface *take away from* the transmembrane voltage, which, as we know, is positive on the outside relative to the inside. It is this transmembrane voltage that is "experienced" by the voltage sensors of voltage-gated membrane ion channels. On the other hand, an intracellular electrode records the voltage between the cytoplasm and a distant reference potential without registering the surface charge). The term *surface charge screening* means that divalent cations latch onto and neutralize the negative residues and so *increase* the membrane polarization (potential difference across the membrane). Surface charge screening therefore reduces the likelihood of the activation of voltage-gated ion channels and dampens excitability. All cations screen surface charges, but divalents are much more effective than univalents (Hille, 2001). Ca^{2+} and Mg^{2+} reinforce each other's stabilizing effect. The physiological levels of $[Ca^{2+}]_o$ and $[Mg^{2+}]_o$ are "calibrated" for optimal function. Deviation downward of either one leads to hyperexcitability, a condition known by clinicians as ***tetany***, while their elevation reduces excitability, causing lethargy, as well as weakness of heart and skeletal muscles. The effects of experimental lowering of $[Ca^{2+}]_o$ are manifested in CNS neurons in depolarization and reduced membrane resistance (Pan and Stringer, 1997).

An additional, possibly very important effect of $[Ca^{2+}]_o$ has been described by Xiong and MacDonald (1999; Xiong et al., 1997). Lowering of $[Ca^{2+}]_o$ apparently opens ***nonspecific cation channels*** that are permeable for monovalent cations without much selection. The result is depolarization. The channel seems to be operated by "sensing" $[Ca^{2+}]_o$ itself, and it is independent of membrane potential. Depending on how widespread this phenomenon is, it could be a major factor in pathological processes. Positive feedback could be initiated by this channel because depolarization can activate voltage-operated calcium channels, and inflow of calcium into cells can further lower $[Ca^{2+}]_o$, with more of the nonspecific channel opening, more depolarization, and more calcium channel activation. We shall return to this problem (Chapter 11: "Drugs acting on voltage-gated ion channels" and Chapter 15: "Not one spreading depression channel . . .").

Ca^{2+}–Mg^{2+} Antagonism: Synaptic Transmitter Release

Unlike the synergism of Ca^{2+} and Mg^{2+} in charge screening, the two divalent cations act antagonistically at all chemically operated synapses. Raising $[Ca^{2+}]_o$ enhances and raising $[Mg^{2+}]_o$ inhibits the release of transmitter substances from presynaptic axon terminals (Del Castillo and Engbaek, 1954). Influx of Ca^{2+} through voltage-gated Ca channels from ISF into presynaptic terminals is an absolute requirement for normal synaptic transmission (Katz, 1966). Mg^{2+} ions block calcium channels, and the Mg^{2+} that is normally present limits the inflow of Ca^{2+}. With $[Mg^{2+}]_o$ constant, transmitter release from axon terminals at central synapses is highly sensitive to changing $[Ca^{2+}]_o$ levels. For example, lowering $[Ca^{2+}]_o$ from 1.2 to 1.0 mM depresses the synaptically transmitted electric signal, fEPSP, by 34% (Fig. 4–4) (Dingledine and Somjen, 1981). Similarly, steep dependence was reported more recently for cerebellar synapses (Mintz et al., 1995) and neocortex (Tsodyks and Markram, 1997).

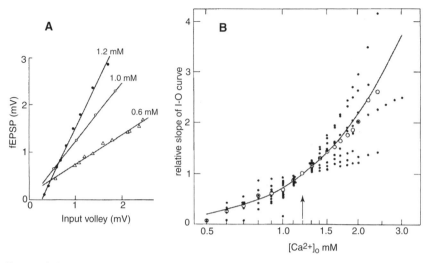

FIGURE 4–4. Dependence of excitatory postsynaptic potentials (EPSPs) on extracellular calcium concentration. **A:** The extracellularly recorded EPSP as function of input volley, at three different concentrations of extracellular calcium in one hippocampal tissue slice, in CA1 stratum radiatum. The straight lines are regression functions. **B:** The slope (regression coefficient) of the EPSP input-output functions (determined as in **A**), as a function of $[Ca^{2+}]_o$ (measured in the tissue with ion-selective microelectrodes), from hippocampal slices. The slope found at the control level of $[Ca^{2+}]_o$ (1.2 mM) was taken as unity. Dots are individual data points; circles are averages. The control $[Ca^{2+}]_o$ of 1.2 mM is marked by the arrow. (Modified from Dingledine and Somjen, 1981.)

In the previous section, we saw that variations in $[K^+]_o$ affect presynaptic transmitter release differently from postsynaptic excitability. Changing $[Ca^{2+}]_o$ also has dual action, because raising it enhances transmitter release but reduces postsynaptic excitability, while lowering it impairs synapses and increases irritability. Also, as with $[K^+]_o$, the contest between the opposing effects is decided by the concentration, and it varies with synapse type. In hippocampal tissue slices, presynaptic transmitter release wins over postsynaptic excitability. Transmission to pyramidal cells in the CA1 sector of such a slice was exaggerated when $[Ca^{2+}]_o$ was raised from 1.2 to 1.8 mM, and it was depressed when $[Ca^{2+}]_o$ was lowered to 0.8 mM (Fig. 4–5) (Balestrino et al., 1986). More drastic lowering of $[Ca^{2+}]_o$ caused synaptic block, as expected (Rausche et al., 1990). In isolated mouse spinal cord, reflexes were maximal when $[Ca^{2+}]_o$ was raised to between 2.4 and 3.6 mM, and they were depressed at 4.8 mM (Czéh and Somjen, 1989).

Both excitability and synaptic transmission are monotonically depressed when $[Mg^{2+}]_o$ is raised, and they are enhanced when $[Mg^{2+}]_o$ is lowered (Czéh and Somjen, 1989; Erulkar et al., 1974; Rausche et al., 1990). In isolated brain tissue slices, reducing bath $[Mg^{2+}]$ can induce epileptiform discharges (Chapter 8: "Cal-

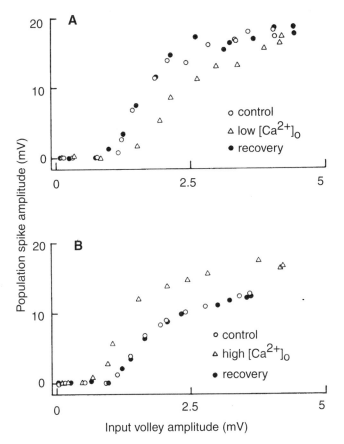

FIGURE 4–5. The influence of extracellular calcium concentration on synaptic transmission. Recording conditions similar to those of Figure 4–2. Control level of $[Ca^{2+}]_o$ was 1.2 mM. **A:** Low $[Ca^{2+}]_o = 0.8$ mM. **B:** High $[Ca^{2+}]_o = 1.8$ mM. (Modified from Balestrino et al., 1986.)

cium, magnesium, and seizures"). By contrast, raising $[Mg^{2+}]_o$ depresses transmitter output and can paralyze skeletal muscle as well as central synapses.

Ca^{2+} and Mg^{2+} antagonize one another in certain physiological functions outside the CNS, for example in blood clotting, and also in the contraction of smooth muscle.

Tetany

Clinically, deficiency of either of the two main divalent cations causes the signs of tetany, a syndrome dominated by muscle cramps. Low-calcium tetany is usually the result of deficient parathyroid function. In earlier days it was also common in children suffering from rickets, but this deficiency disease has become rare, at least in peacetime, in the Western world. Acute, severe magnesium deficiency is less common in people, but more of a potential problem in cattle and horses.

Tetanic cramps are caused by hyperexcitability of peripheral nerves and skeletal muscle. When the blood concentration of Ca^{2+} or Mg^{2+} changes acutely, brain levels change much less, so that the peripheral signs dominate the clinical picture (Fig. 1–3) (Hilmy and Somjen, 1968; Kemény et al., 1961; Somjen et al., 1966, 1987a). Of the competing effects of low $[Ca^{2+}]_o$, impaired transmitter release and increased irritability of nerve and muscle, the latter is clinically manifested. Also, in the laboratory, when $[Ca^{2+}]$ was lowered in the blood by the infusion of a chelating agent such as citrate or EGTA, signs of tetany appeared long before neuromuscular transmission failed (Allen et al., 1985; Somjen et al., 1987a), confirming the greater sensitivity of the surface screening effect on skeletal muscle fibers compared to that on neuromuscular transmission.

The manifold other signs and symptoms of chronic hypo- and hypercalcemia are outside the scope of this volume.

Magnesium Ions Modulate Ion Channels

Both calcium and magnesium interact with and are cofactors of numerous enzymes, but these biochemical effects fall outside the scope of this book. Relevant for our purpose, however, is the manner in which Mg^{2+} modulates ion channels (Hille, 2001). Alone among ligand-gated ion channels, the NMDA-operated channel not only requires glutamate or aspartate (or NMDA) for activation, but it is also *voltage dependent*. As long as the membrane is at resting potential, neither glutamate nor the other glutamate agonists have much effect on the NMDA receptor channel; only when α-amino-3-hydroxy-5-methyl-4-isoxalepropionic acid (AMPA) receptor-mediated synaptic current or other stimulation depolarizes the membrane can the gate of the NMDA channel open. This is because Mg^{2+} ions plug the channel when the membrane potential is strongly negative, but magnesium is removed from the pore of the channel when the membrane depolarizes, allowing ion current to flow. If Mg^{2+} is removed from the cell's environment, the channel is readily opened by NMDA or glutamate, regardless of the prevailing membrane potential (Dingledine et al., 1999; Hille, 2001).

Mg^{2+} is permeable through nicotinic acetylcholine receptor channels, but it moves slowly through the pore and, while it traverses the channel, it slows down the flux of other ions (Hille, 2001). Finally, intracellular Mg^{2+} is responsible for the rectifying property of inwardly rectifying K^+ channels (Hille, 2001).

In conclusion

Seizures are favored by low $[Mg^{2+}]$ for three reasons: (*1*) reduced surface screening, enhancing excitability; (*2*) increased release of transmitter from presynaptic nerve endings; and (*3*) removal of the block from NMDA receptor-controlled channels.

Sodium, chloride, and osmotic effects in the central nervous system

The Sodium Chloride Concentration Is Important for Neurology in at Least Three Ways

First, the NaCl concentration affects intracranial pressure; *second*, osmotic stress influences neuronal function; and *third*, both $[Na^+]_o$ and $[Cl^-]_o$ have direct, specific effects on neuronal function.

In almost all the ECF of the body, NaCl is responsible for by far the largest fraction of osmolarity. Endolymph in the inner ear is the sole exception; there K^+ takes the place of Na^+. In most cases, clinically significant changes in the concentration of Na^+ and Cl^- go hand in hand. The NaCl concentration rises during dehydration and decreases during acute water poisoning. As mentioned (Chapter 3), acute water poisoning causes serious CNS disturbances manifested as convulsions of central origin, delirium, stupor, and coma; if untreated, it can cause death. The rule in the clinic is that danger is imminent if plasma Na^+ drops below 120 mM. Water poisoning affects brain function partly because it raises intracranial pressure, for the BBB is more permeable to water than to ions. In addition to altering intracranial pressure, whenever water moves either into or out of the brain, ISF and CSF become diluted or concentrated, causing osmotic stress of brain cells, which perturbs neuronal function (Chapter 3: "Water poisoning . . .").

A note on technical problems in the unraveling of low [NaCl] effects

In experiments on whole animals, the intracranial pressure and changes in blood circulation confound the direct effects of osmotic pressure on neurons and their synapses, but in experiments on brain slices in vitro there is no such interference. On the other hand, there are other technical pitfalls that can distort extracellular voltage recordings in brain tissue both in situ and in vitro. Because of the high resistance of cell membranes, most of the current that is detected by an extracellular electrode flows in the interstitial spaces, with a smaller but not insignificant fraction flowing through the cells. When cells swell at the expense of interstitial space, extracellular signals appear to be increased, independently of any changes in the physiological currents generated by neurons. This artifact arises because the voltage registered by extracellular microelectrodes is the product of the current times the tissue electric impedance (*Ohm's law*). If cells swell and the interstitial space is compressed, the resistance to extracellular current increases. The current delivered by excited neurons remains (almost) unchanged, because the current *source resistance* is much higher than the *load* (i.e., the extracellular resistance), so that action currents and synaptic currents behave as (almost) constant current sources. If the current stays the same while extracellular resistance increases, the extracellular voltage increases. The interstitial volume fraction (ISVF) and therefore the tissue resistance change markedly during pathophysiological activity and especially during osmotic stress. A further complication is the frequency dependence of the signal. The transcellular current fraction is larger for high-frequency signals because of the capacitive reactance of cell membranes. Finally, the fraction of the total current flowing across cells increases whenever cell membrane resistances are significantly decreased. If the transcellular current flow increases, the fraction flowing in the interstitium decreases, and so does the extracellularly recorded voltage.

Hypotonicity as Well as Iso-Osmotic Low [NaCl]$_o$ Facilitates and Elevation of Osmolarity Depresses Synaptic Transmission

Both acute water poisoning and hypernatremia disturb brain function. Trials on isolated tissues and cells avoid the systemic effects, and also allow testing of low [Na$^+$]$_o$ and low [Cl$^-$]$_o$ independently of reduced osmolarity.

In tissue slices of cerebral neocortex and hippocampal formation, lowering the osmolarity of the bathing fluid enhanced extracellular fEPSPs, while raising osmolarity depressed them (Fig. 4–6) (Chebabo et al., 1995a; Huang and Somjen, 1995; Rosen and Andrew, 1990). According to Ballyk et al. (1991), however, while in cortex synaptic transmission was indeed enhanced by low osmolarity, in hippocampus the extracellular signal seemed to be increased only because of the increased tissue resistance (cf. the technical note above) and intracellular EPSPs were unaffected. Subsequent analysis revealed, however, that the tissue resistance was responsible for only about half of the increase in fEPSPs (Chebabo et al., 1995a).

As a control experiment, we tested the effect of replacing NaCl with sugars. Low [NaCl]$_o$ at normal osmolarity should not have had an effect or, if any, it should have depressed EPSPs by reducing inward Na$^+$ flux. To our surprise, replacing bath NaCl by equiosmolar fructose or mannitol, so that the solution remained isotonic, also boosted fEPSPs. The effect was weaker than that of an unsubstituted (hypotonic) [NaCl] deficiency, but it was still quite marked, reproducible, concentration dependent, and reversible (Chebabo et al., 1995a). The interstitial volume fraction remained constant, proving that cells did not swell when bath [NaCl] was reduced at constant osmolarity. The specific conductivity of NaCl-deficient solution is reduced and this raises tissue resistance somewhat, but much less so than when compression of interstitial space is added to low [NaCl]$_o$.

The recording of synaptic currents from patch-clamped pyramidal neurons convincingly confirmed potentiation of excitatory synapses in the CA1 region of

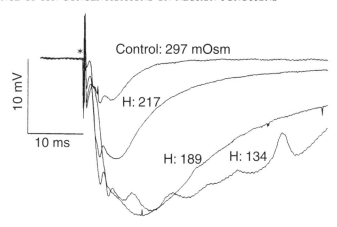

FIGURE 4–6. Hypotonic potentiation of excitatory synaptic transmission. Extracellularly recorded focal excitatory postsynaptic potentials (fEPSPs) in a hippocampal tissue slice CA1 stratum radiatum in control solution and three levels of hypotonia. Osmolarity was lowered by reducing [NaCl] in bathing solution, with other ingredients unchanged. The numbers next to the traces show solution osmolarities measured with an osmometer. Note that fEPSPs not only become larger but also last longer. The undulations of the trace recorded at the lowest osmolarity indicate repetitive firing of neurons. (Modified from Chebabo et al., 1995a.)

hippocampus by both low osmolarity and low $[NaCl]_o$ (Fig. 4–7). Not only excitatory but also inhibitory synaptic currents (both EPSCs and IPSCs) were powerfully enhanced in a concentration-dependent manner when the slices were exposed to hypotonic bathing fluid (Huang et al., 1997). Iso-osmotic lowering of $[NaCl]_o$ again had a similar if somewhat weaker depressant action. Tissue impedance has negligible influence on such whole-cell current measurements. (If it has an effect, it would appear to blunt the observed increase of the EPSC because, from the point of view of whole-cell recording, tissue resistance is *in series* with the current source in the cell membrane.)

Low Osmolarity and Low $[NaCl]_o$ Potentiate the Voltage-Gated
Calcium Current but Depress the Potassium Current

The next question concerns the mechanism by which low osmolarity and low $[NaCl]_o$ enhance synaptic transmission. One obvious candidate is increased release of transmitter from presynaptic axon endings. Since transmitter release is governed by calcium influx into the terminal, potentiation of Ca^{2+} currents could explain the effect. Indeed, in isolated pyramidal neurons, voltage-dependent Ca^{2+} currents were enhanced but K^+ currents were depressed when either bath osmolarity or $[NaCl]_o$ was reduced (Figs. 4–8, 4–9) (Somjen, 1999). Like the increase

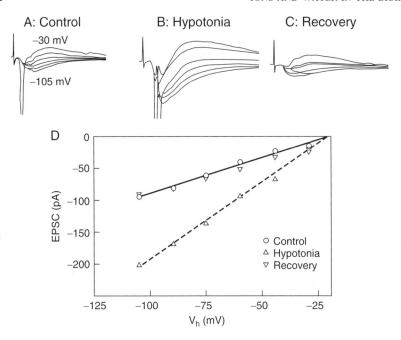

FIGURE 4–7. Hypotonic exposure potentiates synaptic currents. **A–C:** Sample recordings made in a whole-cell configuration from a patch-clamped CA1 pyramidal neuron in a hippocampal slice. Synaptic currents were evoked by stimulating the Schaffer collateral-commissural bundle. Each trace was made at a different holding potential (V_h). The numbers above and below the traces under A show the least and most negative holding potentials in the series. Hypotonia enhanced both the inward and outward components of the synaptic currents (excitatory [EPSC] and inhibitory [IPSC] postsynaptic currents). The osmolarity of the hypotonic solution was 230 mOsm, prepared by reducing [NaCl] by 40 mM in the artificial cerebrospinal fluid of the bath. **D:** The amplitude of the EPSC (measured at a constant time after the stimulus) as a function of the holding potential (V_h), in control solution (301 mOsm) and in hypotonia (230 mOsm). The points are the mean values from five cells in five slices. (Modified from Huang et al., 1997.)

in synaptic currents, the amplitudes of voltage-dependent calcium currents were graded as a function of lowered osmolarity. If calcium currents in synaptic terminals behave like those in isolated pyramidal neurons, that could explain the hypoosmolar enhancement of synaptic transmission. The mechanism of the potentiation of I_{Ca} is not clear, but it could be attributed to reduced surface charge screening (Hille et al., 1975). Surface screening by Na^+ may be feeble compared to screening by Ca^{2+} if the comparison is made ion for ion, but the extracellular Na^+ concentration is about 100 times higher than that of Ca^{2+}, and therefore it is presumably not negligible. However, this leaves the depression of potassium current by low $[NaCl]_o$ unexplained.

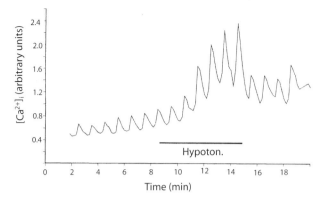

Figure 4–8. Hypotonic exposure causes elevation of intracellular calcium activity and of depolarization-induced $[Ca^{2+}]_i$ responses in an isolated neuron. $[Ca]_i$ was measured as the fluorescence ratio of two indicator dyes, fluo-3/fura-red, in a freshly isolated hippocampal CA1 pyramidal cell. The cell was held in whole-cell patch-clamp condition for the recording of current-voltage functions. The sawtooth pattern resulted from repeated application of constant intensity-depolarizing steps, each of which evoked inward Ca^{2+} current. Hypotonia raised both the baseline $[Ca^{2+}]_i$ and the transient $[Ca^{2+}]_i$ responses. During hypotonia, bath osmolarity was lowered from 296 to 188 mOsm (60 mM NaCl deleted from the bath). (Reproduced from Somjen, 1999.)

Hypotonic Cell Swelling Favors Ephaptic Interaction Among Neurons

The compression of the interstitial space caused by hypotonic swelling contributes to cerebral irritability, regardless of the potentiation of synaptic transmission. As cell swelling pushes neuron membranes closer together, electrical (*ephaptic*) interaction among neurons is accentuated, facilitating the synchronization of discharges (Fig. 7–11) (Dudek et al., 1990; Faber and Korn, 1989; Jefferys, 1981; Snow and Dudek, 1984a; Traub et al., 1985). In electrical terms, the increased interstitial resistance diverts a larger fraction of the synaptic or action currents of one neuron to flow through cell membranes of its neighbors, while less of the current is being shunted through interstitial spaces.

Hypertonicity Depresses All Ion Currents

Voltage-gated Na^+, K^+, and Ca^{2+} currents are all depressed when osmolarity is raised by adding mannitol, fructose, or sucrose to the bath (Huang and Somjen, 1997), and so is synaptic transmission (Huang and Somjen, 1995, 1997; Rosen and Andrew, 1990). Generalized depression can explain the somnolence culminating in coma in severe water loss. It is also worth noting that in many cases of diabetic coma, hyperosmolarity rather than acidosis appears to be the main cause of the CNS depression (Matz, 1997).

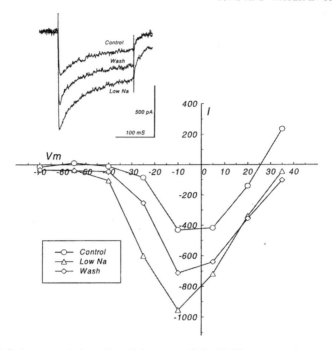

Figure 4–9. Iso-osmotic lowering of the extracellular NaCl concentration augments the voltage-dependent Ca^{2+} current. I-V curves recorded in whole-cell configuration from a patch-clamped, freshly isolated hippocampal CA1 pyramidal cell. The inset shows three superimposed calcium currents, evoked by depolarizing steps from a –110 mV prepulse to –10 mV, in normal solution, in low [NaCl] and during partial recovery by washing with normal solution. The I-V curves are from the same cell in the three conditions. Low NaCl: 60 mM deleted (from 130 mM normal) and substituted for by equiosmolar sucrose. (Reproduced from Somjen, 1999.)

Chloride Has Effects of Its Own

There is one more important factor in the syndrome of low [NaCl]: the effect of low $[Cl^-]_o$ on synaptic inhibition. The primary mechanism of both glycine- and $GABA_A$-operated inhibitory synapses is the opening of anion channels that are selectively permeable to chloride. In most central neurons, $[Cl^-]_i$ is lower than would be expected for equilibrium; in other words, E_{Cl} is more negative than the resting V_m (Table 2–1). $[Cl^-]_i$ is kept low by active outward transport from these cells. The opening of Cl channels causes inflow of Cl^-, and the inward flux of negative charges is equivalent to outward electric current, causing hyperpolarization, which is recorded as the IPSP. Hyperpolarization moves the membrane potential away from the threshold for impulse generation, and that is one of the reasons for inhibiting excitation. But opening Cl^- channels opposes excitation even if Cl^- ions are at equilibrium (that is, $E_{Cl} = V_m$ at rest) for two reasons: (*1*) boosting Cl^- conductance tends to fix the membrane voltage close to E_{Cl}, which, in this case, is equal to the resting potential, and thus it would resist depolarization; (2) any increase in membrane conductance itself acts as an electrical shunt, dissipating the effect of EPSPs. If, however, for any reason $[Cl^-]_o$ becomes much lower or $[Cl^-]_i$ becomes much higher than normal, so that E_{Cl} becomes more positive than the resting potential, then opening Cl^- channels will depolarize the membrane. In this case, inhibitory synapses can be converted to produce an excitatory effect. In fact, this is the normal situation in very early stages of development, at least in rodents, when GABAergic synapses are the main excitatory synapses (Ben-Ari et al., 1997). In some neurons, for example dorsal root ganglion (DRG) cells, even in adults $[Cl^-]_i/[Cl^-]_o$ is normally higher than it would be at equilibrium, so that GABA applied to these cells causes depolarization (Deschenes et al., 1976). This has been known for many years, but its significance is still perplexing because there are no known GABAergic synapses in DRG. It has been assumed that the GABA receptors in the DRG cell somas are identical to those serving presynaptic inhibition at the axon terminals of the same cells in spinal gray matter (Eccles, 1964), but this does not solve the mystery of their presence in the ganglion. More to the point for our purposes is the fact that, under intense synaptic bombardment, cortical and hippocampal neurons can become overloaded with Cl^-, and the opening of $GABA_A$-controlled channels then depolarizes the cell instead of hyperpolarizing it (Andersen et al., 1980; Bracci et al., 2001). The conversion of inhibition into excitation may be important in the induction of seizures by electrical stimulation (Chapter 6: "Malfunctioning inhibitory synapses . . .").

There is another, less well known effect at inhibitory synapses. While Cl^- is the main charge carrier at glycine and $GABA_A$ receptor–operated inhibitory synapses, it is not the only anion involved. There is also a significant added conductance for bicarbonate, which allows HCO_3^- to flow out of cells while Cl^- flows in when GABAergic inhibitory synapses are activated (Kaila et al., 1997). This is because E_{Cl} normally is more negative while E_{HCO3} is more positive than resting V_m. In all cells, probably without exception, HCO_3^- concentrations inside and outside are close, both being about 24 or 25 mM. With $[HCO_3^-]_o$ being nearly the same as $[HCO_3^-]_i$, the equilibrium potential, E_{HCO3}, is not far from zero (Table 2–1). V_m being negative inside, the difference between E_{HCO3} and V_m represents an outward driving force. At the steady state at rest, uphill transport must keep $[HCO_3^-]_i$ constant. Part or most of this transport is performed by a HCO_3^-/Cl^- exchanger that helps to keep $[Cl^-]_i$ lower and $[HCO_3^-]_i$ higher than it would be at equilibrium. Opening a bicarbonate conductance, however, impels the outflow of HCO_3^-. During $GABA_A$-mediated inhibition, outward flow of negatively charged HCO_3^- curtails but cannot overshadow the hyperpolarization achieved by the inflow of Cl^-. Under normal conditions the more intense Cl^- current wins, but at low $[Cl^-]_o$ its advantage is lessened and the depolarizing HCO_3^- current becomes significant.

In Conclusion Concerning Low [NaCl]ₒ Effects

To recapitulate, the hyperexcitability typical of acute hyponatremia has several components: (*1*) raised intracranial pressure, with attendant increased resistance to CBF; (*2* and *3*) low osmolarity and shortage of Na^+ ions, both of which enhance synaptic transmission and augment voltage-gated calcium currents and depress potassium currents; and (*4*) low chloride concentration, which impairs inhibitory synapses. This, then, is the complex pathogenesis of the seizures seen in stokers' cramps and other forms of water poisoning.

Acidosis generally lowers and alkalosis boosts excitability

Alkalotic Tetany Does Not Result from a Reduced Free Calcium Level

Clinical alkalosis causes a condition remarkably similar to the tetany caused by calcium or magnesium deficiency (Grant and Goldman, 1920). Neurological disturbance due to hyperventilation was first recognized around the turn of the twentieth century. Experimenting much of the time on themselves, the pioneer investigators noticed strange buzzing sensations and twitching of their extremities when they deliberately hyperventilated. At around the same time, the similarity was noticed between the cramps caused by calcium deficiency and the so-called hysterical contractures in hands and feet first described by Charcot several decades earlier (Fig. 4–10). A feature of hysterical attacks was prolonged and extreme overbreathing. Pulling these various observations together, investigators have guessed that hyperventilation lowered blood calcium. Disappointingly, when plasma calcium was actually measured during voluntary hyperventilation, it was found to be either normal or slightly elevated. Still, the calcium hypothesis was again revived when it was discovered that pH influences the binding of calcium to plasma proteins (György and Vollmer, 1923) (for other historical references, see Somjen and Tombaugh, 1998). If alveolar ventilation exceeds the metabolic requirement, the CO_2 content of blood is reduced and the pH becomes more alkaline, according to the *Henderson-Hasselbalch* relationship (Eq. 2–2; Chapter 2: "pH is regulated . . ."). Alkalinization of plasma pH favors the binding of calcium to protein and to other chelators such as bicarbonate, thus lowering the free, ionized fraction. Through many editions, textbooks have carried this explanation of hyperventilation-induced tetany, but this appealing explanation turned out to be misleading. As has been said in another context, a beautiful hypothesis was slain by an ugly fact.

While the physical chemistry has been correct in a qualitative sense, the calcium-binding effect of alkalinization turned out to be too weak and the decrease in free Ca^{2+} in circulating blood plasma far too small to explain neuromuscular tetany (Oberleithner et al., 1982; Somjen et al., 1987a). It is the H^+

A

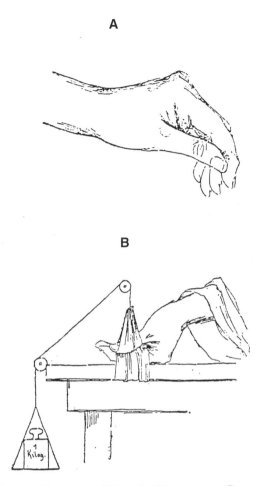

B

FIGURE 4–10. Charcot's illustration of "hysterical" contracture. Cramp of hand muscula-ture (*main d'accoucheur*) resulting from hyperventilation-induced alkalotic tetany. **A:** Position of the fingers in cramp . **B:** Demonstrating the strength of the contracture.

ions themselves that powerfully influence ion channel functions, quite indepen-dently of calcium. The cause of alkalotic tetany is the shortage of protons, not of free Ca^{2+} (Somjen and Tombaugh, 1998; Tombaugh and Somjen, 1998), al-though the concomitant small $[Ca^{2+}]_o$ changes in blood plasma presumably re-inforce the effects of low $[H^+]_o$. In brain tissue $[Ca^{2+}]_o$ remains stable in the face of major pH_o shifts; therefore, in the central effects of acidosis and alkalosis, Ca^{2+} does not play even an ancillary part (Fig. 4–11) (Balestrino and Somjen, 1988). Even though $[Ca^{2+}]_o$ in brain is not affected by pH_o, synaptic transmis-sion is powerfully modulated (Fig. 4–12).

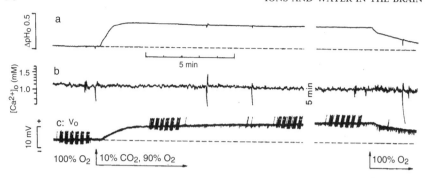

FIGURE 4–11. Effect of inspired CO_2 on hippocampal pH_o and standing voltage, and lack of effect on extracellular calcium concentration. Pen writer (polygraph) recordings from the dentate gyrus of an anesthetized rat. a: Changes in pH_o recorded with an ion-selective microelectrode; low pH plotted up. b: Extracellular calcium concentration recorded with an ion-selective microelectrode. The brief pen deflections are artifacts. c: Extracellular voltage (V_o) recorded from the reference barrel of the pH electrode against ground in the neck muscles. The acid-induced positive shift of V_o is generated at the blood-brain barrier. The groups of deflections are electrical stimulations, such as the ones used to obtain the responses in Figure 4–12. At the break in the traces, 5 min of recordings are deleted. Inspired gas changed at the arrows. (Modified from Balestrino and Somjen, 1988.)

Protons Inhibit All Voltage-Gated Ion Currents That Have Been Tested, but Not to the Same Degree

The acid-base effect on channel function can be quantitated by plotting the amplitude of an ion current evoked by a constant voltage step against the pH of the bathing solution. Alternatively, instead of the measured current, the computed ion conductance may be represented as the dependent variable. Such plots are sigmoid and resemble titration functions (Fig. 4–13B, 4–14) (Hille, 1968; Tombaugh and Somjen, 1996, 1998). A virtual K_D can be defined at the midpoint of the steep part of the curve. If all ion channels were equally affected, then the pH effect on inward currents would be offset by an equal effect on outward currents and overall excitability would remain unchanged. This, however, is not the case. In most nerve cells the K_D for Ca^{2+} current falls in a more acid region than that of Na^+ currents, while K^+ currents are located even further in the alkaline direction. Expressed differently, the sensitivity to protons can be ranked as follows: $I_{Ca} > I_{Na} > I_K$ (Tombaugh and Somjen, 1998). Within the entire pH range compatible with life, K^+ currents are almost fully enabled in most cells. For this reason, pH changes within the physiologically relevant range modulate the inward Ca^{2+} and Na^+ currents much more powerfully than the outward K^+ currents. Therefore alkalinization strongly favors inward currents and enhances excitability, while acid depresses excitability. At synapses the alkalotic effect is amplified because, in addition to

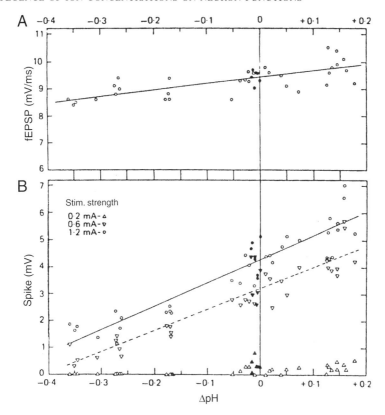

FIGURE 4–12. pH dependence of synaptic transmission. Recordings made from dentate gyrus of an anesthetized rat (as for Fig. 4–11). pH was lowered by raising inspired CO_2, and it was raised by hyperventilation (increased artificial ventilation). pH and electrical responses were measured with a double-barreled ion-selective microelectrode, with stimulation by way of the perforant path (angular bundle). **A:** Focally recorded extracellular excitatory synaptic potential (fEPSP) was measured as the initial steepest rate of change (slope) of the trace. **B:** Synaptically evoked population spike (PS) amplitude evoked at three different stimulus pulse intensities, the weakest of which was just above threshold. The points represent single responses; the straight lines are regression functions. Note that both fEPSP and PS vary with pH, but the effect is much more marked for the PS, indicating strong postsynaptic action. (Modified from (Balestrino and Somjen, 1988.)

the increasing excitability of postsynaptic target cells, the enhanced Ca^{2+} currents boost the release of transmitter substances.

The sigmoid titration curves of Figures 4–13B and 4–14 seem different from the straight regression lines fitted to the data in Figure 4–12. This is because the pH range in Figure 4–12 is barely more than 0.5 unit, limited to the steepest, nearly linear middle part of the "titration" function. The normal pH of the brain is poised where the sensitivity of the pH change is greatest.

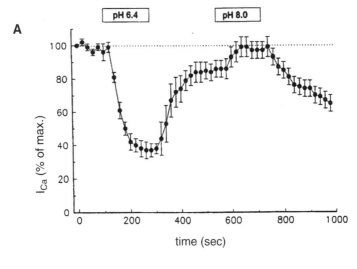

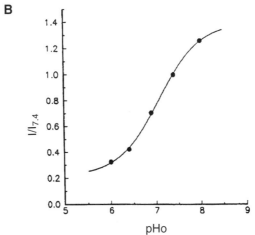

FIGURE 4–13. pH dependence of voltage-gated calcium currents in central neurons. **A:** High-voltage activated (HVA) calcium current amplitudes recorded from freshly isolated rat CA1 pyramidal neurons, evoked at 20 s intervals, in control solution (pH 7.4), at pH 6.4 and pH 8.0. Mean ±S.E.M. data from five cells. Incomplete recovery following exposure to pH 6.4 and pH 8.0 due to "rundown." **B:** The pH dependence of HVA calcium currents. Relative amplitudes, corrected for rundown. Each point represents the mean of at least five cells. (Modified from Tombaugh and Somjen, 1996.)

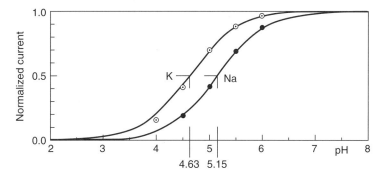

FIGURE 4–14. pH dependence of voltage-gated K^+ and Na^+ currents of the node of Ranvier in frog myelinated axon. pK values for I_K: 4.63 and for I_{Na}: 5.15. Within the pH range compatible with life, I_K is insensitive to pH changes. (Modified from Drouin and The, 1969.)

The pH of the cytosol is slightly more acidic than that of the ISF, and the intracellular pH is regulated to some degree independently of that of the extracellular milieu (Chapter 2: "pH is regulated . . .") (Bevensee and Boron, 1998; Chesler, 1990). As acids are produced by metabolism, if cellular pH regulation fails, the consequence is intracellular acidosis. *Protons inhibit ion channels from the inside as well as from the outside*, but the strength of the effect on the internal and external faces of the channel may differ (see Tombaugh, 1998, and the review by Tombaugh and Somjen, 1998).

While most cells are depressed by acid, there are exceptions. Acid-sensing cells in arterial ***chemoreceptors*** are excited by protons. So are the ***respiratory neurons*** in the brain stem that regulate breathing (Dean et al., 1990) and a few cells in the spinal cord (Speckmann and Caspers, 1974). Acid-induced excitation resides within the membrane of respiratory neurons, and it does not require synaptic transmission (Dean et al., 1990). It could be that in acid-excited cells, K^+ currents are more strongly depressed by H^+ than are Na^+ and Ca^{2+} currents. This hypothesis asks to be tested.

pH Effects on Ligand-Gated Ion Channels

Of the *ligand-gated* ion channels, *glutamate-controlled* excitatory channels are depressed by H^+ ions, just like voltage-gated channels. The pH effects on ligand-gated and voltage-gated ion channels reinforce one another, resulting in powerful modulation of excitatory synaptic transmission (Fig. 4–12). In comparing the slopes of the regression lines of Figures 4–12A and 4–12B, it is apparent that the postsynaptic population spike was more powerfully influenced by pH_o than was the fEPSP. This could be interpreted as meaning that postsynaptic voltage-gated channels were more strongly affected than ligand-gated channels, but this conclusions must be restrained. Both fEPSP and population spike amplitudes are determined by multiple interacting variables, most of which are very nonlinear (see also above: "Input-output functions in the analysis of synaptic efficacy").

Deviating from the general rule, *GABA$_A$ receptor–controlled* inhibitory currents are enhanced by acid pH (Traynelis, 1998). The reciprocal action, depression of EPSPs and enhancement of IPSPs, amplifies the excitation by high pH and the depression by low pH.

Another exception to the general rule, intracellular acidosis boosts the *ATP-controlled potassium channel, K_{ATP}.* Under resting conditions in healthy cells these channels are strongly inhibited by the prevailing ATP, but under metabolic stress, when ATP levels decline, they open (Chapter 18: "Postsynaptic hyperpolarization . . ."). Superimposed on ATP control, protons counteract the inhibition by ATP. Therefore, intracellular acidosis will enhance $I_{K,ATP}$ indirectly, mediated by restraining ATP-dependent inhibition (Davies, 1990).

Key points

Changes in ion distribution alter neuron function. The changed concentration gradient influences membrane potential and alters the driving force of ion currents. It can also have direct effects on ion channel functions.

Potassium distribution, $[K^+]_o/[K^+]_i$, is the most important determinant of resting membrane potential. The Na^+ conductance of resting neuronal membranes is low but not negligible. For this reason, as long as $[K^+]_o$ remains close to its normal level, small changes in $[K^+]_o$ have relatively little influence on V_m.

Moderately elevated $[K^+]_o$ enhances excitatory synaptic transmission. Higher $[K^+]_o$ causes seizures, and even higher $[K^+]_o$ inactivates membranes and silences neurons.

Both Ca^{2+} and Mg^{2+} stabilize excitable membranes by screening fixed negative charges on the outside of ion channels. Too little of either of these divalent ions increases excitability and can cause tetany. Too much reduces excitability.

At chemical synapses, Mg^{2+} acts as an antagonist of Ca^{2+}. Raising $[Ca^{2+}]_o$ boosts synaptic transmission. Elevated Mg^{2+} prevents Ca^{2+} entry into axon terminals and therefore blocks synaptic transmission.

Additionally, Mg^{2+} regulates NMDA receptor–controlled channels. At resting membrane potential, NMDA channels are plugged by Mg^{2+}; depolarization relieves the Mg^{2+} block.

Low osmotic pressure boosts synaptic transmission. In part this is due to the lowering of the NaCl concentration, independently of the osmotic effect. Both low osmolarity and low [NaCl] potentiate voltage-gated Ca^{2+} current, and this could explain the enhanced synaptic transmission.

Protons inhibit voltage-gated and glutamate-operated ion channels but enhance GABA-mediated inhibition. Alkalosis causes tetany, independently of ionized Ca^{2+} levels.

Low $[K^+]_o$ low pH, and high $[Mg^{2+}]_o$ in CSF and cerebral ISF relative to blood plasma synergistically moderate the excitability of CNS tissue.

II

CEREBRAL SEIZURES

5

A Primer of Epileptiform Seizures

Part II reviews the mechanisms of epileptic fits and the role that ions play in causing them. Chapter 5 presents a brief overview of the salient clinical features of seizures, much of which will be familiar to medically trained readers.

Names and notions

There can be no better introduction to a chapter on seizures than a statement written in 1870 by John Hughlings Jackson (1835–1911), whom many call the father of British neurology:

> A convulsion is but a symptom, and implies only that there is an occasional, an excessive, and a disorderly discharge of nerve tissue on muscles. This discharge occurs in all degrees; it occurs with all sorts of conditions of ill health, at all ages, and under innumerable circumstances.
>
> (See Jackson, 1870)

Epilepsy is defined as a chronic condition characterized by *repeated unprovoked seizures*. *Unprovoked* must be precisely defined, for genuinely epileptic seizures can in some cases be precipitated by sensory stimuli such as flashing lights or sudden loud noise (Loiseau, 1998; Puranam and McNamara, 2001). We must therefore distinguish between *precipitated* and *provoked*. An example of provocation is electroconvulsive shock, which produces tonic-clonic seizures in brains that may be perfectly normal. Other insults that can cause seizures in persons who are not epileptic include infections, trauma, a variety of drugs, and even severe sleeplessness. As textbooks have stressed since Jackson's day, epilepsy is not a disease but a disorder, like fever, and it can be caused by many different underlying conditions (Engel and Pedley, 1998a,b). Unlike fever, however, epilepsy can manifest in many very different forms, and once a brain has become epileptic, its propensity to generate seizures usually remains for a long time, sometimes for life. Regardless of the initial cause and variation of overt signs, certain underlying pathophysiological features are common to all types of seizures.

More than 5% of all people are said to suffer at least one epileptiform seizure during their lives, and this number does not include fever-induced (febrile) seizures of infants. The cumulated incidence of epilepsy, that is, the total number of persons who suffer multiple fits over an extended period of time, is about 3 or 4 per 100 person-lifetimes among Americans and 1.3 among Danes. The prevalence—that is, the percentage of persons in the population who actually have epilepsy at any one time—is less, because many cases remit after a few years; it is somewhere between 0.4% and 1.0% in different studies (Hauser, 1998; Hopkins, 1987a). Keeping seizures under control occupies a major fraction of neurological practice.

This chapter is meant to clarify some terms and basic concepts concerning epileptiform seizures, mainly for readers not familiar with the clinical terminology. The voluminous literature on this topic has generated its own vocabulary, replete with synonyms and near-synonyms.

According to Webster's New Collegiate dictionary, *to seize* means to take possession of or to attack or overwhelm. For *seizure* Webster's has several definitions; one of them is "a sudden attack, as of a disease." At one time, epileptic patients were thought to have been *seized* by demons or perhaps by the devil. The Greek word *epilamvanein*, from which *epilepsy* is derived, also means "to be seized" (Engel and Pedley, 1998). Historians credit the text attributed to Hippocrates with dispelling the notion of a supernatural cause of the "falling sickness," but this insight was not universally accepted for many centuries, not even by medical professionals (Temkin, 1971). It is still common to use the words *spell* and *fit* interchangeably, and superstition about this disease has not yet disappeared (Sonnen, 1998). There is no denying that a major epileptic attack is strange and frightening to witness.

Heart attacks are sometimes called *cardiac seizures*, and cerebral seizures were formerly distinguished as being either *hysterical* or *epileptic*. The term *hysterical attack* has been replaced by *psychogenic pseudoseizure* (Kanner and Parra, 1998) in current professional language for seizures without an abnormal EEG. A seized heart stands still, but a seized brain is possessed by uncontrolled neuron discharge. Actually, a heart can also fail to pump blood because it beats too fast, as in *ventricular flutter* or *torsade de pointes* (Chapter 10: "Long Q-T . . ."), or because electrical impulses fail to follow a prescribed course and run instead in wildly disorganized patterns, as in ventricular fibrillation, conditions that could be considered related to cerebral seizures.

In today's usage the word *seizure*, by itself and without qualifiers, has become a generic term for any kind of epileptic event. Webster's dictionary defines a **paroxysm** (derived from the Greek word) as a sudden attack or "any convulsion, as of laughter, rage, sneezing, etc; a fit, a spasm." **Convulsions**, again according to Webster, are "violent and involuntary contractions of muscles." Epileptic seizures need not cause convulsions, and we speak of **convulsive** and **nonconvulsive seizures**. Textbooks define *epileptiform seizures* as involving the *episodic, uncontrolled, excessive, synchronous discharge* of groups of central neurons. How seizures can be distinguished from tremors of central origin, myoclonic movements, or chorea, which at first glance also seem to fit this definition, is a task that must be left to neurology textbooks.

Excessive synaptic excitation, decreased inhibition, or increased activity of both excitatory and inhibitory synapses can result in seizure. Ever since the beginning of modern medical thinking about epilepsy, *hyperexcitability* of cerebral tissue has been a central theme. Often the discussion centered on a balance of excitation and inhibition: either excess of the former or deficiency of the latter could cause epileptic seizures. There is much evidence supporting this notion but, as we shall see in detail later, in many examples of epileptogenesis both synaptic excitation and inhibition are enhanced relative to the norm.

A Note on Synchrony

After the introduction of EEG into clinical practice, *synchronicity* came to be considered one of the cardinal features of epileptic seizures besides excessive excitability. The word *synchronicity*, however, is in need of clarification. It is generally agreed that in order to be detectable in EEG traces, signals of many neurons must coincide. If by synchrony we mean that many neurons must be excited to make a seizure, then this is correct. If, however, we expect phase-locking of action potentials, then this is true in some but by no means all types of seizures. More often synchrony refers to the coincidence of slow potential waves, such as synaptic potentials or slow intrinsic currents. In this form of synchronization the action potentials triggered by the synchronized waves need not be time-locked. During a tonic seizure, impulses of different neurons may be fired at different frequencies and at irregular, quasi-random intervals. Time-locked firing of spikes by many cells does, however, occur during epileptiform bursts and during tonic seizure in the hippocampal formation, at least during experimental seizures. We called this phenomenon **lockstep firing** to emphasize the difference from the more common synchronization of slow potentials (Somjen et al., 1985) (see Fig. 7–8 and Chapter 7: "Hippocampal pyramidal neurons . . . "). The abnormal synchrony of epileptic discharges must be distinguished from normal synchronized slow waves, for example in the α rhythm and sleep spindles seen in EEG.

Normal brain function depends on each neuron performing its particular task. During a seizure, neurons are either firing in an incoherent, random barrage or are forced into a common, regular, but purposeless beat. In the former case we speak of *tonic* discharge and in the latter case of *clonic* discharge. In either case, neurons are prevented from performing their normal function.

Types of seizures

Seizures can be *convulsive* if there is overt twitching or cramping of muscles or *nonconvulsive* in their absence. They can be *partial* if only a limited brain area participates or *generalized* if a major part of both cerebral hemispheres is involved. Partial seizures can be *simple* or *complex*. *Focal seizures* include simple partial seizures but also include asymmetrical but widespread paroxysmal discharges. According to the 1981 revision of the International Classification of Epilepsies, partial seizures are defined as *simple if consciousness is retained and as complex if it is lost or at least impaired* (Engel et al., 1998b). Simple partial seizures arise mostly in neocortex and complex partial seizures in the subcortical temporal lobe structures, namely, the amygdala and hippocampal formation, but this is by no means an absolute rule (Williamson and Engel, 1998). A partial seizure can start small and then engulf larger and larger brain areas, and it may eventually evolve into a *secondary generalized seizure*. Simple partial seizures involving the motor area of the neocortex are also known as *Jacksonian fits* after J. Hughlings Jackson (see also below: "Seizure propagation"). A complex partial seizure mobilizes a sequence of neuron activity that runs a prescribed but abnormal course and can make the patient move and act in odd ways without making him or her fall down in spite of impaired consciousness. Such *automatisms* and stereotyped, unwilled, odd, purposeless, and unwelcome behaviors that include lip smacking, chewing, plucking of clothes, posturing, and, rarely, more complex actions. It is as if a subroutine of programmed behavior was activated without intent by the behaving individual. Because these types of seizures usually originate in structures of the temporal lobe, the underlying condition is described as *temporal lobe epilepsy* (*TLE*) or *mesial temporal lobe epilepsy* (*MTLE*). Milder manifestations of MTLE include motor arrest and staring, known as *temporal lobe absence*. Sometimes MTLE automatisms occur without impaired consciousness and are then considered to be simple partial seizures (Engel et al., 1998b). Following an MTLE seizure psychological disruption can continue far into the postictal period (Leung et al., 2000).

Simple partial seizures, causing convulsions in one limb or in many muscle groups on one side of the body, are sometimes followed by paralysis, called *Todd's palsy* after the physician who described this effect (Szabó and Lüders, 2000). The condition is usually transient and may last for up to 48 hours unless continuous seizures intervene. The muscles that are lamed are typically those that were seized earlier by the convulsions.

Generalized seizures always render the patient unconscious. A generalized seizure can be minor, causing an **absence** or momentary lapse of consciousness, sometimes with minor muscle twitching but no falling down and no major convulsion. Poupart first described the condition in 1705, and later Tissot recognized it in a patient who also had convulsive epilepsy and proposed the relationship between the two syndromes. It was Tissot who introduced the terms *petit accès* (meaning "small attack") to describe the momentary lapses of consciousness and *grand accès* for convulsive seizures. In the jargon of the nineteenth-century French hospitals, these expressions later became **petit mal**, which means "little illness" or "small trouble," and **grand mal**, the "big trouble" of major epilepsy (*mal* being used in the same sense as in *mal de tête* for headache). More historical details may be found in the famous volume by Temkin (1971). Absence epilepsy occurs mainly in childhood. Many but not all children who have suffered absences develop major seizures as adults (Petsche, 1962). *Generalized* or *typical absence* seizures must be distinguished from temporal lobe absence, which is not generalized, as mentioned above.

Upon hearing of epilepsy, most lay persons think of **generalized tonic-clonic convulsions (GTCS)** (the currently approved synonym for *grand mal*). During a classic tonic-clonic fit, the patient loses consciousness and falls to the ground. In the initial, tonic phase there is simultaneous spasm of most or all major skeletal muscle groups, while during the later clonic phase the body jerks rhythmically. Frequently there are signs of autonomic nervous system activation, such as salivation. The convulsions are followed by a period of deep coma, and recovery is gradual and protracted.

Ictus is the Latin word for a blow (it can also mean stroke, cut, sting, wound, and stress), and it is used to refer to any type of major seizure. **Interictal discharges** are brief abnormalities, detected on EEGs, that occur between seizures. In the absence of an EEG record, interictal discharges usually go unnoticed. Epileptic fits can come without warning, but patients sometimes have a premonition of an impending attack. The manifold sensations that can herald a seizure are called **auras**. Perhaps the most famous of all epileptics, Dostoyevsky, wrote of his own aura: "You healthy people, you cannot imagine the joy that fills an epileptic in the second before the attack. . . . I never know whether the moments of pleasure last for an instant or for an hour, but believe me, I would not barter them against all the happiness of a lifetime" (quoted by (Zweig, 1958). Longer passages describing epileptic experiences in Dostoyevsky's works may be found in Temkin (1971).

Unfortunately, few patients share this happy experience. More often, auras are elementary sensations or simple hallucinations such as flashes of light, or the image of a person, or tingling or numbness of the skin, or a strange smell, or peculiar feelings in the viscera, almost always disquieting rather than welcome. Whatever form they take, they arise from the uncalled-for firing of groups of neurons, and the subjective nature of the aura depends on the location in the brain of this uncontrolled discharge. This has been dramatically confirmed in the work of Penfield and colleagues, who used electrical stimulation of the exposed brains of patients during surgery in order to find the epileptogenic focus. The patients were locally anesthetized and conscious. If the stimulus evoked the aura familiar to the patient, the surgeon knew that he has hit the right spot (Penfield and Jasper, 1954).

Status epilepticus has been defined as either continuous or intermittent seizures lasting for 30 minutes or longer (DeLorenzo, 2000; Walton, 1985). Ordinary seizures are self-limiting and are usually followed by a period of depressed excitability. Status epilepticus comes about when the mechanisms that ought to stop the seizure fail (Treiman and Heinemann, 1998) (see Chapter 7: "How do seizures stop?"). Since there are many types of seizures, status epilepticus can take different forms (Lepik, 1990). *Generalized tonic-clonic status epilepticus* is a severe and sometimes life-threatening emergency in which one major convulsion follows another, with only brief periods of quiet interrupting the spasms.

It has been usual to divide the epilepsies into two broad categories, *symptomatic* (synonym: *secondary*) and *essential* (or *idiopathic*). Symptomatic epilepsy is the manifestation of an identifiable brain lesion or disease. *Essential* used to mean, of course, "of unknown origin." It has been suspected for a long time that many essential cases are the result of various complex gene defects (Singh et al., 2002). The genetic basis is now gradually being revealed as definable defects in the molecular structure of ion channels or, using a newly coined term, *channelopathies* (Ashcroft, 2000; Mamelak and Lowenstein, 1998; Noebels et al., 1998; Steinlein, 2001) (see Chapter 10).

This brief summary of the most common forms of epileptic seizures is very far from complete. Comprehensive catalogs may be found in the numerous textbooks and monographs devoted to the subject (Engel et al., 1998a; Hopkins, 1987b; Lüders, 2001).

Electroencephalography

Discovery of the Berger Waves

The first EEG recording ever published was that of the son of the inventor, Hans Berger (1929) (for translations of Berger's papers, see Gloor, 1969). Berger was not the first to record the electrical activity from a brain, but he was the first to register brain waves from the intact human scalp. He was a psychiatrist, and his original goal was to discover the process underlying schizophrenia. In this he did not succeed, but his instrument found other good uses, arguably the most important being the diagnosis of epilepsy.

Berger defined the basic terms to describe EEG activity. He named the *a waves*, regular 8–12 Hz oscillations, best seen with the eyes closed and maximal over the occipital region, typical of relaxed wakefulness, and *β activity*, irregular, low-amplitude, 13–30 Hz oscillations that are most typical of the alert waking state but, as it was realized later, also present in the rapid eye movement (REM) stage of sleep. Berger was the first to see α *blocking* (sometimes called the *Berger effect*), the transition from α to β activity on opening the eyes (Berger, 1930). There was some initial skepticism about whether the feeble electrical oscillations Berger reported were indeed produced by cerebral activity. Adrian, who was among the first to confirm their reality, called them *Berger rhythm* (Adrian and Matthews, 1934) but the term fell into disuse. Berger also described the slow, large-amplitude waves in the 0.5–4 Hz range seen in deep sleep, but he considered these a form of slow α. These slow, irregular waves are now taken to be a distinct category and are named *δ waves*. According to Steriade, there are three distinct patterns that underlie δ activity (Amzica and Steriade, 1998). Low-amplitude, irregular, high-frequency activity is traditionally considered *desynchronized*, assuming that it represents the independent action of individual cells, while the larger α and δ waves are generated by the simultaneous action of larger numbers of cells. This turns out to be only partly true. Beneath what in a scalp EEG appears as low-amplitude, irregularly fluctuating voltage, there can be high-frequency synchronous activity (Steriade and Amzica, 1996).

Frequency Domains of Electroencephalographic Waves

Present day convention defines the following frequency ranges in brain waves: delta: 0.1–3.5 Hz; theta: 4–7.5 Hz; alpha: 8–13 Hz; beta: 14–30 Hz; gamma: more than 30 Hz (usually 30–100 Hz) (Bragin et al., 1995; Buzsáki and Traub, 1998; Niedermeyer, 1999b). Evidently, there is no correlation between frequency and position in the Greek alphabet; instead, the choice of each symbol has historical reasons. Theta waves are prominent in hippocampal recordings in certain mental states. The high gamma frequencies are not visible in conventional EEG tracings and must be extracted by computational techniques (Tallon-Baudry et al., 1998). A better view of the high frequencies is presented by intracranial electroencephalography (iEEG). The opportunity is available when human patients are monitored with implanted electrodes, sometimes for several days, for the accurate mapping of epileptogenic foci in preparation for surgery (reviewed by Kahana et al., 2001). Some investigators consider synchronized gamma oscillations the neural substrate for the "binding" or coherence of neuron excitation required for pattern recognition, while theta oscillations are perhaps associated with higher-level expectations and strategies (Engel et al., 2001; Jefferys et al., 1996; Kahana et al., 2001).

*Electroencephalographic Waves Represent Synaptic Potentials
and "Slow" Intrinsic Currents*

When EEG was new, action potentials were the only known neuronal electric signals. Of course, EEG waves are much slower then nerve impulses, and therefore it has been assumed that the recording instrument averaged the envelope of multiple spikes fired by many neurons. Once EPSPs and IPSPs were discovered, it was easy to conclude that synaptic potentials and not spikes underlie the EEG. Cortical cytoarchitecture suggested that the main generators are the apical dendrites of pyramidal neurons. By and large, this explanation still holds, but it needs certain amendments. Synaptic currents involve not only the dendritic tree but also the cell somas, especially in the case of IPSPs. Also, dendritic membranes are not just passive recipients of synaptic input, but also produce slow "active" current waves generated by voltage-dependent ion channels (Chapter 7: "Dendrites are not passive . . ."), and these can contribute to the EEG trace (Lopes da Silva, 1991). And, finally, while the current registered in the surface EEG trace is indeed generated in the cerebral cortex, the rhythm of the oscillations is often paced by reciprocal synaptic interchange between cortical and subcortical structures (Chapter 7: "In conclusion: Both cortex and thalamus are required . . .").

Electroencephalography in epilepsy

Interictal Discharges

Diagnosing epilepsy from conventional EEG tracings is rarely straightforward, because between fits the pathological signs are subtle and may occur infrequently. To "catch" a seizure, it may be necessary to monitor brain waves for many hours, even days. For obvious reasons, this cannot be a routine procedure. Therefore, neurologists first look for telltale signs on EEG traces taken in seizure-free intervals that might permit a diagnosis or at least arouse suspicion. The common signs apart from seizures are ***interictal discharges*** in the form of ***EEG spikes***, ***sharp waves***, *poly-spikes*, isolated large-amplitude slow waves, and isolated ***spike-wave (SW)*** complexes (Fig 5–1A). The difference between an EEG spike and a sharp wave is timing. A spike lasts for less than 70 ms, a sharp wave for 70–200 ms. To confuse the uninitiated, in cellular electrophysiology *spike* means the main depolarizing phase of an action potential that lasts for 1 or 2 ms, and membrane potential fluctuations on the time scale of EEG spikes are called *waves*. The mechanism of interictal discharges will be discussed in Chapter 7. Multiple interictal discharges may herald the onset of an ictal seizure (Fig. 7–9) (Amzica and Steriade, 2000; Anderson et al., 1986; Jami, 1972; Köhling et al., 2001; Prince et al., 1983), but this is not always the case (Jensen and Yaari, 1988), and the overall frequency of these brief abnormalities during the seizure-free periods does not correlate with

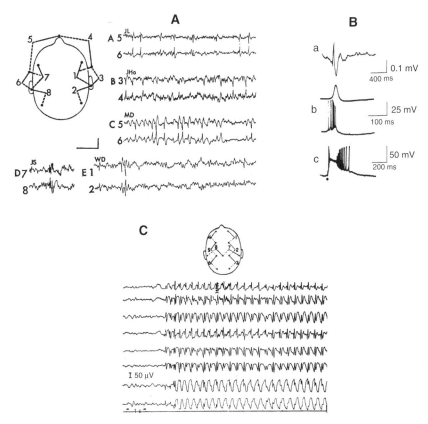

FIGURE 5–1. Interictal discharges (**A** and **B**) and spike-wave seizure (**C**). **A:** Assorted interictal electroencephalographic (EEG) discharges from five different patients. **B:** Interpretation of the EEG "spike". a: Electroencephalographic record from a patient. b: Upper trace: strychnine spike from the cortex of a cat; lower trace: intracellular record of a paroxysmal deplorizing shift (PDS) from a cat cortical neuron during a strychnine spike. c: Intracellular record of PDS from an in vitro slice prepared from epileptogenic cortical tissue of a human patient. **C:** The EEG record of a generalized 3/s spike-wave discharge during absence seizure. (**A** from Engel et al., 1975; **B** from Avoli and Gloor, 1987; **C** from Walton, 1985.)

the severity of the condition (Binnie, 1987). In fact Engel and Ackerman (1980) found a negative correlation between interictal discharge frequency and the inclination for seizure discharges in kindled rats, and suggested that the interictal discharges represent predominantly inhibitory events. Also, in some in vitro models, interictal discharges appear to suppress ictal seizures (Avoli, 2001; Bragdon et al., 1992; Swartzwelder et al., 1987). Reviewing the literature, de Curtis and Avanzini (2001) forcefully argue that interictal and ictal discharges are generated by different cell groups and that the former are not predictive of the latter. On the contrary, they assert that interictal discharges are protective against ictal seizures, and, quoting Gotman (1991), they conclude that interictal discharges are "more a reflection of past seizures than an indication of the likelihood of future ones" (see also Avoli, 2001). Nonetheless, in several types of experimentally induced seizures in brains in situ and brain slices in vitro, there is a striking and unmistakable progression from sporadic to rapidly repeated interictal discharges culminating in full ictal seizures, and there are recordings suggesting that an interictal discharge can trigger a major seizure event (Fig. 7–9) (e.g., Amzica and Steriade, 1999, 2000; Anderson et al., 1986; Gumnit and Takahashi, 1965; Jami, 1972; Jensen and Yaari, 1988; Köhling et al., 2001; Prince et al., 1983). It must be emphasized (again) that a similar appearance of electrical recordings need not always mean identity of underlying mechanisms; similar interictal events may be expressions of different processes.

Electroencephalography in Ictal Events

If recognition of interictal discharges requires training, the EEG manifestations of ictal events are dramatic and unmistakable even to the untutored eye (Risinger, 2000) (Figs. 5–1, 5–2). Without an EEG record, absence seizures can sometimes go unnoticed or be taken for inattention or distraction, but the EEG shows easily recognizable complex waves over wide areas of both hemispheres, repeating at a regular, approximately 3/s (more generally 2–4 Hz) rhythm. This is the frequency in humans and cats (Figs. 5–1C, 7–4). In rodents the frequency is 6–9 Hz except in the "slow-wave epilepsy" mutant mouse, in which the rhythm is 3/s (McCormick and Contreras, 2001; Noebels, 1999; Petsche, 1962). Berger recognized the 3 Hz rhythm as a hallmark of absence seizures, but his equipment did not detect the sharp spike-like component interspersed between the waves. Soon thereafter, Gibbs et al. (1935) saw the entire pattern and named it the *egg-and-dart design*. Their evocative term has unfortunately been replaced by the less picturesque *3 per second spike-and-wave* (or *spike-wave, SW*) discharge.

Generalized *tonic* seizures are characterized by a massive *high-voltage, fast-discharge* pattern, also described as *hypersynchronization*, most often between 15 and 20 Hz but sometimes faster or slower than these limits. During *clonic* convulsions the EEG shows bursts of large-amplitude, high-frequency waves that beat at the same rhythm as the muscle spasms (Fig. 5–2) (Risinger, 2000).

Direct recording from the human cortex with DC-coupled amplification reveals a slow negative shift of the baseline voltage during seizures (Ikeda et al., 1996, 2000). Animal experiments suggest that this sustained negative shift is generated largely by depolarization of glial cells (Ransom, 1974; Somjen, 1973, 1993) (see Chapter 2: "Glial cells regulate . . ." and Chapter 7: "Sustained depolarization . . .").

To produce voltage fluctuations that can be detected by electrodes fastened to the scalp, many nerve cells must cooperate, a process expressed by the term *syn-*

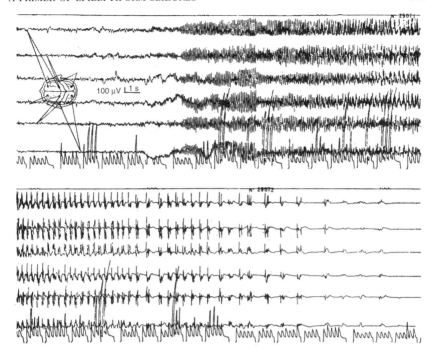

100 µV ⌊1 s

FIGURE 5–2. Electroencephalogram (EEG) of a generalized tonic-clonic seizure. Six EEG traces and, on the seventh (bottom) trace, repeated frequency spectra derived from the sixth (left temporo-occipital) EEG record. On the upper panel the preictal normal EEG is followed by the tonic phase of the seizure, with the EEG dominated by high-amplitude 9–10 Hz waves. The lower panel shows the clonic phase followed by postictal EEG silence. The patient was partially paralyzed by curare, eliminating muscle artifacts. (Reproduced from Gastaut and Broughton, 1972)

chronization. We should stress that "large-amplitude" or "high-voltage" EEG waves recorded from the scalp are rarely more than about 500 µV, almost always smaller than the QRS complex of the normal EKG. Voltages get larger when recorded from the cortical surface (electrocorticogram, ECoG) instead of the scalp, larger yet from microelectrodes within the cerebral gray matter, and even larger from microelectrodes inserted into individual neurons. Yet even the strongest biological currents are far too weak to light the bulb of a flashlight.

For diagnostic purpose, seizures may be provoked during EEG recording sessions by requiring the subject to *hyperventilate* or by optical stimulation with repeated *light flashes* (Takahashi, 1999). The pioneer neurosurgeon Foerster (1924) first reported that hyperventilation can provoke a seizure in an epileptic patient and suggested its use as a diagnostic tool. As we have seen (Chapter 2: "The special case ... pH gradient"), hyperventilation causes ***respiratory alkalosis***, and alkalosis potentiates voltage-gated as well as glutamate-regulated ion channels.

Flickering light or other sensory stimuli activate some but by no means all types of epilepsy (Loiseau, 1998; Takahashi, 1999). It probably acts by evoking a rhythmic, synchronized discharge in large numbers of neurons in the visual receiving areas of the forebrain. What may be surprising at first is that sleep sometimes reveals seizures in EEG tracings that are scarce in the waking state (Contreras and Steriade, 1995; Degen, 1980; Steriade and Amzica, 1998). This again may be explained by the rhythmic, synchronized activity of neurons (sleep spindles) that occurs in certain stages of sleep. While desynchronized activity of the waking brain can repress a seizure, synchronized activity in sleep can favor it (Amzica and Steriade, 2000; Coulter, 1998; Steriade et al., 1994).

To "catch" a spontaneous attack, patients in major clinical centers are often monitored around the clock with combined EEG and video recording to document seizures. If the patient is a candidate for surgery, multiple electrodes are implanted in the brain region suspected to be the epileptogenic focus. These probes may be left in place for several days or even weeks and monitored continuously, assisting in the accurate localization of the site of origin of the seizures.

Seizures of focal origin that do not respond to drug treatment and seriously impair the patient, whether partial or secondarily generalized, can often be cured by surgical ablation of the primary focus (Ojemann, 1987; Penfield and Jasper, 1954). For the person to be eligible for surgery, several spontaneous seizures should be seen to arise from a consistent focus, as detected by implanted electrodes during prolonged monitoring. During surgery, precise localization of the focus may be aided by electrical stimulation of the exposed brain. Weak electrical stimulation of the right spot evokes either the aura or the actual electrical seizure pattern that is typical of the patient's fits.

Seizure propagation

The "March" of Jacksonian Seizures

In the title of a volume of collected essays, epilepsy has been called *Epilepsy: A Window to Brain Mechanisms* (Lockard and Ward, 1980). Nowhere is this more true than in the case of simple partial motor seizures, with a focus in the primary motor area of the precentral gyrus. J. Hughlings Jackson described these fits first and, on the suggestion of Charcot, they have come to be known as *Jacksonian seizures*. Generated in the motor area of the neocortex, they typically begin with twitching in an extremity, most often the hand and sometimes the foot, and then they "march" up the arm or the leg. The spasms can then spread further to involve most of the muscles of one side of the body. Other patterns are also common. With remarkable insight, Jackson recognized that the progression of the spasm from one muscle group to another expresses the propagation of an abnormal nerve discharge within a region of the brain where the control of muscles is represented in a spatially ordered fashion. On Jackson's part, this was just a brilliant guess. The anatomical location of the motor area was discovered later (Fritsch and Hitzig, 1870) (Chapter 6: "Mrs. Hitzig's historical dressing table"). The predilection of Jacksonian fits to begin in the hand region has been attributed to the relatively large representation of this body part in the motor cortex (Kotagal and Lüders, 1998).

The unanswered question is, how do the fits propagate in the cortex? The sequence of the spasms is congruent with the layout of the representation of the body's muscles in the motor cortex, but this does not explain how seizure discharges move from one neuron group to the next. Some of the possible mechanisms have been discussed by Jasper (1969) and Purpura (1969). The possible answers include the following. (*1*) The march could be routed by way of **synaptic connections**. Excitation could be conveyed through short axons in the superficial cortical neuropil or by way of U-shaped fiber connections in white matter, or else it could take the long route of circular reverberation going one way by corticothalamic fibers and returning through thalamocortical connections. The rate of spread is much slower than axonal conduction, but the delay could be explained because at each next group of cells, excitation would have to build up gradually to the trigger level at which paroxysmal firing would erupt. Seizure-like events can, however, propagate in gray matter, at least in vitro, even when synapses are not functioning (Konnerth et al., 1983; Pan and Stringer, 1996). (*2*) The seizure discharges could propagate by electrical interaction among neurons, either (*a*) through *gap junctions* among neurons or (*b*) through electric current flowing from one cell to the next, crossing the plasma membrane of both cells, known as **ephaptic interaction** (Fig. 7–11) (Dudek et al., 1983; Haas and Jefferys, 1984). (*3*) The spread could be mediated *chemically* by **volume transmission** by way of interstitial spaces bypassing synaptic connections. The excitant agent, spilled from seized neurons, would diffuse in the interstitial space and excite neighboring cells to recruit them into the seizure. The agent could be, for example, potassium (Amzica et al., 2002; Lian et al., 2001) or glutamate, the two likely substances mediating the propagation of spreading depression (Chapter 15: "Van Harreveld's dual hypothesis"). Decades ago, Van Harreveld and Stamm (1953b) compared *spreading depression* to *spreading convulsions*, implying a similar mechanism for the propagation of both. (*4*) Another candidate for a nonsynaptic mechanism for seizure propagation could be the network of **astrocytes**. (*a*) K^+ ions can be forwarded through gap junctions and spread over the quasi-syncytial glial net in the spatial buffer mechanism (Chapter 2: "The spatial buffer concept") (Heinemann et al., 1991; Lux et al., 1986). (*b*) Alternatively, calcium waves could mediate the propagation. Among cultured astrocytes and among glial cells in brain tissue slices, calcium waves can be triggered by a variety of stimuli, and these can propagate by way of gap junctions among the glial cells (Dani et al.,

1992; Finkbeiner, 1992). Elevated calcium appears to cause the release of glutamate from the astrocytes, inducing glutamate receptor-mediated inward current in adjacent neurons (Nedergaard, 1994; Parri et al., 2001; Rose and Konnerth, 2001a).

There is, to my knowledge, no recent work that could help to choose among these several possible synaptic or nonsynaptic mechanisms to explain the Jacksonian march of simple partial seizures. In brain tissue slices maintained in low-Ca^{2+} bathing solution, spontaneous bursts arise that do propagate without the benefit of synapses (Haas and Jefferys, 1984; Konnerth et al., 1983). Heinemann et al. (1995) emphasized the broadcasting of K^+ through the glial gap junctional network as a means of propagating seizure-like events bypassing synaptic transmission. Bikson et al. (1999) also found evidence for the role of gap junctions in the formation and propagation of epileptiform bursts, while the observations of Lian et al. (2001) seem to suggest the diffusion of a humoral mediator. Still, what works in hippocampal tissue slices in vitro need not necessarily be relevant to motor cortex in intact brains. Therein lies an excellent topic for a future Ph.D. dissertation.

Seizures Spread Over Longer Distances Through Fiber Tracts

Jacksonian seizures march over contiguous territory, from one locus in the motor cortex to its neighbor. Partial seizures that are initially limited to one locality can, however, ignite seizures at distant foci and eventually become generalized. Long-distance spread is mediated by the bombardment conveyed from an active seizure focus by way of fiber tracts and synaptic connections (e.g., Bertram et al., 1998; Lothman et al., 1985a; for review, see Lothman et al., 1991). Repeated, intense excitation is, however, not sufficient for the provocation of a seizure. The target area must be ready to respond with paroxysmal discharge. Conditions that enable paroxysmal activity include not only the membrane properties of the neurons but also the arrangement of their interconnections, the properties of the glial tissue, and the interstitial space.

Key points

Epileptiform seizures are episodic, correlated, yet nonfunctional responses of cerebral neuron populations that transiently disrupt the normal functioning of brain tissue.

The first sections of this chapter present standard definitions of some of the most often used clinical terms relating to epileptic seizures and to EEG.

Seizures can be induced in healthy brains.

The CNS of many epileptic patients functions normally between seizures. The anomaly underlying the attacks may be subtle, critically poised, in a state like an unstable equilibrium, so that seizures erupt when the balance is upset.

Partial (focal) seizures are restricted to a region of the brain. Generalized seizures involve large parts of both cerebral hemispheres. Partial seizures can but need not cause clouding of consciousness, while generalized seizures always suppress consciousness.

Seizures often do but need not cause overt muscle cramps; that is, seizures can be convulsive or nonconvulsive, depending on whether brain regions of motor function are involved. Complex partial seizures induce unwilled automatic movement patterns, with impaired consciousness.

Normal EEG waves are generated by the slow currents of neurons, mainly synaptic and intrinsic currents in the apical dendrites of neocortical pyramidal cells.

Interictal discharges are diagnostic signs seen in EEG recordings of epileptic patients. Without an EEG trace, they go unnoticed.

Absence seizures are accompanied by a 3/s SW EEG pattern. Tonic seizures are characterized by high-frequency, high-amplitude, irregular activity, clonic seizures by bursts of high-amplitude waves.

Jacksonian-type simple partial motor seizures in their classical form begin as convulsive movements in a hand and progressively extend into the affected arm. Eventually they can become generalized. The march of Jacksonian fits maps the representation of body parts in the motor cortex. The mechanism of cortical propagation is not known; it could be synaptic or nonsynaptic.

6

Experimental Seizures

Animal models of the human condition are necessary to elucidate the mechanisms of epileptic seizures and to develop drugs that can control them. Over the decades, experimental conditions have been created that present interictal discharges, absence seizures, simple and complex partial seizures with or without secondary generalization, and tonic-clonic convulsive seizures. These will now be described.

Epileptiform seizures can be provoked in normal brains

Mrs. Hitzig's Historical Dressing Table

Until 1870 the majority of physiologists believed that the cerebral cortex acts as a single system, with no discernible specialization among regions. It was also widely held that, unlike peripheral nerves and skeletal muscle, the forebrain, or at least the cortex, could not be excited by electric current (Brazier, 1988). There have been sporadic reports of muscular twitching provoked by electrical stimulation of exposed brains of animals, but these were dismissed as artifacts and were explained as caused by the spread of the current into the nerves or muscles of the face or into the spinal roots (Finger, 2000). These widely held views were dispelled by Gustav Fritsch and Eduard Hitzig, two young and as yet unknown surgeons, recently demobilized from the Prussian army (Fritsch and Hitzig, 1870).

Since they held no academic position at the time, they performed the most momentous experiments in cerebral physiology of the nineteenth century in a Berlin home, on the dressing table of Mrs Hitzig. According to a secondhand account, Fritsch had made an earlier chance observation. When dressing the skull wound of a soldier, he noticed that irritation of the exposed brain caused twitching of muscles on the contralateral side of the body (Wieser, 2000). There is no documentation of this, but opportunities were doubtless abundant on the battlefields of the wars of Prussia. In the famous paper (Fritsch and Hitzig, 1870), Hitzig mentions that he had earlier evoked muscle twitching by applying electricity to the head of a man, but this involved current through the intact scalp and skull and, as he admitted, it therefore was inconclusive. The main experiments were conducted on anesthetized dogs. Stimulating a well-circumscribed area of the brain with galvanic current through closely spaced bipolar electrodes, Fritsch and Hitzig evoked movement of the muscles of the opposite side of the body. When they used just-threshold stimuli, the contractions were limited to a small group of muscles, and when they moved the electrodes to a nearby spot, a different group of muscles was excited. Large areas of the cortex were, however, unresponsive to stimulation. In their paper there is a drawing of a dog's brain, with the spots marked where stimulation elicited contralateral movement; this was the first such map, to be followed by many. Most importantly, the sensitive spots were in the same region in all dogs. The authors wrote, "Ein Theil der Convexität des grossen Hirnes ist motorisch, ein anderer Theil ist nicht motorisch" (One part of the cerebral convexity is motor, the other part is not). These results proved, first, that the cortex was in fact electrically excitable, and second, that it was not functionally homogeneous but had specialized regions.

For our narrative, of special importance is the discovery by Fritsch and Hitzig of electrically triggered seizures. Using interrupted (tetanic) current, they saw muscle contractions that outlasted the stimulation (*Nachbewegungen*, evidently the result of *afterdischarge*), and when they turned up the stimulating current, they provoked generalized epileptiform convulsions. To make sure that this was not a manifestation of preexisting epilepsy, they questioned the former mistress of one of the dogs, who confirmed that in the 6 preceding years the dog had never had a seizure (Fritsch and Hitzig, 1870).

Two quotes now come to mind, both heard in lectures in long bygone student days, their sources sadly forgotten. One was "*Jedermann ist epilepsiefähig*," which means "everybody is capable of epilepsy." The other was "Convulsibility is the price paid for neuronal complexity." I should be grateful to any reader who can identify the authors of these two epigrams, which aptly address a stunning peculiarity of the mammalian cerebrum. The point about neuronal complexity needs comment, though. Flies with relatively unsophisticated nervous systems can also convulse in ways that are somewhat reminiscent of epileptic mammals (Lee and Wu, 2002). Moreover, seizure-like discharges occur in single-neuron microcultures (Segal, 1991) and can also be generated in computer models representing a single neuron (Kager et al., 2002b, and Chapter 9). The real issue is, however, not complexity but this: if seizures can be provoked in perfectly normal brains, then the question "why are some people epileptic?" can be turned around: "why are not all people epileptic?" Or, as Jung and Tönnies (1950) asked more than half a century ago: "Why are normal nervous systems not overcome by an epileptic attack each morning at the moment of awakening?"

The pages that follow deal with these and related problems and introduce some of the ways in which epileptiform seizures can be provoked in normal brains.

Shock Therapy Triggers Epileptiform Convulsions

Under various names, such as *electroconvulsive therapy* (*ECT*), *shock therapy*, and *metrazol shock*, epileptiform seizures have been used in psychiatric practice. The inspiration for this procedure was a perceived antagonism between epilepsy and schizophrenia (see also Starr, 1996). Nyirö and Jablonszky, of the State Neurological and Mental Hospital at Lipótmezö in Budapest, saw epilepsy improve in some patients when they developed schizophrenia (recounted by de Meduna, 1936). Subsequently G. Müller observed the reverse: two of his catatonic schizophrenic patients improved when they became epileptic (also quoted by de Meduna, without giving the literature reference). Impressed by these anecdotal observations, de Meduna, also working in Budapest, began to induce epileptiform convulsions to treat schizophrenia. At first he used camphor and later pentylenetetrazol as the convulsant drug (known earlier as *cardiazol, metrazol*, or *pentetrazol* [PTZ]). Insulin shock treatment was introduced in 1933 by M. Sakel. Insulin usually causes a more peaceful coma, sometimes with muscle twitching but with no violent convulsion. After the introduction of antipsychotic drugs, metrazol and insulin shock treatments were largely abandoned. Electroconvulsive therapy was introduced in 1938 by U. Cerletti and L. Bini to treat intractable psychotic depression, and it is still used for that purpose, but no longer to treat schizophrenia. Convulsions during ECT are now prevented by sedation and muscle relaxant drugs, but it is considered necessary to provoke a generalized tonic-clonic cortical electrical discharge in the brain in order for the treatment to be effective.

Local Electrical Stimulation Can Provoke a Seizure-Like Afterdischarge

Stimulation through electrodes applied to the exposed surface or an afferent pathway to the neocortex or the hippocampus, or to brain slices in vitro, can trigger a paroxysmal afterdischarge that outlasts the stimulus and resembles other types of seizure discharges (Gloor et al., 1961; Jung and Tönnies, 1950; Kandel and Spencer, 1961b). To induce a seizure, the frequency of stimulation has to be high enough and the train of pulses must last for a critical length of time (Somjen et al., 1985).

In intact brain, such locally induced seizures can expand into other areas if the stimulation is intensive enough.

Elevated Temperature

In hippocampal slices prepared from the brains of immature rats, raising the temperature within the moderate, clinical fever range altered the synaptically evoked responses. Instead of the normal EPSP with a single spike, feverish slices responded with impulse bursts resembling interictal discharges. Tissue slices from adult rats did not show such temperature-dependent burst firing (Tancredi et al., 1992). Temperature-induced hyperexcitability was interpreted to be a model of infantile *febrile seizures*.

Increased excitation and decreased inhibition, but also the simultaneous increase in both, can render brain tissue prone to seizures

Ever since Jackson defined the substrate for epileptic seizures as the "excessive and disorderly discharge of nerve tissue," many have assumed that paroxysmal activity represents pathologically excessive excitation. If normal function requires a balance of excitation and inhibition, then either an excess of the former or a deficit of the latter could cause a seizure. Since glutamate is the principal excitatory transmitter and GABA is the main inhibitory transmitter in the brain, much effort has been expended to find either potentiation of glutamatergic transmission or a failure of GABAergic inhibition in clinical and experimental epilepsy (reviews in Meldrum et al., 1999; Treiman, 2001).

Yet it turns out that inhibitory synapses are not always weakened, and sometimes they are strengthened, together with excitatory synapses (Avoli, 1984; Giaretta et al., 1985; Lothman et al., 1992; Tuff et al., 1983). Even more remarkably, after suppression of all glutamatergic excitatory synaptic transmission, the blockade of potassium channels induces spontaneous discharges in hippocampal slices, and these are triggered and synchronized by $GABA_A$ receptor–mediated inhibitory synaptic activity (Avoli et al., 1996).

Jackson's characterization of seizure discharges as *disorderly* may be as important as and sometimes more important than *excessive*. Even *disorderly* needs amending. As we shall soon see, in spike-wave and clonic seizure discharges there is regular, rhythmic, synchronous beating of massed impulse volleys. Excessive, inappropriate "order" can disrupt the normal activity of brain cells as much as does chaos. Similarly to seizures, electrical stimulation can also impose inappropriate synchrony on neuron populations and so interfere with normal function. When the cortex of conscious human patients is stimulated prior to ablating an offending lesion, the stimulation can elicit positive or negative responses. Among the positive responses are unwilled muscle contractions, various sensations, or even images of remembered events. Among the negative responses are the arrest, or laming, of voluntary movement by stimulation of so-called *negative motor areas* (Lüders et al., 1998). Similarly, stimulating the language areas of the neocortex renders patients temporarily speechless (Dinner and Lüders, 1998; Ojemann, 1980). Neurosurgeons use this phenomenon to find the borders of cortical speech areas, which they must not injure (Ojemann, 1987).

The point is this: electrical stimulation evokes synchronized neuron discharges, which can disrupt normal function just epileptic fits do. Hypersynchronization can be achieved by excitatory volleys, but also by inhibitory volleys followed by postinhibitory rebound excitation (Chapter 7: "Rebound excitation . . .")

Seizures induced by stimulant poisons

Pentylenetetrazol

***Pentylenetetrazol* (PTZ, metrazol)** is one of numerous poisons capable of causing seizures. The mode of action of PTZ in mammals is not clear (Ajmone-Marsan, 2000). In molluscan ganglia it reduced chloride-dependent inhibitory synaptic currents (Pellmar and Wilson, 1977) and induced the firing of impulse bursts in normally silent neurons (David et al., 1974). Also, in *Aplysia* neurons, rectifier potassium current was inhibited (Klee et al., 1973). In cloned potassium channels from rat brain, it reduced open probability at depolarized membrane potentials but increased open probability at negative voltages, changes whose possible effect on seizure generation is difficult to predict (Madeja et al., 1996). The problem in interpreting the results of such experiments is not only that the "models" are very unlike real brain tissue, but also that the concentrations used to elicit effects are usually much higher than the epileptogenic levels in intact mammals.

Blocking Synaptic Inhibition Can Induce Seizures

Some of the other convulsant drugs have better-defined pharmacological actions. Many act by tipping the balance between synaptic excitation and inhibition in favor of the former, either by blocking inhibitory synapses or by stimulating excitatory synapses. ***Bicuculline*** and ***picrotoxin*** (PTX) block $GABA_A$ receptors that mediate the fast action of GABA, the main inhibitory transmitter in the cerebrum and cerebellum. Penicillin has a weaker, similar action, but that is not the complete explanation of its ability to induce seizures (see below: "Penicillin induces seizures . . ."). Blocking $GABA_A$-mediated inhibition in brain slices induces spontaneous burst discharges, and it transforms stimulus-induced, synaptically transmitted responses into seizure-like events (Connors, 1984; Hwa et al., 1991; Jones, 1988; Masukawa et al., 1989; Telfeian and Connors, 1998; Traub and Jefferys, 1994). In patients being prepared for surgery, GABA levels measured by microdialysis were lower while glutamate was higher in the epileptogenic hippocampus than in the inert contralateral structure. During seizures, GABA increased on both sides but more so in the inactive side (During and Spencer, 1993).

Strychnine blocks glycine-operated synaptic receptors. Glycine is the main inhibitory transmitter in the spinal cord; accordingly, strychnine convulsions originate in spinal gray matter. The glycine-binding site of the NMDA receptor is, however, not affected by strychnine. Death by strychnine poisoning is horrible because the victim does not immediately lose consciousness. The drug causes violent generalized muscle spasms, and death follows by suffocation as respiratory muscles become incapacitated. Because they do not originate from the brain, strychnine seizures are not considered epileptiform. Nonetheless, high concentrations of strychnine applied directly to the cortical surface do induce localized seizure-like activity in the exposed region of the neocortex (Bremer, 1936; Pollen and Lux, 1966; Towe et al., 1981). This could be an illustration of Gaddum's first rule of pharmacology, which states that "enough of anything will block anything," but Pollen and Lux (1966) concluded that the cortical effect is due to a shift in the equilibrium potential of the IPSP, not to blockade of the receptor. A shift of the equilibrium potential of the IPSPs is expected if a neuron acquires too much chloride (see below: "Malfunctioning inhibitory synapses . . ."). Towe et al. (1981) interpreted current source density analysis of strychnine-induced EEG "spikes" as composites of exaggerated EPSPs plus dendritic calcium currents. Strychnine is also capable of exciting neurons isolated from invertebrate nervous systems, independently of all synapses, inhibitory or excitatory, indicating a direct influence on intrinsic membrane currents (Klee et al., 1973).

Sudden Drug Withdrawal

Terminating chronic administration of a depressant drug can induce seizures. Examples include drugs that bolster the action of GABA-mediated inhibition, such as **barbiturates** and **benzodiazepines**.

When GABA itself was infused by a mini-pump locally into the cerebral cortex and the infusion was stopped, a seizure focus was created, resulting in a partial epilepsy that lasted for days or weeks (Brailowsky et al., 1987; Silva-Barrat et al., 2000). The hyperexcitability is also detectable in tissue slices prepared from the previously in situ-treated cortical area; it can also be created by exposing slices to GABA in vitro. The epileptogenic withdrawal effect has been attributed to *down-regulation of GABA_A receptors* during prolonged exposure to excess GABA (Casasola et al., 2002).

Malfunctioning Inhibitory Synapses Could Change into Excitatory Synapses

γ-Aminobutyric acid, acting on $GABA_A$ receptors, is an excitatory transmitter in newborn animals (Ben-Ari et al., 1997). Also, GABA applied directly to DRG cells at any age causes depolarization (Deschenes et al., 1976). In these neurons the chloride equilibrium potential (E_{Cl}) is more positive than the resting membrane potential, so that opening Cl^--permeable channels causes efflux instead of influx of Cl^-, and efflux of Cl^- generates inward instead of outward electric current. In adult brains, the usually hyperpolarizing $GABA_A$-mediated IPSP could, theoretically, become a depolarizing signal if the neuron accumulates excess Cl^- (Chapter 4: "Chloride has effects of its own"). Prolonged exposure to GABA itself has been shown to raise $[Cl^-]_i$ because, if enough of the GABA-operated Cl^- channels stay open for a long enough time, the removal of Cl^- from the cell cannot keep up with its accumulation (Thompson and Gähwiler, 1989a, 1989b). γ-Aminobutyric acid–induced influx can raise $[Cl^-]_i$ only to the level where it reaches the electrochemical equilibrium. This explains (in part) the fading of long-lasting GABA-induced hyperpolarization (the other reason being receptor *desensitization*), but this will not convert inhibition into excitation, nor will it eliminate synaptic inhibition completely. In the Cl-equilibrated state, $GABA_A$ receptor activation no longer alters V_m. Nonetheless, inhibition remains effective, if reduced (Chapter 4: "Chloride has effects of its own").

To raise $[Cl^-]_i$ above its equilibrium level, something has to go drastically wrong with one of the manifold transport mechanisms. Most forebrain neurons keep $[Cl^-]_i$ below equilibrium by the action of an ATP-dependent Cl^- pump assisted by other carriers (Inagaki et al., 1998). By contrast, in cultured glial cells, a furosemide-sensitive carrier, probably the Na/K/2Cl cotransporter, moves Cl^- inward and maintains $[Cl^-]_i$ well above its equilibrium level (Walz, 1995). Neurons do have the Na/K/2Cl as well as the K/Cl cotransporter. The former tends to move Cl^- in, causing a positive E_{Cl} shift; the latter moves Cl^- out, causing a negative E_{Cl} shift (Kaila, 1994). Furosemide, which inhibits both carriers, shifts the equilibrium potential of IPSPs in the depolarizing (positive) direction. This shows that the normal net effect of the neuronal Cl cotransporters is to move Cl^- outward (Thompson and Gähwiler, 1989b), unlike in glial cells, where they predominantly favor influx. Nonetheless, furosemide inhibits seizures as well as SD and HSD (Gutschmidt et al., 1999; Müller, 2000; Read et al., 1997; Schwartzkroin et al., 1998). This can be explained by the effect of pathologically high $[K^+]_o$ during seizure and even higher during SD. Elevated $[K^+]_o$ hinders efflux mediated by the K/Cl cotransporter and favors influx by the Na/K/2Cl cotransporter. As a result, $[Cl^-]_i$ could be raised to the point where IPSPs would invert and became excitatory signals. This inversion of IPSPs would be prevented by furosemide, which would block the influx of Cl^-, carried by the cotransporters.

In conclusion

We do not know whether Cl⁻ accumulation figures in epileptogenesis and, if it does, how it happens. However, the possibility exists.

There is, however, yet another way in which GABA could become an excitatory agent. Besides chloride, the $GABA_A$ receptor–controlled channel is also permeable to bicarbonate. The hyperpolarizing effect of the Cl⁻ influx is blunted by the depolarizing efflux of HCO_3^-. Because the Cl⁻ current is normally much larger than the HCO_3^- current, the IPSP normally is a hyperpolarizing signal. The effect of the HCO_3^- current is detected only by the fact that the reversal potential of the IPSP (E_{GABA-A}) is not quite as negative as E_{Cl}. Experimental conditions can be created, however, in which the HCO_3^- current initiates a complex reaction sequence resulting in powerful excitation (Kaila et al., 1997; Voipio and Kaila, 2000). A brief high-frequency stimulation of inhibitory input to hippocampal neurons first evokes the expected hyperpolarizing IPSP, but this is followed by a large depolarizing wave that outlasts the stimulation by a couple of seconds. Kaila and colleagues called this depolarization first the GABA-mediated depolarizing postsynaptic potential (GDPSP) and later the ***GABA-mediated depolarizing nonsynaptic potential*** (GDNSP) to emphasize its peculiar genesis. Key to the scheme proposed by these authors to explain the GDNSP is the intensive activation of a network of inhibitory interneurons, resulting in an accumulation of extracellular K⁺. Rising $[K^+]_o$ has two effects. It inhibits the Cl⁻ efflux mediated by the K/Cl cotransport, thus reducing the GABA receptor–mediated Cl⁻ current (see above) and shifting the balance in favor of the (depolarizing) bicarbonate current. Additionally, the high $[K^+]_o$ depolarizes neurons directly. As K⁺ spreads by diffusion, it causes depolarization of adjacent cells' membranes, not originally affected by the GABA (Voipio and Kaila, 2000). Whether this mechanism is relevant for seizures and for their propagation is not known but is worth investigation.

Are Inhibitory Synapses Failing in Clinical Epilepsy?

There may be genetic causes for the malfunctioning of inhibitory synapses. Failure of inhibitory synapses due to genetic or acquired causes may be important in some forms of clinical epilepsy and their experimental models. Defective inhibition was a feature of the electrophysiology of some brain tissue slices prepared from temporal lobes of patients during epilepsy surgery (Masukawa et al., 1989; Uruno et al., 1994). The GABA concentration was lower and the glutamate concentration was higher in dialysate from epileptogenic foci than from the contralateral homologous site in human patients (During and Spencer, 1993). Also, *fast-kindling* rats, which are genetically more susceptible to kindled seizures, have reduced GABAergic function compared to rats that kindle more slowly (McIntyre et al., 2002). Yet it is important to reiterate that suppression of inhibition is not a universal requirement for the generation of seizures or for the development of clinical epilepsy (Avoli and Olivier, 1989; Bernard et al., 2000; De Deyn et al., 1990; Olsen and Avoli, 1997). In fact, in some forms of seizure, the activity of both inhibitory and excitatory neurons is enhanced. Increased inhibitory function and rebound excitation may be important for the synchronization of bursts (Andersen and Andersson, 1968; Prince and Jacobs, 1998) (Chapter 7: "rebound excitation . . ."). During clonic convulsions, synaptic inhibition contributes to the arrest of the discharges during the relaxed moments between spasms. Also, as will become clear in Chapter 7 ("Spike-wave seizures . . ."), IPSPs dominate under the "dome" of spike-and-wave EEG complexes.

In conclusion

The answer to the question "Are inhibitory synapses failing in clinical epilepsy?" is both yes and no, depending on the seizure type.

Seizures Induced by Agonists of Excitatory Synaptic Receptors

Kainic acid, a poison derived from a seaweed, stimulates a class of glutamate receptors named after it, **kainate receptors**, which contribute to the fast phase of normal glutamatergic synaptic excitation. Kainate receptors are expressed in high desnity in the hippocampal formation, especially in the CA3 and CA4 regions (Okazaki and Nadler, 1988). This explains why kainic acid poisoning induces complex partial seizures of the temporal lobe type. Besides its immediate action, kainate can cause a persistent epileptic state in experimental animals, which outlasts the presence of the drug in the body (see below: "Kainic acid").

The muscarinic cholinergic agents, **carbachol** and **pilocarpine**, can also cause seizures (Turski et al., 1989). Like kainate, pilocarpine treatment can cause status epilepticus, which is usually followed after a latent period by a permanently epileptic condition.

Penicillin Induces Seizures by Multiple Actions

When penicillin was new, it was given intrathecally (by injection into the arachnoid space) to patients suffering from bacterial meningitis. Many of them developed violent convulsions. At first, it was not clear whether the seizures were caused by the disease or by the treatment, but then it became obvious that penicillin is, in fact, a convulsant drug. It is safe when given in the usual dosage by the usual parenteral routes only because it passes the BBB sparingly. Its exclusion from the CNS is, however, not absolute, and large systemic doses do induce seizures in experimental animals (Prince and Farrell, 1969). Intravenous or intramuscular administration of toxic amounts of penicillin induces absence seizures with 3/s spike-wave EEG discharges, a condition called **feline generalized penicillin epi-**

lepsy (FGPE) (Gloor, 1984). Large doses cause convulsions of spinal origin as well (Lothman and Somjen, 1976b; Schwindt and Crill, 1984). A small amount injected into or applied to the surface of the neocortex or the hippocampal formation causes localized interictal discharges. In the forebrain, penicillin antagonizes GABAergic inhibitory synapses, and this was assumed to account for its convulsant action. The blockade of GABAergic inhibition by penicillin is, however, not complete. Intramuscular administration of the dose that induces FGPE did not affect cortical inhibition at all (Giaretta et al., 1985). In the spinal cord penicillin induces both interictal and ictal-like discharges, but it has no detectable effect on glycinergic inhibitory synapses (Lothman and Somjen, 1976c). It suppresses the so-called negative dorsal root potentials, also known as the *DR-IV*, which are believed to reflect presynaptic inhibition. There is, however, no correlation between the spinal seizures induced by penicillin and the suppression of presynaptic inhibition as assessed by the testing of reflexes (Kinnes et al., 1980). In hippocampal slices, low concentrations of penicillin enhanced EPSPs and only high concentrations depressed IPSPs (Avoli, 1984). One must inevitably conclude that suppression of synaptic inhibition does not explain the seizures caused by this drug. Penicillin can induce repetitive firing at axon terminals, causing excessive release of transmitter substance, and this may be the most important clue to its convulsant action (Gutnick and Prince, 1972; Lothman and Somjen, 1976a; Stasheff et al., 1993).

Drugs That Block Potassium Channels

4-Aminopyridine (4-AP) and *tetraethylammonium (TEA)* also induce spontaneous epileptiform activity in brain tissue slices (Perreault and Avoli, 1991; Rutecki et al., 1990). This can take the form of either interictal or ictal discharges. Inhibition of K^+ currents affects neuron function in several ways. Action potential duration increases because the repolarization is delayed, and the postspike subnormal period of excitability is lessened as hyperpolarizing afterpotentials are depressed or eliminated. The latter effect favors high-frequency firing. At relatively low concentrations of the K^+ channel blockers, the main effect is increased transmission at both excitatory and inhibitory synapses (Rutecki et al., 1990). This is probably caused by the prolongation of presynaptic action potentials that keeps Ca^{2+} channels open for a longer time, boosting the release of transmitter substances (Perreault and Avoli, 1991).

Drugs That Boost Sodium Current

Certain alkaloids derived from plants alter the properties of voltage-gated channels, shifting activation or reducing inactivation. The most-studied one is *veratridine*, which favors the open state of the Na^+ channel, making neurons hyperexcitable.

Hille (2001) calls it an "agonist" of the channel, implying the existence of a specific binding site, even though the channel is not ligand-operated. Tissue slices exposed to veratridine become spontaneously active, and neurons in such slices generate a seizure-like discharge (Alkadhi and Tian, 1996; Otoom et al., 1998).

Ion Imbalance

Besides specific poisons, too much or too little of the ions that are essential to brain function can also become convulsants. Too much K^+ or too little Ca^{2+}, Mg^{2+}, Cl^-, or H^+ in ECF can have this effect. These will be discussed in detail in Chapter 8.

Nonsynaptic Epileptogenesis

Several teams discovered at about the same time (or rediscovered, after Sabbatani, 1901) that depriving brain tissue slices of calcium induces spontaneous synchronized burst discharges that resemble interictal activity and sometimes ictal seizures (Jefferys and Haas, 1982; Taylor and Dudek, 1982; Yaari et al., 1983). Since low external calcium blocks all chemical synapses, the synchronization of the discharge must be mediated by nonsynaptic mechanisms. Removal of surface screening explains hyperexcitability but not synchronization. Among the possible synchronizers of nonsynaptic seizures could be ephaptic interaction, gap junctions, and the release into the interstitial space of ions or of neuroactive substances acting at extrasynaptic receptors (Bikson et al., 2002; Dudek et al., 1983; Jefferys, 1995; Lian et al., 2001; Yaari et al., 1986). Decalcified tissue slices are far removed from brain pathology, but nonsynaptic ictal seizures demonstrably occur in intact brains too. In baboons, during reflex seizures provoked by flashing lights, interstitial calcium levels decreased so much that synaptic transmission must have been interrupted, yet intense seizure activity continued (Pumain et al., 1985) (see also Chapter 8: "Seizures in real brains can proceed with synapses blocked").

Neuron loss can lead to epilepsy, while excessive epileptic seizures can decimate neurons

Neuron Loss, Neuron Proliferation, and Gliosis Are Evident in Epileptogenic Tissue

In biopsy or autopsy material taken from epileptogenic brain areas, brain damage and disordered cytoarchitecture are common (Dam and Meencke, 1999; Najm et al., 2000). A frequent pathological finding is a ***gliotic scar***, resulting from past *trauma, bleeding, or localized ischemic episode* that killed off much of the neuron population. The same condition is seen in experimental ***freeze lesions***. If located in the hemispheric convexity, such lesions give rise to simple partial epilepsy. In the majority of surgically treated complex partial seizures, the underlying pathology appears to be ***Ammon's horn* (or *mesial temporal*) *sclerosis***, a gliotic hardening in parts of the temporal lobe found in the majority of cases of *temporal lobe epilepsy* (TLE). Selective loss of the pyramidal cells in part of the hippocampus was first described in detail by Sommer (1880) (Fig. 17–2), and the preferentially affected area is sometimes referred to as *Sommer's sector*—CA1 in Lorente de Nó's classification. Sommer acknowledged an 1825 publication by Bouchet and Cazauvieilh as the first one to mention the hardening and atrophy of Ammon's horn in cases of epilepsy (see also reviews by Babb, 1999; Engel, 1998b; Gloor, 1997; Mathern et al., 1998). Another neuron population preferentially destroyed in temporal lobe epilepsy is layer III of the entorhinal cortex (Scharfman, 2000; Schwarcz et al., 2000).

Causality works two ways in selective cell loss, because primary lesions that kill neurons can cause epilepsy, but repeated intense, prolonged excitation can cause neuron loss even in nonepileptic brain (Meldrum, 2002b; Sloviter, 1983, 1999; Sloviter and Damiano, 1981). The possibility of a self-reinforcing vicious circle is evident. Status epilepticus induced by kainate or pilocarpine causes severe cell loss (Fig. 6–1), and the cell loss is blamed for the permanent epileptic state that can result from kainate and pilocarpine treatment (see below: "Kainic acid" and "Pilocarpine")

Yet seizures can induce ***neuron proliferation*** as well, at least in rats (Parent and Lowenstein, 2002). New cells do not take the place of the lost ones, but rather tend to take abnormal positions and make abnormal connections. Madsen and colleagues (2000) found evidence of *neurogenesis* after a single electroconvulsive shock treatment, and the number of neurons in mitosis increased with repetition of the convulsive shocks. Also, after pilocarpine poisoning, which causes lasting epilepsy in rats, dentate granule cells proliferate (Parent and Lowenstein, 2002; Parent et al., 1997). Yet, while granule cells multiply, CA3 pyramidal cells and neurons in amygdala, thalamus, substantia nigra, and a few other areas die in large numbers after pilocarpine poisoning (Turski et al., 1989). It could be guessed that the dentate granule cells, which proliferate, are the source, while CA3 pyramidal neurons, which succumb, were the target of the seizure discharges. This simple reasoning is not satisfactory, however, for freshly sprouted connections target the granule cells themselves, and through these abnormal recurrent excitatory connections, the granule cells are also heavily bombarded by seizures (Molnár and Nadler, 1999; Okazaki et al., 1999) (see below: "Artificial epileptogenic foci . . .").

Five Ideas Contend to Explain Epileptogenesis at Gliotic Scars

In the core of a brain scar, if all the neurons have been replaced by reactive fibrous astrocytes and invading fibroblasts, there can only be electrical silence.

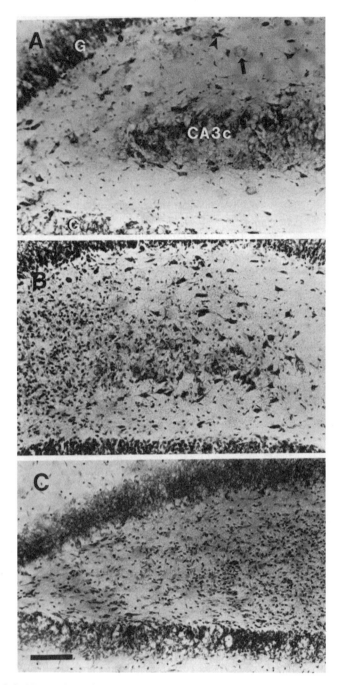

Figure 6–1. Neuron loss after kainic acid treatment. Stained sections from rat hippocampal formation. **A:** Saline-treated control. **B, C:** Two to three weeks after intravenous kainic acid administration. In panel A, "G" marks the dentate granule cell layer, "CA3c" the end of the hippocampal CA3 pyramidal cell layer within the hilus of the dentate gyrus. **B:** Neuron loss from CA3 and CA4 in the dentate hilus. **C:** Shrinkage and gliosis in the dentate hilus. The dentate granule cells remain intact. The calibration bar shows 0.1 mm. (Reproduced from Tauck and Nadler, 1985.)

Seizure activity arises from the transitional border areas, where surviving neurons mingle with reactive glial cells. Several competing but not necessarily mutually exclusive hypotheses have been proposed over the years to explain how gliotic tissue emits uncontrolled discharges.

1. *Mechanical stimulation.* Retracting gliotic scar tissue can pull on dendritic trees of nearby surviving neurons, producing either a "windblown" or a "parasol" deformity (Scheibel, 1980). Mechanical stress can excite the neurons. Over time, however, the neuron membrane is likely to adapt, as do mechanoreceptors of the skin. This idea therefore has little appeal.

2. *Deafferentation.* With the death of some cells and the disappearance of their axons, synaptic sites on the surviving nerve cells become vacant. This has given rise to the ***deafferentation*** hypothesis (Ward, 1969) and the related concept of ***denervation supersensitivity*** (Sharpless, 1969), echoing ideas first formulated by Walter Cannon (1939). After motor nerve injury, skeletal muscle fibers develop abnormal excitability and spontaneous twitching known as ***fibrillations***. A major factor in the denervation syndrome of muscle is the spreading of nicotinic acetylcholine (ACh) receptors into the entire surface membrane of the fiber. Normally, the receptors are restricted to the neuromuscular endplate. Excess receptors are only part of the explanation, because denervated muscle in vitro tends to twitch even in the absence of ACh. Depriving a slab of neocortex of its major input by undercutting the white matter beneath the gray causes the gradual evolution of seizure-like discharges, which increase over several days and could be compared to the behavior of denervated muscle (Hoffman et al., 1994; Prince et al., 1997; Sharpless, 1969). In the epileptogenic borders of cortical scars the neurons that no longer have neighbors are also partially denervated, and their hyperexcitable state could be attributed to the absence of synaptic input. There are morphological abnormalities of neurons in epileptogenic foci, such as greatly reduced numbers of dendritic spines and atrophy of dendrites, which can be the morphological reaction of the target cells to the vanishing of synaptic boutons (Meldrum and Corsellis, 1984; Scheibel, 1980; Ward, 1969).

    In line with this trend of thought, after the partial deafferentation of dentate granule cells by local microinjection of kainic acid into the dentate hilus, the density of NMDA receptors (NR1) first decreases and then increases considerably, starting on the seventh day and lasting for at least 160 days (Mikuni et al., 2000). Also possibly relevant is that neuron cultures, which have been grown in the presence of antagonist drugs that blocked all synaptic transmission, develop spontaneous seizures when the blockers are removed (Furshpan and Potter, 1989). This also suggests that depriving neurons of synaptic input makes them seizure-prone. Input deprivation works even with a ***microculture*** containing just one neuron (Segal, 1991). The neuron in such single-cell microcultures grows recurrent excitatory connections upon itself, termed *autapses*. After analyzing the seizure-like activity of such single-cell cultures, Segal (1994, 2002) came to the conclusion that PDS-type bursts depend mainly on synaptic activity in the autapse, while a prolonged ictal-like discharge is based on the activation of persistent inward current.

3. *Loss of inhibitory interneurons.* Early histological examination of epileptogenic tissue specimens suggested selective loss of short-axon interneurons. These were thought to serve inhibition. Subsequently, it became clear that not all short-axon neurons are inhibitory in function. Moreover, inhibitory cells often survive excitatory cells in epileptogenic foci.

4. *Sprouting of new excitatory connections.* Over the years, the emphasis shifted from denervation and cell loss to the secondary *sprouting* and chaotic reorganization of aberrant synaptic connections that replace lost connections (Babb, 1999; Isokawa et al., 1993; Lehmann et al., 2000; Louis et al., 1998; Sloviter, 1992; Tauck and Nadler, 1985; Wuarin and Dudek, 2001). Where surviving neurons are bereft of synapses, the vacant sites can be colonized by newly formed connections. Absent a purposeful wiring diagram, the cells in the new net may interact in disordered quasi-random patterns, and seizures evolve. Alternatively, the new connections can reinforce recurrent excitation that favors the positive feedback required for self-sustaining seizures (Molnár and Nadler, 1999; Nadler et al., 1980; Sloviter, 1991; Wuarin and Dudek, 2001). As mentioned above, self-reexciting recurrent axons that make autapses in single-neuron cultures are formed if and only if the microculture was maintained in a solution that blocked all synaptic activity (Segal, 1991, 1994). This observation reinforces the idea of an inherent causal link between denervation and sprouting.

   In epileptogenic tissue there is an upregulation of growth factors, especially *brain-derived neurotrophic factor (BDNF), nerve growth factor (NGF)*, and NT-3. On the one hand, these agents protect neurons against ischemic injury and against the cell damage that follows pilocarpine treatment (Biagini et al., 2001). On the other hand, they foster the sprouting of axons, and if the argument is correct, sprouting is a major factor in making gliotic tissue epileptogenic. Binder et al. (2001a) contend that there can be "too much of a good thing" (see also Scharfman et al., 2002; Vezzani et al., 1999a) (see below: "Artificial epileptogenic foci . . .").

5. *The potassium hypothesis.* The potassium hypothesis of seizure generation had its ups and downs over the years (Chapter 8). It has been suggested that the fibrous reactive astrocytes in gliotic scars fail to regulate $[K^+]_o$, a function that normal astrocytes perform in healthy brain tissue (Chapter 2: "Glial cells regulate ion levels . . ."). K^+ released by surviving active neurons would then accumulate in interstitial spaces and excite the same neurons that dis-

charged as well as their neighbors, creating cascading reexcitation culminating in seizure. There is good reason to believe that K^+ ions have a major role in shaping seizures, but this does not necessarily put the blame on reactive astrocytes. The idea of the incompetence of reactive astrocytes in glial scars had early support (Pollen and Trachtenberg, 1970); it then fell into disfavor (Glötzner, 1973; Heinemann and Dietzel, 1984; Pollen and Richardson, 1972) but was revived by recent evidence (Kivi et al., 2000) (see also Chapter 8: "Is impaired potassium buffering . . . ?").

Epileptogenic Scars: What Is the Cause and What Is the Effect?
Self-Destruction of Neurons

Summing up the cumulated data, Meldrum (1997, 2002b) emphasized that brain damage can be both a consequence and a cause of seizures (see also the editorial comment by Sutula and Pitkänen, 2001). Sommer (1880) is usually credited with describing Ammon's horn sclerosis and making the connection between this lesion and epilepsy, but Sommer himself quotes Meynert, and an even earlier thesis by Bouchet and Cazauvieilh that appeared in 1825, as having already reported both the lesion and its frequent presence in epileptics (also quoted by Liberson and Cadilhac, 1954). In his long classical essay, Sommer did emphasize the selective loss of neurons in the area now known as CA1 and often referred to as *Sommer's sector*. A long debate ensued in which one side held that the gliosis caused the seizures and the other side maintained that the seizures caused the neuron loss that led to gliosis. The history of this dispute is reviewed by Gloor in his monumental volume *The Temporal Lobe and Limbic System* (1997, pp. 677–691). Judging by current reports, both views could be right, and sometimes one and sometimes the other is applicable (Mathern et al., 1998). An entire volume is dedicated to the question "Do seizures damage the brain" (Sutula and Pitkänen, 2002). One of the contributions concerned the pathology that evolves during the chronically epileptic state that occurs after electrically induced status epilepticus (Pitkänen et al., 2002). The authors found no correlation between the severity of cell loss and the frequency and severity of spontaneous seizures that occurred over the weeks and months after status epilepticus. They concluded that the damage was done by the original status epilepticus itself and not by the spontaneous seizures that followed. Yet other chapters, some based on animal experiments and others on human clinical observation, did indicate that at least certain types of spontaneous seizures do cause neuron loss. Summing up, Engel (2002) called for more research to define when a seizure does and does not kill nerve cells. This, then, is not a very satisfactory state for guiding therapy and prevention. The clinical consensus seems to be that it is wise to assume that oft-repeated seizures can aggravate the condition.

The Shared Causes of Ischemic and Epileptic Neuron Injury:
Metabolic Failure or Excitotoxicity?

The next question is, then, how do nerve cells injure themselves? At first, pathologists found similarity between neurons dying after status epilepticus and the neurons killed by ischemia (Spielmeyer, 1927). Based on this similarity, they speculated that an epileptic discharge is either accompanied by or actually caused by vasospasm of cerebral vessels. Refuting the idea, Meldrum and Brierly (Meldrum, 2002b; Meldrum and Brierley, 1973) showed that CBF increases during seizures, and concluded that a prolonged, excessive discharge itself is injurious to neurons. This conclusion was supported by Sloviter and Damiano (1981), who produced neuron loss by prolonged, intensive electrical stimulation without the use of drugs.

According to Kreisman et al. (1981) and Leniger-Follert (1984), tissue oxygenation actually increases initially during repeated seizures, suggesting an oversupply of oxygen, as the blood flow increase exceeds the demand. The oxidation of mitochondrial NADH and cytochrome a,a_3 also increases, conforming to the elevated tissue P_{O_2} (Jöbsis et al., 1971; Kreisman et al., 1981, 1983a; Lothman et al., 1975; O'Connor et al., 1972, and other references in these papers). During oft-repeated seizures, however, with time, CBF gradually falls short of demand and tissue P_{O_2} decreases, at least in anesthetized rats, so that tissue P_{O_2} falls and mitochondrial enzyme levels are reduced (Kreisman et al., 1981). Moreover, if the rats are hypoxic, then the mitochondrial NAD becomes reduced to NADH during seizures (O'Connor et al., 1972). Jöbsis et al. concluded that hypoxia neither initiated nor terminated the seizures. It also appears that if the circulation is marginal, then the extra energy demand of a seizure worsens the chances of neuron survival. This is especially so during status epilepticus.

In conclusion

As long as the heart, lungs, and blood vessels are in good condition, the supply of oxygen to seized tissues is more than adequate, and neuron loss cannot be blamed on energy shortage. If the circulation is marginal, the energy stress of seizures can tip the balance and kill cells.

When brain tissue is maintained in vitro, the supply of oxygen is invariant. Heinemann et al. (2002a) recorded the changes in NADH fluorescence and calcium levels in hippocampal organotypic cultures during seizures and correlated these changes with neuron injury. With the oxygen supply constant, seizure discharges were accompanied by initial oxidation followed by reduction of the NAD(P)H/NAD(P)+ system. While in intact brain the superabundant blood flow raised tissue P_{O_2}, causing oxidation of NAD(P)H, with the supply of oxygen remaining fixed in the organ culture, the increased energy metabolism drove the NAD(P)H/NAD(P)+ ratio in the reduced direction (see also Chapter 2: "Keeping ions in their place . . ."). As the tissue lapsed into a status epilepticus–like condition, the NADH fluorescence signals became progressively more feeble; at the same time, free radical levels increased and so did the number of damaged and dying cells. Damage could be mitigated by the radical scavenger α-tocopherol. The authors conclude that cell injury during status epilepticus is caused by reactive oxygen species produced by failure of mitochondrial function (Heinemann et al., 2002a).

The similar appearance of neurons succumbing to ischemia and those injured in an epileptic discharge may be explained if, in both conditions, calcium overloading of mitochondria is the cause of cell death (Meldrum, 2002b). Most probably, epileptic neurons commit suicide by *excitotoxicity*, a mechanism first proposed by Olney (1969) and Rothman (1983) (Chapter 19: "Is excitotoxicity causing . . . ?"). While firing action potentials, neurons open voltage-gated calcium channels; perhaps more importantly, prolonged high-frequency bombardment by glutamatergic excitatory synapses activates NMDA receptor–gated channels. Opening both sets of channels floods the cytosol with Ca^{2+}. If the influx of Ca^{2+} exceeds the cell's ability to remove and sequester the ion, the elevated $[Ca^{2+}]_i$ initiates processes that lead to the demise of the cell. The calcium overload activates a mitochondrial permeability transition (Fig. 2–3), which, if it persists, is lethal (Duchen, 2000; Zoratti and Szabó, 1995).

In summary

The available evidence suggests that seizure discharges are capable of causing neuron death even if the supply of oxygen and oxidizable substrate is adequate. The hazard of excitotoxic cell injury increases if the metabolic energy supply cannot meet the extra demand of a seizure.

The several ways in which excess intracellular calcium can initiate cell injury will be discussed in Chapter 19, "Adoptosis and Neurosis."

*Selective Loss of Inhibitory Interneurons Is Common but Is Not
Necessary for Epileptogenesis; Do Inhibitory Cells Fall Asleep?*

Since neuron loss is a feature in epileptogenic foci and since failing inhibition can cause seizures, it was a small step to assume that the loss of inhibitory interneurons could explain all cases of epileptogenic lesions. Reduced inhibition has been attributed to the selective loss of inhibitory interneurons. When it became possible to identify GABAergic cells in tissue sections by histochemical marking, it appeared, however, that inhibitory interneurons are not necessarily lost in greater numbers than excitatory neurons. Sloviter (1987) reported that GABAergic basket cells in the dentate hilus were spared, while excitatory interneurons succumbed after repeated intensive seizure activity equivalent to status epilepticus. Yet even though the inhibitory neurons survived, GABAergic synaptic inhibition was depressed. To reconcile these seemingly contradictory findings—on the one hand, decreased synaptic inhibition, as tested in physiological experiments; on the other hand, the survival of inhibitory interneurons, as seen in histological specimens—Sloviter (1987, 1991) proposed the **dormant basket cell** hypothesis. He concluded that inhibitory interneurons became inactive because they were functionally disconnected from input that would normally excite them. In the words of Jefferys and Traub (1998), the inhibitory cells "are not lost but fail to perform adequately." The result is disinhibition of the neurons that are the normal targets of the "sleeping" cells. A proclivity for seizures is the result. The idea aroused both support and controversy. It seems valid in at least some forms of experimentally induced seizures (Bekenstein and Lothman, 1993; Bernard et al., 1998; Jefferys and Traub, 1998).

Artificial epileptogenic foci in experimental animals

Neocortical Experimental Epileptogenic Foci

Epileptogenic gliotic scars can be created by destructive lesions, for example by implanting a small amount of *alumina cream* or *cobalt* powder; by microinjection of *tetanus toxin*; or by *freezing* a small area of the cortex. Following a variable latent period, the first electrical abnormalities to appear after such lesions are local interictal discharges. Then, eventually, ictal seizures sometimes evolve. A *functionally isolated cortical slab*, created by cutting the white matter underneath a cortical area, is initially silent unless stimulated (Burns, 1958), but after a few days it generates localized spontaneous discharges. This too has been taken to be an example of deafferentation-induced paroxysmal activity (Sharpless, 1969). Having lived in their place inside the skull for a while, such functionally isolated slabs retain their inclination for seizures discharges in vitro after being sliced and placed in a dish (Hoffman et al., 1994).

Kainic Acid

Some systemically administered chemical agents can create localized epileptogenic lesions. Kainic acid, obtained from a certain seaweed, is one of them. In rats, the fits caused by kainate start with motionless staring, followed by chewing movements, head nodding and head jerking, then "wet-dog shakes," and finally, rearing on the hind limbs, falling, and generalized motor convulsions. This pattern is considered to be the rodent equivalent of temporal lobe epilepsy with secondary generalization. In many cases the final picture is *status epilepticus*. Remarkably, the syndrome is similar whether the kainate was given intravenously or injected into the lateral ventricle or into the gray matter of the amygdala or hippocampal formation. It appears that the kainic acid, even if administered systemically, finds its primary target where there is the largest concentration of high-affinity receptors, in the subcortical temporal lobe structures. Cell loss is maximal in hippocampal CA3 and CA4 areas (Fig. 6–1) (Nadler et al., 1981; Okazaki and Nadler, 1988). The animals that survive the kainate-induced status epilepticus appear normal for several days, but after this latent period they develop spontaneous seizures; in other words, they become epileptic (Treiman and Heinemann, 1998). The pattern of the spontaneous seizures resembles the ones the drug had caused in the first place. Interictal discharges appear in EEG recordings before the spontaneous seizures.

Histological examination of brain tissue taken from kainate-treated animals shows marked pathology. At first there is cerebral edema, especially in the temporal lobe. Soon thereafter, cell injury is evident in the neurons that have been involved in the epileptic discharge. During the latent period, neurons are seen to die off in the vulnerable region. In the final state, characterized by epilepsy, there is profuse sprouting of abnormal excitatory fibers, originating from granule cells of the dentate gyrus and ending in CA3, as well as within the same layer of dentate granule cells where they have their origin. The axons of dentate granule cells form the *mossy fibers* that normally connect the dentate gyrus to the pyramidal cells of the CA3 segment of the hippocampus. These fibers are easily traced because they contain more than usual amounts of zinc, which can be stained to stand out in a histological preparation by a process named *Timm's stain*. Zn^{2+} is stored in synaptic vesicles and is released with glutamate during activation of mossy fibers. Its contribution to synaptic transmission is to dampen the effect of glutamate on NMDA receptors (Vogt et al., 2000). Timm's stain has been used to trace these fibers in both normal and pathological preparations. Rampant proliferation of mossy fibers has been known for some time as a feature of *Ammon' horn sclerosis* in human hippocampus (Fig. 6–2) (Babb, 1997). A very similar picture became apparent in rats made epileptic by inducing status epilepticus either by kainate or by pilocarpine treatment (Esclapez et al., 1999; Lynch and Sutula, 2000; Nadler et al., 1980; Tauck and Nadler, 1985; Wenzel et al., 2000).

Following kainic acid treatment, the freshly sprouted mossy fibers innervate not only CA3 pyramidal cells but also granule cells in the same layer whence they originate (Buckmaster and Dudek, 1999; Lynch and Sutula, 2000; Molnár and Nadler, 1999; Okazaki et al., 1999; Wenzel et al., 2000). Such *recurrent excitatory connections* from granule cells to granule cells are also found in normal brain, but only a few. As their numbers increase, so does their electrophysiological efficiency (Buckmaster and Dudek, 1999; Lynch and Sutula, 2000). It is easy to imagine that reverberating excitation in such a circuit would favor seizure discharges. Moreover, interrupting the mossy fiber pathway by a lesion inflicted prior to kainic acid treatment reduced the sprouting and attenuated the neuronal degeneration and seizures that usually follow kainic acid administration (Okazaki and Nadler, 1988; Okazaki et al., 1988). In a recent paper, Zhang et al. (2002) report that the cell loss and reor-

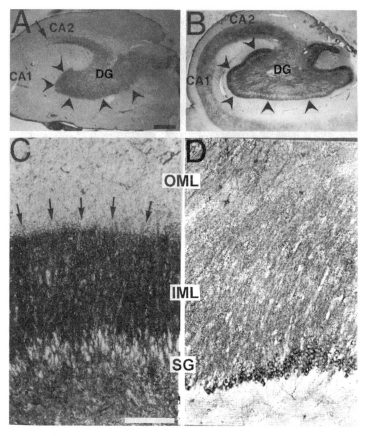

FIGURE 6–2. Mossy fiber sprouting in temporal lobe epilepsy. A: Normal human hippocampal formation, stained for zinc (Timm stain). B: Intensive Timm stain indicated by arrowheads in a specimen from an epileptic human patient in an area where none is seen in the normal tissue. C: Higher magnification illustrating darkly stained aberrant mossy fibers. D: Increased AMPA receptor densities demonstrated by immunocytochemistry in another section from the same specimen as B and C. OML: outer molecular layer. IML: inner molecular layer. SG: stratum granulosum of the dentate gyrus (DG). Calibration bars 1 mm for A and B, 200 μm for C and D. (Modified from Babb, 1997.)

ganization of synaptic connections that usually follow kainate treatment are not necessary for the establishment of recurrent spontaneous seizures, but that the attacks are much more severe in animals in which the pathological anatomy is evident than in animals without such morphological changes.

Pilocarpine

Pilocarpine, a muscarinic cholinergic agent, also induces status epilepticus that brings in its wake a lasting epileptic syndrome similar to the one seen in kainate-treated animals (Avanzini et al., 1998; Mello et al., 1993; Okazaki et al., 1999). The acute seizure is probably related to the immediate effect in **muscarinic receptors**, which, in the brain, are predominantly excitatory (Krnjević, 1975). The muscarinic effect of ACh in brain neurons consists of inhibiting the so-called **M-current**. The ion channels mediating the M-current, the M-channels, contribute a substantial fraction of the resting K^+ conductance of central neurons and therefore regulate the resting membrane potential. Inhibiting the M-current by ACh or its muscarinic analog agonists causes slow depolarization (Brown and Adams, 1980).

Spontaneous seizures begin after a latent period of about 2 weeks following pilocarpine-induced status epilepticus, and appear to be the consequence of neuron loss in the hippocampus and the sprouting of mossy fibers (Mello et al., 1993; Okazaki et al., 1999), reminiscent of kainate-induced pathology. Dentate granule cells proliferate after pilocarpine treatment, at least in rats (Parent et al., 1997). What is even more remarkable, it is the newborn cells whose axons form many, if not all, of the new recurrent abnormal mossy fiber connections that target the supragranular inner molecular layer of the dentate gyrus, plus the stratum oriens of the CA3 sector. Not only pilocarpine treatment but also electrically induced status epilepticus stimulates the proliferation of new dentate granule cells (Parent et al., 1997). Whether or not there is neurogenesis in dentate gyrus of mature human brains is still a subject of controversy (Parent et al., 1997; Rakic, 2002).

Other Epileptogenic Pathologies

An epileptic condition can also result from **teratogenic** brain damage in rats during intrauterine development (reviewed by Jacobs et al., 1999). Here again the morphological substrate appears to be aberrant neuronal connections. One distinct type of such malformation is **microgyria**, in which an area of the neocortex is either devoid of neurons or has fewer than the usual six cell layers. According to Jacobs et al. (1999), the microgyrus receives less than its normal share of thalamic input fibers. The thalamocortical axons that find no target erroneously innervate the surrounding paramicrogyral zone, rendering it hyperexcitable.

The Role of Growth Factors

The pathological morphological changes seen in experimentally induced chronic epileptic foci, whether caused by physical or chemical injury, have this in common: where neurons have been decimated, the vacated synaptic sites on the surviving neurons are recolonized by inappropriate freshly sprouted axon terminals that germinate either from other surviving neurons in the injured region or from cells in more distant intact tissue. Abnormal connections can sprout, however, even if there is no antecedent cell loss. There is much evidence that newly formed connections can become the morphological substrate for the uncontrolled discharge of epileptic seizures. Axon sprouting is probably stimulated by the enhanced production of neurotrophic chemical attractants, including NGF and especially BDNF. This, in the already quoted words of Binder et al. (2001a), is "too much of a good thing" (see also Scharfman et al., 2002, and Vezzani et al., 1999a). Glial cells that proliferate in the damaged tissue may cooperate with neurons in producing additional neurotrophic factors. Brain-derived neurotrophic factor is epileptogenic in more than one way; besides stimulating axon sprouting, it also potentiates NMDA receptor–controlled currents and synaptic excitation, and it facilitates acute seizures in hippocampal slices as well as in intact hippocampus (Jarvis et al., 1997; Scharfman et al., 2002).

Yet BDNF is good as well as bad, for it is also believed to protect neurons from injury and it may perhaps become useful in therapy aimed at appropriate reinnervation after injury (Shetty and Turner, 1999).

Epilepsy can be learned: Long-term potentiation and kindling

Two notable independent yet related studies were performed in the 1960s and early 1970s. One concerned *long-term potentiation* (*LTP*) of synaptic transmission (Bliss and Gardner-Medwin, 1973; Lømo, 1971) (Fig. 6–3), the other the induction of an epileptic state by repeated, initially innocuous stimulation, discovered by Delgado and Sevillano (1961) and Goddard (1967), later dubbed *kindling* (Goddard, 1983) (Fig. 6–4). Common to the two phenomena is the method. In both procedures, repetitive so-called *tetanic* electrical stimulation is applied in order to cause aftereffects of extended duration.

Long-Term Potentiation Is a Prototype of Synaptic Plasticity

Before LTP, there was *posttetanic potentiation* (*PTP*) of spinal synapses (Lloyd, 1949). A brief train of high-frequency electrical stimuli delivered to a spinal dorsal root or to a peripheral nerve innervating skeletal muscle brings in its wake a marked enhancement of the transmission of monosynaptic reflexes. The difference between PTP and LTP is that the former lasts for minutes, whereas the latter lasts for hours in vitro and days in hippocampus in situ (Bliss and Gardner-Medwin, 1973). Long-term potentiation can be induced in many forebrain structures, but it is particularly strong in the synapses of the hippocampus (Racine et al., 1975, 1983). In neocortex it is readily produced in the somatosensory area that has granular cytoarchitecture but not in the agranular primary motor cortex (Castro-Alamancos and Connors, 1996). While some of the very first experiments were done on brains of live animals (Bliss and Gardner-Medwin, 1973), in much of the subsequent work hippocampal tissue slices were used. Long-term potentiation has its counterpart in *long-term depression* (*LTD*). Both are produced by electrical

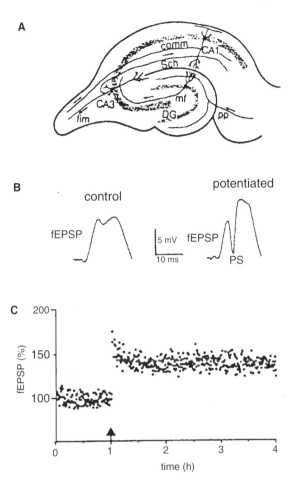

Figure 6–3. Long-term potentiation (LTP). **A:** Diagram of a cross section of the hippocampal formation of a rat showing the main excitatory connections (interneurons omitted). DG: dentate gyrus. CA1, CA3: sectors in hippocampus proper (syn. cornu ammonis). pp: perforant path containing afferent fibers from entorhinal cortex. mf: mossy fiber axons of dentate granule cells addressed to CA3 pyramidal neurons. Sch: Schaffer collaterals, branches of the axons of CA3 pyramidal cells, making excitatory synapses with CA1 pyramidal cells. comm: commissural fibers originating from contralateral hippocampus. fim: fimbria, a major output and input pathway of the hippocampus. **B:** Sample potentials evoked by stimulation of pp and recorded in DG in stratum granulosum (cell body layer) of an anesthetized rat before and after potentiating stimulus train. **C:** Extracellular excitatory postsynaptic potential (fEPSP) as a percentage of control, measured as the steepest rate of rise (initial slope) of traces such as the ones shown in **B**. The arrow marks a brief potentiating tetanic stimulus (250 Hz for 0.2 s). Note that the modest (less than 50%) average increase in the fEPSP slope is associated with a huge increase in the population spike (PS) (see **B**), which is an index of the number of neurons firing in near-synchrony. (Modified from Bliss and Collingridge, 1993.)

stimulation of afferent pathways, but the pattern and timing of the stimulus trains are different.

Many investigators regard LTP and LTD as neurophysiological models for short-term or medium-term learning. This is not the place to enter into a discussion of this somewhat controversial concept. Whatever their exact place in normal brain function, LTP and LTD are remarkable examples of the functional plasticity of certain synapses.

The mechanism of LTP has been assiduously studied in many laboratories. While not all the details are clear, there is general agreement on several of the basic features (reviewed by Baudry and Lynch, 2001; Larkman and Jack, 1995). The activation of NMDA receptors is critical for inducing LTP, for if their activation is prevented or if the influx of Ca^{2+} through NMDA receptor–controlled channels is blocked, LTP cannot take place (Melchers et al., 1988). Single-shock stimulation activates mainly AMPA receptors, and the channels opened by these receptors are almost completely impermeable to calcium. Repetitive stimulation activates AMPA receptor channels long enough to achieve the depolarization that is required to remove the magnesium block of the NMDA channels (see Chapter 4: "Magnesium ions modulate ion channels"). Inward flow of Ca^{2+} through NMDA receptor–controlled gates is the key to the induction of LTP. Once Ca^{2+} is inside the plasma membrane, it initiates cascades of events leading to the long-term change in synaptic efficacy (Rose and Konnerth, 2001b). In experiments, LTP is recognized as the growth of the EPSPs that are evoked by single shock stimulation (Fig. 6–3), and such EPSPs are generated by AMPA receptor-controlled synaptic current. It appears that the calcium signal mediated by NMDA receptor channels during the train stimulus initiates a lasting enhancement of the AMPA receptor-mediated currents. The boost of AMPA currents has been attributed to the incorporation of additional AMPA receptors into the subsynaptic membrane (Baudry and Lynch, 2001).

Electron microscopy reveals subtle morphological changes. One study suggested that synapses are remodeled so that initially many more than usual have multiple transmission zones on individual dendritic spines. Later the spines are seen to be retracted so that synapses become attached to the dendritic shafts (Geinisman et al., 1998). Others reported that dendritic spines become enlarged and their neck widened, improving the electrotonic coupling of synapses on the spines to the dendritic shaft (reviewed by Yuste and Bonhoefer, 2001).

Unlike LTP, LTD may be initiated by the cooperation of AMPA and metabotropic glutamate receptors secondarily activating Ca^{2+} gates of ER (Rose and Konnerth, 2001b).

The various changes listed in the preceding paragraphs concern the postsynaptic target cells. There was, however, also evidence of a presynaptic mechanism, namely, that the increased release of transmitter from axon terminals is responsible for LTP (Davies et al., 1989). The debate between partisans of the presynaptic and postsynaptic hypotheses has been lively. In a recent review, Malenka and Nicoll (1999) forcefully argued in favor of a predominantly postsynaptic explanation. One of the arguments in favor of a presynaptic mechanism was an apparent increase in the quantal content of EPSPs, but Malenka and Nicoll (1999) contended that the recruitment of AMPA receptors could be mistaken for an increase in quantal release.

Other Forms of Long-Term Enhancement of Synaptic Transmission

Transient sublethal hypoxia of brain tissue slices reversibly suppresses synaptic transmission (Chapter 18). After reoxygenation, the hypoxic episode is frequently followed by long-lasting enhancement of synaptic transmission (Schiff and Somjen, 1985). This phenomenon has also been called *anoxic LTP* (Hammond et al., 1994). It may be responsible for epilepsy that sometimes follows an ischemic episode (Hopkins, 1987b; Lüders, 2001).

Exposing hippocampal tissue slices for a limited time to *2-deoxyglucose (2–DG)*, which blocks the metabolism of glucose, also depresses synapses and, after recovery, potentiates not just excitatory but also inhibitory transmission (Krnjević and Zhao, 2000). Even though these two examples of temporary energy failure, hypoxia and 2-DG exposure, have long-term consequences resembling those of stimulus-evoked LTP, the details of the mechanism are not the same. Anoxic LTP enhances principally the NMDA receptor–mediated component, not the AMPA-dependent EPSP (Hammond et al., 1994). Brief 2-DG exposure causes hyperpolarization of neurons, while repetitive stimulation causes depolarization. Moreover, although $[Ca^{2+}]_i$ is raised by 2-DG treatment, the 2-DG-induced LTP is independent of the increase in $[Ca^{2+}]_i$ (Tekkök et al., 1999; Zhao and Krnjević, 2000).

The Small Flame That Lights a Firestorm

Similarly to LTP, kindling is induced by tetanic stimulus trains. Unlike LTP, kindling requires repetition of the stimulation. Many sites in the brain can be stimulated for this purpose, but the most effective sites are the piriform cortex and the amygdala, followed closely by the angular bundle, which is a major input to the hippocampal formation. These sites are also capable of LTP. It has long been known that in these structures seizures are especially easily provoked (Gibbs and Gibbs, 1936; Liberson and Cadilhac, 1954) but, for kindling, the intensity is kept below the threshold required to trigger a seizure in an otherwise untreated brain. The stimulations have to be repeated daily for a number of days or weeks to achieve the fully kindled state. The number of treatments depends on the species of animal, its age, and the site in the brain . In the first trial, the stimulus is adjusted to produce a brief afterdischarge that evokes no overt, observable change in behavior. Then, during the subsequent days, as the same stimulus train is repeated, the afterdischarge gets longer and more intense and the animal starts to show increasingly obvious epileptiform signs (Fig. 6–4) (review by McNamara et al., 1980).

Racine (1972), one of the pioneers of kindling research, distinguished five stages in this evolution. In rats in *stage 1* the eyes blink and the face twitches; *stage 2* involves chewing movements and head nodding; *stage 3* is marked by clonic spasms of the forelimbs; in *stage 4* the animal rears on its hind limbs; and in *stage 5* there is falling down and generalized convulsion. Some kindled animals develop spontaneous interictal discharges, which can continue for up to 6 weeks following cessation of the daily stimulations. If daily treatments are stopped after stage 5 is reached and the animal is tested by a similar stimulus a year later, at first it shows no overt seizure but it can be rekindled much more rapidly than originally. If stimulations are continued much beyond stage 5, some rats eventually show spontaneous ictal seizures; in other words, they become genuinely epileptic. This condition is no longer reversible: even if stimulations cease, the animal remains epileptic for the remainder of its life. Baboons require many more stimulations to kindle but, once kindled, are more prone to become epileptic than are rats. In rats, McIntyre and associates (2002) created two strains by selective breeding, one in which kindling can achieved rapidly and another in which it proceeds unusually slowly.

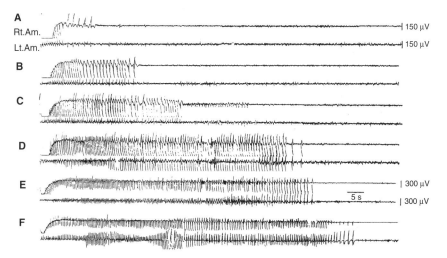

FIGURE 6–4. Kindling. Increasing afterdischarges recorded from right and left amygdala and evoked by daily stimulations of the right amygdala of an awake rat. The same implanted electrode pair served for bipolar stimulation and recording; recording commenced after the end of the stimulus train (60 Hz for 1 s). **A:** Second day. **B:** Fourth day. **C:** Fifth day. **D:** Eighth day (class 1 motor seizure). **E:** Tenth day (class 3 seizure). **F:** Fourteenth day (class 5 seizure). The stimulus intensity was reduced from 50 to 25 μA in the course of the treatment. Note the changing frequency and waveform of the discharge and the increasing participation of the left (unstimulated) amygdala. (Reproduced from Racine, 1972.)

The striking fact is that epilepsy can be induced without creating a scar, without the administration of a poison, and without inducing a genetic defect. (For reviews, see Goddard, 1983; McIntyre et al., 2002; McNamara and Wada, 1998).

Over the years, variants of the original protocol have been developed. For example, there is *rapid kindling*, in which stage 5 is reached in 1 or 2 days by more intensive and more frequent stimulation (Lothman et al., 1985b). Then there is *chemical kindling*, in which repeated administration of a subconvulsive dose of a stimulant drug eventually provokes seizures (Croucher et al., 1995). In brain slices in vitro, a state resembling kindled epilepsy can be induced by repeated stimulation, described as *stimulus-induced bursting (STIB)* (Stasheff et al., 1985). Another in vitro variant of kindling involves exposing piriform cortex tissue slices to a solution in which Cl⁻ was replaced by the impermeant anion isethionate for 30–70 min, followed by normal ACSF. The low-chloride-induced spontaneous epileptiform discharges continued indefinitely after restoration of the normal bath composition (Demir et al., 1998).

The Relationship Between Long-Term Potentiation and Kindling Is Not Simple

Similar but not identical tetanic electrical stimulation is used to induce kindling and LTP, and it was not farfetched to seek a link between the two (Racine et al., 1975, 1983). It seemed that, with repetition of the stimulation, the sphere of influence of the LTP expanded from the first synapse "downstream" to other synapses. It was thought that as LTP spread, the kindling progressed through its successive stages until the entire network became hyperexcitable. In line with this idea, prior LTP facilitated kindling. Also, potentiated synaptic transmission could be demonstrated in previously kindled brain structures (Racine et al., 1975, 1983). Subsequently, it appeared, however, that the link between the two processes is not invariant. We found that kindling can be achieved by trains of pulses applied to the angular bundle without potentiating the responses to single-pulse stimulation of the same pathway (Giacchino et al., 1984). In a similar study, Maru et al. (1982) found that fEPSPs evoked by single shocks increased during the initial stages of kindling, but then they subsided and, by the time kindling was completed, they did not differ from control levels. In some of the kindled animals, the population spike was large in spite of the modest size of the fEPSP, suggesting increased excitability of the postsynaptic target cells. This is quite different from LTP. Then Racine et al. (1983) recorded synaptic responses before and after kindling stimulation of several brain sites. While EPSPs did grow when the lateral olfactory tract or amygdala was stimulated, at other targets early growth was followed by a decrease, confirming the report of Maru et al. (1982). One could argue, of course that, in trials with negative results, LTP may have occurred, but was not observed, at synapses in the net where there were no recording electrodes.

In conclusion

Long-term potentiation and kindling have too much in common to dismiss the similarities as irrelevant. It is probable that LTP assists in kindling, but the kindled state is not simply "LTP overdone."

*Kindling Usually Involves the Sprouting of New Connections without
Massive Loss of Neurons, but Sprouting Is Not Necessary for Kindling*

In the first years after the discovery of kindling, diligent search by many did not turn up any obvious remodeling of morphology (McNamara et al., 1980). Whether or not kindling stimulation causes cell loss has long been debated, and evidence for and against neuron injury seemed to ebb and flood. Reviews of this issue may be summed up as follows: while cells do not disappear on a massive scale, there is selective loss in restricted areas (Bengzon et al., 1997; Bertram and Lothman, 1993; Binder and McNamara, 1998; Cavazos et al., 1994).

Even though neurons do not succumb in large numbers in the early stages of kindling, new excitatory connections do grow (Lynch and Sutula, 2000; Sutula et al., 1988). The sprouting of mossy fibers in the dentate gyrus in kindled brains resembles the lasting effect of kainic acid and of status epilepticus, except that kindling-induced sprouting does not require antecedent cell loss.

The sprouting of new axons is apparently stimulated by an increase in several trophic factors. It has long been suspected that BDNF is the chief actor (Binder et al., 2001a; Lindvall et al., 1998) but *glia-derived nerve growth factor* (*GDNF*), *NGF*, and NT-3 are also candidates (Lindvall et al., 1998).

In normal adult brains there is very little of these growth stimulators, but they are apparently produced during kindling under the influence of freshly expressed immediate early genes, especially c-*fos* (Binder and McNamara, 1998). One of the several receptors on which BDNF acts, *trkB*, seems to be selectively involved. McNamara's group reviewed evidence suggesting that the expression of immediate early genes, especially but not exclusively c-*fos*, is required for kindling (Binder and McNamara, 1998). Repeated afterdischarges induce the expression of the following early genes, listed in order of intensity: *NGFI-A*, c-*fos*, c-*jun*, and *NGFI-B*. The activation of NMDA receptors seems to be the stimulus for the induction. In mutant mice with c-*fos* knocked out, kindling was retarded and attenuated but not abolished, demonstrating that c-*fos* is not the only agent of kindling.

While BDNF has been blamed for fostering kindling epileptogenesis, others contend that it actually protects against epilepsy. Reibel et al. (1998) considerably retarded the evolution of kindling when they infused BDNF into the lateral ventricle during the procedure. On the other hand, when the endogenous BDNF was rendered ineffective by introducing competing "decoy" compounds in the form of false receptor bodies into the lateral ventricle, kindling was greatly retarded

(Binder et al., 1999). Thus, both exogenous BDNF and neutralizing endogenous BDNF reportedly work against kindling evolution, leaving us perplexed.

The discovery of mossy fiber sprouting in the brains of kindled animals naturally led to the conclusion that the new connections were responsible for the propensity for seizures, but here again, doubt grew with added data. Fast kindling is possible within a day, which is much too short a time for the growth of new mossy fibers (Lothman et al., 1985b). At a meeting in 1996, both Racine and Corcoran contended that the sprouting of new connections is neither necessary nor sufficient for the evolution of the kindled state (Corcoran et al., 1998; Racine et al., 1998).

Conclusions from morphological evidence

On balance, the best evidence is that neither cell loss nor sprouting is essential for establishing the kindled state (Dalby and Mody, 2001). Yet the morphological changes could be the cause of the spontaneous seizures that represent true epilepsy, which requires continuation of repeated stimulation beyond the stimulus-induced stage 5 seizures. If so, this would make this form of experimental epilepsy comparable to those caused by focal alumina cream or freeze lesions and pilocarpine and kainic acid treatments.

N-methyl-D-aspartate Channel Activation Facilitates Kindling

There is much evidence that glutamate receptors, especially those controlled by NMDA, are somehow involved in kindling (Mody, 1999) but, again, their exact role is not yet entirely clear. Forty-eight hours after completion of kindling, the NMDA receptor–mediated component of EPSPs is greatly increased relative to the AMPA-mediated component, but 4 weeks later, the proportions return to control levels (Behr et al., 2000; Mody and Heinemann, 1987). Kindling can be retarded but not prevented by blocking NMDA channels (Holmes et al., 1990; McNamara et al., 1988). This is different from LTP, for which influx of Ca^{2+} through NMDA-controlled channels is an absolute requirement (Baudry and Lynch, 2001). The slowing of kindling by NMDA antagonists is not specific; AMPA and kainate receptor antagonists also inhibit the progression of kindling (Cain et al., 1988; Rogawski et al., 2001). However, when drug administration is stopped and stimulations are continued, the rate of kindling rebounds into overdrive and the process is completed in record time. For this reason, Rogawski et al. (2001) contend that the underlying changes progress even though overt seizures are suppressed. They concluded that AMPA receptors "are involved in the expression but not the development" of kindling.

During kindling, the NMDA receptors of hippocampal neurons respond excessively to exogenous glutamate (Martin et al., 1992; Mody et al., 1988), and single NMDA-operated channels are more likely to open when exposed to NMDA (Köhr and Mody, 1994; Mody and Lieberman, 1998). Also, glutamate receptor density is upregulated by kindling (Meldrum et al., 1999; Mody, 1998). The glutamate level increases in several brain regions, and glutamate is released in excess amounts from neurons in the amygdala of kindled animals (Kaura et al., 1995). Repeated microinjections of small, normally subconvulsive amounts of NMDA into the amygdala can achieve chemical kindling, with an end result similar to that produced by electrical kindling (Croucher et al., 1995).

Repetitive stimulation of afferent pathways lowers the interstitial calcium concentration due to the inflow of Ca^{2+} into neurons through synaptically activated and voltage-gated ion channels (see Chapter 2: "Neuronal activity alters ion distributions"). In tissue slices from kindled rats, $\Delta[Ca^{2+}]_o$ responses are enhanced, and they become detectable in cytoarchitectonic layers where they are normally absent (Wadman et al., 1985). The exaggerated influx of Ca^{2+} could reflect enhanced responsiveness of NMDA receptor–controlled channels as well as voltage-gated Ca^{2+} channels (see below: "Kindling alters voltage-gated ion channels").

In an intriguing parallel to kindling, in tissue slices cut from surgically removed neocortex or hippocampus of human patients, some neurons generated EPSPs that had a marked NMDA-mediated component (Avoli and Olivier, 1989; Mody and Lieberman, 1998; Urban et al., 1990a). In brain tissue slices from normal experimental animals, such an NMDA component is absent unless bath $[Mg^{2+}]$ is reduced. Comparing human biopsy specimens to control tissue of healthy animals is, of course, not strictly *lege artis*, but human control material is hard to find. Still, the prominent NMDA response could indicate a role in clinical epileptogenesis.

The Role of N-methyl-D-aspartate Receptors in Maintaining the Fully Kindled State Is Not Settled

The above findings all indicate that the activation of NMDA receptors contributes to the establishment of the kindled state and also that kindling potentiates NMDA-induced responses. There is less unanimity about the role of NMDA receptors in maintaining the kindled state once it has been established. While NMDA receptor–blocking drugs slowed the process of kindling, they proved to be disappointing anticonvulsants against seizures in fully kindled animals (Löscher and Hönack, 1991; McNamara et al., 1988) even though they are effective against some other types of experimental seizures (Meldrum et al., 1999). The low efficacy of NMDA antagonists suggested that NMDA receptors are not involved in the generation of seizures in fully kindled animals. Similarly, the induction of STIB in hippocampal tissue slices could be prevented by blocking NMDA receptors but, once STIB was established, the same blocking drug did not stop the burst discharges (Anderson et al., 1987).

Yet Mody and Heinemann (1987; Mody et al., 1988) found that synaptically transmitted NMDA responses remain potentiated for at least 6 weeks after the last evoked seizure. Moreover, NMDA-operated single channels from kindled animals were much more likely to remain open when exposed to NMDA than were similar channels from control animals, and this change persisted for 60 days following the last kindled seizure (Mody and Lieberman, 1998). Even more remarkably, the response to NMDA of the kindled channels from rats was quite similar to the responses of NMDA channels from human biopsy material, removed during surgery from patients with temporal lobe epilepsy (Mody and Lieberman, 1998). But then the same team, using a different experimental approach, found that NMDA-mediated facilitation of transmission to the dentate gyrus is transient and is no longer present 28 days after completion of kindling (Behr et al., 2001). I. Mody (personal communication) suggests that the discrepancy is due, in part, to different methods: the cell-attached patch-clamp technique was used in the single-channel study of Mody and Lieberman, and whole-cell patch clamp recording was done in the recent trials by Behr et al. The cell-attached method leaves cells intact, while the whole-cell method leaches the cytoplasm and may have removed an intracellular mediator of the enhanced response. But in the study by Behr et al. (2001), NMDA-dependent facilitation of repetitive responses recorded with extracellular electrodes was also transient, present immediately after kindling but absent 28 days later. Behr et al., concluded that the increased NMDA response is required for the "acute throughput" of excitation from entorhinal cortex through dentate gyrus to the CA3 region in the course of kindling, enabling the kindling process, but not for the long-term maintenance of the kindled state. It appears that some NMDA-dependent effects are permanently changed by kindling and others only transiently.

Some of the seeming contradictions may be removed by the different approach taken by McNamara and Nadler and associates (Nadler et al., 1994). The latter group discovered that kindling reduces the sensitivity of CA3 pyramidal cells for NMDA receptor antagonists, and this could explain the low efficacy of these drugs as anticonvulsants even if NMDA receptors were responsible for seizure generation in the fully kindled state. The same team found evidence for the induction of a novel type of NMDA receptor by kindling that is not present in normal hippocampus (Kraus et al., 1994). While "normal" NMDA receptor subunits were not increased 28 days after completion of kindling (Kraus and McNamara, 1998), the "new" kindling-induced NMDA receptor remained expressed for an extended period of time (Kraus et al., 1994). It is at least possible, that this unconventional kindled NMDA receptor, which has no affinity for the NMDA antagonist drugs, is the one that maintains the kindled state.

In conclusion

N-methyl-D-aspartate receptors and kindling. About the following two points there is unanimous agreement: (1) NMDA receptor–controlled responses are potentiated in the course of kindling and (2) activation of normal NMDA receptors facilitates the establishment of the kindled state but is not absolutely required for it.

The role of NMDA receptors in maintaining the kindled state after the completion of treatment is not yet clear. It may be that newly induced, modified NMDA receptors are the ones important for maintaining the fully kindled state.

AMPA Receptors and Kindling

The next question is whether AMPA or kainate receptors have something to do with kindling. This question cannot be approached in the same way as the one concerning NMDA receptors, for blocking AMPA and kainate receptors would abolish excitatory synaptic transmission and thwart the procedure. (Nor is complete absence of glutamate synaptic transmission compatible with survival.) Partial blocking of AMPA receptors did not slow kindling, but it reduced seizure intensity in the fully kindled state (Dürmüller et al., 1994). It is to be expected that damping excitatory transmission should inhibit seizures, regardless of the agent, and the role of AMPA and kainate receptors remains uncertain.

Metabotropic Glutamate Receptors and Kindling

The metabotropic glutamate receptor III (mGluR III) is a presynaptic receptor with inhibitory function. Its activation modulates presynaptic calcium channels, resulting in reduced transmitter output. Klapstein et al. (1999) report a long-lasting decrease in the efficacy of an mGluR III agonist in dentate gyrus in brain slices of kindled rats, suggesting downregulation of the receptor. This contrasts with the increased effectiveness of mGluR II and III agonists in the amygdala of amygdala-kindled rats. A more recent report also suggests that activation of mGluRI and mGluRV receptors does promote bicuculline and 4-AP-induced seizures in hippocampal (not kindled) slices (Lee et al., 2002). The significance of these findings is not immediately obvious, but they may mean that presynaptic mGluRs counteract and postsynaptic mGluRs promote seizures.

Conclusions about glutamate and seizures, kindled and other

There is no question that excess glutamate can cause seizures. Exogenous glutamate can initiate seizures, and seizures ensue whenever the transporters whose job is to remove glutamate from synapses become incompetent (Meldrum et al., 1999). Potentiation of NMDA receptors does assist the evolution of the kindled state. Whether the seizures of fully kindled animals or any of the naturally occurring epilepsies are caused by the excess production or the deficient elimination of glutamate, or by pathological sensitization or modification of any of its receptor types, remains to be seen.

The Effects of Kindling on γ-Aminobutyric Acid–Mediated Inhibition

Several teams have demonstrated changes in the efficacy of GABAergic inhibition that develop in the course of kindling and persist beyond completion of the kindling process. In rapid kindling, for example, synaptic inhibition is reduced (Kapur and Lothman, 1989; Kapur et al., 1989). What makes interpretation of the results difficult is that both increased and decreased inhibition have been reported. Often the same teams found opposite effects in different synaptic circuits or at different stages of the kindling process (Kamphuis et al., 1987, 1991; Lopes da Silva et al., 1998; Sankar et al., 2000). In the hands of Racine et al. (1998), paired pulse inhibition appeared to be powerfully and paradoxically augmented in dentate gyrus, and the enhancement decayed slowly but was not fully recovered 10 weeks after the last kindled seizure. During the oral discussion of this paper, Racine said that his group found paired pulse inhibition augmented in amygdala, piriform cortex, entorhinal cortex, and several other areas. Inhibition diminished only in hippocampal CA1. The loss of inhibition in CA1 may be a factor in the establishment of the kindled state, while the increased inhibition elsewhere could be a compensatory or defensive response, yet neither change reveals the essential mechanism required for kindling.

In conclusion

The role of changing inhibitory synaptic function in kindling has not been firmly established.

Kindling Alters Voltage-Gated Ion Channels

As already mentioned ("*N*-methyl-D-aspartate channel activation facilitates kindling"), in hippocampal tissue slices taken from previously kindled animals, the laminar profile of the stimulus-induced decrease in $[Ca^{2+}]_o$ is altered in a way that indicates greatly enhanced Ca^{2+} influx in regions where it normally is feeble (Wadman et al., 1985). Increased uptake into neurons could occur through NMDA receptor–operated or voltage-gated channels.

Exaggerated operation of voltage-gated *Ca^{2+} currents* was confirmed in isolated neurons harvested from kindled rats (Vreugdenhil and Wadman, 1992, 1994). Similarly upregulated Ca^{2+} currents were found in hippocampal neurons from rats made epileptic by kainate treatment, and also in cells from human brain tissue removed in surgical treatment for temporal lobe epilepsy (Beck et al., 1998). The calbindin content of dentate granule cells is reduced after kindling and, as a result, both the activation and the inactivation of high-voltage activated calcium currents accelerate (Köhr and Mody, 1991).

Small but significant enhancement of *Na^+ currents* was also found in kindled rats, and it persisted for at least 5 weeks after the last kindling stimulation. In CA1 neurons from kindled rats, the steady-state inactivation ($h\infty$) function shifted slightly in the more depolarized direction and the maximal current amplitude also increased moderately (Vreugdenhil et al., 1998). A small shift of $h\infty$ is functionally significant because it opens wider the *window* range of membrane voltages where activation and inactivation functions overlap. When the membrane potential is within the window range, the Na^+ channel is slightly activated, and it is not inactivating. This permits a small inward current to continue indefinitely, and it favors repetitive excitation (Steinhäuser et al., 1990). The window range is also widened in the epileptic state induced by status epilepticus, but in this case it is the activation function (m^3) that is shifted in the more hyperpolarized direction (Ketelaars et al., 2001) (see below: "Epilepsy following electrically induced status epilepticus"). By contrast, *K^+ currents* were essentially unchanged by kindling (Vreugdenhil and Wadman, 1995).

The mirror focus and related phenomena

As W.R. Gowers wrote in 1881, "seizures beget seizures" (quoted by Lothman, 1998; see also Theodore and Wasterlain, 1999). Before the discovery of kindling, the phenomenon known as the *mirror focus* or *secondary epileptogenic lesion (SEL)* was already known (Morrell, 1969). After establishment of an experimental epileptogenic focus, for example by injecting alumina cream into the cortex or by freezing a small cortical area, after a period of time seizure discharges were frequently recorded, not only from the vicinity of the original lesion but also from areas to which it has strong connections, especially its homolog on the contralateral hemisphere. This became known as a *mirror focus*. At first, a secondary focus is driven by the discharges of the primary lesion. At this stage, ablation of the primary focus stills the epileptiform discharges emanating from both the primary and mirror foci. If, however, the primary focus remains untreated for a long enough time, the contralateral secondary focus becomes autonomous. Once autonomy is established, removal of the primary lesion no longer cures the epilepsy of the secondary site. The similarity to kindling is obvious: recurrent bombardment of the originally healthy area by the discharges of the primary focus apparently kindles an epileptic condition in the contralateral secondary focus. The two conditions have recently been compared by McIntyre and Poulter (2001), who found much in common between the two but are reluctant to pronounce them identical until more is known about the underlying molecular mechanisms.

For neurosurgical practice, there is a most unfortunate corollary to these observations. In cases where preoperative diagnostic exploration reveals bilaterally symmetrical epileptiform EEG activity, the question is whether the secondary focus has already become autonomous. Besides, in patients with bitemporal foci, there frequently is also bilateral damage, and it is difficult to determine whether the process has been bilateral to begin with or whether there is a mirror focus. In fact, it is considered rare to have a secondary (mirror) focus evolve without some degree of preexisting damage. In cases where autonomous epileptogenic foci exist on both sides, surgical removal of one does not guarantee a cure. Bilaterally symmetrical ablations are avoided if possible, because neurological deficits are usually more devastating when homologous areas on both sides are removed than after unilateral lesions are excised.

Epilepsy following electrically induced status epilepticus

We have discussed the epileptic condition caused by chemically induced status epilepticus (involving kainate and pilorcarpine). Chronic epilepsy can also be caused by status epilepticus induced by electrical stimulation. This procedure is superficially similar to kindling, but it differs in important ways. While the stimulus trains used for kindling are mild and initially do not change the animal's behavior, to cause post–status epilepticus epilepsy the stimulation must be powerful enough to provoke generalized seizures from the start. Lothman et al. (1989, 1990) stimulated the rat hippocampus almost continuously for extended periods at a pulse frequency of 50 Hz, the pulse trains being interrupted only by brief pauses to detect the beginnings of interstimulus, self-sustained discharges. With this treatment the seizures eventually become self-sustaining, that is, they continue even when the stimulation was stopped. If the self-sustaining seizures are allowed to go unchecked, some of the rats die, but death can be prevented if the seizures are stopped by anticonvulsant drugs. Similarly to pilocarpine and kainate treatment, the rats that have undergone electrically induced status epilepticus appear relatively normal for 1–4 weeks, but then they begin to suffer spontaneous seizures (Lopes da Silva and Wadman, 1999).

Unlike the gentle stimulation used in kindling, status epilepticus always kills many neurons. The cell loss is similar to that of kainate- and pilocarpine-induced chronic epilepsy, and it is probably one of the pathogenic factors. The difference is that in electrically induced status epilepticus the neurons are not killed by a poison but, so to speak, "commit suicide" in the electric storm of their own making. As already mentioned, after both pilocarpine- and electrically induced status epilepticus, while neurons die in hippocampus proper, granule cells in dentate gyrus proliferate, at least in rats (Parent et al., 1997).

Besides morphological changes, intrinsic biophysical properties are also affected in the aftermath of status epilepticus. Ketelaars et al. (2001) report that in hippocampal neurons isolated from rats suffering from status epilepticus–induced epilepsy, the voltage dependence of the activation of Na^+ current (m^3) shifted to a more negative (hyperpolarized) level, while steady-state inactivation (h) shifted to a slightly more positive (depolarized) level, so that the **window current** grew much larger. The maximal amplitude of the Na^+ current was only slightly augmented. In the window the Na^+ current can continue without inactivation, favoring protracted depolarization, and its enhancement may be more important in rendering neurons seizure-prone than is the absolute amplitude of the Na^+ current.

Conclusion Relating to Kindling and Similar Conditions

Not long ago, Racine et al. (1998) began a review of the kindling phenomenon with the statement that "the underlying mechanisms continue to elude us" and proceeded to contest all the then extant theoretical explanations (see also Dalby and Mody, 2001). Nonetheless, some points, mostly negative, have been settled. Cell loss and sprouting occur in kindled animals but are not essential for the establishment of the kindled state. Upregulation of NMDA receptors advances the kindling process, but its role in maintaining the kindled state is uncertain. Voltage-gated ion channels are altered in kindling. Again, their importance in establishing and maintaining the kindled state remains to be clarified.

Key points

A wide variety of insults can cause seizures in brains that are not epileptic. Among them are electrical current, trauma, fever, and stimulant poisons.

Increased excitation, decreased inhibition, but also the simultaneous increase in both can induce acute seizures. So can the boosting of Na^+ channels or the blockade of K^+ channels.

The $GABA_A$ receptor–controlled inhibitory synapses can become less effective or can even convert to excitatory action if neurons fill up with Cl^-. Low $[Cl^-]_o$ causes seizures in isolated brain tissue slices.

In isolated brain tissue slices, seizure-like spontaneous activity can be induced by withdrawing Ca^{2+} from the bath, even though all synaptic transmission is abolished.

Low $[Mg^{2+}]_o$ also induces seizures in brain tissue slices. The main reason is unblocking of NMDA receptor–controlled channels, assisted by reduced surface charge screening and generally enhanced synaptic transmission.

Gliotic scars can become chronic epileptogenic foci. Among the possible etiological factors are cell loss, especially in inhibitory interneurons; partial denervation inducing aberrant reinnervation by newly sprouted connections targeting vacated synaptic sites; and impaired clearing of excess extracellular K^+. Growth factors, especially BDNF, are suspected of stimulating the sprouting of anomalous connections.

Neuron loss can be both the cause and the effect of seizures. Neuron loss resulting from seizures is not usually caused by metabolic insufficiency, but more probably by excitotoxicity.

Kindling is a procedure in which repeated mild tetanic stimulation of certain sites in the brain establishes a seizure-prone state. The amygdala and hippocampus are especially prone to kindling and produce seizures considered to be a model of human temporal lobe epilepsy. Kindling can cause true epilepsy, that is, recurrent spontaneous seizures. Long-term potentiation occurs in some synapses during kindling. Upregulation of NMDA receptors probably has a role in establishing the kindled state, as it also has in LTP. Inhibition mediated by GABA is changed in the course of kindling in different ways in various pathways. Voltage-gated Ca^{2+} and Na^+ channels are also altered by kindling.

A chronically epileptic state frequently follows experimentally induced status epilepticus, whether induced by electric stimulation, kainate, or pilocarpine. Epilepsy evolves after a latent period during which morphological changes take place.

7

Electrophysiology of Seizures

Ictal events appear on EEG traces as electrical storms. Microphysiological techniques reveal the ways in which the normal finely-tuned yet stable-patterned activity of healthy neurons can be perverted during seizures.

Chapter 7 explores in detail the electrophysiology of epileptiform discharges and their relationship to the normal electrical function of brain cells.

Impulse bursts, "epileptic neurons," and paroxysmal depolarizing shift

Unusual Firing Patterns in Experimental and Clinical Epileptic Foci

One of the hotly debated issues in the early days of electrophysiological research in epilepsy has been whether a single neuron could be epileptic. The concept implied that epilepsy resulted from an abnormality of the neuron membrane. According to the competing view, an epileptic discharge is always generated by assemblies of synaptically connected neurons, and the fault lies in the properties of the network, not the pathology of its members. In retrospect, this debate may have been more about emphasis than about principle. For there can be little doubt that seizure discharges represent the synchronized activity of a sizable population of neurons, yet it is hard to imagine that such a discharge could arise without some pathology in at least some members of the seized population.

Calvin, Ward, and associates called *epileptic* the neurons that fired brief high-frequency bursts of action potentials in the vicinity of epileptogenic foci in patients and in experimental animals (Fig. 7–1) (Calvin et al., 1968, 1973; Ward, 1969; Wyler and Ward, 1980). There are neurons that fire spike bursts quite normally, and these will be discussed in the next section. To be considered epileptic, according to Ward's criteria, a cell had to be found in an epileptogenic zone, and it had to fire high-frequency bursts not usually seen in the normal condition of the same cell population. In addition to resulting from chronic gliotic lesions, abnormal spontaneous burst firing can be induced acutely by the local injection of penicillin and a number of other stimulants. Calvin found different patterns of abnormal firing and classified them according to certain specific criteria. His two chief categories were the "high-frequency only" and the "long first interval high-frequency burst" patterns (Calvin et al., 1968; 1973). The reality of the recordings has never been in doubt but there were two questions, still only partially answered. One was whether or not these firing patterns are indeed pathognomonic for epileptogenic foci (debated at a meeting by Rayport, 1972, and Calvin, 1972); the other concerned the mechanism of their generation (Ogata, 1976, and see below).

Firing Spike Bursts by Normal Neurons

Very generally, when neurons are artificially depolarized for a few seconds by current injected through an intracellular microelectrode, three different patterns of response may be recorded (Figs. 7–2, 7–3, 9–2, 9–3). The cell may fire action potentials one after the other, as long as the stimulus lasts, known as a ***regular firing pattern***. In regular firing, (*1*) the frequency may be more or less constant or (*2*) it may be initially higher than it is later. The deceleration of frequency is called ***spike frequency adaptation***, a phenomenon related to *accommodation* and *refractoriness*, which are the result of inactivation of sodium conductance and activation of potassium conductance. Strongly adapting (or accommodating) cells might fire one or a few spikes and then stop in spite of continued stimulation. Unlike regularly firing cells, some neurons respond to steady depolarization by groups

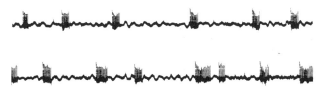

FIGURE 7–1. High-frequency burst firing of an "epileptic" neuron. Extracellular recording of the impulse discharge of a neuron obtained during surgery of a human patient within the epileptogenic focus in the parietal cortex. Impulse frequency within each burst 280–400 Hz. (Reproduced from Ward, 1969.)

of high-frequency spikes separated by longer periods of silence (Connors and Gutnick, 1990). This last pattern is called (*3*) ***burst firing*** or sometimes *bursting*, although no explosion is implied (Figs. 7–2, 7–3, 9–3, 9–4). According to Lisman (1997), burst firing serves to make transmission more secure. There are neurons that insist on firing in one of these basic modes, but some switch from regular to burst firing, depending on the type of synaptic input they receive. Other neurons can be induced to change their habit, for example by altering the ionic environment or exposure to certain drugs.

The Mechanisms of Burst Firing

Burst firing was first studied in detail in neurons in the nervous systems of invertebrates, mostly snails and slugs. ***Pacemaker cells*** are spontaneously active and generate rhythmically repeated slow waves of depolarization on which multiple action potentials "ride." Some pacemaker cells are active in the absence of input from synapses, even when physically isolated from their peers. Others must be challenged by synaptic excitation or a brief electric pulse. Some snail cells in central ***pattern generator*** circuits produce strongly depolarizing plateau potentials with high-frequency showers of action potentials that inactivate as the depolarization progresses (Straub et al., 2002). Without a figure legend, these voltage traces could easily be mistaken for epileptiform bursts in seized mammalian neurons: (see below: "Interictal epileptiform impulse bursts . . .").

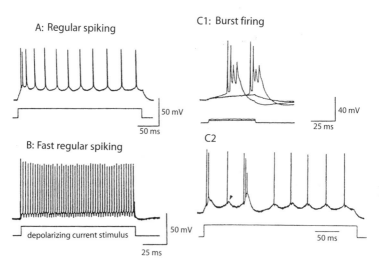

FIGURE 7–2. Firing patterns of neocortical neurons. Intracellular recordings from neurons in brain tissue slices in vitro stimulated by intracellular current injection. A, B, C1: From guinea pig, C2: From mouse cortex. (Modified from Connors and Gutnick, 1990.)

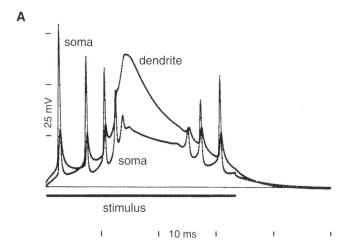

A

soma

dendrite

25 mV

soma

stimulus

10 ms

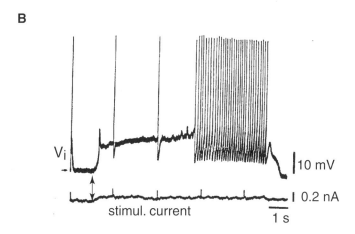

B

V$_i$

10 mV

0.2 nA

stimul. current

1 s

FIGURE 7–3. Burst firing can be generated by persistent depolarization of dendrites or of the neuron soma. **A:** Simulated dendritic and somatic potentials generated by a computer model of a hippocampal pyramidal cell. The dendritic response is dominated by a slow calcium-mediated spike; the soma fires sodium-dependent action potentials. **B:** Intracellular recording from a neuron in a thalamic tissue slice in vitro. The two-headed arrow marks the start of a very small depolarizing current injected into the cell soma. The disproportionately large, sustained depolarization response is attributed to the activation of a persistent sodium current ($I_{Na,P}$). (**A** modified from Traub and Llinas, 1979; **B** from Jahnsen and Llinas, 1984a.)

Pacemaker potentials are generated by slow voltage-gated inward Na^+, Ca^{2+}, or mixed cation currents that activate and inactivate more slowly than the fast Hodgkin-Huxley-type transient Na^+ current ($I_{Na,T}$). In the range of voltages within which such slow currents are active, the membrane behaves as if it were a *negative resistance* (Lux, 1984; Wilson and Wachtel, 1974). This term implies that, instead of resisting, the membrane assists the depolarization imposed on it. Stated differently, depolarizing current injected by an outside generator activates a voltage-controlled inward current that intensifies the depolarization by the stimulus itself. The voltage-gated slow Na^+ or Ca^{2+} channels that assist depolarization vary among different burst-firing cells. The slow depolarization is terminated by hyperpolarization, caused in part by the eventual slow inactivation of the inward currents and in part by voltage-gated and calcium-dependent outward K^+ currents. Then, as Ca^{2+} is removed from hyperpolarized cells, the K^+ current abates and the next round of slow depolarization can once more take over and produce the next pacemaker potential. The mechanism of pacemaking can be quite complex, involving numerous interacting channel types. Figures 9–2 to 9–7 show computer simulations of various types of rhythmic firing.

Some neurons in mammalian nervous systems, for example neuroendocrine cells, respiratory neurons in the brain stem, and thalamic cells fire spontaneous bursts of spikes using similar mechanisms (e.g., Steriade et al., 2001; Suter et al., 2000). Respiratory pacemaker neurons continue rhythmic burst firing even when synapses are blocked, which proves that the bursts are generated by intrinsic membrane mechanisms (Dean et al., 1990). Some other neurons that are not spontaneously active respond to stimulation with brief bursts of high-frequency firing. In neocortex of rodents some neurons fire only "regularly" spaced single spikes, but many of the pyramidal cells in layers IV or V tend to respond with bursts when stimulated (Connors and Gutnick, 1990; Connors and Telfeian, 2002). In recordings from hippocampal neurons, Kandel and Spencer (1961a) found that action potentials fired by some cells ended in a *depolarizing afterpotential (DAP)* (or *afterdepolarization, ADP*), a small wave following the spike. The same cells that produced DAPs were also inclined to fire spike bursts, and Kandel and Spencer suggested that the large, slow depolarizing wave on which the spikes of a burst ride arises by coalescence of successive DAPs. More than one type of ion current could generate DAPs. The possibilities include *dendritic calcium currents* and somatic or dendritic *persistent Na^+ current*, $I_{Na,P}$ (Figs. 7–2, 7–3) (Crill, 1996; Deisz, 1996; Traub and Llinas, 1979).

Among the neurons that can switch from burst mode to regular firing mode are the cerebellar Purkinje cells. These respond to input from the inferior olivary nucleus, conveyed by climbing fibers, with spike bursts that ride on large depolarizing waves, termed *complex spikes*, but they generate single, *simple spikes* when stimulated by way of parallel fibers that originate from cerebellar granule cells (Eccles et al., 1966a). Llinas and Sugimori (1980a, 1980b) analyzed the responses of cerebellar Purkinje cells and concluded that plateau-like depolarizations are generated by dendritic calcium current as well as by somatic persistent sodium current. Pyramidal cells in the somatosensory *barrel* area of the neocortex can also generate complex spikes in response to normal physiological input evoked by the bending of facial whiskers (Helmchen et al., 1999; see also Buzsáki and Traub, 1998). The intracellular voltage trajectories of complex spikes, which are normal, and ***paroxysmal depolarizing shifts (PDSs)***, which are signs of epilepsy, look remarkably alike (Figs. 5–1, 7–3A) (see below: "Interictal epileptiform impulse bursts . . ."). Entorhinal cortex layer II cells respond with membrane potential oscillations and spike clusters when exposed to muscarinic agonists (Klink and Alonso, 1997).

Moreover, cells that normally always fire regularly can be transformed into burst generators by pathology or by drugs. Under normal conditions, only a minority of CA1 pyramidal cells fire spike bursts. The majority belongs to the regular firing neuron type, but they too can be converted to the burst firing pattern. The K^+ channel blocking compound, 4-aminopyridine (4-AP), induces bursting by facilitating dendritic Ca^{2+} current in these cells, similarly to several other cell types (Magee and Carruth, 1999). Pilocarpine and veratridine induce burst firing by different mechanisms. So do elevated $[K^+]_o$, alkalinization, and lowering of $[Ca^{2+}]_o$ (Alkadhi and Tian, 1996; Church and Baimbridge, 1991; Jensen and Yaari, 1997; Sanabria et al., 2001; Su et al., 2001).

Among the neurons that normally can change their firing mode are thalamic cells. These can fire either regularly or in bursts, depending on their holding potential (Jahnsen and Llinas, 1984a,b). In hippocampus, pyramidal cells in the CA3 sector are much more likely to generate bursts than are the pyramidal cells of CA1. In piriform cortex, neurons respond to single-shock input from various nuclei of the amygdaloid complex with all-or-none impulse bursts riding on large, depolarizing waves (McIntyre and Wong, 1986). In neocortical burst firing cells, Purkinje cells, and CA3 pyramidal cells, the slow, depolarizing wave of the complex spikes is generated by inward current mainly through voltage-controlled calcium channels in apical dendrites (Fig. 7–3A) (Connors and Telfeian, 2002; Llinas and Sugimori, 1980a; Traub and Llinas, 1979; Wong et al., 1979). The fast spikes that are triggered by and appear to ride on the crest of the slow wave are, however, common sodium action potentials, and they are generated in the membrane of the cell soma and the initial segment of the axon.

Computer analysis of the currents underlying burst firing are presented in Chapter 9: "Features of the spike burst response."

Dendrites Are Not Passive Conductors of Synaptic Input

Before the discovery of voltage-controlled dendritic ion channels, many neuroscientists regarded the dendritic tree of central neurons as a passive receiver of synaptic input, incapable of generating action potentials or other active responses (Grundfest, 1957). Transmitter released from excitatory presynaptic terminals was thought to depolarize the subsynaptic membrane, and if many such synapses were simultaneously active, the depolarization was conducted by passive *electrotonus* to the cell body and to the initial segment of the axon, where nerve impulses were born. Inhibitory synapses, usually closer to the cell body or actually on the soma membrane, could intercept excitatory synaptic depolarization and prevent firing. In this theoretical construct, input seemed heavily biased in favor of synapses close to the cell soma. It was hard to see what purpose was served by synapses near the tips of dendrites far from the initial segment of the axon. The actual electrotonic distance spanned by the apical dendrites of hippocampal pyramidal cells turns out to be not much greater than 1, allowing passive conduction of distant EPSPs with 30%–40% efficacy (Turner and Schwartzkroin, 1980). In addition, the concept of purely passive dendrites was challenged even at its inception, and by now it is quite clear that there are many voltage-dependent conductances in dendritic membranes (Llinas and Sugimori, 1980a; Purpura et al., 1966; Tank et al., 1988). Dendritic voltage-dependent inward Na^+ and Ca^{2+} currents have at least two functions. Active inward currents assist the conveyance of input from the farthest synapses at the tips of dendrites to the cell body (Herreras, 1990). But these currents do more than simply amplify input. Active dendritic currents generate slow depolarization and shape the impulse bursts, the impulses themselves being fired by the neuron soma and axon (Figs. 7–3, 9–3, 9–4) (Ross et al., 1993; Traub and Llinas, 1979; Wong et al., 1979). The existence of an assortment of Na^+, Ca^{2+}, and K^+ channels in dendritic membranes is no longer in doubt. Not yet complete is the much more tedious job of determining, which channels are present in which neurons' dendrites.

Somatic Bursts, Distinct from Dendritic Complex Spikes,
Depend on a Persistent Sodium Current

Superficially similar spike bursts can be produced, however, by very different mechanisms. Llinas and Sugimori (1980b) first proposed the existence of slowly inactivating Na^+ current in cerebellar Purkinje cell soma (Fig. 7–3B). They contrasted the somatic location of this slow Na^+ current with the predominance of Ca^{2+}-dependent currents in the dendrites (Llinas and Sugimori, 1980a). Veratridine is a poison that can cause hippocampal cells to fire prolonged high-frequency spike bursts riding on large depolarizing waves, either spontaneously or in response to brief stimulus pulses (Alkadhi and Tian, 1996). These discharges need no synaptic input, but they are suppressed by low concentrations of *tetrodotoxin (TTX)*. The responsible intrinsic current is apparently a persistent (i.e., slowly inactivating) *sodium current, $I_{Na,P}$*. Even without veratridine, such a current can be detected in many types of central neurons but normally it is quite small (Crill, 1996).

Whether this normal small current is generated by a channel different from the one responsible for the large, rapidly inactivating Na^+ current ($I_{Na,T}$), or whether it represents incomplete inactivation of a minority of the conventional Na^+ channels, is not entirely clear. Mutated variants of the Na^+ channel with defective inactivation have been created, and animals bearing such mutated genes suffer from epilepsy (Kearney et al., 2001; Noebels, 2002). Persistent inward current also appears to be the main driver of ictal-like discharges of single neurons grown in *microculture* with synaptic transmission blocked (Segal, 2002) (see also Chapter 6: "Five ideas . . ."). Besides veratridine administration, other manipulations can substantially enhance $I_{Na,P}$ and induce burst firing initiated mainly in the soma membrane. Replacing most of the Ca^{2+} by Mn^{2+} or Mg^{2+} effectively blocks inward calcium currents, yet it promotes the firing of spike bursts in CA1 pyramidal neurons (Su et al., 2001). Several tests have identified the current responsible for the low-calcium burst firing as $I_{Na,P}$ (see also Bikson et al., 2002). We shall meet the persistent Na^+ current repeatedly, as it appears to be important in a number of pathological reactions. Besides low $[Ca^{2+}]_o$, elevated $[K^+]_o$ also enhances $I_{Na,P}$ (Somjen and Müller, 2000), and so does hypoxia (Hammarström and Gage, 1998). These effects are prominent in seizures, SD, and hypoxia.

$I_{Na,P}$ is sensitive to lower concentrations of TTX than is $I_{Na,T}$ (Alkadhi and Tian, 1996). Several investigators, however, also described a persistent voltage-gated current carried by Na^+ that is not blocked by TTX (Deisz, 1996; Hoehn et al., 1993; White et al., 1993). Others have challenged the existence of such a TTX-insensitive Na^+ current, claiming that it is a laboratory curiosity, not manifest under normal conditions (Chao and Alzheimer, 1995a). New support for its existence came from in situ hybridization, which showed the presence of a channel apparently identical to a TTX-resistant cardiac channel (SCN5A) in brain (Hartmann et al., 1999; Noebels, 2002). This channel is preferentially expressed in limbic structures prone to oscillating activity.

In conclusion

It is important to remember that slow depolarizing waves supporting burst firing behavior can be generated by more than one ionic mechanism. Simple inspection of intracellular recordings cannot always distinguish among them.

*Interictal Epileptiform Impulse Bursts Resemble Normal
Burst Firing, but Are They the Same?*

Intracellular recordings from "epileptic" neurons also reveal waves of depolarization on which rides a group of closely spaced action potentials, usually but not invariably of decreasing amplitude (Figs. 5–1B, 7–9a) (Ayala et al., 1973; de Curtis et al., 1999; Lopantsev and Avoli, 1998; Prince, 1968b). The slow membrane potential wave is called a ***paroxysmal depolarizing shift (PDS)*** by some and a *depolarizing shift (DS)* by others. The groups of action potentials triggered by the PDS are the intracellular counterparts of the impulse bursts detected by extracellular microelectrodes near epileptic neurons. Superficially, they look alike in epileptogenic foci created by various means in neocortex and in the hippocampal formation. Often but not always, PDSs are followed by prolonged afterpotentials. Such an afterpotential can consist of a prolonged low-amplitude depolarization, a hyperpolarizing undershoot, or a sequence of depolarizations followed by hyperpolarization (de Curtis et al., 1999). The structure of the long first interval burst of Calvin et al. (1968) (and see above: "Epileptic neurons") is also illuminated by intracellular recordings and computer simulation. In this pattern, the first spike is a synaptically triggered action potential fired just prior to the slow wave. The high-frequency burst follows a little later, riding on a wave of intrinsic inward current triggered by the preceding EPSP (Ogata, 1976; Traub et al., 1993). When the PDSs of many epileptic neurons are synchronized, they give rise to extracellular current that can be detected on a surface EEG as the interictal discharges called *sharp waves* or *spikes* in EEG parlance (Chapter 5: "Electroencephalography in epilepsy") (Figs. 5–1A,B, 7–9a, 8–1A). As we have noted, what is called a *slow* wave on intracellular records corresponds to the *spike* or *sharp wave* of the EEG trace.

Paroxysmal depolarizing shifts have been explained in two competing ways: they may be either *synaptically* evoked or generated by *intrinsic membrane currents*—or more probably a combination of both. Several investigators suggested that they represent *giant EPSPs* (Ayala et al., 1973; Connors and Gutnick, 1984; Johnston and Brown, 1981). In favor of this interpretation, blocking synaptic transmission, or just the NMDA-dependent component of EPSPs, abolished the PDSs induced by penicillin or low magnesium (Johnston and Brown, 1981; Tancredi et al., 1990). In general, PDSs are composed of an initial fast depolarization followed by a slow wave of depolarization and are often terminated by hyperpolarization. It has been suggested that the early depolarizing component is generated by AMPA receptor–mediated glutamatergic excitation, and the later slow wave follows as NMDA receptors become activated (Meldrum et al., 1999).

In an early paper Prince (1968a, 1968b) suggested that the PDS (called by him the DS) is a giant synaptic potential that is bolstered by a membrane abnormality, and it is followed by hyperpolarization generated by an IPSP. Later, Prince and colleagues (Prince and Connors, 1984; Prince and Schwartzkroin, 1978) demonstrated that hyperpolarization of neurons blocks the PDSs. An EPSP would be exaggerated by hyperpolarization because its reversal potential is near zero volts. Based on these findings, Prince proposed a dual mechanism: giant EPSPs triggering intrinsic voltage-gated currents. Adding to the confusion, PDSs seemed all-or-none events in some trials, supporting the idea that they are generated by voltage-gated currents (Gutnick et al., 1982), but in other reports they were said to be graded, which would make synaptic generation more likely (Matsumoto et al., 1969). In hippocampal slices treated with 4-AP, the reversal potential of

PDSs was either –26 mV (under current clamp) or –14 mV (under voltage clamp) (Rutecki et al., 1987). This suggests generation by a mixture of several currents. Wong and Traub (1983) concluded that under the influence of penicillin or bicuculline, PDS-based bursts are initiated by intrinsic currents in the CA2–CA3 region but are then transmitted synaptically to the CA3 region.

Most strikingly, it turned out that PDS-like events can occur in preparations where synaptic transmission has been abolished (see also Chapter 6: "Nonsynaptic epileptogenesis"). For example, in brain slices bathed in a low-calcium solution synaptic transmission is blocked, yet spontaneous synchronized interictal-like discharges arise over time, and their intracellular counterpart resembles PDSs (Albrecht and Heinemann, 1989; Haas and Jefferys, 1984). Pan and Stringer (1996, 1997) emphasized the similarity of PDS-like events in hippocampal slices bathed in low calcium (with synapses incapacitated) to those induced by kainate (with excitatory synapses in good working order).

In hippocampal slices prepared from rats previously rendered epileptic by pilocarpine treatment (see Chapter 6: "Pilocarpine"), synchronized interictal discharges and PDSs can be recorded in CA1 pyramidal cells that normally do not generate impulse bursts. These postpilocarpine PDSs also have the characteristics of all-or-none intrinsic responses but require triggering by glutamatergic synaptic input (Sanabria et al., 2001). Reviewing current source density analyses of interictal discharges by several teams, Mitzdorf (1985) also concluded that they arise as exaggerated synaptic potentials augmented by intrinsic Ca^{2+} currents. According to a reverse interpretation, bicuculline-induced PDSs start as intrinsic depolarizing waves in one neuron, which then recruits its neighbors through recurrent excitatory synaptic connections (de Curtis et al., 1998, 1999).

The role of GABAergic inhibition is equally ambiguous. Köhling et al. (1998, 1999) recorded spontaneous interictal-like (sharp wave) activity in slices of epileptogenic temporal neocortex taken in surgery from human patients. The activity was GABA-dependent because it was abolished by bicuculline. Current source density analysis identified the initial sink in layer II and the border of layers II and III, a region known as *supragranular*. The authors concluded that the spontaneous sharp waves were initiated by some pathological alteration of synapses in these layers.

If we accept that giant EPSPs initiate PDSs, which then activate intrinsic currents, the pathologically exaggerated size of the EPSP remains to be explained. Again, competing explanations have been proposed. Suppressed inhibition could amplify excitation. In line with this, penicillin subdues GABA-dependent IPSPs in the cerebral cortex without completely eliminating them (see Chapter 6: "Penicillin induces seizures . . ."). In spinal cord, however, penicillin does not interfere with glycine-dependent synaptic inhibition; nevertheless, it induces PDS-like events (Lothman and Somjen, 1976b). Perhaps a more general mechanism may be exaggerated release of transmitter. This can result from prolonged presynaptic action potentials, for example under the influence of 4-AP (Perreault and Avoli, 1991), or ectopic spike generation causing multiple firing of presynaptic terminals. Abnormal spike firing in presynaptic terminals has been demonstrated in several types of experimental seizures by antidromic recording from afferent axons, and was also confirmed by the so-called impulse collision technique (Gutnick and Prince, 1972; Lothman and Somjen, 1976a; Scobey and Gabor, 1975; Stasheff et al, 1993). The importance of such ectopic spike generation was supported by computer simulation (Traub et al., 1996a). The biophysical mechanism of the ectopic action potential generation (in the absence of K^+ channel blockers) has not been explored.

Paroxysmal Depolarizing Shifts Are Generated by Different Mechanisms in Different Models

These various findings compel the conclusion that there is more than one way to make a PDS, even if superficially they all look alike. The problem then is, which of the models best resembles the interictal events of clinical epilepsy—or are there also several types in human patients? The currently prevailing synthesis of diverse findings is that (most?) PDSs are initiated by exaggerated excitatory synaptic potentials, which then secondarily trigger intrinsic membrane currents, mainly dendritic Ca^{2+} currents. Ectopic spikes backfired from the axon, especially its terminals, can complicate the picture. The depolarizing wave may or may not be followed by hyperpolarization produced by a combination of IPSP and intrinsic K^+ current.

In the Hippocampus Paroxysmal Depolarizing Shifts Originate from the CA3 Sector

Pyramidal cells in the CA3 segment are endowed with the ability to generate impulse bursts. To trigger these bursts, the potassium concentration in the bathing fluid must be raised to 5 mM. In many studies, 5 or 5.5 mM K^+ has been used for normal ACSF. By contrast, CA1 cells are less likely to fire spike bursts even at such (moderately) elevated levels of $[K^+]_o$. This difference between CA1 and CA3 pyramidal cells probably explains why interictal discharges originate, as a rule, from CA3 and are conducted by way of synapses to CA1 pyramidal cells (Lothman et al., 1981; Prince et al., 1983; Wong and Traub, 1983). The CA1 cells produce interictal discharges if and only if they are compelled to do so by input from CA3.

Not only CA3 pyramidal cells but also the neurons in piriform cortex have an innate inclination for burst generation (McIntyre and Wong, 1986). This property is probably a factor in the propensity of these regions to become epileptogenic during kindling.

Spike-wave seizures are a pathological variant of oscillating brain activity

The Contrast of Petit Mal and Grand Mal

The characteristic seizures of *primary generalized absence epilepsy* consist of brief spells during which the patient loses consciousness but does not fall to the ground. It has several forms, with or without muscle twitching or jerking, but they all have in common a synchronized, bilateral 2.5–4 Hz SW pattern of EEG discharges (Figs. 5–1C, 7–4) (Niedermeyer, 1999a; Petsche, 1962).

Absence seizures differ from major convulsive disorders not just in their clinical manifestations but also, most strikingly, in their pharmacology. Some drugs, notably those that augment GABAergic inhibition, that are effective anticonvulsants in other forms of epilepsy, actually aggravate SW seizures (Coenen et al., 1995), while those that can control absence epilepsy are useless against major convulsive disorders (Leresche et al., 1998) (see Chapter 11). One might wonder whether petit mal and grand mal have anything in common. Yet there are also clear links between the two conditions (Lüders, 2001; Petsche, 1962). Some patients have both absence episodes and major convulsive seizures. Some children, who in their early years suffer only from absences, develop tonic-clonic epileptic seizures later in life. Therefore, even though the mechanisms of the SW phenomenon and the tonic-clonic seizures are different, some genetic defects seem to predispose to both types of disorders.

Four questions arise: (*1*) What is the biophysical nature of the SW format? (*2*) What drives the rhythmic repetition? (*3*) How is the discharge synchronized within and among widely spaced areas? (*4*) Why does the discharge stop? In the paragraphs that follow, we will try to find answers to these questions. First, however, we address the more general concepts of central rhythm generators. Then we explore the similarities and differences between normal and pathological brain oscillations.

Alpha Waves and Sleep Spindles

Alpha waves were among the earliest discoveries of Hans Berger (1929). In 1968, Andersen and Andersson published a monograph with the ambitious goal to explain rhythmic brain activity. Even though they titled their book *Physiological Basis of the Alpha Rhythm*, almost all of their experimental observations concerned spindle oscillations that are common during barbiturate anesthesia. They felt justified in equating alpha waves with spindles mainly because of the similar frequency range, the regular sinusoidal course of the oscillations, and the similar, mainly dendritic, generator of the surface potentials detected by EEG and ECoG recordings. Probably few investigators completely accept this premise today (Niedermeyer, 1999b) even if there are some general similarities among various types of synchronized oscillations. Rhythmic depolarization-hyperpolarization sequences underlie them all, but neither the rhythm generators nor the membrane currents need be the same. The Andersen-Andersson monograph presented a pioneering approach, combining experimental work with theory and computer simulation. It contains the first detailed and explicit proposal based on the biophysics and synaptic connections of neuron populations as these were then known, and some elements of their analysis do survive in the more complex explanations that have evolved since.

Thalamic Nuclei Coordinate Normal Cortical Rhythms

Andersen and Andersson (1968) trace the evolution of the main ideas concerning the mechanism of cortical rhythms. The historical background of brain rhythms is also reviewed in the volume by Steriade et al. (1990). There have been two main competing basic ideas. One assumed cellular autorhythmicity, based on **intrinsic pacemaker mechanisms** in central neurons, and the other proposed that impulses **reverberate** in **recurrent pathways** in a circular motion among interconnected neurons. Both ideas were, to some degree, inspired by the then known electrophysiology of the heart. The sinoatrial node is, of course, a cellular pacemaker par excellence. Myocardial fibrillation provided a model for reexcitation by circular movement of excitation (Carmeliet, 1999).

The concept of autorhythmicity residing in cortical pacemakers was weakened when it turned out that interrupting input to the cortex by undercutting white matter abolished α waves and sleep spindles (Burns, 1958). The idea regained some credence when such isolated cortical slabs were allowed to survive for an extended period. In this chronic state, the isolated cortex developed a rhythmic activity, albeit of an abnormal type (Sharpless, 1969) (see also Chapter 6: "Neocortical experimental epileptogenic foci"). Rhythmic reverberation of waves of excitation was thought to occur between thalamus and cortex. Morison and Dempsey (1942, also Dempsey and Morison, 1962) discovered the diffuse thalamocortical projection system next to the specific relay nuclei and demonstrated that rhythmic cortical waves can be evoked by stimulation of the thalamus.

Rebound Excitation and Its Role in Pacemaking

Classical electrophysiology recognized a phenomenon called **anode-break excitation**, named more poetically *postanodal exaltation* by Erlanger and Gasser (1937). It was then already well known that hyperpolarization reduces excitability and that the termination of a sufficiently long hyperpolarizing pulse (*anode break*) can trigger an action potential. Hodgkin and Huxley (1952) provided the explanation. In the squid giant axon at rest, voltage-dependent Na^+ conductance is partially inactivated. Hyperpolarization removes the inactivation. Allowing the membrane potential to fall back from a hyperpolarized level to its resting potential activates the sodium channels and triggers an action potential. The transient T-type (inactivating) calcium currents ($I_{Ca,T}$) can similarly be turned on by the cessation of hyperpolarization.

Rebound excitation in the wake of IPSPs has been observed in many neurons in the CNS (Kandel and Spencer, 1961a), especially in thalamic neurons (Steriade et al., 1990). Because of the slower kinetics of activation and inactivation of calcium channels, postinhibitory rebound excitation of central neurons is primarily caused by disinactivation of calcium rather than sodium channels (Fig. 7–7) (Coulter, 1998; Steriade et al., 1990).

Postinhibitory rebound excitation was central to the theory proposed by Andersen and Andersson (1968) to explain the rhythmicity of the thalamic pacemaker circuit. In 1968 the neuronal Ca^{2+} channels had not yet been discovered, and Andersen and Andersson assumed that Na^+ channels were responsible for the rebound excitation. In their scheme, action potentials fired by thalamic cells excite inhibitory interneurons in a recurrent inhibitory loop that resides in the thalamus and requires no cortical connection. When a thalamic neuron fires an impulse, it excites an inhibitory interneuron, which then sends an IPSP by way of the recurrent loop back to it. At the termination of the IPSP, the cell undergoes postinhibitory rebound excitation, which once more excites the inhibitory interneurons and repeats the cycle. Branching axons of the inhibitory neurons could recruit additional cells into the oscillations. Andersen and Andersson constructed a computer model to demonstrate how such a neuron assembly could produce synchronized beating. Thalamocortical connections would impose the rhythm on the cortex, but the pace would be set within the thalamus. In their view, this scheme explains α rhythm as well as sleep spindles, but they did not address the presence of consciousness in the one condition and its absence in the other. In later decades the basic idea proved correct, but the scheme was considerably expanded and modified in the light of newer biophysical and morphological data. The mechanisms of the α rhythm and sleep spindles are no longer considered to be identical (Steriade et al., 1990).

The Spike-Wave Complex Corresponds to Depolarization-Hyperpolarization Sequences in Pyramidal Neurons

The SW EEG pattern of absence seizures has been investigated in great detail and with considerable success. It is fair to say that in broad outline it is well understood, even if there is some difference of opinion concerning the details.

Rhythmical SW oscillations are typical of absence seizures, but isolated or repeated SW complexes are also seen in some other conditions (Petsche, 1962; Risinger, 2000). Interictal discharges can take the form of isolated SW complexes as well as sharp waves and EEG spikes. At least superficially, these isolated events resemble the SW patterns that are repeated with a 3/sec rhythm during absence seizures.

Absence seizures are imitated in animal models such as feline generalized penicillin epilepsy (see Chapter 6: "Penicillin induces . . .") (Gloor, 1984; Prince and Farrell, 1969) and in several lines of epileptic mice and rats (Burgess and Noebels, 1999; Danober et al. 1998; Midzianovskaia et al., 2001; Noebels, 1984) (see below: "Genetic models of absence epilepsy"). In rodents the rhythm is usually faster, 6–11 Hz (McCormick and Contreras, 2001; Midzianovskaia et al., 2001). In addition, in ketamine-xylazine anesthetized cats, the normal sleep pattern is from time to time interrupted by spontaneous seizure-like discharges of the SW pattern, either at 3–6 Hz or in "runs" at an unusually high frequency of 10–20 Hz (Neckelmann et al., 2000; Steriade and Contreras, 1995) Amzica et al. (2002) called attention to the similarity of the fast runs in these cats to the EEG seizures seen during sleep in children with Lennox-Gastaut syndrome.

The SW pattern appears to represent a stereotyped, basic form of pathological discharge. Both the spike and the wave are predominantly negative when recorded from the surface of the hemisphere against ground, and the spike remains negative but the wave turns positive when recorded deep within cortical gray matter (Destexhe, 1998; McCormick and Contreras, 2001; Mitzdorf, 1985). Examination of the waveform recorded from different cytoarchitectonic layers of the neocortex (*laminar analysis*) explained this voltage profile. The spike that is uniformly negative wherever it is recorded represents current that flows inward over a wide expanse of the surface of pyramidal neurons. By contrast, current flows during the wave outward from cell bodies, and perhaps also from basal dendrites or the most proximal segment of apical dendritic trunks, but inward into the widely spreading branches of the apical dendrites of pyramidal cells. Intracellular electrodes inserted in the cell bodies of pyramidal neurons of the neocortex record *depolarization during the extracellular spike, followed by hyperpolarization during the extracellular wave* (Avoli and Kostopoulos, 1982). Neurons discharge action potentials at high frequency during the spike and are silenced during the wave (Kandel and Buzsáki, 1997).

Similarly to PDS, SW complexes could theoretically be generated either by synaptic inputs, specifically as an EPSP-IPSP sequence (Jefferys and Roberts, 1987), or by successively activated inward and outward intrinsic membrane currents, or as a combination of the two types of mechanisms. During absence seizures, when the SW discharges appear to be synchronized and generalized over wide areas of both hemispheres, coordination must be achieved by the concerted action of synaptic circuits. At shorter distances nonsynaptic mechanisms, especially ion fluxes, can also synchronize SW activity (Amzica et al., 2002). Perhaps synaptic circuits set the general pace, and synaptic potentials trigger the intrinsic currents and resulting ion fluxes that shape and phase-lock at short distance the discharge of individual cells. This, in fact, is probably the essence of the phenomenon.

The Hypothesis of Intracortical Synchronization

From the beginning, there was disagreement on whether the neocortex or subcortical centers fashion the SW rhythm. Gloor (1984) quotes Gibbs and Gibbs as the first proponents of the *diffuse cortical hypothesis*, suggesting that the widespread synchronized discharge is generated within the neocortex, without assistance from subcortical structures. Two key observations supported their contention. First, convulsant drugs applied to the surface of the brain induced typical SW discharges. Second, lesions cutting the connections between cortex and subcortical nuclei but sparing the interhemispheric callosal connections did not prevent the eruption of bilaterally synchronous SWs (quoted by Gloor, 1984). Recent work with cortical and thalamocortical tissue slices demonstrated the possibility of synchronization among intracortical interneuron networks achieved by excitatory gap junctional coupling and inhibitory synaptic linkage (Amitai et al., 2002; Gibson et al., 1999). Other evidence emphasizes the importance of the neocortex in initiating SW activity, but it does not support true autonomy of the cortex (Meeren et al., 2002; Neckelmann et al., 1998).

The Centrencephalic Hypothesis

Against a *cortical generator* of generalized SW seizures, Penfield and Jasper proposed a **centrencephalic** pacemaker (Jasper and Drooglever-Fortuyn, 1947; Penfield and Jasper, 1954). The idea was partly inspired by Moruzzi and Magoun's (1949) and Morison and Dempsey's (1942) work demonstrating the influence of subcortical input on the electrical activity of the cortex. Penfield and Jasper suggested that the "highest level of neural integration" is to be found in subcortical nuclear masses including the *nonspecific nuclei of the thalamus* and parts of the basal ganglia. If one assumes that consciousness is maintained by these nuclei, supported by input from the upper brain stem (Moruzzi and Magoun's **ascending reticular system**), then consciousness is expected to be switched off whenever seizures erupt there. Diffuse, bilateral projections from this central gray matter mass to both hemispheres of the neocortex could explain how seizure discharges originating here can start simultaneously over much of both cerebral hemispheres and remain tightly synchronized during the entire seizure. The precise synchrony suggested a single pacemaker. This idea was reinforced when Jasper and colleagues evoked an SW discharge by rhythmic stimulation in the reticular nucleus of the thalamus (Jasper and Drooglever-Fortuyn, 1947).

Gloor (1968) attempted to synthesize the two competing views. Based on injections of sodium amytal and metrazol (PTZ) into either the carotid or the vertebral artery of patients with generalized SW seizures, he concluded that generalized seizures were generated by abnormal interaction of cortical and subcortical mechanisms. The results of subsequent animal experiments were taken to support this view (Avoli et al., 1983; Gloor, 1984; Gloor and Fariello, 1988). As summarized recently by Kostopoulos (2000), SW discharges develop in the same circuits that govern sleep spindles, but with an important difference. Pathologically increased cortical excitability converts the normal rhythm into a seizure. Increased excitability is shown by the increasing propensity for spike firing by cortical cells prior to the onset of an SW seizure. The rhythm of the SW waves (3–4 Hz) is one-half or one-third that of spindles (9–11 Hz). The spike of the SW discharge is but an exaggerated excitatory spindle wave that brings in its wake the wave, which represents inhibition. The recruitment of inhibitory waves suppresses the impending next spindle wave or two. As spindle waves go missing, the 9–11 Hz spindle frequency is converted into the 3–4 Hz SW rhythm (Fig. 7–4) (Kostopoulos, 2000; McLachlan et al., 1984). Gloor's ideas were based mainly on EEG and single-neuron recordings in penicillin-induced SW discharges in anesthetized cats (FGPE). Out of a large number of experimental observations, two early ones were especially salient. While intramuscular injection of a large dose of penicillin could covert the EEG spindles into SW discharges, microinjection of penicillin into the thalamus could not. On the other hand, silencing the thalamus by microinjection of KCl solution stopped both sleep spindles and SW discharges. The inference—that enhanced cortical excitability was responsible for the transition from spindles to an SW discharge—was reinforced by the demonstrations that ongoing SW discharges reverted to spindles when cortical excitability was depressed. Extensive use of multiple recordings from cortical and thalamic neurons by several teams supported the basic concept of mutual thalamocortical interactions in rhythm generation (Fig. 7–5, 7–6, 7–7) (Avoli et al., 1983; Coulter, 1998).

In conclusion

Both cortex and thalamus are required for spike-wave discharge. Cortical source-sink distributions are similar during sleep spindles and SW discharges, indicating that the same cortical neuron populations participate in the two types of activity (Kandel and Buzsáki, 1997), but the rhythm generator of the two patterns is not the same. The thalamic nuclei are autonomous pacemakers of sleep spindles, but both the neocortex and the thalamus are required to produce SW seizures.

Genetic Models of Absence Epilepsy

Penicillin-induced seizures are no longer considered the best animal model for absence epilepsy. They have been replaced by inbred and/or mutant strains of rodents, the most intensively studied of which are GAERS, which stands for *genetic absence epilepsy, rat from Strasbourg* (Avanzini et al., 1996; Danober et al., 1998) and the WAG/Rij strain from the Netherlands (Midzianovskaia et al., 2001; Peeters et al., 1992).

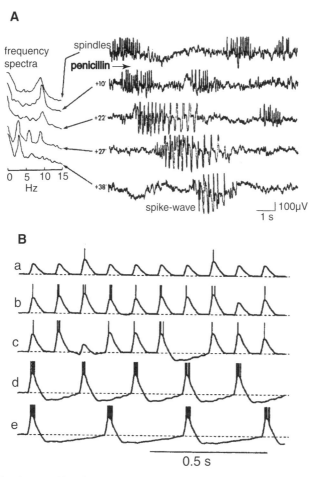

Figure 7–4. The transition from electroencephalographic (EEG) spindles to spike-wave (SW) discharges (the Gloor-Kostopoulos hypothesis). **A:** Electroencephalographic tracings before and after the intramuscular administration of a convulsant dose of penicillin. Cat neocortex. The numbers to the left of the EEG traces show times in minutes after the penicillin administration. The insets show frequency spectra for each EEG trace. Note the abrupt switch of the dominant frequency from 9 Hz (spindles) to a triple peak of 9, 5, and 3 Hz and then to 3 Hz (spike-wave [SW] discharge). **B:** Schematic representation of the proposed mechanism of the transition from spindle waves to SW discharge, inferred from intracellular recordings in thalamus and cortex. a: Before penicillin administration, showing rhythmic excitatory postsynaptic potential (EPSP) waves. b–e: After penicillin administration. In b, EPSPs are increased. Then, in c, occasional waves drop out due to increasing inhibition. In d every second wave and in e two out of every three waves are suppressed, stabilizing the rhythm at one-third of the original frequency. The SW discharge results from augmented EPSP-IPSP sequences. IPSP: inhibitory postsynaptic potential. (Modified from Kostopoulos, 2000.)

The Roles of Thalamic Relay Nuclei and the Reticular Nucleaus

The choreography of the SW oscillations engages three main actors: the ***thalamus proper*** (or *relay nuclei*), the ***reticular nucleus of the thalamus*** (*nucleus reticularis thalamu, NRT*) (Figs. 7–5, 7–6), and the ***neocortex***. This much is agreed on; only the details of the interaction are not completely settled. One scheme devised to explain thalamocortical rhythmicity is shown in Figure 7–7. A short summary of some of the ideas follows.

Thalamic neurons are unusually richly endowed with two ion channel types: low-threshold transient Ca^{2+} channels that generate the ***T-current*** (I$_{Ca,T}$) (also known as ***low voltage-activated [LVA]*** calcium channels) and the ***hyperpolarization-activated nonspecific cation current (I$_h$)***, and both are instrumental in bringing about thalamic oscillations. While the animal is alert, the resting potential of thalamic cells is around –60 or –65 mV, and neither of these two currents is active. As a result, the cells are in a nonoscillating state. I$_{Ca,T}$ is inactivated at this voltage, and I$_h$ requires a more negative voltage to be activated (McCormick and Huguenard, 1992). This level of *alerted resting potential* is stabilized by cholinergic and monoaminergic input from the brain stem, that is, by the *ascending alert-*

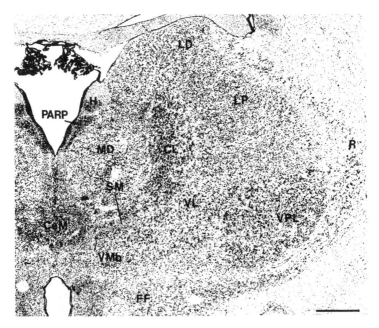

FIGURE 7–5. Cytoarchitecture of the dorsal thalamus of a cat. R: reticular nucleus, which surrounds the relay and intrinsic nuclei like a shell. VPL: ventroposterolateral nucleus (n.). VL: ventrolateral n.; LP: lateroposterior n. LD: lateral dorsal n. MD: dorsomedial n. CL: central lateral n. CeM: centromedian n. H: habenular n. FF: fields of Forel. PARP: posterior pararentricular n. of epithalamus. (Reproduced from Steriade et al., 1990.)

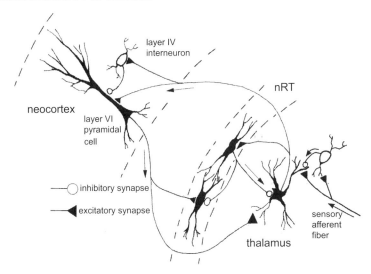

Figure 7–6. Synaptic connections involved in thalamocortical rhythm generation. Schematic representation of the basic thalamocortical circuit. nRT: nucleus reticularis thalami (reticular nucleus). The cells in the reticular nucleus are inhibitory neurons, acting on each other as well as on the thalamocortical relay cells. Note the reciprocity of the thalamocortical and corticothalamic connections, the anatomical substrate of the feedback loops. (Modified from Coulter, 1998.)

ing system. In this alert state, action potentials can normally be produced by sodium and potassium currents and the thalamic neurons in the various specialized nuclei can carry on with their daily task, processing information arriving either from sensory receptors to be sent on to neocortex or from the neocortex to be shaped into motor commands.

During slow-wave sleep and absence seizures, thalamic neurons engage in synchronized oscillations that suppress their patterned, purposeful waking activity, in essence disconnecting the cerebral cortex from the "lower" parts of the CNS. Slaght and colleagues (2002) recently proposed a detailed scenario for the thalamocortical oscillations as seen in the genetic absence epilepsy strain from Strasbourg (GAERS) rats (see also (Danober et al., 1998). The oscillations are shaped by the two slow currents, $I_{Ca,T}$ and I_h. A peculiarity of thalamic neurons is the presence of an appreciable "window" current of the T-type calcium channels resulting from overlap of the domains of activation and steady-state inactivation (Hughes et al., 1999). To start an oscillatory cycle, the neurons must first be hyperpolarized. The hyperpolarization turns off the activation and removes the inactivation of $I_{Ca,T}$ (moves V_m out of the window) (Slaght et al., 2002). At the same time, it activates I_h. The mixed cation current of I_h flows inward and starts a slow depolarizing slide of the membrane toward or just below its resting level. Since the inactivation has

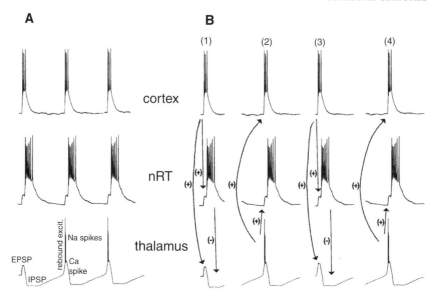

FIGURE 7-7. Interpretation of thalamocortical oscillations. To follow this set of diagrams, refer to Figure 7–6. **A:** Intracellular recordings from the principal players: neocortex (neuron giving rise to the corticothalamic axon with excitatory connections to both nucleus reticularis thalami (nRT) and thalamic relay cell), reticular (nRT) cell (inhibitory neuron) and thalamus (thalamocortical relay cell, sending excitatory connections to both cortex and nRT). **B:** The back-and-forth exchange that generates the rhythmically repeating activity. Labels next to the arrows: (+) means excitatory volley; (–) means inhibition. (1): An impulse burst in the cortical cell initiates the cycle by evoking excitatory postsynaptic potentials (EPSPs) in both the nRT and the thalamic neuron. The nRT cell then sends a powerful inhibitory postsynaptic potential (IPSP) to the thalamic cell. (2): In the wake of the IPSP, rebound excitation in the thalamic relay cell generates a calcium spike, which triggers a burst of impulses, which then send EPSPs to nRT and cortical neurons. (3): The excited cortical cell returns a volley of excitatory impulses to nRT and thalamic relay neurons, while the nRT cell sends IPSPs to the thalamus. (4): Rebound excitation in thalamus starts the next cycle. (Modified from Coulter, 1998.)

been removed from the $I_{Ca,T}$ during the preceding hyperpolarization, $I_{Ca,T}$ is activated and it accelerates the already ongoing depolarization. This, then, is ***rebound excitation*** initiated by I_h and completed by $I_{Ca,T}$. At the height of the depolarization, the thalamic cells fire a burst of action potentials that are conducted to both the neocortex and the NRT. Burst-firing neurons in both the cortex and the NRT respond with a calcium-mediated slow wave that triggers a burst of impulses. The impulses are then conducted back to both the NRT and the thalamus proper. The output from the NRT is GABAergic, and it hyperpolarizes the thalamic cells, preparing them for the next wave. When the glutamatergic volley from the cortex arrives in the thalamus, it boosts the already ongoing depolarization, which triggers the next burst of spikes.

The primary, genetically determined abnormality distinguishing GAERS rats from normals has been blamed on nothing more than enhanced $I_{Ca,T}$ in neurons of the NRT (Avanzini et al., 1996; Tsakiridou et al., 1995). Computer simulation suggested that enhanced $I_{Ca,T}$ causes a phase shift enabling reticular neurons to entrain the firing of the thalamocortical neurons that drive the cortex (Thomas and Grisar, 2000). The result is hypersynchrony among widespread populations. Supporting this concept, mutated mice deficient in the T-type channel are resistant to absence seizures, and their thalamocortical neurons do not show the normal propensity for burst firing (Kim et al., 2001).

Alternative explanations of SW discharges have been reviewed (Danober et al., 1998; Destexhe, 1998; McCormick and Contreras, 2001; Steriade and Contreras, 1995) (Figs. 7–5, 7–6, 7–7). A computer model incorporating the three actors— thalamus, neocortex, and NRT—has been presented by Destexhe (2000). All of these proposals attempt to explain both sleep spindles and SW oscillations. They all assign the major roles to the three areas—neocortex, thalamic relay nuclei, and NRT. The oscillations are governed by feedback combining recurrent excitation with recurrent inhibition and rebound excitation. The period is influenced by the time it takes to complete the circular motion in the feedback lines, as well as the activation and inactivation kinetics of the currents involved.

Primacy of the Neocortex Restored?

Using equipment that today seems primitive but was advanced for its time, Petsche (1962) followed the appearance of spikes and waves among eight EEG electrodes recording from human patients. One surprise was that spikes and waves sometimes moved independently over the surface. But, more importantly, the rhythm of the discharge was dictated by a primary, presumably cortical, zone, and the waves traveled from this cortical pacemaker to other regions. Petsche named the phenomenon *roaming waves* (*Wanderwellen*). The waves propagated with a velocity in the meters-per-second range. Recently, Petsche's concept received new support. Lopes da Silva and colleagues (Meeren et al., 2002) implanted arrays of electrodes in the cortex and thalamus of unanesthetized, freely moving rats of the WAG/Rij absence epilepsy strain. Precise recording disclosed that in the initial half second of SW seizure the cortical discharge was ahead of the thalamic discharge. Moreover, there existed a stable cortical focus from which the SW activity spread to the other cortical areas at a velocity of about 1.3 m/s, the same order of magnitude found by Petsche (1962) in sick children. These speeds are compatible with synapse-to-synapse propagation. The initial focus was in the facial area of the somatosensory cortex, and, indeed, during the absence attack, the whiskers and snout of the rats twitched. Later, beyond the initial half second, the rhythm was interactive between cortex and thalamus, with no consistent leader. Phase shifts back and forth between thalamus and cortex were also observed by Petsche (1962). The seemingly perfect synchrony of SW discharges, as they appear on clinical EEG, is, according to Meeren et al. (2002), an illusion, because the conventional EEG method does not resolve the propagating wave in time or in space.

Brief Summary of Cortical and Thalamic Oscillations

Many thalamic and some cortical neurons normally have the propensity to fire in rhythmically recurring bursts. Rhythmic repetition of the bursts is initiated by a priming stimulus. Subsequent synchronization of the bursts among a population of neurons and between distant areas is mediated by synaptic pathways. Synchronized rhythmicity can be normal, generating the α rhythm and sleep spindles, or abnormal, resulting in the SW pattern of generalized absence seizures. The transition from the normal to the pathological pattern may be caused by enhanced excitability of the neocortex.

The thalamic nuclei are autonomous pacemakers of sleep spindles, but both the neocortex and the thalamus are required to produce SW seizures. The reticular and relay nuclei of the thalamus coordinate and pace the sleep spindles, while the δ waves originate mostly in neocortex. The neocortex may be the initiator of SW seizures, but eventually the rhythm becomes a joint function as the corticothalamic and thalamocortical circuits become phase-locked. Slow-wave sleep and SW seizures have this in common: the widely synchronized neuron activity makes patterned input impossible, and it effectively disconnects the forebrain from sensory input.

The Pharmacology of Spike-Wave Absence Epilepsy Differs from That of Other Ictal (Convulsive) Disorders

Strikingly, some drugs that suppress ictal seizures are either ineffective or actually worsen SW absence seizures. An exception is valproate, which is useful against absence seizures as well as other forms of epilepsy (Holmes and Riviello, 2001; McNamara, 2001). It is to be expected that drugs that enhance GABA receptor–controlled currents could aggravate absence seizures, because IPSPs and post-inhibitory rebound are essential steps in the generation of SW seizures (Chapter 11: "Drugs that modify synaptic transmission") (Coenen et al., 1995). On the other hand, ethosuximide, which is the drug of first choice for absence epilepsy, is useless in major convulsive cases (Holmes and Riviello, 2001; Leresche et al., 1998). A likely explanation is that ethosuximide in low concentration inhibits T-type calcium current, persistent Na$^+$ current, and calcium-dependent K$^+$ current, but has no effect on $I_{Na,T}$ and favors regular firing while suppressing impulse bursts (Leresche et al., 1998).

Sustained depolarization of neuron somas generates (some or all?) tonic seizures

The Cellular Mechanism of Tonic-Clonic Seizures Differs from That of Spike-Wave Seizures

Individual neurons fire action potentials at regular or irregular intervals throughout a tonic seizure discharge, but some cells tend to cease firing occasionally for short periods. The neuron population as a whole is excited as long as the seizure lasts, but individual members may pause, so to speak, to catch their breath. The pause in firing is caused by inactivation of sodium channels in the cell soma, which is strongly depolarized during tonic seizures (see below, "Hippocampal tonic seizures . . ." and Figures 7–9, 7–10, 8–1, 9–5). As already emphasized by Kandel and Spencer (1961b), however, even when the spike generator in the cell soma is inactivated, the axon can continue to fire action potentials that are conducted normally to target synapses. The impulses can be generated in a region of the axon that is close enough to the soma to be depolarized to a level above firing threshold, but far enough so that the sodium channels are not inactivated. In different cells the amplitude of the intracellularly recorded action potentials can either decrease steadily as depolarization progresses until firing stops, or irregular impulse firing can continue, with the spikes varying in size and frequency, apparently at random, with occasional gaps in the series (Fig. 7–9a). The variations in amplitude are also due to partial *inactivation of Na+ channels*. In many recordings made during tonic paroxysmal activity from the cell soma, miniature spikes replace for a while the full-sized impulses; this is attributable to action potential generation at a distance from the recording point, probably the axon. As the tonic phase nears its end and the membrane begins to repolarize, spikes can regain their normal amplitude. In the hippocampal formation the firing of pyramidal or granule cells is more precisely synchronized than in neocortex, giving rise to large-amplitude population spikes in extracellular recordings not seen in neocortex (see below) (Fig. 7–8).

Intracellular recordings nevertheless do look alike, whether from neocortex, entorhinal cortex or hippocampus, or even spinal motoneurons (Fig. 7–9). The key point is that the action potentials ride on a sustained depolarization instead of a series of EPSP waves, and between spikes, the voltage does not return to baseline but remains depolarized (Glötzner and Grüsser, 1968; Jensen and Yaari, 1997; Kandel and Spencer, 1961b, 1961c; Lopantsev and Avoli, 1998; Lothman and Somjen, 1976c; Sawa et al., 1963; Somjen et al., 1985; Sugaya et al., 1964). Some have called the sustained tonic depolarization a *paroxysmal depolarizing shift*, implying identity with the depolarizing wave of interictal discharges. There is no a priori reason to assume that the two kinds of depolarization are generated by the

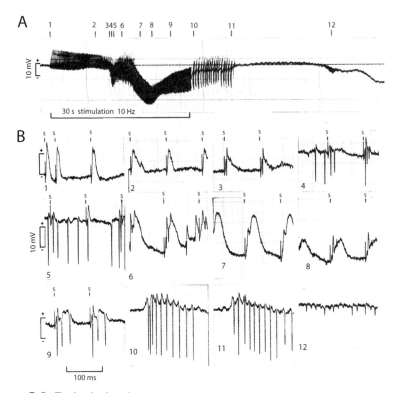

FIGURE 7–8. Tonic-clonic seizure provoked by electrical stimulation in the hippocampal formation. Extracellular recording from the granule cell layer of the dentate gyrus of an anesthetized rat. Stimulation of the perforant path (angular bundle). **A:** Continuous taped record (DC-coupled) traced by a pen recorder. Note the very large negative shift of the baseline about halfway during the stimulation. The late negative shift toward the end of the trace is the start of spreading depression (SD). **B:** Expanded segments from the tape recording played back on a digital oscilloscope. The numbers below the frames correspond to the numbers above the ink trace of A. Small "s" marks stimulus pulses. The positive waves evoked by each stimulus in frames 1–3 and 6–8 are focally recorded excitatory postsynaptic potentials (fEPSPs). Sharp negative spikes are population spikes (PSs). In frame 4, PSs appear to have been fired independently from the stimuli. In frame 5 the free-running PSs (intercurrent discharge) are more frequent and very large (lockstep firing). In frame 8 the stimulus-evoked PSs are inverted (positive), probably because the cell somas are depolarized and inactivated and the impulses are fired in the axons at a distance from the recording electrode. Frames 10 and 11 show clonic bursts. Frame 12 shows irregular firing heralding the oncoming SD. (Reproduced from Somjen et al., 1985.)

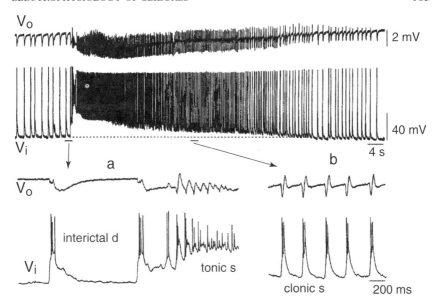

FIGURE 7–9. Interictal and tonic-clonic discharge in entorhinal cortex. Extracellular (V_o) and intracellular (V_i) recording from a neuron in layer V of lateral entorhinal cortex in a rat brain tissue slice. Epileptiform activity was induced by 4-aminopyridine (4-AP), which blocks certain K^+ channels. a and b: Expanded segments of the continuous record. The tonic seizure is initiated by an interictal discharge. The cell remains depolarized during the tonic phase (no repolarization between impulses) and during the initial part of the clonic discharge. Initially during the tonic phase the action potentials are reduced in size due to inactivation. The extracellular potential is negatively shifted, while the V_i remains depolarized. (Modified from Lopantsev and Avoli, 1998.)

same mechanism; in fact, evidence strongly suggests that the two are different. As we have seen (see above: "Interictal epileptiform bursts . . ."), the principal generator of the PDS of interictal discharges is usually in the dendritic tree, while tonic depolarization during ictal events is generated by sustained inward current in the neuron soma (Fig. 7–10). In hippocampal stratum pyramidale (cell body layer), extracellular recording of low-Mg^{2+}-induced synchronized *PDS takes the form of a positive wave* with a burst of negative population spikes (Tancredi et al., 1990). By contrast, during low-Mg^{2+}-induced ictal events, the extracellular *voltage shifts in the negative direction*, with prolonged repetitive negative population spikes. The transition from interictal to ictal discharges clearly demonstrates this contrast (Anderson et al., 1986). In other words, for the PDS, the cell somas are current *sources*; for the ictal depolarization, they are *sinks*. Before further discussion of tonic seizures, we must consider the morphology required for meaningful analysis of electrophysiological data.

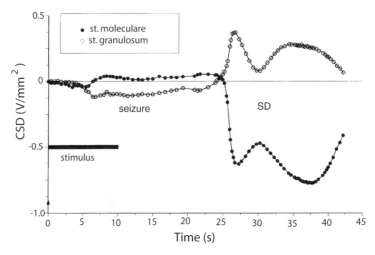

Figure 7–10. Current source density (CSD) analysis of the sustained potential shifts during seizure and spreading depression (SD). Recording from dentate gyrus (DG) of an anesthetized rat. A 16-contact miniature array of nonpolarizable electrodes was inserted in the hippocampal formation; the CSD was derived from the recordings from points within DG. Potentials were sampled at times between population spikes to obtain the CSD of the DC baseline shift. The seizure (similar to that of Fig. 7–8) and the ensuing SD were provoked by 10 s 10 Hz stimulation of the angular bundle. St. granulosum: granule cell body layer. St. moleculare: layer of apical dendrites. The points of the graph show the computed CSD of the DC baseline between discharges. Current sink plotted as negative, source as positive deflection. During the seizure, a steady current sink is maintained in the cell body layer. During SD a much larger sink develops among the dendrites. (Modified from Wadman et al., 1992.)

Cytoarchitecture of the Hippocampal Formation Favors Analysis of the Electrophysiology of Seizures

The hippocampus is a useful tissue to study epileptiform discharges, not only because it is the structure most prone to be seized, but also because of the simple arrangement of the neurons. The somas of the main neurons types, pyramidal cells in hippocampus proper and granule cells in dentate gyrus, are tightly packed in a single layer, the hippocampal stratum (st.) pyramidale and dentate st. granulosum. In these soma layers there are no dendritic trees, only thin lamellae of glial processes separating neuron cell bodies, and neuron membranes are sometimes directly apposed (Green, 1964). This is not so in neocortex, where numerous axons, dendrites, and glial processes traverse the five cell layers and the cell bodies lie farther apart. The dendritic layers of the hippocampal formation consist mainly of neuropil, a felt work of dendritic processes and axons, with many synapses plus interspersed glial tissue and only scattered interneuron cell bodies. Because of this simple architecture, extracellular recording and current source density analysis in the hippocampal formation can provide more information than the same techniques applied to neocortex or subcortical gray matter nuclei.

A note on naming

In some anatomy texts (e.g., Fig. 18–14 in *Human Neuroanatomy*, by Carpenter and Sutin, 1983), the hippocampal CA1 layer called *st. radiatum* is shown limited to the zone nearest the cell soma, containing the shafts of the apical dendrites and the commissural axons with their terminations on the dendrites. The zone where the apical dendrites divide into their main branches, and where the Schaffer collaterals and the input from septum and raphe arrive, is designated *st. lacunosum*, and the terminal branches of the dendrites form the *st. moleculare*. Following the somewhat different nomenclature of Lorente de Nó (1934), those of us who record electrical potentials from hippocampus mean by *stratum radiatum* the entire zone in which commissural fibers as well as Schaffer collaterals make excitatory connections to pyramidal cells, containing the main trunk as well as the larger branches of the apical dendrites of hippocampal pyramidal cells. Only the outermost layer, containing the final ramification of the dendritic tree, is designated the *stratum moleculare-lacunosum*. (See also Rosene and van Hoesen, 1987, for comparison of rat and primate). In electrophysiological experiments on intact brains, we find the boundaries of the layers guided by the shape of the complex potential waves evoked by electric pulses delivered to defined sites where afferent fiber bundles are known to be found (Andersen et al., 1966). The electrode locations may be confirmed later by histological tracing of the electrode tract, but the appearances of the voltage responses are so characteristic that this is not always required. In hippocampal slices, electrode placement is guided by vision through the dissecting microscope but, ultimately, the electric signal confirms the exact position (Dingledine et al., 1980).

Another note: Membranes may be depolarized by active inward currents or by passive outward currents

Membrane potentials can be depolarized or hyperpolarized by the opening of ion channels, either voltage-gated or ligand-controlled. *Inward* current through ion channels *depolarizes* and *outward* current *hyperpolarizes* neurons. The membrane potential can also be altered by current generated by an extrinsic source. The membrane then behaves passively. The source of the current imposed on a passive membrane can be an electronic stimulator, or the generator can be an active process in another part of the cell, conducted to the passive membrane by electrotonus. In either case, the *imposed current* has to flow *outward* in order to *depolarize* a passive membrane. It may be baffling at first to hear that both inward and outward currents depolarize a membrane. Here is the explanation. The direction of current flow is conventionally defined as the direction in which *positive charge moves*—which is, of course, opposite to the flow of negative charge. At rest, the membrane is positively charged on the outside relative to the inside. When Na^+ or Ca^{2+} *channels open, the inward flow of cations brings positive charge into the cell* and the standing resting membrane potential dissipates: this, by definition, is inward current. When, however, depolarization is imposed on a passive membrane by an external source, the standing charges must be neutralized. Therefore, either an intracellular electrode must *put positive charge into the* (*originally electronegative*) *inside* or an external electrode must put *negative charge on the outside*; either way, the depolarizing current imposed on a passive membrane flows outward. To hyperpolarize cells, the reverse applies. Active hyperpolarization requires the opening of channels that conduct current outward, while an external generator must supply an inward current to make the inside more negative. In other words, depolarization occurs when membrane channels *dissipate* the existing charge or when external current generators *neutralize* the existing charge.

When excitatory synapses depolarize dendrites, the entire neuron depolarizes, but more so near the synapses than farther away. At the active site, under the synaptic endings, current flows inward. In the cell body region where there are usually no or few excitatory synapses, the passive depolarizing current flows outward. When inhibitory synapses are active at or near the neuron soma, the active hyperpolarizing current flows outward and the passive current flows inward at the distal dendrites. But synaptic inhibition works not just by shifting V_m but also by increased membrane conductance, shunting excitatory current (see Chapter 6: "Malfunctioning inhibitory synapses . . .").

Current Source Density Analysis

Current source density (CSD) analysis *can accurately locate the regions where current is flowing into cells (sinks) and the regions where current emerges from cells (sources), but it does not distinguish between active and passive generators* (Howland et al., 1955; Mitzdorf, 1985; Nicholson and Freeman, 1975). Another limitation of CSD analysis is that it cannot unravel individual components when more than one current flows among the cells. In live, healthy brain under natural conditions this is, of course, the case most of the time. Current source density analysis is a powerful tool if and only if many cells in a regular geometric array are active synchronously and in the same sense, and if they dominate concomitant interference by lesser players. The regular and relatively simple cytoarchitecture of the hippocampal formation is especially suited for CSD analysis. In st. pyramidale and st. granulosum of hippocampus and dentate gyrus, extracellular signals can reliably be assumed to be generated by neuron cell bodies, while those recorded in the layers containing apical dendrites are dominated by synaptic current fields. In gray matter with more complicated architecture such as neocortex and subcortical gray matter nuclei, extracellular currents from various generators mingle, and it is hard to tune in to one of the several simultaneous broadcasters.

There are technical pitfalls to CSD studies. If recording points are spaced too far apart, sharply localized focal areas may be missed. If tissue resistance between electrode pairs varies and is not corrected for, quite erroneous maps can be derived. If many successive events are averaged, variations among individual discrete events may be missed.

Hippocampal Tonic Seizures Are Sustained by Inward Current in Neuron Somas

As we have seen, the hippocampal formation is one of the most seizure-prone structures in the brain (Gibbs and Gibbs, 1936; Kandel and Spencer, 1961c). Liberson and Cadilhac (1954) were the first to use DC-coupled amplifiers to record tonic seizure discharges in hippocampus and were able to see the "moving baseline" (*décharges sur une base mouvant*), which had escaped earlier detection because the commonly used EEG amplifiers filter out the DC component. Gloor and associates (1961, 1964) then discovered that the sustained paroxysmal voltage shift is negative in the cell body layers and positive in the layers containing apical dendrites. The polarity of the sustained voltage shifts was not only a new finding but also odd, because extracellularly recorded excitatory synaptic potentials (fEPSPs) appear as negative waves among the dendrites where the synapses are located and generate inward currents, and as positive waves among cell bodies that act as passive sources, completing the extracellular loop of the synaptic current. So-called ***population spikes***, extracellular signals representing the aggregate or ***compound action potential*** fired by a number of granule cells, have the opposite polarity of fEPSP, negative in st. granulosum (and st. pyramidale) and positive in st. granulosum (or st. radiatum) (Fig. 6–3B). This corresponds to the site of generation of action potentials at the cell soma and the initial segment of the axon. The polarity of the seizure-related DC shift was therefore opposite to that caused by synaptic excitation and parallel to the population spike. It follows that the paroxysmal DC shift had to be generated by a mechanism other than synaptic activation. Gloor's observation was largely ignored for a while, perhaps because it did not fit the general thinking prevalent at the time, which blamed seizures on excessive synaptic excitation. It is important to note that the ΔV_o during seizure-like activity induced in the absence of functioning synapses by low

$[Ca^{2+}]_o$ in hippocampal slices is also negative in st. pyramidale and positive in st. radiatum (Haas and Jefferys, 1984).

In the hippocampal formation of normal anesthetized rats, seizure-like discharges can be provoked by prolonged, repetitive stimulation of afferent pathways (Kandel and Spencer, 1961b; Purpura et al., 1966). We utilized the simplicity of the hippocampal formation to analyze the shifts in voltage and ion distribution during seizures, and we rediscovered Gloor's negative ΔV_o shift in cell soma layers (Somjen et al., 1985). (Fortunately, we came across Gloor's papers before going to press.) To provoke seizures, we stimulated the angular bundle, an easily accessible section of the perforant path connecting the entorhinal cortex to the dentate gyrus. The first few stimuli in a train evoke the expected positive fEPSP in st. granulosum (cell body layer) of the dentate gyrus (Fig. 7–8B, detail 1). If the stimulus is strong enough, then the positive fEPSP wave is interrupted by a negative population spike. After a normal fEPSP, the extracellular voltage returns to its resting or baseline level. If the stimulus is repeated at a frequency between 5 and 20 Hz, the evoked potentials soon begin to change configuration (Fig. 7–8B). The fEPSP becomes smaller, but instead of a single population spike, two or more are triggered by each stimulus pulse. If stimulation is continued for 10 or more seconds, population spikes begin to appear between the stimuli and unrelated to them. These spikes, which we termed *intercurrent*, take off on their own, independently of the stimulus-evoked fEPSPs (Fig. 7–8B, details 4–5) (Somjen et al., 1985). Coincidently with the appearance of intercurrent firing, the DC baseline in st. granulosum shifts by several millivolts in the negative direction (Fig. 7–8A), as reported earlier by Gloor et al. (1961) and confirmed again by Stringer and Lothman (1989), who termed it *maximal dentate activation* (*MDA*). Stimulus trains that are strong and long enough to provoke a negative DC shift and intercurrent population spike firing in the soma layers are often followed by a paroxysmal afterdischarge. This could be tonic in the beginning, followed by repeated clonic bursts of population spikes (Figs. 7–8, 8–2, 8–3). During the clonic bursts, the negative DC in st. granulosum (or CA1 st. pyramidale) gradually declines, and each burst of negative population spikes is superimposed on a brief positive wave (Fig. 7–8A,B, details 10, 11).

The population spikes that are fired between stimuli (intercurrently) are grafted onto the displaced baseline potential, without the benefit of EPSPs. The polarity of the sustained DC shift suggests current flowing inward into the neuron cell bodies. Current source density analysis has confirmed the presence of a *sustained sink* during tonic seizure in the *soma layer* of st. granulosum, matched by a sustained source among apical dendrites in st. moleculare (Fig. 7–10) (Wadman et al., 1992). Intracellular recording from CA1 pyramidal neurons in hippocampal slices disclosed sustained depolarization during electrically provoked seizure discharges (Somjen et al., 1985). Taken together, these convergent data confirm that the seized neurons were depolarized by steady inward current through channels in the membrane of neuron cell bodies. The apical dendrites served as mere passive sources, completing the current loop. The current flow maintaining the tonic paroxysmal firing is therefore clearly different from the PDS of interictal discharges, as well as from normal EPSPs, since in both, CSD detects the active sinks among the dendrites (Mitzdorf, 1985; Pockberger et al., 1984). In agreement with the somatic inward current generator, Gluckman et al. (1996) were able to suppress high $[K^+]_o$-induced seizure-like events in hippocampal slices by an electric field imposed on the tissue, oriented in such a way as to hyperpolarize the soma and depolarize the dendrites of the seized pyramidal cells.

The mechanism of the somatic inward current was not immediately obvious. The generators could be either synaptic or voltage-operated channels. Synapses on hippocampal pyramidal cell somas are, however, for the most part GABA-operated and inhibitory (Andersen et al., 1964). Ordinarily, the activation of GABA receptor–operated synapses induces hyperpolarization. As already mentioned, the Cl^--dependent $GABA_A$ effect can turn into depolarization if the equilibrium potential, E_{Cl}, shifts to a more positive level than the resting potential (see Chapter 6: "Malfunctioning inhibitory synapses . . .") (Andersen et al., 1980). Much earlier, Purpura et al. (1966) noted that both EPSPs and IPSPs tend to subside during repetitive afferent stimulation (see also Whittington et al., 1995). We (Somjen et al., 1985) speculated that during the repetitive activation the pyramidal cells could have become loaded with Cl^-, causing a positive shift of E_{Cl} . But the fading of IPSPs could also be explained by desensitization of the GABA receptors. Ben-Ari and Krnjević (1981) favored this explanation because they found that the GABA-induced conductance change was suppressed together with the hyperpolarizing IPSP. Choking $GABA_A$-operated channels would suppress IPSPs but would not depolarize the cell. Nonetheless, more recently, Bracci et al. (1999) attributed the steady depolarization of hippocampal neurons following tetanic stimulation to $GABA_A$-mediated "inverted" inhibition. Bracci et al. term this phenomenon *post-tetanic γ activity*, but they also conclude that this "may well have more to do with epilepsy than with cognition."

The steady depolarization of neuron somas could also be due to sustained voltage-gated inward current provided, for example, by a persistent Na^+ current, $I_{Na,P}$, or any of the nonspecific cation currents, possibly also assisted by window current of $I_{Na,T}$ or $I_{Ca,T}$. Rising $[K^+]_o$ can enhance $I_{Na,P}$ (Somjen and Müller, 2000) and, of course, $[K^+]_o$ does increase during repetitive afferent stimulation (Fig. 8–2) (Somjen and Giacchino, 1985). In this scenario, $I_{Na,P}$ would be sufficiently activated to trigger a self-sustained afterdischarge when both depolarization of V_m and the rise of $[K^+]_o$ reaches critical levels. Computer simulation shows that such a cooperative action of ΔV_m , $\Delta [K^+]_o$, and $I_{Na,P}$ could indeed result in tonic paroxysmal firing (Fig. 9–5) (Kager et al., 2001, and Chapter 9).

Hippocampal Pyramidal Neurons Fire in Lockstep during Seizures

The nature of the free-running population spikes seen during paroxysmal discharge was puzzling (Fig. 7–8B, details 4, 5). These reliably appear in recordings of hippocampal tonic paroxysmal seizures in st. granulosum of DG or st. pyramidale of CA1 (Bracci et al., 1999; Gloor et al., 1961; Somjen et al., 1985; Stringer et al., 1989). During prolonged, repetitive stimulation, these large-amplitude compound action potentials appear in between the stimulus-induced responses when the negative shift of the DC baseline starts, and they can continue during the afterdischarge. Having unusual amplitudes of 10–30 mV and a duration of 2–3 ms, they must represent the near-simultaneous firing of many of the tightly packed neuron cells bodies. Most puzzling was the absence of a discernible synaptic potential that could have triggered and synchronized the spikes. There are no known examples of similarly large-amplitude, extracellularly recorded compound action potentials elsewhere in brain tissue. We called this exceptional temporal coordination *lockstep firing* (Somjen et al., 1985). Only electrical interaction among the cells could explain the temporal locking of their excitation. Electrical coupling can come about in two ways. If two cells lie close enough, the current of action of one can penetrate the membrane of the other sufficiently to influence the timing of the excitation of the second cell, a mechanism known as *ephaptic interaction* (Fig. 7–11) (Dudek et al., 1986; Jefferys, 1995; Snow and Dudek, 1984a). Neuron somas are packed close enough in the hippocampal formation, especially in st. pyramidale of the CA1 sector, to enable the injection of a significant fraction of the action current of one neuron into the membrane of its neighbor, and there is experimental evidence for ephaptic interaction among hippocampal neurons during low calcium-induced (synapse-free) as well as picrotoxin-induced (synaptically sustained) seizures (Jefferys, 1995; Snow and Dudek, 1984a). Alternatively, the phase locking may be achieved by *gap junctions* between neurons (Dudek et al., 1983; Köhling et al., 2001; Rash et al., 2001).

Gap Junctions among Neurons Are Important for Seizure Generation

Gap junctions exist among neurons in the hippocampal formation and in neocortex. Even though their number diminishes with age, they never disappear (Connors et al., 1983; Dudek et al., 1983; Kandler and Katz, 1995; Knowles et al., 1982; MacVicar and Dudek, 1980; Rash et al., 2001). Most reports concern gap junctions among neuron dendrites, but recently Schmitz et al. (2001) reported that gap junctions also couple the axons of hippocampal pyramidal neurons. They point out that it is sufficient for each axon is joined to one or two of its neighbors in order to generate a tightly coupled mass discharge in a population. They also speculate that gap junctions may be modulated by messenger substances as well as internal pH. Lockstep firing could result from the wide opening of such junctions

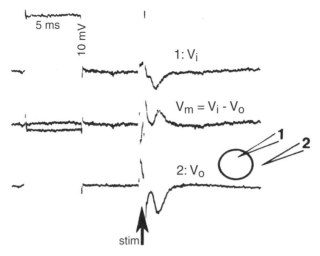

FIGURE 7–11. Ephaptic interaction among neurons. Simultaneous recording from inside (V_i) and immediately outside (V_o) a CA1 pyramidal cell in a rat hippocampal slice. Synaptic transmission was blocked by low $[Ca^{2+}]$ and Mn^{2+}. The stimulus was an antidromic volley below threshold for the axon of the recorded cell but above threshold for some of its neighbors. The middle trace shows the true membrane potential change obtained by subtracting V_i from V_o. Note that the 10 mV calibration pulse seen at the beginning of the V_i and V_o traces disappears in the subtracted trace. The small positive wave after the stimulus artifact on the V_m trace is caused by ephaptic current generated by the action potential of adjacent cells traversing the recorded cell's membrane. Even though the ephaptic wave is small, if it is superimposed on other sources of excitation (such as tonic paroxysmal depolarization), it could force the phase-locking of the action potentials fired by the neuron population. (Modified from Taylor and Dudek, 1984.)

during seizures. Traub et al. (2001) found support for this concept in both experiments and computer simulations. Earlier, Herreras et al. (1994) proposed a similar mechanism for the impulse showers that propagate ahead of a wave of SD (see also Chapter 16: "Mechanisms of spreading depression propagation").

Gap junctions probably serve to synchronize the impulse bursts that erupt in brain slices when extracellular Ca^{2+} is removed, for in the absence of Ca^{2+}, synapses cease to operate (Haas and Jefferys, 1984; Chapter 6: "Nonsynaptic epileptogenesis"). Closing such junctions, either by intracellular acidification or by selectively acting drugs, suppresses seizures in brain tissue slices even in the presence of functioning synapses, underscoring the importance of gap junctions for seizure generation. Recently, Köhling et al. (2001) showed that drugs that block gap junctions prevent the transition from interictal to ictal activity in hippocampal slices bathed in zero magnesium solution. In another study, Jahromi et al. (2002) reduced epileptiform afterdischarges evoked by trains of electrical stimuli in the presence of moderately elevated $[K^+]_o$ by blocking gap junctions. Importantly, they also showed that closing the gap junctions did not reduce the electrical excitability of the neurons. Rather, neuron input impedance increased as the electrical communication between neurons was blocked. Consequently, excitability, as gauged from the number of spikes fired in response to a depolarizing pulse, actually increased; nonetheless epileptiform activity decreased.

Neurons in Neocortex Depolarize Similarly to Hippocampal
Pyramidal Cells During Tonic Seizure Discharge

During tonic seizure neurons in neocortex, like those in hippocampus, fire action potentials that are triggered from a steadily depolarized baseline membrane potential (Fig. 7–9). The depolarization can become strong enough to inactivate the action potentials intermittently. During the clonic phase, the membrane potential fluctuates in synchrony with the EEG. After the seizure, during the postictal EEG silence, the membrane potential is usually hyperpolarized (Glötzner and Grüsser, 1968). The sustained depolarization is similar to that seen in hippocampal neurons, but there is no lockstep synchronization of impulses (Fig. 7–9). Only the slow paroxysmal waves underlying the PDS and the rhythmic clonic depolarizations are synchronized among cells, not the spikes that ride the crests of the slow waves.

Are Posttetanic γ-β Oscillations a Form of Paroxysmal Afterdischarge?

Synchronized EEG waves recorded in healthy brains have received much attention recently, because they are thought to be essential for pattern recognition and other cognitive functions and perhaps for the conscious state (Engel et al., 1999, 2001; Joliot et al., 1994). Finely patterned synchrony is described as *binding* the activities of anatomically separated neuron groups. Roughly translated, neuron *ensembles* tuned to the same oscillatory frequency together represent, or map, cogent cognitive content. In particular, rhythms in the γ (30–100 Hz) and θ (4–7.5 Hz) range (Niedermeyer et al., 1999) demand attention—and have provoked controversy (Joliot et al., 1994). The γ frequency activity can be detected using advanced analysis in the hippocampus of unanesthetized, freely moving rats (Bragin et al., 1995) and anesthetized cats (Steriade and Amzica, 1996) and cortical EEG of humans (Joliot et al., 1994; Tallon-Baudry et al., 1999).

Regular, high-frequency synchronized activity can be triggered in hippocampal slices by electrical stimulation, and it seemed at first that analysis of this activity could elucidate the mechanism of the physiological γ oscillations (Jefferys et al., 1996; Traub et al., 1997). In the wake of patterned tetanic stimulus trains, the hippocampal slice generates reproducible extended sequences of large-amplitude population spikes, attesting to the precise synchronization of the firing of many neurons, rather similar to the lockstep firing seen in a paroxysmal afterdischarge (Somjen et al., 1985) (Fig. 7–8). The posttetanic γ afterdischarge starts at a high frequency, which then declines. This has been described as the γ-β *transition*, because the initial rate is >30 Hz and the final rate 10–25 Hz (Bracci et al., 2001; Traub et al., 1999b). The transition can be sudden when pyramidal cells start to "miss alternate beats." At this β phase, subliminal V_m oscillations (presumably synaptic potentials) still continue at the initial γ frequency, but only every second of these oscillations triggers an action potential, so that the "output" frequency is halved and it drops into the β range. With other stimulus parameters, however, a different pattern ensues in which the decline in frequency is not abrupt but smooth and gradual, and the dividing line between the γ and β phases seems arbitrary (Bracci et al., 1999). In either case, the extracellular oscillations and population spikes ride on a steady ΔV_o that is negative in st. pyramidale, and the intracellular traces show oscillations superimposed on a sustained depolarization. Based on experiments in hippocampal slices as well as computer simulations, Traub, Jefferys, and colleagues conclude that the posttetanic γ phenomenon requires (*1*) a steady depolarizing influence on pyramidal neurons, presumably glutamatergic, and (*2*) synchronous oscillating IPSPs generated by synaptically interconnected populations of inhibitory interneurons pacing the rhythm that entrains the pyramidal cells. Pyramidal neurons either fire at the rebound of each IPSP (Fig. 7–7) or, in other cases, the IPSPs invert into depolarizing potentials, perhaps due to the Cl⁻ loading of the cells (Bracci et al., 2001; Traub et al., 1996b; 1999b).

It is, of course, not at all certain that the hard-to-detect γ frequency ripples of the EEG of alert human subjects have the same biophysical basis as the fast oscillations in the cortex of anesthetized cats (Steriade and Amzica, 1996) or the high-frequency population spikes evoked by stimulus trains in hippocampal slices (Traub et al., 1996b). The published illustrations of the in vitro γ phenomenon look very much like recordings from hippocampus in seizure (Gloor et al., 1961; Liberson and Cadilhac, 1954; Somjen et al., 1985, 1986). Surveying their data, Bracci et al. (1999) also came to the conclusion that "post-tetanic gamma discharge may turn out to have more to do with epilepsy than with cognition." Moreover, high-frequency EEG oscillations, even faster than the γ rhythm, can herald the onset of major seizures in human patients (Traub et al., 2001).

Clonic Repeating Bursts Can Be Generated by Synaptic Interaction or by an Interplay of Intrinsic Currents and Ion Shifts

In classical generalized tonic-clonic or grand mal seizures, tonic spasm of much of the skeletal musculature is followed by a series of repeated brief clonic convulsions. The electrophysiological counterpart of clonic muscle convulsions is a series of repeated synchronized impulse bursts. In experimentally induced seizures such repeated bursts can follow tonic seizure discharge, or they can arise without an antecedent tonic seizure. In intracellular recordings from central neurons, groups of action potentials ride the crest of waves of depolarization that resemble repeating PDSs (Figs. 5–1B, 7–9 b). The entire series of depolarizing waves may be superimposed on a gradually declining depolarized baseline, which is the "tail" of the preceding tonic depolarization, or else the clonic waves can erupt from a normal resting or even a hyperpolarized baseline membrane potential (Figs. 7–8, 7–9) (Somjen et al., 1985; Traub et al., 1996a).

How Much Do Glial Cells Contribute to the Paroxysmal Extracellular Direct Current Shifts?

During a tonic seizure the EEG fluctuates irregularly at relatively high frequency and large amplitude (Fig. 5–2) (Chapter 5: "Electroencephalography in epilepsy"). Direct current recording from the cortical surface shows a sustained negative shift of the baseline voltage on which the voltage fluctuations ride (Figs. 7–9, 8–4) (Gumnit and Takahashi, 1965; Ikeda et al., 1996, 1999; Lothman et al., 1975; O'Leary and Goldring, 1964; Sugaya et al., 1964). In clinical DC-coupled EEG recordings, a sustained negative voltage shift may be recorded during SW absence episodes as well as during tonic-clonic seizures (Ikeda et al., 1999, 2000; Petsche, 1962).

The DC-EEG voltage shifts recorded during seizures from the scalp or the cortical surface were at first attributed to inward current in apical neuron dendrites, but O'Leary and Goldring (1964) speculated about a possible glial component (see also Ikeda et al., 1999; Speckmann and Elger, 1999). Scalp recordings provide no clue to the possibly multiple interfering processes that generate the voltage shift. The skin is not only a long way from the brain, but is also separated from it by many layers of tissue. Besides neurons and glia, there are also epithelial and endothelial (BBB) as well as blood flow-born streaming potentials to be considered (Voipio et al., 2003). A negative scalp ΔV during the tonic phase of a seizure, even if cerebral in origin, is more likely to be of glial than neuronal origin, because distal apical dendrites probably supply positive (source) extracellular current during tonic seizures (Fig. 7–10) (see above: "Hippocampal tonic seizures . . .").

Intracellular recordings made from neurons in neocortex and spinal cord during tonic-clonic seizures are quite similar to those from hippocampal pyramidal cells. Direct current–coupled extracellular recordings are, however, different. Paroxysmal **sustained potential shifts** (SP shifts, ΔV_o) in the spinal cord and the neocortex are negative through the entire depth of gray matter, albeit not to an equal degree in all layers (Ikeda et al., 2000; Lothman and Somjen, 1976b, 1976c; Lothman et al., 1975), while in the hippocampal formation the cell body layers become negative but the apical dendritic layers either remain unchanged or shift in the positive direction (Gloor et al., 1961; Somjen et al., 1985) (Figs. 7–8, 8–2, 8–3). For reasons mentioned, interpretation of extracellular voltages and CSD of neocortex is not unambiguous. There is, however, much evidence that the glial contribution is greater in neocortex than it is in the hippocampal formation (Ransom, 1974; Somjen, 1993).

Some of the earliest intracellular recordings from presumed glial cells were made during experimentally induced acute seizures (Glötzner and Grüsser, 1968; Ransom, 1974) and electrical stimulation of the tissue (Ransom and Goldring, 1973b; Somjen, 1970). Prior to their positive identification, the cells were called, cautiously, *silent* or *unresponsive* or *presumed glia*. At first it seemed possible that these were nonspiking neurons or even unresponsive passive neuron dendritic processes, but intracellular marking and postmortem histology identified them unambiguously as glia, usually astrocytes. What these recordings had in common was, first, a resting potential on average more negative than that of neurons; second, the absence of action potentials, synaptic potentials, or any others sign of active membrane responses; and third, a slow depolarization during excitation of neurons in the neighborhood, with no change in the input resistance of the glial cells themselves. The absence of a membrane resistance response indicated passive depolarization due to elevated $[K^+]_o$, in line with the earlier discoveries of Kuffler and collaborators on glia in cold-blooded creatures (Kuffler and Nicholls, 1966) (see Chapter 2: "The plasma membrane of astrocytes").

Observations on *Necturus* optic nerve (Orkand et al., 1966) reinforced the suspicion (O'Leary and Goldring, 1964) that depolarization of glial cells can generate DC shift in CNSs. Glial generation of ΔV_o shifts in spinal cord was confirmed by recordings from spinal cords. Repetitive stimulation of spinal dorsal roots or afferent nerves causes a remarkably large, stable, and reproducible negative shift of the extracellular voltage that permeates the entire gray matter of the spinal segments served by the afferent input (Somjen, 1970). This sustained potential shift was clearly correlated with depolarization of glial cells, and not at all with the activity of neurons. A three-way correlation was later established between extracellular ΔV_o shift, glial depolarization, and transient increase of $[K^+]_o$ in spinal gray matter (Fig. 7–9) (Lothman and Somjen, 1975). As far as neocortex is concerned, others have found the correlation of $[K^+]_o$ and glial membrane potential (Castellucci and Goldring, 1970; Ransom and Goldring, 1973b), and we have established the correlation of $[K^+]_o$ and sustained extracellular potential shifts, during electrical stimulation of normal cortex as well as during seizures (see reviews by Somjen, 1973, 1993). The effect of K^+-induced glial depolarization dominates the ΔV_o shift most closely in spinal cord and somewhat less so but still strongly in neocortex. $[K^+]_o$ increases when many neurons are simultaneously excited, and they dump K^+ ions into the interstitium faster than they can be removed by reuptake by the neuronal 3Na/2K-stimulated ATPase plus the glial buffer System (see Fig. 2–7, Chapter 2). Glial depolarization is detected by extracellular electrodes if and only if different regions of the glial electrical net (or quasi-syncytium) are depolarized unequally (Fig. 2–10) (Dietzel et al., 1989; Joyner and

Somjen, 1973). Uniform depolarization does not generate current in the extracellular medium.

The question then is, what about the contribution of glial tissue in hippocampus? Is it reasonable that we have ignored glia in the interpretation of CSD data from hippocampus (Fig. 7–10), as if the signal was produced exclusively by neurons? It appears that in the hippocampal formation glial tissue contributes little or nothing to extracellular DC. This is so in spite of the fact that, similarly to neocortex and spinal cord, repetitive afferent stimulation causes glial cells in hippocampus to depolarize. Yet unlike neocortex, the glial depolarization in hippocampus is not accompanied by a correlated extracellular voltage shift (Casullo and Krnjević, 1987). Also, laminar analysis of DC shifts and $[K^+]_o$ changes during seizure discharges led to the conclusion that the sustained potential shifts were of neuronal rather than glial origin (Somjen and Giacchino, 1985; Somjen et al., 1985). The likely explanation is that glial processes are sparse in hippocampal formation compared to neocortex or other parts of the CNS. Green (1964) commented on the scarcity of glial tissue in the cell body layers of the hippocampal formation. Kuffler, (1967) and Kuffler and Nicholls (1966) estimated that about 50% of the volume of gray matter in mammalian neocortex and cerebellum is occupied by glial processes. Casual inspection of published illustrations of hippocampus (e.g., Westrum and Blackstad, 1962) and of electron micrographs kindly provided some years ago by colleagues in pathology and pharmacology suggest that in hippocampus the glia/neuron volume ratio must be much lower than 1:1. There are more glial elements in neuropil than in cell body layers, but even among the dendrites there do not appear to be nearly enough glia to fill 50% of the total volume. I can find no published quantitative analysis comparing the glial volume fraction in neocortex and hippocampus. Clearly, this matter asks for quantitative work, even if the effort is dauntingly tedious.

In conclusion

High $[K^+]_o$-induced depolarization of astrocytes is mainly responsible for sustained extracellular potentials shifts in the spinal cord; it contributes a major fraction to such potentials in neocortex, but adds little to the extracellular DC shifts in hippocampal formation. This is of practical interest for the interpretation of DC-coupled extracellular electrical recordings.

How do seizures stop?

What stops a seizure is as much a problem as what starts it. If the process is self-sustaining, why does it not go on forever? According to Treiman and Heinemann (1998), the mechanisms of seizure termination are poorly understood.

In general, ictal seizures are followed by a prolonged depressed state. In human patients, tonic-clonic fits are followed by ***postictal coma*** and an extended period of exhaustion. Over the years several explanations have emerged, and each could be valid in some but not all cases.

1. *Depolarization-induced inactivation* was perhaps the first proposal to explain the ultimate extinction of epileptic attacks and the inexcitable state that follows them (Fertziger and Ranck, 1970). Intracellular recordings seemed to refute this contention because, instead of depolarization, at the end of a seizure neurons usually are hyperpolarized and remain so for a while (Glötzner and Grüsser, 1968; Kandel and Spencer, 1961b). Yet sometimes experimentally induced seizures are terminated by SD (Fig. 7–10). Spreading depression involves nearly complete depolarization of neurons, it extinguishes all neuronal activity, and its recovery is followed by strong hyperpolarization and prolonged inexcitability (see also Part III). Bragin et al. (1997) addressed the mechanism of the termination of electrically provoked paroxysmal afterdischarges in anesthetized rats. In their work, the end of afterdischarges was heralded by high-frequency oscillations in the cell body layer generated by depolarizing waves of pyramidal cells, which they termed *afterdischarge termination oscillations* (*ATOs*). The oscillations were followed by a very large negative shift of the extracellular potential in the dendritic layers, whose intracellular counterpart was major depolarization and inactivation of the firing of neurons. The depolarization propagated slowly and had all the other characteristics of SD waves. The authors suggested that the propagating depolarization was primarily caused by K^+ spilled by neurons, and that it was conducted by interaction among glial cells and neurons.

   Whether or not SD-like depolarization plays a part in human epilepsy is not known. However, it seems plausible that it does occur, especially in generalized status epilepticus.

2. *Postictal hyperpolarization* is most frequently seen in intracellular recordings at the termination of the discharge of seized neurons (Glötzner and Grüsser, 1968; Kandel and Spencer, 1961b). It is generated by a combination of IPSPs and voltage-gated and calcium-controlled K^+ currents, assisted by the electrogenic 3Na/2K ATP-fueled ion pump (Jefferys and Roberts, 1987).

3. *Metabolic processes* may play a role. Simple depletion of the readily available transmitter pool may be a factor. Also, acidification of ECF due to accumulation of lactic acid and CO_2 can reduce neuronal excitability (Chapter 4: "Protons inhibit . . ."). Elevated levels of lactate have been measured in human patients during and after seizures (During et al., 1994).

Key points

Sustained depolarization evokes in some neurons regular spiking and in others recurrent high-frequency spike bursts separated by silent intervals. Burst firing can be governed by Ca^{2+} current, usually in dendrites, or by persistent Na^+ current, usually in cell soma.

Sporadic abnormal burst firing by neurons underlies interictal EEG discharges. Interictal bursts are the result of PDSs in neurons that, in most cases, are started by "giant" EPSPs, which then trigger dendritic Ca^{2+} currents. The EPSPs that initiate the PDS may be exaggerated by multiple firing in presynaptic axon terminals. However, not all PDSs are produced by the same mechanism.

Spike-wave seizures result from the abnormal functioning of thalamocortical rhythm generators. The EEG spike represents depolarization; the wave, hyperpolarization of individual neurons. Synaptic and intrinsic currents interact in producing the pattern. Rebound excitation following hyperpolarizing waves is essential for setting the rhythm. The primacy of cortex or thalamus is disputed, but both are required for the complete pattern.

During SW absence seizures the patient's awareness of the surrounding is interrupted, because the rhythmic burst discharges of thalamic neuron populations interdict receipt and processing of sensory signals.

Sustained depolarization of neuron somas underlies the tonic seizure discharge. The tonic depolarization is not generated by excitatory synapses and its mechanism differs from that of PDSs. In hippocampal formation (but not in neocortex) the action potentials of many neurons are strictly synchronized in a lockstep pattern, probably achieved through ephaptic interaction.

Sustained extracellular voltage shifts evoked by repetitive electrical stimulation and accompanying seizure discharges are generated mostly by glial depolarization in spinal cord, in part by glia in neocortex, but mostly by neurons in the hippocampal formation.

Major epileptic attacks end in postictal coma followed by a prolonged period of exhaustion. Experimentally induced seizure discharges are usually stopped by hyperpolarization of the participating neurons. The hyperpolarization results from K^+ current and the electrogenic effect of ion pumps. Less commonly, SD interrupts seizures. Metabolic acidosis and exhaustion of transmitters and their precursors perhaps play a part in the clinical postictal depressed state.

8

Ions and Seizures

During seizure discharges the concentration of potassium in cerebral ISF increases, and the concentrations of calcium and sodium decrease (Figs. 8–2, 8–3, 8–4) (Heinemann et al., 1977; Hotson et al., 1973; Lothman et al., 1975; Lux and Heinemann, 1978; Somjen, 1980; Somjen and Giacchino, 1985; Somjen et al., 1986). These changes in extracellular concentration are due to the release of K^+ from and the influx of Na^+ and Ca^{2+} into excited neurons. On balance, more ions enter than leave cells, glia as well as neurons. Because of the net gain of osmotic equivalents, cells swell and the interstitial volume fraction ((ISVF) decreases (Lux et al., 1986). Even though some of the Cl^- ions also leave the interstitial space, $[Cl^-]_o$ usually increases slightly, because water is moving from the extracellular to the intracellular compartment faster than are Cl^- ions (Dietzel et al., 1980, 1982). At the start of a seizure the pH of the ECF becomes alkaline; then a slow acidosis takes over. According to Kaila and Chesler (1998), two membrane transports produce the alkalinization, a Ca^{2+}-dependent uptake of H^+ into cells, and the $GABA_A$-induced outflow of HCO_3 (see Chapter 6: "Malfunctioning inhibitory synapses . . ."). The slow acidosis is produced by metabolic processes. Some of these changes, high $[K^+]_o$, low $[Ca^{2+}]_o$, alkalinization and osmotically induced cell swelling, facilitate paroxysmal discharge and could be factors in keeping seizures going (Andrew, 1991; Korn et al., 1987; McBain, 1994). Only the late acidosis could assist in stopping seizures (Chapter 7: "How do seizures stop?"). In the following pages, we shall examine the significance of each ion for epileptiform discharge.

Potassium and seizures

Too Much Extracellular Potassium Can Induce Seizures

Feldberg and Sherwood (1957) injected small amounts of a KCl solution into the lateral ventricle of cats through a permanently implanted cannula. The animals were seized by epileptiform convulsions. More than a decade later, Zuckerman and Glaser (1968, 1970a) perfused the lateral ventricle with artificial CSF in which the K^+ concentration was elevated and recorded electrographic seizure activity in the hippocampus. Subsequently, they also recorded the DC shift that accompanied the K^+-induced seizure and suggested that this sustained negative potential represented depolarization of neurons by the excess K^+ (Zuckermann and Glaser, 1970b).

With the widespread use of isolated slices of brain tissue, it became possible to study the conditions for K^+-induced seizures more precisely. Modest elevation of $[K^+]$ in the bathing fluid facilitated the triggering of electrically induced paroxysmal activity (Somjen et al., 1985). With 5.5 mM $[K^+]$ in the bath, the concentration used as the normal control by some laboratories, it was easier to provoke seizure-like afterdischarges than at the true normal concentration of 3–3.5 mM. Between 7 and 8 mM $[K^+]_o$ spontaneous activity erupts (Jensen and Yaari, 1997; Korn et al., 1987; Rutecki et al., 1985; Traynelis and Dingledine, 1988), and it can take the form of brief interictal discharges or more prolonged ictal events (Fig. 8–1). Several of the effects of high $[K^+]_o$ described in Chapter 4 ("Changing potassium levels . . .") can promote epileptiform activity. Moderate depolarization of neurons brings the membrane closer to the firing threshold, and stronger depolarization can induce firing. Excessive depolarization, on the other hand, suppresses excitation, as Na^+ channels are inactivated and the cell becomes inexcitable. Added to the directly exciting effect of high $[K^+]_o$ is the depolarization of presynaptic terminals that can trigger uncalled-for firing of action potentials and activation of voltage-gated calcium channels, causing inappropriate release of transmitter substances. As a third effect, excess $[K^+]_o$ forces the uptake of Cl^-, which renders $GABA_A$-mediated synaptic inhibition less effective (Chamberlin and Dingledine, 1988; Korn et al., 1987). Finally, high $[K^+]_o$ potentiates $I_{Na,P}$ (Somjen and Müller, 2000).

Adding interest (or perhaps confusion?) to the story, too low $[K^+]_o$ can also cause seizure-like discharges (Gorji et al., 2001) or favor ictal over interictal activity (Bragdon et al., 1992).

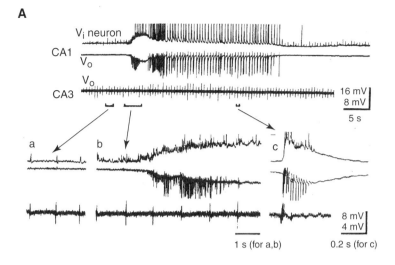

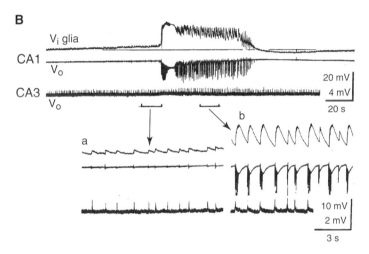

Figure 8–1. Tonic-clonic seizures induced by elevated extracellular potassium. Spontaneous seizures erupt in rat hippocampal slices bathed in fluid containing 8.5 mM K+. **A:** Recording from a CA1 pyramidal cell (V_i), from its extracellular neighborhood (V_o), and from the CA3. The 8 mV calibration is for V_o, the 16 mV for V_i. a–c: Expanded portions of the continuous traces. a: Before the ictal event, CA3 generated brief interictal discharges synaptically transmitted to CA1. b: CA3 does not participate in the ictal seizure of CA1. The profound depolarization of the CA1 neuron during the tonic phase and the start of the clonic discharge is accompanied by a negative shift of V_o, similar to dentate gyrus stratum granulosum in Figures 7–8, 8–2B. c: A clonic burst. **B:** Intracellular potential of a glial cell in CA1 and V_o in CA1 and CA3 recorded simultaneously. **a:** Before seizure onset the glial cell slowly depolarizes, with small superimposed transients coinciding with interictal discharges. This premonitory slow depolarization indicates a gradual increase of $[K^+]_o$. A much larger, sudden depolarization marks the onset of the ictal seizure. **b:** Waves of glial depolarization with each clonic impulse burst. (Modified from Traynelis and Dingledine, 1988.)

The Potassium Hypothesis of Seizure Generation

Based on meager facts, Green (1964) proposed that K^+ ions released from excited neurons and accumulating in narrow interstitial spaces could cause epileptiform seizures. It was, however, the paper by Fertziger and Ranck (1970) that clearly formalized the *potassium hypothesis of seizure generation*. The authors envisioned a positive feedback loop, or vicious circle, in which overexcited neurons discharged excess K^+ into the interstitium, which then reinforced the excitation and rendered a seizure self-sustaining. According to their scheme, seizures terminated when K^+-induced depolarization eventually inactivated Na^+ currents, stopping the discharge and terminating the release of more K^+ (Fig. 9–8B).

Potassium Accumulates in Interstitial Fluid during Seizures

To accept the potassium hypothesis, it was necessary to demonstrate that excess K^+ accumulates in ECF during seizures. Fertziger and Ranck (1970) measured the K^+ concentration at the surface of the brain and found that excess potassium was oozing from the surface during seizures. Recordings of the depolarization of so-called *idle cells* (correctly assumed to be glia) confirmed that $[K^+]_o$ increases during seizures (Sugaya and Karahashi, 1971) (Fig. 8–1B). Finally, the introduction of potassium-selective microelectrodes enabled direct recording of potassium levels in interstitial spaces (Vyskocil et al., 1972; Walker, 1971). Using these probes, several laboratories recorded the impressive rise of $[K^+]_o$ during seizures (Figs. 8–2, 8–4). During interictal discharges, brief modest increases were seen, but a much larger elevation was consistently recorded during many different types of ictal events (Amzica et al., 2002; Lehmenkühler, 1988; Lothman and Somjen, 1976a; Lothman et al., 1975; Lux, 1973; Moody et al., 1974; Prince et al., 1973; Sypert and Ward, 1974; Vern et al., 1979). During sustained seizures $[K^+]_o$ reached or at least approached the "ceiling" of 8–12 mM (Heinemann and Lux, 1977; Moody et al., 1974). The level of $[K^+]_o$ reached during seizures is sufficient to induce seizures in isolated brain slice preparations, a key requirement for the acceptance of the potassium hypothesis (Jensen and Yaari, 1997; Korn et al., 1987; Rutecki et al., 1985; Schweitzer and Williamson, 1995; Traynelis and Dingledine, 1988).

The main route by which K^+ leaves seized neurons is via voltage-gated and Ca^{2+}-stimulated K^+ channels. In hippocampus, $[K^+]_o$ reaches considerably higher levels in cell body layers than in the layers containing dendrites and neuropil (Figs. 8–2, 8–3D) (Somjen and Giacchino, 1985). There are two reasons: the interstitial spaces are narrower here, although not by very much (McBain et al., 1990), and the currents related to impulses and their afterpotentials are maximally dense through the membranes of cell body and axons (Wadman et al., 1992). Still, smaller but not negligible contributions probably come through synaptic currents. The $GABA_B$

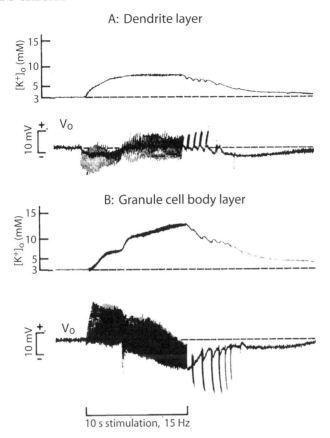

FIGURE 8–2. Extracellular potassium level during seizure. Recording with a double-barreled ion-selective electrode from dentate gyrus, stimulation of the angular bundle, in an anesthetized rat (similar to Fig. 7–8). A and B from the same animal at different times. $[K^+]_o$ starts to increase as soon as stimulation begins. At the onset of the seizure, $[K^+]_o$ gets an extra boost in the granule cell body layer, but it remains flat among the dendrites. A large negative shift of the V_o baseline marks the seizure in stratum granulosum, but at the same time in the dendrite layer, V_o shifts in the positive direction. Note also opposite polarities of the V_o deflections in the two layers during clonic afterdischarge. (Modified from Somjen and Giacchino, 1985.)

receptor–controlled channels are selectively permeable to K^+ ions. Perhaps more importantly, glutamate-induced EPSPs are generated by channels permeable to both Na^+ and K^+. The more the membrane depolarizes, the greater the driving force pushing K^+ out; on the other hand, growth of the ratio $[K^+]_o/[K^+]_i$ slows the outward flow. Depolarization diminishes the driving force moving Na^+ into the cell.

The steady ceiling level to which $[K^+]_o$ rises during prolonged ictal seizures is established when a balance is reached between the outflow from and uptake into

DG, dendrite layer

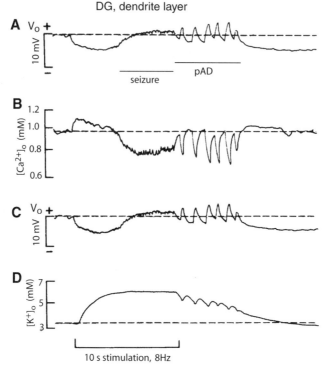

FIGURE 8–3. Extracellular calcium and potassium level changes during seizure compared. Simultaneous recording with two double-barreled ion-selective electrodes in the stratum moleculare of the dentate gyrus of an anesthetized rat. Stimulation of angular bundle. The recordings were low-pass filtered to emphasize sustained changes. **B.** At the beginning of stimulation $[Ca^{2+}]_o$ increased, but then it markedly decreased during the tonic seizure and during each wave of clonic afterdischarge. **C** and **D** are similar to Figure 8–2A. pAD: paraoxysmal afterdischarge.

cells. Some of the K^+ ions are being pumped back into the same excited neurons that lost them and others are taken up by glial cells, probably mainly astrocytes (Fig. 2–7) (Chapter 2). Glial cells accumulate excess K^+ both actively and passively, fulfilling their function as K^+-buffers. The glial membrane 3Na/2K pump is stimulated by elevated $[K^+]_o$, releasing Na^+ while taking in K^+. Some of the passive K^+ flux equalizes the electric charge imbalance created by the 3Na/2K pump and some of it drives the "spatial buffer" (Chapter 2: "Glial cells . . .") (Figs. 2–7, 2–10). Some of the entering K^+ is accompanied by Cl^-, causing osmotic swelling of glia (see below).

Recordings of $[K^+]_o$ Lead to the Rejection of the Potassium
Hypothesis—Perhaps Prematurely

With ion-selective electrodes, it became possible to follow the magnitude and time course of ion concentration changes (Lothman and Somjen, 1976a; Lothman et al., 1975; Lux, 1973, 1974; Prince et al., 1973). In spite of the consistently impressive levels of $[K^+]_o$ recorded during seizures, such measurements have led several investigators (alas, including me) to reject the potassium hypothesis (Benninger et al., 1980; Futamachi et al., 1974; Lux, 1974; Lux and Heinemann, 1978; Pedley et al., 1976; Somjen et al., 1986). There were three main arguments against the notion that K^+ ions induce seizures triggered by electrical stimulation or by drugs (other than K^+ itself). First, the hypothesis predicted that there should be a fixed threshold of $[K^+]_o$ at which seizures are triggered, by analogy to a threshold potential for nerve impulses, but no such threshold level of $[K^+]_o$ could be defined (except according to Sypert and Ward, 1974). The second problem was that the increase in $[K^+]_o$ seemed to lag slightly behind the eruption of the electrographic seizures instead of leading them or at least rising concurrently. Third, and perhaps most importantly, electrical stimulation of healthy CNS gray matter sometimes drove $[K^+]_o$ to levels equal to those seen in seizures without necessarily triggering one. Nonetheless, it was clear that the 8–12 mM concentration of $[K^+]_o$ reached during a seizure cannot fail to have a strong effect on the neurons and synapses that produced the rise in the first place (Hablitz and Heinemann, 1987, 1989; Heinemann et al., 1990b; Lux, 1973; Somjen et al., 1986). Therefore, potassium had to have a hand in shaping the course of the discharge, if not its initiation.

At closer scrutiny, none of the three arguments is completely compelling. A technical flaw weakens them. The joined tips of double-barreled microelectrodes at their smallest diameter measure about 2×5 μm and often more, which is much larger than the spaces between cells in undisturbed CNS. The probe inevitably creates a small, liquid-filled cavity in the tissue where the K^+ released from neurons is diluted and its increase is slowed. In the defense of potassium-selective microelectrodes, the trajectory of the depolarization of glial cells closely tracked the voltage of the electrodes (Lothman and Somjen, 1975; Lux, 1974). As far as the third argument is concerned, it is true that the ranges of $[K^+]_o$ seen during stimulations that do and do not provoke seizures overlap. If, however, one follows the $[K^+]_o$ levels as they rise in the course of one trial before and after seizure onset, a different picture emerges. At first, prolonged, repetitive stimulation before paroxysms erupt causes $[K^+]_o$ in the cell soma layers to rise to an apparently steady ceiling. Then, when seizure-like activity begins, there is a second increase, reaching a higher steady ceiling level (Fig. 8–2B) (Somjen and Giacchino, 1985; Stringer and Lothman, 1989; Stringer et al., 1989).

In conclusion

The onset of seizure activity is marked by an increase in $[K^+]_o$ well above the ceiling attained in the seizure-free condition.

Potassium and the Interictal-to-Ictal Transition

Dichter et al. (1972) proposed a variant of the potassium hypothesis. They attributed to K^+ accumulation the transition from interictal discharges to ictal seizures. This version of the potassium hypothesis was also challenged (Pedley et al., 1976). Nonetheless, measurements in at least one preparation convincingly showed the interictal-ictal transition to be mediated by $[K^+]_o$ (Jensen and Yaari, 1997). When the bath potassium concentration was raised to 7.5 mM, all hippocampal slices developed repeating, brief, spontaneous spike bursts. In fewer than half of the slices, ictal episodes occurred as well. Ictal seizures were preceded by a slow rise of $[K^+]_o$ in the tissue, and the seizure erupted from a definite threshold $[K^+]_o$ level. More recently, Borck and Jefferys (1999) induced seizure activity by blocking $GABA_A$-mediated inhibition, and they too concluded that elevation of $[K^+]_o$ was important for converting brief interictal discharges into seizure-like events. And, as we shall see in Chapter 9, true-to-life computer simulation suggests that this could indeed be possible.

Is Impaired Potassium Buffering by Reactive Astrocytes Responsible for Chronic Epilepsy Foci?

Not long after the potassium hypothesis of seizures and the glial potassium buffering hypothesis were launched, Pollen and Trachtenberg (1970) combined the two to explain epileptic seizures originating from the periphery of glial scars. They suggested that the fibrous astrocytes in and around glial scars differ from their normal protoplasmic progenitors in that they are rendered incompetent to regulate $[K^+]_o$. An unbridled rise of $[K^+]_o$ could explain the epileptogenicity of the scar (see also: Chapter 6: "Neuron loss . . ."). Two corollaries follow from the glial impairment hypothesis. The biophysical properties of reactive astrocytes must differ from their normal counterparts, and in the vicinity of epileptogenic scars, excess $[K^+]_o$ must be cleared more slowly than in normal tissue. When these predictions were tested, the results were at first negative or ambiguous (Glötzner, 1973; Pollen and Richardson, 1972). More recently, Walz and Wuttke (1999) examined reactive astrocytes in gliotic hippocampal slices prepared from rats previously treated with kainic acid. The astrocytes in the gliotic tissue slices vigorously accumulated K^+ when $[K^+]_o$ was raised, similarly to cultured protoplasmic astrocytes, suggesting that they have the capacity to regulate $[K^+]_o$ in their environment (see also Heinemann et al., 1995).

However, working with specimens from both guinea pigs and human patients, Picker et al. (1981) found that the membrane potential of reactive astrocytes from epileptogenic human brain tissue is less sensitive to elevated $[K^+]_o$ than the membrane potential of normal human or guinea pig glia. And quite recently Heinemann et al., (2000; Kivi et al., 2000) also found evidence that glial cells in epileptogenic tissue from human patients do not buffer excess K^+ well. Normally, the accumulation of excess $[K^+]_o$ is greatly augmented by blocking glial K^+ channels with barium, but this ion had no such effect in sclerotic human tissue. The studies of both Picker et al. (1981) and Heinemann et al. (2000) are remarkable in that they used biopsy material from human patients. While the findings do not directly demonstrate a connection between failing K^+ buffer function and seizures, they do suggest that, in some epileptogenic foci, this could, after all, be a factor.

Calcium, magnesium, and seizures

Electrophysiology of Low Extracellular Calcium–Induced Paroxysmal Activity

As already noted, Regoli and Sabbatani (Sabbatani, 1901) applied citrate and oxalate to the exposed cerebral cortex and induced epileptiform convulsions. Sabbatani correctly concluded that chelation of the calcium normally present in brain tissue caused the seizures, not the anions themselves. As we have also seen, the common clinical signs of low-calcium tetany are muscle spasms of peripheral origin, but seizures generated in the CNS can also occur (see Chapter 4: "Tetany").

Exposing hippocampal or neocortical tissue slices to a bath from which Ca^{2+} has been omitted causes the appearance of spontaneous, synchronized impulse bursts similar to interictal discharges (see also Chapter 6: "Nonsynaptic epileptogenesis") (Agopyan and Avoli, 1988; Haas and Jefferys, 1984; Jefferys and Haas, 1982; Konnerth et al., 1983, 1986; Snow and Dudek, 1984b). Spontaneous firing is readily explained by the removal of the surface charge screening (see Chapter 4: "Calcium and magnesium"), but the synchronization among the excited neurons at first seems baffling because, in the absence of Ca^{2+}, all synaptic communication is interdicted. The only explanation of the synchrony can be electrical interaction, either ephaptic or by way of gap junctions. Electrical coupling is also the likely reason for the lockstep firing of action potentials during hippocampal seizures, even when synapses are operational (Fig. 7–8, see Chapter 7: "Sustained Depolarization . . .").

Pan and Stringer (1996, 1997) compared low-calcium-induced interictal PDSs with those caused by kainate and pointed to the similarities. Analyzing low-calcium-induced spontaneous discharges in computer simulation, Nelken and Yaari (1987) concluded that the extracellular accumulation of K^+ provides the positive feedback making these synchronized discharges possible without the assistance of functioning synapses.

During Seizures, Calcium Is Taken Up by Neurons from the Extracellular Fluid

Repetitive electrical stimulation of afferent pathways invariably drives up $[K^+]_o$ levels among the target neurons. The behavior of $[Ca^{2+}]_o$ during electrical stimulation of normal spinal gray matter or cerebral cortex is less predictable. Depending on the location within the tissue, $[Ca^{2+}]_o$ can increase, decrease, or show biphasic changes (Heinemann et al., 1986; Somjen, 1980) (see also Chapter 2: "Extracellular calcium responses"). During seizure discharges $[Ca^{2+}]_o$ behaves more consistently than it does during nonparoxysmal responses. It usually decreases from its normal level of 1.0–1.4 mM by 0.2–0.4 mM in cat and rat neocortex and hippocampal formation and by 0.6–0.8 mM in hippocampal slice culture (Kovács et al., 2001; Lux et al., 1986) (Fig.8–3B). These changes are much greater than those seen during electrical stimulation in the absence of seizures (Hablitz and Heinemann, 1987; Heinemann and Konnerth, 1980; Heinemann et al., 1986; Kovács et al., 2000; Somjen and Giacchino, 1985). The difference between seized and normal responses stimulated speculation about a causal role for $\Delta[Ca^{2+}]_o$ in seizure generation, especially since, in some recordings, $[Ca^{2+}]_o$ appeared to start declining before $[K^+]_o$ began to increase (Heinemann et al., 1978; Pumain et al., 1983).

The decrease in extracellular calcium level indicates a substantial surge into cells. The likely ports of entry into cells include not only voltage-gated Ca^{2+} channels and NMDA receptor–controlled channels but perhaps also the Na^+/Ca^{2+} exchanger operating in "reverse" or "Ca^{2+} enter" mode (Figs. 2–4, 16–4) (Blaustein and Lederer, 1999). If all the 0.4 mM of Ca^{2+} missing from the interstitium during a tonic seizure ended up freely dissolved in the cytosol of neurons, then $[Ca^{2+}]_i$ would increase by about 120 μM. This calculation took into account the low end of the possible range, assuming that neurons occupy on average about 50% of the total volume of the tissue, and assigning 15% to ISVF and 35% to glia. If the ISVF is 20%, and/or the fractional neuron volume is smaller than 50%, or the $\Delta[Ca^{2+}]_o$ is more than 0.4 mM, then $\Delta[Ca]_i$ must be even greater. This much Ca^{2+} in cytosol would be lethal for the cell. In fact, measurement in neuron cell cultures by fluorescent indicator dye during low-Mg^{2+}-induced in vitro status epilepticus registered a rise of only 0.4 μM (Pal et al., 1999). While a cell culture is certainly not an intact brain, the order of magnitude of the recorded response is probably representative of real seizures. The difference between the calculated and actual increase in $[Ca^{2+}]_i$ is accounted for by binding to calcium-binding proteins and sequestration in organelles, mainly ER and mitochondria (see Chapter 2: "Intracellular calcium activity . . .") (Kovács et al., 2001). After a seizure $[Ca^{2+}]_o$ returns slowly to the control level. Bound calcium may, however, not necessarily be rendered harmless. According to some investigators (reviewed by Solà et al., 2001), the binding of calcium by calmodulin starts a cascade that eventually leads to hyperexcitability of neurons and long-term epileptogenesis. During low-$[Mg^{2+}]_o$-induced seizures in hippocampal slice cultures $[Ca^{2+}]_i$ shows large fluctuations superimposed on an elevated baseline (Kovács et al., 2000, 2001).

Seizures in Real Brains Can Proceed with Synapses Blocked or Weakend

The international record for the seizure-related decrease of $[Ca^{2+}]_o$ was reached in neocortex of baboons suffering from photosensitive reflex epilepsy (Pumain et al., 1985). During tonic seizures induced by visual stimulation, $[Ca^{2+}]_o$ decreased on average by 0.9 mM and sometimes more, at which level synaptic transmission must have ceased; nonetheless, the electrically recorded seizure proceeded with full force. This is the more remarkable, because it was not in an in vitro model system but in the intact brain of a primate suffering from a clinical condition. Moreover, the seizures were not just interictal-like burst discharges but full ictal events. It does not follow that synapses are irrelevant to seizures in other forms of epilepsy, but it does prove that they are not absolutely necessary.

Even the more moderate drop in $[Ca^{2+}]_o$ of 0.2–0.4 mM usually registered during tonic seizures (see above) weakens synaptic transmission, if not abolishes it. Remarkably, in the course of ictal seizures, $[K^+]_o$ also rises to a level where synaptic transmission begins to be depressed (see Chapter 4: "Changing potassium levels . . ."). Added to the effect of low $[Ca^{2+}]_o$ and high $[K^+]_o$, there may be depletion of available transmitters in synaptic boutons. Thus, prolonged major seizures proceed while synapses are gradually being weakened for more than one reason. Any satisfactory theoretical explanation of seizure generation must take this into account.

Seizures Induced by Low External Magnesium

Hippocampal slices bathed in ACSF from which Mg^{2+} is omitted produce not only interictal discharges but also ictal events that resemble high $[K^+]_o$ and electrically induced seizures (Anderson et al., 1986). Paroxysmal activity does not start immediately after Mg^{2+} deprivation but evolves over time. At first, sporadic interictal discharges appear; then they increase in frequency. In many but not all slices, prolonged ictal seizures eventually erupt. Ictal events are often but not always preceded by increasingly frequent interictal discharges (Anderson et al., 1986). Similar seizures occur in Mg^{2+}-deprived hippocampal slice cultures (Kovács et al., 2001). Neocortical slices bathed in zero $[Mg^{2+}]_o$ generated repeated bursts represented in extracellular recordings by an initial sharp wave followed, after a pause, by a series of negative waves at 8–12 Hz that were paced by oscillations generated within layer 5 (Flint and Connors, 1996). Low $[Mg^{2+}]_o$ also favored SD (Mody et al., 1987).

Low $[Mg^{2+}]_o$ promotes seizures for three reasons: (*1*) reduced surface screening, which enhances excitability; (*2*) increased release of transmitter from presynaptic nerve endings; and (*3*) removal of the magnesium block from NMDA receptor–controlled channels (Chapter 4: "Calcium and magnesium"). As we saw earlier, Mg^{2+} shares with Ca^{2+} the membrane-stabilizing action of screening surface charges. For the generation of seizures, however, the effect of low $[Mg^{2+}]_o$ on synapses is more important. With $[Ca^{2+}]_o$ remaining normal, removing $[Mg^{2+}]_o$ promotes the influx of Ca^{2+} through voltage-gated channels and therefore potentiates the release of transmitters from presynaptic terminals. It also enhances current through dendritic Ca^{2+} channels. Finally, and perhaps most importantly, removing Mg^{2+} removes the obstruction from normally plugged NMDA-controlled channels (Hille, 2001). The removal of surface charges by itself favors spontaneous firing, but the synchronization of the discharges is mediated by augmented synaptic transmission, especially by the prolonged synaptic excitation through unplugged NMDA receptor channels. The importance of NMDA channels is underscored by the suppression of low-$[Mg^{2+}]_o$-induced seizures by NMDA antagonist drugs (Avoli et al., 1991; Mody et al., 1987).

Unlike low-$[Ca^{2+}]_o$-induced seizure-like activity, which proceeds without synaptic function, low-$[Mg^{2+}]_o$-induced seizures require functioning synapses.

Compared to other ions, we know little about the membrane transport of Mg^{2+}, or about the behavior of this ion during normal function or during seizures. Liquid ion exchangers that are sensitive to magnesium are also sensitive to calcium and therefore are hard to use in microprobes. There is no evidence that redistribution of magnesium ions plays a role in experimental seizures—other than those induced by lowering $[Mg^{2+}]$—or in human epilepsy. However, as they say, the absence of evidence is not the same as the evidence of absence.

Na+, Cl-, and cell volume changes in seizures

Evidence that both hypotonicity and iso-osmotic low $[NaCl]_o$ bolster synaptic transmission was reviewed in Chapter 4 ("Sodium, chloride, and osmotic effects . . ."). The likely mechanism is upregulation of voltage-gated Ca^{2+} channels. Low osmolarity and low $[NaCl]_o$ also facilitate seizures, in part because of the potentiation of excitatory synaptic transmission and also for other reasons.

Low $[Cl-]_o$ Is Epileptogenic

Yamamoto and Kawai (1968) were the first to induce epileptiform discharges in an in vitro brain slice. They did this by removing Cl- from the bathing solution and replacing it with propionate, which does not penetrate the channel that is opened by $GABA_A$ receptors. Washing the surface of an exposed cortex of an otherwise intact brain with Cl^--free solution leaches Cl^- from the tissue; this procedure also induces seizures (Ransom, 1974). In low $[Cl^-]_o$, IPSPs are depressed as the driving force on Cl^- ions decreases. When $[Cl^-]_o$ is very low, the $GABA_A$-induced current actually inverts, causing depolarization instead of hyperpolarization and therefore excitation instead of inhibition (see Chapter 6: "Malfunctioning inhibitory synapses . . ."). Seizure-like evoked and spontaneous events were analyzed by Avoli and colleagues (1990), who concluded that the current underlying the prolonged paroxysmal depolarization was a mixture of inverted $GABA_A$-dependent inhibitory and NMDA-dependent excitatory currents. It should be added that the recordings of Avoli et al.'s long bursts show extreme depolarization with complete inactivation of spike firing, which are features more like those of SD than of tonic seizures (see Part III). Their short bursts do resemble the PDS of interictal discharges. In addition, in the absence of the Cl^--mediated IPSP, the influence of the depolarization caused by the outflow of HCO_3^- through the $GABA_A$-operated anion channel is felt (Voipio and Kaila, 2000).

Changes in $[Cl^-]_o$ During Seizures

During interictal discharges, the extracellular concentration of Cl^- first decreases and then increases. During ictal events $[Cl^-]_o$ usually increases slightly (Dietzel et al., 1982; Lehmenkühler et al., 1982a). The increase is attributed to the shrinkage of the interstitial volume fraction. Nonetheless, there is evidence that some Cl^- leaves the interstitial fluid and enters both glial cells and neurons during seizures. Some Cl^- is forced into glial cells, coupled to K^+ ions that are taken up due to the elevated $[K^+]_o$. Uptake of K^+ takes place, as we have seen, as glial cells fulfill their functions as regulators of $[K^+]_o$ (Chapter 2: "Glial cells regulate . . .") (Walz, 2000b). The uptake of Cl^- is coupled to K^+ through electric force, and it can go through the parallel pathways of selective potassium and chloride channels, as well as through the K/Cl and Na/K/2Cl cotransporters (Bourke et al., 1978; Boyle and Conway, 1941; Kimelberg, 1990). The simultaneous uptake of K^+ and Cl^- causes swelling of glial cells.

Technical note

The exchanger usually used in ion-selective microelectrodes for measuring Cl^- is not nearly as selective as the ones available for various cations. Interference by other anions is a problem (Nicholson and Rice, 1988). Because there is much more Cl^- in ECF than any of the other ions, it is assumed that the electrode registers mainly Cl^-. However, if there were substantial fluxes of HCO_3^-, this could modify the measurement.

That Cl$^-$ is not only admitted into astrocytes but is also taken up by neurons has been inferred from the shift of the reversal potential of GABA-induced IPSPs that occurs during seizures (Chamberlin and Dingledine, 1988; Korn et al., 1987). Cl$^-$ can enter through GABA$_A$-controlled channels. It follows that powerful and prolonged activation of GABA$_A$ inhibition can, in the long run, throttle its own inhibitory Cl$^-$ current. As E$_{Cl}$ is only slightly more negative than the resting potential, if [Cl$^-$]$_i$ builds up, equilibrium is soon approached and the driving force for Cl$^-$ vanishes. Additionally, Cl$^-$ may be exchanged for HCO$_3$$^-$, and some of it may accompany the influx of Na$^+$ into neurons. The loading of neurons with excess Cl$^-$ makes inhibitory synapses less effective and favors continuation of tonic seizures (see also Chapter 6: "Seizures induced by stimulant poisons").

During Seizures [Na$^+$]$_o$ Decreases

Seizure-induced decrease of [Na$^+$]$_o$ is consistently observed, but it is moderate, between 9–15 mM, amounting to at most 10% of the normal 145 mM (Lux et al., 1986). The main reason is the inward Na$^+$ current that generates action potentials, plus influx of Na$^+$ with excitatory synaptic potentials. Just as the rise of [K$^+$]$_o$ is limited by the combined action of reuptake by neurons and uptake by glial cells, the drop of Na$^+$ is mitigated by the same 3Na$^+$/2K$^+$ membrane pumps in neuron as well as glial membranes. Neurons get rid of the excess they gained, and glial cells temporarily release some of the reserve in their cytosol to replenish the depleted interstitial fluid.

Osmotic Cell Swelling During Seizures Facilitates Ephaptic Interaction Among Neurons

As we have just seen, glial cells take up KCl when confronted with high [K$^+$]$_o$, necessitating osmotic water inflow and swelling. In neurons the release and uptake of ions are probably not balanced, and they too swell. Judged by intrinsic optical signals (IOSs), osmotic and activity-induced cell swelling occurs mainly in dendritic layers, largely sparing cell body layers (Fayuk et al., 2002). Of course, IOSs do not distinguish glial from neuronal signals, but theoretical calculation and computer simulation suggest that, besides astrocytes, neuronal dendrites also expand slightly during seizures (Dietzel et al., 1982; Kager et al., 2002b). The combined swelling of neurons and glial cells squeezes the interstitial spaces (Dietzel and Heinemann, 1986). As the interstitium shrinks, neuron membranes become more closely apposed and interstitial tissue resistance increases, favoring ephaptic interaction and synchronization (Andrew et al., 1989; Dudek et al., 1986; Traub et al., 1985).

Maintaining a ceiling of the K^+ concentration during seizures and restoring ion distributions thereafter costs energy

The *ceiling* of the elevation of $[K^+]_o$ during a seizure (Heinemann and Lux, 1977) (Figs. 8–2, 8–3B, 9–5A) represents a balance between the rate of K^+ release from neurons and the rate of its clearing from the interstitium. To achieve this balance, the clearing must be stimulated sufficiently to "catch up" with the release. The clearing of K^+ is achieved by the combined action of reuptake into neurons, dispersion by glial spatial buffer and siphoning, and active uptake by glial cells (Fig. 2–7). The increased workload of active pumping by both neurons and astrocytes requires extra metabolic energy, needed especially to supply ATP to the 3Na/2K ATPase ion pumps. Extra work is required not only during the seizure but also after its termination to restore the disturbed distributions of K^+, Na^+, Ca^{2+}, H^+, Cl^- and HCO_3^-. The extra energy demand could strain the cells' resources.

As described in Chapter 2 ("Keeping ions in their place . . .") Chance, Jöbsis, and associates (Chance et al., 1962; Jöbsis et al., 1971; Rosenthal and Jöbsis, 1971) pioneered the use of fluorometry for assaying the redox state of NADH/NAD$^+$ to gauge energy metabolism in intact cells and in intact organs, including brain (Fig. 2–12). Later, Jöbsis et al. (1977) introduced differential reflectance spectrophotometry to assess the redox state of mitochondrial cytochromes a,a$_3$. To recapitulate the main points: in brain in situ with normal blood flow, intramitochondrial enzymes invariably become oxidized during seizures (Fig. 8–4) (Jöbsis et al., 1971; Lewis and Schuette, 1975; Lewis et al., 1974; Lothman et al., 1975). Blood flow also increases, and so does tissue partial pressure of oxygen, indicating that in the brains of otherwise healthy individuals, the increased blood supply exceeds the metabolic demand. Only if inspired oxygen is reduced or the cerebral circulation fails do the signals invert, showing reduction of NADH/NAD$^+$ and the cytochromes. The brain becomes, as it were, "short of breath."

In vitro brain preparations have no cardiovascular regulation, so the supply of oxygen does not change with the demand. In these systems NAD(P)H and FAD initially become oxidized but then are reduced during seizure discharges (Fig. 2–13) (Heinemann et al., 2002b; Schuchmann et al., 1999), D. Fayuk and D.A. Turner, personal communication). (For details and more references, see Chapter 2: "Keeping ions in their place . . .".)

Key points

High $[K^+]_o$ can induce seizures, and during seizures induced by other agents $[K^+]_o$ increases, providing for positive feedback (Fig. 9–8). High K^+ probably rarely if ever initiates seizures, but it is important for the evolution and maintenance of self-regenerating seizures.

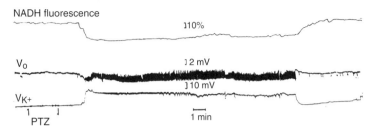

FIGURE 8–4. Oxidation of reduced nicotinamide adenine dinucleotide (NADH) and elevation of extracellular [K+] during cortical seizure. Recording from the neocortex of a cat *cerveau isolé* preparation. Fluorescence was recorded from a small area of the epi-illuminated cortex through a microscope and appropriate optical filters, and it was corrected for changes in reflected light. The seizure was induced by the intravenous injection of pentylenetetrazol (PTZ). During the prolonged seizure, the corrected NADH fluorescence trace indicated steady oxidation of NADH. V_o: extracellular potential from the reference barrel of the ion-selective electrode; V_{K+}: voltage of the K+ selective electrode. The double barreled ion-selective microelectrode was inserted at the edge of the area of optical recording (see also FIG. 2–12). (Modified from Lothman et al., 1975.)

Leaching either Ca^{2+} or Mg^{2+} from in vitro brain slices induces spontaneous seizure-like discharges. In low $[Ca^{2+}]_o$ these synchronized events proceed without the benefit of synaptic transmission. In low $[Mg^{2+}]_o$ they depend on NMDA receptors. During seizures $[Ca^{2+}]_o$ decreases. The behavior of $[Mg^{2+}]_o$ is not known. In at least one naturally occurring epileptic condition in baboons, $[Ca^{2+}]_o$ was seen to drop to levels where synapses must have been paralyzed, yet seizures continued.

The combined effects of low $[Ca^{2+}]_o$, high $[K^+]_o$, and the depletion of transmitters from presynaptic axon endings weakens synaptic transmission as tonic seizures progress. Seizure discharge appears to be prolonged by non-synaptic factors.

Cells swell during seizures. $[Na^+]_o$ decreases but $[Cl^-]_o$ usually increases slightly. Most of the Na^+ that leaves the interstitium is exchanged with K^+ released from neurons. The increase in $[Cl^-]_o$ is attributed to concentration due to shrinkage of the interstitial space. The cells that swell are probably mainly astrocytes, which take up KCl. There is evidence that Cl^- also enters neurons. A true, complete balance sheet for all ion movements has not yet been compiled.

Substituting Cl^- by impermeant anions in the bath fluid induces seizure-like discharges in brain tissue slices. The cause is probably failure of $GABA_A$ receptor–mediated inhibition.

In intact brains of live animals, mitochondrial respiratory enzymes become oxidized during seizures, except if the blood flow is insufficient, in which case they become reduced. In brain tissue preparations in vitro, initial oxidation is followed by reduction of respiratory enzymes.

9

Solving Seizure Mechanisms by Simulations

Computers cannot discover what *is*, but they can define what *may be*—provided, of course, that the parameters incorporated in the program are congruent with reality. Most of our problems in cerebral biophysics are too complex and difficult to solve analytically, but they can be approached with numerical simulations. In view of the multitude of interacting variables governing brain function, when slide rules and adding machines are inadequate, digital computers are needed. The development of desktop computing power has brought realistic simulations within the reach of neuroscientists.

The first neural computer models consisted of connected nets of simple units, each capable of no more than a yes/no choice in response to the sum of the inputs from other members of the population. Over the years, the algorithms became much more sophisticated. Today model cells can have complex shapes and membranes with synaptically activated and voltage-dependent ion channels. Different sets of channels may be represented in different regions of each cell. In the history of neural computation there has been a fork in the road, with one branch leading to the design of artificial intelligence, another to analysis of normal brain function, and yet another branch to the simulation of cerebral pathology. Computers naturally lend themselves to the simulation of seizures (Dichter and Spencer, 1969; Kager et al., 2000, 2001, 2002b; Lewis and Rinzel, 2000; Lytton et al., 1998; McCormick and Contreras, 2001; Traub et al., 1987, 1999a, 2001; Traub and Llinas, 1979).

Computer analysis of normal firing patterns

To understand paroxysmal discharge, it is necessary to first examine the role of various membrane ion currents in shaping normal firing patterns. Voltage changes are readily recorded from live cells, but ion currents can be recorded only if the membrane potential is clamped to a constant level and pharmacological or other interventions suppress all but one of the currents. Computer simulation is the only method that enables visualization of several different ion currents while the model cell is generating active responses. Using computer simulation, one can ask whether a given hypothetical combination of parameters can produce the expected membrane voltage response. To repeat: not whether it *does* but whether *it can*.

Notes for the uninitiated

In live tissue, a microelectrode inserted into an electrically excitable cell can be used to stimulate the cell by injecting depolarizing (electrode tip positive) current and to record the response of the membrane potential. This simple procedure is known in laboratory jargon as ***current clamp***, a somewhat misleading expression. *Clamp* (as used correctly in *voltage clamp*) implies imposed constancy, but while the current issuing from the microelectrode may indeed be constant, the current triggered in the cell membrane is not—unless the cell is dead. A stimulating current of extended duration and sufficient strength applied to a neuron under current clamp can evoke the repetitive firing of action potentials. The pattern of firing can be broadly subdivided into two classes: ***regular spiking*** and ***intrinsically burst firing*** (Connors and Telfeian, 2002). The former produces a series of individual impulses; the latter generates groups of closely spaced spikes separated by longer intervals of silence (see also Chapter 7: "Firing spike bursts by normal neurons").

For readers not used to the conventions of the diagrams illustrating membrane biophysics, here are some guidelines. In representations of voltage, positive is plotted up. In representations of current, inward current is shown down. This may be confusing at first, because inward ion currents (plotted down) depolarize membranes (voltage plotted up), while outward currents (up) re- or hyperpolarize (voltage down). The use of positive and negative signs for current is arbitrary because, for example, an outward ion current (plotted as positive) arises when positive ions flow out of the cell but also when negative ions (e.g., Cl^-) flow into the cell.

Another source of confusion comes from the contrast in the (conventionally designated) directions of active membrane ion currents versus externally imposed passive stimulating currents This was discussed in Chapter 7 ("Another note: Membranes may be depolarized by active inward current or by passive outward current"). Here we must add this: which ions carry charge across the membrane when an extrinsic current is imposed on a membrane depends on which channels happen to open. As voltage-gated channels open, the driving force of the imposed stimulating voltage is summed with the driving potential of the ions whose channels are being activated. The driving potential of an ion is the difference between its equilibrium potential and the prevailing membrane potential.

Our Model

Figures 9–1 – 9–7 were produced by a computer model created with the help of the "Neuron" simulation environment devised by Hines, Moore, and Carnevale (Hines and Carnevale, 1997). The model itself is illustrated in Figure 9–1 (Kager et al., 2002a, 2002b; Kager, et al., unpublished). It represents a neuron hav-ing a soma with basal and apical dendrites attached, surrounded by an interstitial space, which in turn is enveloped by a glia-endothelial "ion buffer system." Na^+, K^+, Ca^{2+}, and Cl^- concentrations were computed. Inside the neuron and the "glia" compartment, impermeant anions were also represented. The membranes of the neuron and the glia were endowed with a variety of Na^+, K^+, Ca^{2+}, and Cl^- conductances and transporters that maintained a steady state in the unstimulated resting condition. Free Ca^{2+} inside the neuron was regulated by a buffer system.

Two types of simulated firing patterns of the computer model neuron

Computer simulation is useful to reveal the ion currents that might create the two firing types, *regular* and *burst firing*, described in Chapter 7 ("Firing spike bursts by normal neurons"). Figure 9–2 shows regular spiking, and Figures 9–3 and 9–4 show a repeating burst pattern, both firing patterns having been evoked by a constant depolarizing current. The main difference between the two behaviors lies in the voltage-dependent calcium conductances and the calcium-dependent K^+ conductance, which were adjusted to be large for the bursting condition but small for the regularly firing condition.

Features of Regular Spiking

In the examples of regular spiking, real and simulated, shown in Figures 7–2A and 9–2, the intervals between the action potentials are short at first and longer later, demonstrating spike frequency adaptation. The driving force that energizes K^+ currents is represented by the distance in Figure 9–2A between the dotted line labeled "E_K" and the solid line representing the membrane potential, V_m. The shift of E_K is caused by the flux of K^+ from neurons into the interstitial space.

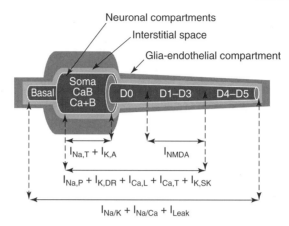

FIGURE 9–1. Schematic representation of the computer model (not to scale). This model was used for the simulations of Figures 9–2 to 9–7 and 16–1 to 16–4. The "neuron" consists of a cell soma with apical and basal dendrites attached. The neuron was surrounded by interstitial space and that, in turn, was enveloped in a glia-endothelial compartment. Initial concentrations were set for Na^+, K^+, Ca^{2+}, Cl^- and for intracellular impermeant anions to conform to known physiological data. Passive (leak) conductances for Na^+, K^+, Ca^{2+}, and Cl^-, and active pump currents ($I_{Na/K}$, transporting 3Na against 2K) were present in the entire surface membrane of the neuron and glial compartments. Neuronal calcium was regulated by the intracellular buffer (CaB), a 3Na/Ca exchange port ($I_{Na/Ca}$) (see also Fig. 2–4), and an active Ca^{2+} extrusion pump (not shown). Voltage-dependent conductances were present in the cell soma and apical dendritic segments D0–D3. $I_{Na,T}$: transient (Hodgkin-Huxley type) Na^+ current; $I_{Na,P}$: persistent Na^+ current; $I_{K,DR}$: delayed rectifier (persistent) K^+ current; $I_{K,A}$: A-type (transient) K^+ current; $I_{K,SK}$: Ca^{2+} dependent SK-type K^+ current; I_{NMDA}: N-methyl-D-aspartate (NMDA) receptor–operated current, permeable to Na^+, K^+, and Ca^{2+} and governed jointly by V_m and $[K^+]_o$. $I_{Ca,L}$: L-type, high-voltage activated, persistent Ca^{2+} current; $I_{Ca,T}$: T-type low-voltage activated transient Ca^{2+} current. (This figure and Figures 9–2 to 9–7 represent unpublished work of H. Kager, W.J. Wadman, and G.G. Somjen.)

Figures 9–2B and 9–2C show the currents that generate the action potentials of Figure 9–2A. When the stimulating current is turned on, at first the membrane potential, V_m, shifts toward a more positive level passively as the membrane capacitance is filled (Fig. 9–2A). The first spike is generated when the inward transient Na^+ current, $I_{Na,T}$, is activated in the neuron soma (Fig. 9–2B). The spike ends and V_m repolarizes when $I_{Na,T}$ becomes inactivated and the two outward currents, the delayed rectifier K^+ current, $I_{K,DR}$, and the smaller A current, $I_{K,A}$, become active (Fig. 9–2B,C). The two K^+ currents then drive V_m in the negative direction, approaching E_K, and cause V_m to sink below its rest level, producing the hyperpolarizing afterpotential. A sluggish, small inward current, the persistent Na^+ current $I_{Na,P}$, is turned on during the spike, and it persists beyond termination of the spike. The continued stimulus current plus $I_{Na,P}$, ensures that a new

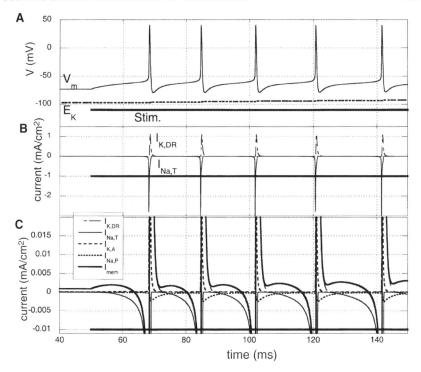

FIGURE 9–2. Computer simulation of regular firing. **A:** Membrane potential (V_m) and equilibrium potential of K^+ (E_K). The horizontal bar shows the timing of the stimulation (Stim.) by depolarizing current applied to soma of the neuron. Note the increasing intervals between action potentials (spike frequency adaptation). E_K is slightly elevated with each spike. **B:** The main Hodgkin-Huxley-type currents generating the spikes. Outward current is shown as positive deflection. **C:** Currents shown on an expanded scale to illustrate the small but important contributions of $I_{K,A}$ and $I_{Na,P}$. I_{mem}: the net (aggregate) membrane current (for abbreviations, see legend to Fig. 9–1). The pump current ($I_{Na/K}$), which is not shown to avoid crowding the figure, contributes to the outward currents producing the afterhyperpolarizations, and it is responsible for spike frequency adaptation.

depolarization starts. When inactivation of $I_{Na,T}$ has been removed by the repolarization, $I_{Na,T}$ is reactivated and initiates the next spike.

In a real nervous system, neurons are stimulated by excitatory synaptic input. Excitatory synapses are usually located in the dendrites. Experimentally, neurons can be excited by current injected into the neuron soma, which is analogous to the manner in which we stimulated our model cell. The dendrite behaved largely passively under these simulated conditions. Although a small, persistent Na^+ current, $I_{Na,P}$, and a low-threshold Ca^{2+} current were activated in the dendrite (not illustrated), these inward currents were too small to produce a dendritic action potential. The next paragraph describes burst firing, which is governed by the apical dendrite.

Features of the Spike Burst Response

The most important actors that produce the striking burst patterns of Figures 9–3 and 9–4 are a sizeable low threshold Ca^{2+} current $I_{Ca,T}$, and a Ca^{2+} dependent K^+ current $I_{K,SK}$ that is turned on by elevation of $[Ca^{2+}]_i$. Bursts began with the firing of an action potential in the neuron soma, followed closely by a small spikelet in the dendrite (Fig. 9–4A). The dendrite had no $I_{Na,T}$ in this simulation and therefore it generated no Na^+ dependent action potential. The small dendritic spikelets seen riding on the slower depolarizing waves (Fig. 9–3, 9–4A) were produced by electrotonic conduction from the soma to the dendrite. In its turn, the dendrite also influenced the soma through electrotonic conduction. The slow waves that govern the timing of the bursts as seen in Figure 9–4A were mainly generated in the dendrite, by the activation of $I_{Ca,T}$ assisted by a small $I_{Na,P}$ (Fig. 9–4C). The active dendritic depolarization is often referred to as a ***calcium spike*** even though it is a much slower response than the Na^+ dependent spikes

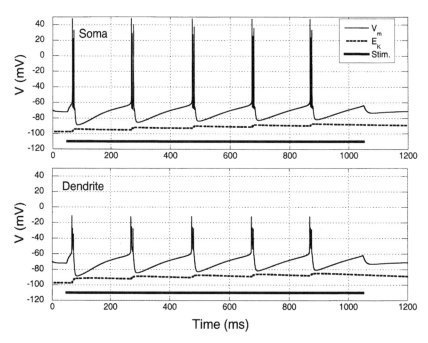

FIGURE 9–3. Simulated burst firing. V_m and E_K as in Figure 9–2A. Top: From the neuron soma. Bottom: From dendritic segment D2 (see Fig. 9–1). The Na^+-dependent spikes are generated in the soma and are passively (electrotonically) conducted into the dendrite, but the slow depolarizations that govern the spike bursts are generated by active currents in the dendrite. The stepwise positive shifts of E_K progressively limit the afterhyperpolarizations following each burst, resulting in shortening of the interburst intervals.

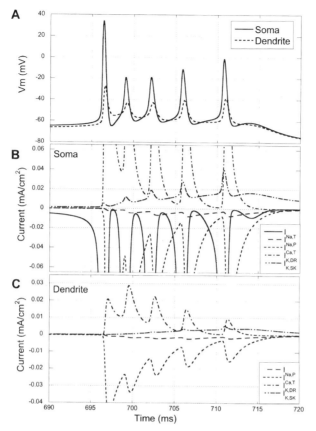

FIGURE 9–4. Analysis of simulated burst firing. **A:** Superimposed tracings of the membrane potential in soma and D2 dendrite during a stimulus-evoked spike burst. The small spikelets in the dendrite are electrotonically conducted from the soma and are therefore slightly delayed relative to the soma spikes. The burst is kept alive by the calcium-dependent slow, active depolarization of the dendrite. **B:** The main currents generating the spike burst in the soma. **C:** The main currents in the D2 dendritic segment. The T-type low-threshold Ca^{2+} current I$_{Ca,T}$ dominates the slow depolarizing wave that governs the burst. I$_{K,SK}$ is a [Ca^{2+}]$_i$ -dependent K$^+$ current, and it builds up as Ca^{2+} accumulates in the dendrite. (Different trial from Figure 9–3.).

of axons and neuron somas. The conductance of I$_{Ca,T}$ was adjusted so as to be higher for the apical dendrite than for the soma, because published data suggest a higher channel density in the dendritic tree of pyramidal neurons (Karst et al. 1993 ; Magee et al. 1998). Nonetheless, the large Na-dependent action potentials in the soma caused intense surges of Ca^{2+} by way of maximally activating I$_{Ca,T}$ in the soma membrane as well (Fig. 9–4B). Still, the slow waves that controlled the course of the bursts were dominated by the depolarization in the dendrite (Fig. 9–4A). It is also notable that the step-wise positive shifts of E_K, caused by the efflux of K$^+$ during each burst, are larger at the dendrite than at the soma (Fig. 9–3). An important factor is the *surface/volume ratio*, which is greater the farther one moves along the tapering dendrite, so that even for equal flux, the concentration changes are larger farther out. After the first action potential the subsequent spikes in a burst were triggered by "pacemaker potentials" generated by the oscillating interplay of inward and outward currents in the cell soma ($I_{Na,T} + I_{Na,P} + I_{Ca,T}$ versus $I_{K,DR} + I_{K,SK} + I_{K,A}$; see Figure 9–4B, where the small $I_{K,A}$ has been deleted to avoid crowding the graph). The prolonged, marked hyperpolarizing afterpotentials that separate the bursts were generated by $I_{K,DR}$ plus $I_{K,SK}$, assisted by the ion pumps (ion pump currents are not illustrated.). The dendritic hyperpolarizing afterpotentials reinforced, by way of electrotonic conduction, the hyperpolarizing afterpotentials of the soma.

Parenthetically, it should be mentioned that it is possible to simulate burst firing in a single-compartment model, that is a "soma" without dendrites. Dendritic dominance of burst firing is, however, closer to the behavior of real live neurons.

Seizure-like self-sustaining and self-limiting afterdischarges analyzed by a neuron model

Analysis of Tonic (Regularly Spiking) Afterdischarge

The model neuron was able to produce afterdischarges, which means that it could continue to fire impulses after the depolarizing stimulating current has ended (Fig. 9–5). To continue tonic firing, two conditions had to be satisfied. $[K^+]_o$ had to have risen to a high enough level during the stimulation to limit repolarization when the stimulus ceased, and an inward current had to remain active after the end of the last spike to initiate renewed depolarization. In our simulation, this role was played by the persistent (slowly inactivating) Na$^+$ current, $I_{Na,P}$. Such a persistent Na$^+$ current is present in most hippocampal CA1 pyramidal cells and in many other central neurons (see Chapter 7: "Somatic bursts . . .") (Crill, 1996; French et al., 1990; Hammarström and Gage, 1998; Somjen and Müller, 2000).

Two kinds of regularly spiking afterdischarge were generated: simple and self-regenerating. During a simple afterdischarge, the firing frequency started at a high rate and then it declined. The length of simple afterdischarges depended on the level of $[K^+]_o$ reached at the end of the stimulus; $[K^+]_o$ and firing decreased together. The afterdischarge became self-regenerating when $[K^+]_o$ remained high or increased slightly after the stimulus ended. Firing frequency dropped abruptly when the stimulating current was turned off, but then it picked up again before

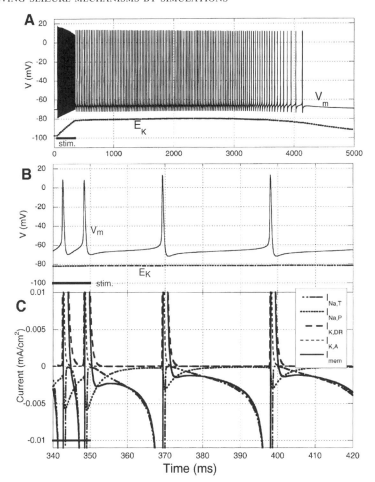

FIGURE 9–5. Simulated self-regenerative tonic paroxysmal afterdischarge. **A:** V_m and E_K as in Figures 9–3 and 9–4. Firing is maintained by depolarization due to the elevated E_K. **B:** Part A on an expanded time scale to illustrate the transition from stimulus-evoked firing to self-regenerative afterdischarge. **C:** The main currents generating the firing. Abbreviations as in Figures 9–1 and 9–2. Note that I_{mem} is inward between spikes, while it was outward between spikes in Figure 9–2. Inward flow of net somatic current is essential for self-regenerating seizures (Fig. 7–10). The presence of $I_{Na,P}$ following each spike ensures reactivation of $I_{Na,T}$ for the next spike. Firing stops when E_K has subsided so that V_m falls below threshold.

finally slowing down and stopping. Figure 9–5 illustrates such a self-regenerating afterdischarge.

Analysis of the underlying currents and ion concentrations clarifies the mechanism that forces prolonged impulse firing in the absence of an extrinsic stimulus. Figure 9–5C shows the most important ion currents operating toward the end of the stimulation and during the start of the afterdischarge. During each spike $I_{Na,P}$

was activated, and it lingered well past the termination of each spike. As $I_{Na,P}$ subsided, $I_{Na,T}$ was reborn, and it gave rise to the next spike. After each spike V_m repolarized; then it slid slowly in the depolarizing direction, resembling a pacemaker potential. The repolarization was the work of $I_{K,DR}$, the pacemaker potential the combined result of the subsidence of $I_{K,DR}$, the residual $I_{Na,P}$ and the gradual reactivation of $I_{Na,T}$. It is important that the sum of all currents, I_{mem}, remained inward between spikes. Each spike injected a small dose of K^+ into the interstitium. High $[K^+]_o$ was sustained as long as its clearing from the interstitium did not exceed its release from neurons. Yet $[K^+]_o$ did not rise boundlessly but reached a maximum or ceiling (Fig. 9–5A), just as it does in live CNS tissue (Heinemann and Lux, 1977; Moody et al., 1974). The ceiling was reached when glial uptake and the neuron ion pump became sufficiently stimulated to "catch up" with the release of K^+ from the neurons, achieving a new steady state. When this balance is upset, SD can ensue, as discussed in Part III (Figs. 16–5, 16–6).

It may be said that, during the afterdischarge, the elevated $[K^+]_o/[K^+]_i$ ratio took over the role that the stimulating current played earlier: it ensured the continued depolarization. Yet in itself, it would not have been sufficient. High $[K^+]_o$ could maintain firing by stimulating the complex interplay of the several voltage-gated currents that produced the *pacemaker-like potentials* between spikes (Fig. 9–5B,C) that triggered each next action potential. The net membrane current, I_{mem}, remained inward between spikes, in agreement with the current source density data of Figure 7–10, which demonstrated a sustained current sink (inward current) in the layer of neuron somas during the seizure (Wadman et al., 1992). The CSD of Figure 7–10 was computed from baseline data points between population spikes and therefore it represented the sustained current, neglecting the action currents.

$I_{Na,P}$ is potentiated by high $[K]_o$ (Somjen and Müller, 2000). This feature was not incorporated in the simulation of Figure 9–5. Such modulation probably reinforces the positive feedback required for seizure-like behavior in a live brain.

The simulated afterdischarge was not only self-sustained but also self-limiting, because slowly but surely, $I_{Na,P}$ was inactivated, and the 3Na/2K ion pump and the glial buffer overcame K^+ accumulation in the interstitium. V_m hyperpolarized and $[K^+]_o$ dived below its resting level in the wake of the afterdischarges, as they do also after seizures in real brains. It was possible to influence the threshold and duration of afterdischarges by adjusting the simulated conductances of the various modeled ion channels.

Analysis of Clonic (Burst-Type) Afterdischarge

Inserting a sizable low-threshold Ca^{2+} conductance in the apical dendrite membrane converted tonic, regular spiking into intermittent, clonic firing (Figs. 9–3, 9–4). Slowing the clearing of $[K^+]_o$ and adjusting ion conductances produced a clonic, bursting afterdischarge (Figs. 9–6, 9–7). The mechanism of the seizure-

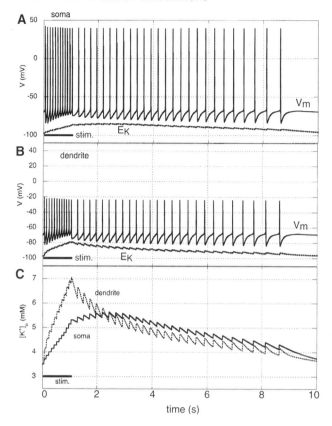

FIGURE 9–6. Simulated clonic paroxysmal afterdischarge. **A, B:** V_m and E_K in soma and dendrite D2. Individual spikes within each burst are not resolved on this compressed time scale, but see the expanded scale in Figure 9–7A. **C:** Extracellular potassium concentration around dendrite D2 and soma.

like clonic afterdischarge was in several respects similar to the one creating the normal burst pattern of Figure 9–4. In both cases, the dendrite imposed its rhythm on the soma. This leading role of the dendrite is underscored by comparing the courses of $[K^+]_o$ during tonic and clonic afterdischarge. During tonic firing, $[K^+]_o$ rose much higher at the soma than at the dendrite and remained so until the discharge terminated. In the case of clonic firing, $[K^+]_o$ at the apical dendrite rapidly shot up higher than at the soma. Later it subsided to slightly below the soma level, but the "sawtooth" oscillations of $[K^+]_o$ were of consistently larger amplitude at the dendrite than at the soma (Fig. 9–6C).

Yet the dendrite is not sovereign, but interacts with the soma in creating the burst pattern. Figure 9–7 compares V_m and ion currents in soma and dendrites for one burst in the middle of the clonic afterdischarge. Figure 9–7A makes it clear that the first impulse in a burst was triggered in the soma very slightly before the

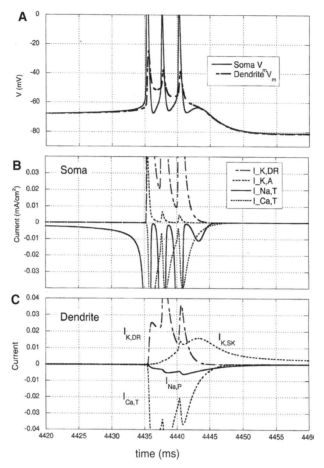

FIGURE 9–7. Analysis of a simulated clonic burst. From the middle part of the clonic after-discharge illustrated in Figure 9–6, on an expanded scale. **A:** V_m during a burst superimposed on the soma and the D2 dendrite segment. The slow depolarizing wave that is responsible for the burst occurs in the dendrite (compare with Fig. 7–3A). **B:** Currents in the soma. **C:** Currents in the dendrite. $I_{Ca,T}$ is the main inward current generating the dendritic slow wave.

response in the dendrite began. Shortly thereafter, the passive spikelet in the dendrite activated the dendritic T-type Ca^{2+} current, $I_{Ca,T}$, plus the small, persistent Na^+ current, $I_{Na,P}$ (Fig. 9–7C). These two dendritic inward currents produced a slow dendritic Ca^{2+} spike. The electrotonically conducted effect of the dendritic active response added to the depolarization of the soma and reignited the somatic $I_{Na,T}$, resulting in the brief burst of three Na^+ action potentials (Fig. 9–7A,B). Other somatic inward currents, $I_{Ca,T}$ and the (in this case) very small $I_{Na,P}$ (which is not shown in Fig. 9–7B), slightly augmented the somatic impulses. The Ca^{2+}-dependent K^+ current, $I_{K,SK}$, had a curiously double-edged effect. Being an outward current, it aided repolarization. Since, however, it continued to flow throughout the interburst intervals, it continued to add K^+ to the ECF, helping to maintain depolarization of both soma and dendritic membranes (Fig. 9–6C).

A Brief Discussion: What Do These Simulations Mean?

These simulations suggest that the concerted action of high $[K^+]_o$ and intrinsic membrane currents can generate a self-sustained afterdischarge in a single neuron without synaptic input. The simulated *tonic afterdischarge* resembled neuron behavior during a *tonic seizure* in living brain tissue, as reported in the literature. Simulated $[K^+]_o$ rose to a maximal or ceiling level, as it does in real life (Heinemann and Lux, 1977; Moody et al., 1974). The rise in $[K^+]_o$ during a tonic seizure was maximal around the soma, as it is during tonic paroxysmal firing in hippocampus (Somjen and Giacchino, 1985) (Fig. 8–2). The membrane potential remained depolarized throughout self-sustained discharges (Figs. 7–9, 8–1A). In the more intense simulated afterdischarges, firing was temporarily interrupted by depolarization-induced inactivation (not illustrated). These features are typical of intracellular recordings from hippocampal and neocortical neurons during seizures (Glötzner and Grüsser, 1968; Kandel and Spencer, 1961c; Somjen et al., 1985; Steriade et al., 1998). During seizures in hippocampal formation, current source density analysis demonstrated a sustained inward current in the soma layers (Wadman et al., 1992) (Fig. 7–10). In the model neuron soma, during self-regenerating afterdischarge, the net membrane current, I_m, was inward in between action potentials (Fig. 9–5C).

The simulations have also shown that firing of a neuron can add enough K^+ to the interstitium to sustain the depolarization that keeps the firing going. In other words, the neuron can keep reexciting itself by means of the K^+ it releases (Fig. 9–8C). The culprit is not K^+ by itself, but excess $[K^+]_o$ acting in concert with intrinsic ion currents. In the simulation of Figure 9–5C, the critical intrinsic current was $I_{Na,P}$, and in Figure 9–7C it was $I_{Ca,T}$ assisted by $I_{Na,P}$. Other intrinsic inward currents could, theoretically, substitute for $I_{Na,P}$, provided that they have the proper cellular distribution and activation and inactivation characteristics. An example is the **calcium-sensing nonselective cation channel** (*csNSC*) (Xiong and MacDonald, 1996) (see also Chapter 15: "Not one spreading depression channel but the cooperation of several . . .").

As in the experiments on live brain tissue, in our simulations there was no single fixed threshold level of $[K^+]_o$ for evoking an afterdischarge. The trigger level of $[K^+]_o$ varied according to other conditions imposed on the model. To initiate afterdischarge, a sufficiently powerful stimulus was first needed to elevate $[K^+]_o$. This is in line with the experimental observation that the rise of $[K^+]_o$ lags slightly behind the onset of paroxysmal firing. K^+ *is not the initial stimulus for a seizure, yet it does govern its evolution.* This recalls the suggestion that the accumulation of K^+ causes the transition from interictal to ictal discharge (Borck and Jefferys, 1999; Dichter et al., 1972). As we have seen, the exact role of interictal discharges in epilepsy is controversial (Binnie, 1987) (Chapter 5: "Interictal discharges"), and our simulations do not speak to that controversy. Our model experiments do emphasize the importance of an initial triggering event that starts the positive feedback that renders the seizure self-sustaining. In clinical epilepsy, this initial stimulus probably requires synaptic interaction among many neurons and therefore could not be incorporated in our single-neuron model.

To produce clonic afterdischarge, sufficiently intense low-threshold voltage-gated Ca^{2+} currents were inserted in the dendritic membrane. Neither the dendritic location nor the choice of cation is essential. The key to repeated burst firing is the presence of a slow inward current that brings in its wake an even slower outward current, producing the typical depolarization-hyperpolarization sequence.

Elementary seizure-like discharges can occur without functioning synapses. However, to initiate and orchestrate a complete clinical epileptic seizure, synaptic connections are required.

Multiunit, synaptically connected model systems

Traub and collaborators labored for many years to unravel the tangled skeins of interacting variables that produce seizure-like events, devising more and more complex and sophisticated computer models (Traub and Jefferys, 1998; Traub and Llinas, 1979; Traub et al., 2001). The earliest versions imitated penicillin-induced burst discharges and consisted of limited numbers of elements. The number of model cells interconnected by excitatory and inhibitory synapses grew, and by 1990 one model representing high $[K^+]_o$-induced epileptiform activity consisted of 9000 excitatory and 900 inhibitory cells (Traub and Dingledine, 1990). This giant system was designed to imitate conditions in elevated $[K^+]_o$ in the CA3 region of hippocampal slices. Both E_{Cl} and E_K were assumed to have shifted in the depolarizing direction, but ion levels were assumed to remain constant and fluxes were not computed. In general, in all these quasi-random networks, triggered or spontaneous synchronized bursts of impulses, PDSs, and clonic repeating discharges depended on reducing inhibition and emphasizing recurrent excitatory connections (see also Miles et al., 1988). Other models incorporated intrinsic slow voltage-gated currents, and electrical interactions were added to synaptically mediated signals (Lewis and Rinzel, 2000; Traub and Llinas, 1979; Traub et al., 1985, 2001). Thalamocortical SW oscillations were simulated by Lytton et al. (1997) and Destexhe (2000).

Two recent papers have attempted realistic analyses of complex problems. One tackles the distinctions in the generation of ictal compared to interictal discharges (Traub et al., 1996a). The other asks what separates normal from pathological synchronized oscillations (Traub et al., 1999a). Traub et al. (1996a) analyzed recordings from hippocampal tissue slices by comparing the behavior of the live tissue to computer simulations. The tissue slices were made quasi-epileptic either by blocking K^+ currents with 4–amino-pyridine (4-AP) or by blocking $GABA_A$ inhibition by bicuculline, and they were primed for epileptiform behavior by slightly elevated $[K^+]_o$ (5 mM) and $[Ca^{2+}]_o$ (2 mM). The recordings were made from CA3 pyramidal neurons, which have a natural propensity for burst firing and interictal discharges but, in the absence of convulsant drugs, rarely if ever generate tonic-clonic seizures (Avoli, 2001; Heinemann et al., 1992; Jensen and Yaari, 1988; Lothman et al., 1991) except in tissue slices from very young rats (Calcagnotto et al., 2000). The computer model featured 192 neurons, each of which received excitatory input from 20 of the other, randomly chosen units. The computerized model neurons had soma and dendritic compartments, and they were endowed with voltage-dependent Na^+-, K^+-, Ca^{2+}-, and Ca^{2+}- dependent K^+ conductances, as well as AMPA and NMDA-style synaptically controlled currents. y-Aminobutyric acid–dependent inhibition was absent in the model, as it was in the bicuculline-induced seizures in live slices. To imitate spontaneous ectopic presynaptic firing (Gutnick and Prince, 1972; Stasheff et al., 1993), random (Poisson function) spikes were generated in the model axons. Neurons in both the tissue slices and the model generated ictal-like discharges. Traub et al. (1996a) defined three successive phases within the ictus. An initial discharge of brief tonic activity, consisting of a major depolarization and rapidly inactivating spikes lasting for less than 0.5 s, was called the *primary burst*. This was followed by *secondary burst discharges* on a declining depolarized baseline membrane potential, followed by *tertiary bursts* of depolarizing waves similar to repeated PDSs, each triggering a few high-frequency spikes. The PDS-like depolarizations of the tertiary bursts arose from a normal or hyperpolarized baseline membrane potential.

All the simulated ictal events in this study (Traub et al., 1996a) were driven by dendritic depolarization. The primary and secondary discharges depended on synaptically mediated activation of dendritic NMDA-dependent and intrinsic (voltage-gated) currents. The NMDA-induced depolarization decayed because of built-in desensitization. Neurons were recruited into synchronized bursts by excitation spread through random interconnections. The tertiary discharge was driven by the ongoing firing of ectopic presynaptic impulses, and it also became synchronized by the excitatory synaptic connections among neurons,

In a more recent major paper Traub et al. (1999a) address the question "What is the difference between functionally relevant and functionally disruptive synchronized oscillations in the γ frequency range (around 40 Hz)?" Signals in this range can be picked up in healthy brains in the course of normal function, as well as during seizures (see Chapter 7: "Are posttetanic γ-β oscillations a form of paroxysmal afterdischarge?"). Discussing the relation of normal and pathological signals, Bracci et al. (1999) pointed out that γ oscillations detected by electrodes inserted in normal brains are feeble compared to the massive signals recorded as posttetanic γ, evoked by trains of electric stimulation in hippocampal slices. The faintness of the normal signal means that only a few of the many neurons are bound into a synchronous rhythm in the course of normal operation, while masses are phase-locked in a seizure. Bracci et al. concluded that their recordings may be more relevant to epilepsy than to cognition. Traub et al. (1999a) concluded that the difference between a coherent discharge during normal function and during seizures can be recognized by comparing the timing in the two cases. Synchrony for achieving perceptual *binding* requires the phase lag to be less than 1 ms over sizable distances. Seizure-related discharges are synchronized an order of magnitude less precisely, and this degree of "sloppiness" disrupts normal function. Traub et al. proposed that the functional oscillatory patterns are degraded into disruptive, sloppy oscillation when synaptic inhibition weakens.

My interpretation differs from the definition of Traub, Jefferys, and Whittington (Traub et al., 1999a). I would say that *normal function is transacted in meaningful, subtle, and precise patterns, but* pathological firing overwhelms large populations and obliterates normal patterns.

Two general conclusions

Two general conclusions emerge at this point:

1. *Seizure-like discharges can be a final common path of many convergent roads.* There does not appear to be a unique solution to the seizure problem. The multiplicity of the events that can lead to seizures has been emphasized by Traub et al. (1996a).
2. *Convulsive behavior requires no sophistication.* One or a few simplified model cells can simulate behaviors that convincingly resemble real seizure discharges.

This is because during the seizure large assemblies of neurons behave in (nearly) identical fashion.

Synapses or Ion Fluxes: Which Are More Important?

We have come back to our opening sentence to this chapter: computers cannot discover what *is*, but they can define what *may be*. We have seen that a single model neuron can produce life-like seizure discharges without synaptic connections if ion fluxes are taken into account. We have also seen that appropriate arrangements of synaptic connections among multiple model neurons can imitate epileptiform behavior even if ion shifts are not computed. Evidently, in real brains, when many neurons fire simultaneously, ion levels change and synapses are also activated—except that maximal seizure discharges apparently can deplete interstitial fluid of Ca^{2+} to the point where synapses become unoperational (Pumain et al., 1985). But this condition arises only during the seizure, not during its initiation.

Clearly, to fully describe epileptic seizures, it will be necessary to combine in one model synaptic connections as well as the fluxes of ions into and out of neurons and astrocytes.

Key points

A computer model of a single neuron, surrounded by interstitial space and a glial envelope, can generate a seizure-like afterdischarge that is both self-regenerative

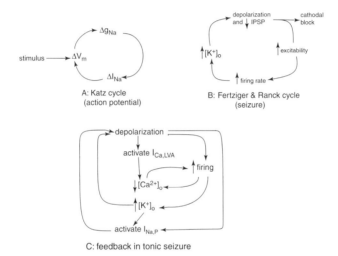

FIGURE 9–8. Positive feedback in biophysics. **A:** Conceptual diagram by Bernard Katz of the generation of the upstroke of an action potential. Depolarization (ΔV_m) opens Na^+ channels, causing increasing Na^+ conductance (Δg_{Na}), resulting in increased inward Na^+ current (ΔI_{Na}), resulting in more depolarization. The cycle stops when Na^+ channels are inactivated, and repolarization is hastened when K^+ channels open. **B:** Fertziger and Ranck's historically influential diagram of the role of elevated extracellular K^+ concentration in self-regenerating seizure discharges. Elevated $[K^+]_o$ causes neuron depolarization and supposedly reduces the efficacy of synaptic inhibition (assumed because of a hypothetical influx of Cl^- into neurons), raising excitability, increasing the firing rate and hence reinforcing the increase in $[K^+]_o$. The seizure is supposed to be arrested when depolarization progresses to the level where Na^+ channels are inactivated (cathodal block). **C:** Ion shifts that influence the course of seizures. Depolarization activates Ca^{2+} currents, resulting in lowering of $[Ca^{2+}]_o$, which, in turn, enhances neuronal excitability and hence contributes to the increased firing rate. Elevation of $[K^+]_o$ reinforces depolarization and potentiates persistent Na^+ current ($I_{Na,P}$), which further augments depolarization. (A modified from Katz, 1966; B modified from Fertziger and Ranck, 1970)

and self-limiting. The model needs life-like ion currents and continuous computation of the ion fluxes and concentration changes.

A simulated tonic afterdischarge requires sustained rise of the $[K^+]_o/[K^+]_i$ ratio to a ceiling level and the operation of a small, persistent inward current, for example a slowly inactivating Na^+ current ($I_{Na,P}$) in the neuron soma.

The afterdischarge becomes clonic when a low-voltage activated Ca^{2+} current ($I_{Ca,T}$) and a calcium-dependent K^+ current are inserted in the dendritic membrane. The courses of $[K^+]_o$ and $[Ca^{2+}]_i$ interact with ion channels to produce the clonic seizure.

Several large, multiunit, synaptically connected computer model systems have been described that can generate seizure-like events. In these models, ion fluxes and ion concentration changes have not been computed. A realistic system will require simulation of both, synapses and ion shifts.

Data from live brains as well as computer simulations suggest that *uncontrolled, recurrent excitation in synaptic circuits starts seizures, while ion shifts maintain and shape them* (Fig. 9–8).

10

Seizures, Channels, Genes

The problem in most, if not all, clinical epileptic conditions is defective ion channel or ion transporter function. The fault can be inherited or acquired, and it can lie in either ligand-operated or voltage-gated ion channels, or in exchangers or ion pumps. The malfunction can affect neurons or glial cells. The result can be excessive inward ion current, too little outward current, or too much of both, or the abnormal distribution of ions.

The new name for biphysical disorders is ***channelopathy*** (Ashcroft, 2000; Masson, 2002; Ptacek and Fu, 2001). Research into clinically relevant defects in channel function is in its infancy, but rapidly growing. In this chapter I can do no more than to introduce some of the discoveries currently in the center of attention. The emphasis will be on cases where altered channel function can plausibly be linked to the generation of seizures.

Finding the links between mutant genes and disease

In ***idiopathic*** epilepsies the channel disease is genetically determined, but the pattern of heredity is often hard to unravel because of variable penetrance and complexity of multiple gene defects. The inherited abnormal genes can either enhance (***gain-of-function***) or suppress (***loss-of-function***) the expression of the channels, or they can cause some more subtle disorder such as altered voltage dependence of activation or delayed inactivation.

Acquired channelopathies can be caused by many insults. In some of the acquired (*symptomatic*) epilepsies, clinical or experimental, the pathogenic ion channel anomalies have been identified, but it is not always clear what has degraded the channel's function. In some cases, this could be an acquired modulation of gene expression; in others, the ion channels are damaged by toxins or other noxious influences—for example, autoimmune disease (Waxman, 2001; Whitney and McNamara, 1999). Berkovic and Scheffer (2001) emphasized that, even in evidently acquired cases, a genetic predisposition may play an important part.

The superfamily of ion channels comprises many families, subfamilies, and sub-subfamilies. Small variations in subunit amino acid composition account for significant variations in the way the channels function. Differences can alter in subtle yet important ways the voltage dependence or the kinetics of activation or inactivation and other properties. In Waxman's (2002) words: "channel diversity . . . [enables] . . . different types of neurons to sing different songs or at least produce music in different keys." The rapidly growing genetics literature is outside the scope of this book. For reviews, the reader is referred to Ashcroft (2000), Hille (2001), and Pulst (2000), Bock and Goode (2002).

Research into the molecular mechanisms of epileptogenesis is accelerating, but a comprehensive picture has not yet emerged. For now, the most striking feature is the multitude of mutations that can affect the same gene, and the multitude of genes and their products causing widely varying channel disorders that nonetheless can cause similar types of seizures (Malafosse and Moulard, 2002). Sizable catalogs of suspected genes have been compiled, and the list is growing so rapidly that review publications are almost obsolete by the time they are printed. Recent surveys may be found in the following references: Crunelli and Leresche (2002), Hirose et al. (2002), Malafosse and Moulard (2002), Pulst (2000), and Steinlein and Noebels (2000). Instead of adopting the separate, hard-to-learn nomenclatures of genes and of channel proteins, for our purpose it will be sufficient to refer to channel types, as we have so far, by the main functional properties of their currents.

Human genetic research begins with a survey of the genetic material of patients with a known pedigree. The epidemiology of epilepsy is such that the best-studied cases are rare syndromes that have easily traced Mendelian genealogies. The inheritance patterns of the more common forms of the disease are often obscure, the affected genes are hard to identify, and the molecular basis of the disease is even harder to discover. Whenever a suspected gene is identified, the next task is to find its protein transcript, then to identify the malfunction of that protein, and finally, to trace the way in which a faulty channel or other malformed protein causes the clinical disorder.

Pathogenic genes can also be hunted in animals suffering from inherited epilepsies, either natural or artificial. For example, selective breeding has produced the Strasbourg strain of rats with absence epilepsy (GAERS; see Chapter 7: "The roles of thalamic relay nuclei . . ."). Other models have been created by inducing mutations or by the deliberate insertion of preselected faulty genes, most often in mice. As in human genetic studies, identifying the mutated, abnormal, missing, or nonfunctional gene(s) responsible for a disease is but the first step. Also, as in human genetics, in animal strains, establishing the causal link between bad gene and bad function is rarely simple.

Linking the gene product(s) to the clinical syndrome is further complicated when the immediate cause of an overt disease sign is the secondary or tertiary consequence of the primary, genetically determined defect. An example is a knockout mutant mouse lacking a K^+ channel protein, which normally is expressed in fast-spiking inhibitory neurons of deep neocortical layers (Lau et al., 2000). The defective interneurons lose the ability to fire rapidly, resulting in diminished inhibition of their synaptic target neurons. The primary defect is located in a K^+ channel, but the enhanced susceptibility to seizures is caused secondarily by reduced GABAergic function.

Selected examples of genetic abnormalities of pathogenic channels will now be briefly presented.

Lessons from inherited skeletal and cardiac muscle channelopathies

Myotonia Congenita

Before we discuss epileptogenic channel defects, a brief digression may be helpful. The earliest discovered channelopathy was one that causes a hereditary muscle disease, *myotonia congenita*. As reported by Bryant (1969) and retold by Ashcroft (2000), the story began with a certain family of goats that regularly fell down in the field whenever they were frightened by a passing train and tried to run away. The goats' exercise-induced muscle cramp was similar to the main disorder in human myotonia. The chief complaint in this disease is the inability to normally relax a contracted muscle, a form of pathological *afterdischarge*. Electrophysiological examination of skeletal muscle in biopsy material, first from goats and later from humans, showed the defect to be greatly reduced chloride conductance of the muscle fiber membrane. In healthy muscle fibers the Cl^- conductance of the membrane is high, and Cl^- is passively distributed so that at rest its concentration is near its electrochemical equilibrium (E_{Cl}). When the muscle fiber is depolarized, either naturally by the endplate potential or artificially by the experimenter, the membrane potential moves away from E_{Cl}, and excitation is limited by the inward surge of Cl^- ions that slows the depolarization, acting, as it were, as an "inertial brake." Reduced Cl^- conductance (g_{Cl}) favors excitation in two ways. The resting membrane resistance is reduced, and as a result, a smaller current causes greater depolarization. In addition, the inertial brake fails so that excitation continues in afterdischarge, causing the unrelenting cramp. K^+ ions accumulating in T-tubules cooperate in maintaining the depolarization of the myotonic sarcolemma. In normal fibers, depolarization within the T-tubule is shunted by the high g_{Cl}, preventing spread of the depolarization and unwanted action potential firing, but the shunt is absent in myotonic muscle fibers. The sick genes of both autosomal dominant and autosomal recessive forms of human myotonia congenita have been identified (Ashcroft, 2000; Pulst, 2000).

There are other forms of myotonia caused by other inborn channelopathies. Also well analyzed is **hyperkalemic periodic paralysis**. In this disease, any moderate increase in blood plasma K^+ concentration, as may occur during moderate exercise or even the eating of bananas, causes first myotonic cramp and then paralysis. The underlying channel anomaly is incomplete inactivation of Na^+ channels (Ashcroft, 2000; Masson, 2002). Persistent Na^+ current ($I_{Na,P}$) is potentiated by high $[K^+]_o$ in muscle (Barchi, 1995; Hoffman et al., 1995), as it is in central neurons (Somjen and Müller, 2000) (see Chapter 4: "Potassium on persistent Na^+ current"), and excitation of the muscle fibers adds to the already elevated interstitial $[K^+]_o$, resulting in uncalled-for, long-lasting excitation. Eventually the sustained depolarization allows slow inactivation to take hold, and hence the cramp ends in depolarization-induced paralysis. One could call myotonic cramps *muscle seizures*, and one is tempted to compare the sequence of myotonia followed by paralysis to an ictal cerebral seizure followed by SD.

Long Q-T and Torsade de Pointes

A form of cardiac seizure is known as *torsade de pointes* ("twisting of the spikes") because of the ECG sign of the condition, a waxing and waning of now upright and then inverted high-frequency QRS complexes (see, e.g., Ashcroft, 2000). The resulting paroxysmal tachycardia seriously impairs cardiac output. Torsade de pointes can be due either to deficient K^+ current or to enhanced, persistent Na^+ current, both of which counteract repolarization. Mutation in any of several genes governing different components of subunits of potassium or sodium channels can be involved in producing this syndrome. This is a typical example of very different channel disorders causing the same clinical picture. A milder manifestation of the same channel anomalies is a prolongation of the cardiac action potential, detected on ECGs as the *long Q-T interval* (*LQT*) sign (Ashcroft, 2000; Lester and Karschin, 2000; Robertson, 2000).

The pathogenesis of the myotonias and of myocardial arrhythmias is instructive because of their similarity to brain disorders. In neurons, resting Cl^- conductance is usually quite low, but impaired $GABA_A$-induced Cl^- conductance is a factor in certain cerebral seizures. In various other types of epilepsy the abnormal function of K^+ channels or enhanced, persistent Na^+ currents are important. Also, elevated $[K^+]_o$ is an important link in the chain of events in disturbed heart and muscle as well as brain function.

In conclusion

The channelopathies causing hyperexcitation of the myocardium and of skeletal muscle seem to be first cousins of those of epileptic cerebral tissue.

Examples of channelopathies that cause epilepsy

Mutations in Genes Coding Sodium Channels

An autosomal dominant form of epilepsy that begins with febrile seizures in early childhood, known as ***generalized epilepsy with febrile seizures plus* (GEFS+)**, is associated with mutations in Na^+ channel genes (Berkovic and Scheffer, 2001). Spampanato et al. (2001) created mutations in rat chromosomes at loci corresponding to the two known mutations in GEFS+ patients and used these to express defective Na^+ channels in *Xenopus* oocytes. One of the mutations showed markedly accelerated recovery from inactivation in the diseased channel, enabling rapidly repeated activation and reduced use-dependent depression. This means, presumably, that neurons carrying the affected channel are able to fire at higher frequency than do their counterparts in healthy brains. It is easy to imagine that more rapid firing could cause fast increase in $[K^+]_o$, which, as we have seen, favors seizure generation. The effect of the other mutation examined in this study is less easily understood. It did not produce the same defect; in fact, it showed enhanced inactivation and use-dependent depression. This is undoubtedly a technically very impressive study that stimulates interesting speculation. Whether these defects fully explain the GEFS+ syndrome remains to be seen.

Delayed inactivation of mutated Na^+ channels caused a variety of neurological disorders, including epilepsy in mice (Kearney et al., 2001; Noebels, 2002). In one study, animals that had mostly a mutated gene died early, but those in which expression was only 20%, while 80% of the channels had wild-type properties, survived but were severely disabled (Meisler et al., 2002).

For several short reviews of the neurological consequences of mutated sodium channels, see Bock and Goode (2002).

Calcium Channels and Absence Seizures

Because of the many functions of calcium ions, anomalies of *calcium channels* could potentially wreak havoc in many ways. Not long ago, Steinlein and Noebels (2000) summed up the then available data, stating that several human neurological conditions have been associated with mutations in Ca^{2+} channels but that none concerned epilepsies. They contrasted the absence of identified human mutants with the four inbred *mouse* strains that show *absence epilepsy*, all four with mutations of different subunits of voltage-gated Ca^{2+} channels (see also Burgess and Noebels, 1999; Crunelli and Leresche, 2002; Lester and Karschin, 2000).

Not entirely surprisingly, a short time after the review by Steinlein and Noebels (2000), Jouvenceau et al. (2001) described a child with both absence and tonic-clonic seizures, as well as ataxia and other problems, who had a mutation of the gene encoding the P/Q-type Ca^{2+} channel. When the mutated gene was coexpressed with the corresponding wild-type gene in *Xenopus* oocytes, the conductance of the resulting hybrid channel was severely depressed. This is reminiscent of the defect in *tottering* mice, which have absence seizures and show loss of cerebellar Purkinje cells and depressed P-type Ca^{2+} currents in the surviving Purkinje cells (Lester and Karschin, 2000; Steinlein and Noebels, 2000). Purkinje cells are GABAergic, and electrical stimulation of the cerebellum can inhibit experimental seizures. Loss of Purkinje cell–mediated inhibition could perhaps underlie seizure susceptibility. Another group (Escayg et al., 2000) identified mutant candidate genes encoding other components of Ca^{2+} channels in several other cases of generalized epilepsy with episodic ataxia, but the functional significance of these mutations is uncertain.

Potassium Channel Anomalies

The numerous and varied potassium channels serve to stabilize the resting potential and to repolarize neurons after impulse discharge. In doing so, they are responsible for the release of K^+ from excited neurons. Like Ca^{2+} channels, their malfunction could jeopardize neurons in various ways. Mutations in a variety of genes coding various subunits of various K^+ channels have been found to be associated with absence epilepsies and myoclonic epilepsies (Crunelli and Leresche, 2002; Gardiner, 1999). The myocardial K^+ channel whose mutation is implicated in the long Q-T syndrome (see above) has relatives in the brain. The cerebral variants encode the ***M-channel***, which contributes to the K^+ conductance responsible for the resting potential. The M-channel is inhibited by muscarinic ACh agonists, resulting in slow depolarization. This channel is expressed in largest concentration in structures involved in synchronous network oscillations (Cooper et al., 2001). Various mutations of the M-channel have been associated with ***benign familial neonatal convulsions*** (***BFNC***), an autosomal dominant condition.

Defective γ-Aminobutyric Acid–Mediated Inhibition

Reduced IPSP is the suspected cause of several types of epilepsy, the type being determined by the specific GABAergic neuron population that is most affected. The excitatory function of GABA in the earliest postnatal developmental stages (Ben-Ari et al., 1997) has been blamed for the high susceptibility of infants to seizures (DeLorey and Olsen, 1999).

Two different mutations of GABA channel genes have been found to be associated with childhood absence epilepsy in two well-studied families. In one, the bezodiazepine receptor of the GABA channel did not function; in the other, GABA output at inhibitory synapses was reduced (Crunelli and Leresche, 2002).

Angleman's syndrome is a severe, complex developmental disorder with signs that include mental retardation and epilepsy. The chromosome defect causing the disease in the majority of the patients has been identified (Ashcroft, 2000). DeLorey and Olsen (1999) described a mouse strain with an analogous chromosome defect, and attributed the epilepsy in both human and mouse to the deficiency in GABAergic function.

Several other animal epilepsy models have reduced GABA function. Besides the gain-of-function defect in $I_{Ca,T}$, this is one of the defects in the *Strasbourg rat strain of absence epilepsy* (*GAERS*, see Chapter 7: "Spike-wave seizures") and also in the *tottering* and *lethargic* mouse strains, which develop seizures as well as other neurological disorders (DeLorey and Olsen, 1999). Mentioned above is the mouse strain in which knockout of potassium channels of inhibitory interneurons caused, as a secondary consequence, disinhibition of target neurons (Lau et al., 2000).

Nicotinic Acetylcholine Receptors

Nicotinic acetylcholine receptors (nAChRs) have been implicated in *autosomal dominant nocturnal frontal lobe epilepsy* (*ADFNLE*) (Berkovic and Scheffer, 2001; Hirose et al., 2002; Lerche et al., 2001). Several mutations have been found in different patients. When one type of defective gene derived from human patients was inserted in *Xenopus* oocytes, the transcribed channel showed faster desensitization and slower recovery than wild-type channels. In other trials there was use-dependent potentiation of channel current, which is not manifest with control genetic material from healthy individuals. The latter anomaly could conceivably cause buildup of excitation leading to seizure, but the finding of opposite genetically determined channel function changes associated with the same disease condition is confusing.

There is, to my knowledge, no report of abnormal genes coding glutamate receptors being involved in the pathogenesis of human epilepsy.

The consequences of defective channel function detected in human epileptic brain tissue

Electrophysiological properties of neurons and synapses of epileptic individuals show the signs of diseased ion channels. Much of the experimental work relating to epileptogenic channels concerned brain tissue from experimental animals. For the clinician, the most important question remains, to what degree do these models represent human conditions, and which of the models is closest to which form of natural disease? Searching for answers, clinicians teamed up with laboratory scientists to explore, as much as possible, the epileptic human brain.

Opportunities to explore the electrophysiology of diseased human brains occur during surgery and while patients are monitored with implanted probes in preparation for surgery (Engel, 1998a). Besides recordings made at the time of surgery in the operating room, specimens removed from patients have been studied in much the same way as brain tissue slices prepared from experimental animals. A perennial problem in human studies is the absence of directly comparable healthy control material. Three ways around this obstacle have been found. One was to compare data from epileptic patients with those obtained from healthy animals and sometimes also from epileptic animals. Another was to compare epileptogenic with nonepileptogenic specimens, usually from the tissue surrounding and inevitably removed together with brain tumors or other lesions. Finally, for certain purposes, such as biochemical and molecular neuropathological studies, human postmortem material can serve as a control (Blümcke et al., 1999; Lombardo et al., 1996).

Observations in Intact Brains

We have already encountered the work of Calvin, Ward, and colleagues, who explored with microelectrodes the exposed neocortex of patients undergoing surgery for epilepsy (see Chapter 7, "Impulse bursts, 'Epileptic neurons'") (Fig. 7–1). The anomalous behavior of neurons in epileptic foci suggested to Calvin and Ward that there was something inherently wrong with these cells (Calvin et al., 1968, 1973)—in today's terminology, that intrinsic membrane properties caused epileptic neuron behavior. Recent work on biopsy specimens from human patients as well as from mutant epileptic animals indeed points to defects in transmitter receptor and ion channel functions (see below).

Besides electrical recording, microdialysis with implanted probes has been applied to patients during preoperative diagnostic observation. During and Spencer (1993) found glutamate to be higher and GABA lower in the epileptogenic hippocampus than in the contralateral inert region. They, as well as Wilson et al. (1996), reported a striking increase in glutamate, aspartate, GABA, and taurine release during seizures. This was similar to findings in rats with kainate-induced epilepsy, in contrast to the very small release of amino acids during electrical stimulation of nonepileptic control rats.

Brain Tissues of Epileptic Patients Show Anomalies
of Receptors and Channels

When the surgeon removes a bit of a human brain in one piece, there is an opportunity to examine the specimen while it is still (more or less) alive. Thin slices can be cut and maintained in vitro, much like those harvested from rats. The main features of the electrophysiological recordings from human biopsy material are very similar to those of brain slices from animals. If the tissue comes from a clinically proven epileptogenic focus, then subtle differences are found. One of these anomalous signs, among the earliest detected, was the presence of a marked *NMDA receptor–dependent component in the EPSPs*. This was reported for tissue samples from both neocortical and hippocampal epileptogenic foci (Avoli and Olivier, 1989; Hwa and Avoli, 1992; Hwa et al., 1991; Urban et al., 1990a) (see also Chapter 6: "*N*-methyl-D-aspartate channel activation facilitates kindling").

Lieberman and Mody (1999; Mody and Lieberman, 1998) recorded single NMDA channels of dentate granule cells isolated from surgical specimens of temporal lobe epilepsy patients using the cell-attached patch clamp method. The human epileptic neurons had prolonged channel open times, similar to those found in cells of kindled rat but not in control cells of healthy rats. The authors attributed the difference to a loss of *calcineurin* and *calmodulin* in the epileptic cells, because these proteins modulate NMDA receptor function. In another study, Mody and associates found *calbindin* also reduced in surviving granule cells in sclerotic human temporal lobes (Nägerl et al., 2000). They considered the loss of calbindin as promoting neuron survival, because the resulting enhanced inactivation of voltage-gated Ca^{2+} channels is expected to limit Ca^{2+} uptake.

Also, in hippocampal slices from human epileptics, single stimuli applied to the perforant path evoked multiple population spikes in dentate granule cells. In normal rat slices, similar stimuli evoke a single spike, but after inhibitory synaptic effects were reduced with bicuculline, the rat slices responded similarly to those of epileptic humans (Masukawa et al., 1989). The authors suggested that insufficient GABAergic synapses could have caused the epilepsy.

Isolated individual neurons from surgical biopsy samples were examined in a whole-cell patch-clamp by M. Vreugdenhil and W.J. Wadman (personal communication), who found that cells from epileptic human subiculum generated unusually large, *persistent Na$^+$ currents*. The $I_{Na,P}$ in the cells from the patients was large compared to that in normal rat subicular cells. In spite of the absence of human controls, this finding is powerfully suggestive because, as we have repeatedly seen, $I_{Na,P}$ is potentially important in seizure generation.

Key points

Many forms of epilepsy result from the malfunction of ion channels. Channelopathies can be inherited or acquired. Different channel anomalies can cause similar clinical manifestations. Ligand-operated or voltage-gated channels, or both, may be involved. Sometimes clinical conditions are caused by simultaneous subtle degradation in several different gene products, none of which by itself would necessarily be pathogenic.

Channelopathies were identified as causes of muscle and heart diseases before being identified in brain diseases. Myotonia congenita results from defective Cl^- conductance in skeletal muscle fibers. Hyperkalemic periodic paralysis is attributed to gain of function in persistent voltage-gated Na^+ current. Either persistent Na^+ or impaired K^+ current can cause a long Q-T interval and torsade de pointes in cardiac ventricles.

Defective inactivation of voltage-gated Na^+ channels is associated with some epileptic conditions, including generalized epilepsy with febrile seizures, and several forms of epilepsy in mice.

Ca^{2+} channel defects have been implicated in absence epilepsy of people and mice. In addition, some absence syndromes are associated with reduced function of GABA receptor channels.

Defects of the muscarine receptor–controlled K^+ channel (mediating the M-current) are linked with benign familial neonatal convulsions.

In epileptic foci of human patients, microdialysis demonstrated glutamate overflow.

In brain tissue slices from human epileptics, EPSPs had a marked NMDA receptor–mediated component that is not normally present in tissue of healthy animals.

Persistent Na^+ current is abnormally intense in neurons from epileptic human subiculum.

11

Mechanisms of Action of Antiepileptic Drugs

To cure epilepsy, one should repair the defective channels. While no longer considered beyond the realm of the possible, attainment of this ideal goal is some time in the future. Meanwhile, clinicians do what they can to alleviate the suffering of patients with seizure disorders. To stress the obvious, seizures could, of course, be completely suppressed by blocking Na^+ channels, but this is incompatible with survival. Nonetheless, most of the routinely used anticonvulsants are indeed channel or receptor antagonists or modulators. Such treatment amounts to balancing one malfunction by inducing another, opposing malfunction. For this reason, all of the therapeutic agents have side effects (Meldrum, 2002a). Schachter (2002) emphasized that currently available drugs are "anti-ictal, not anti-epileptic," treating the symptom, not the disease. Yet Leite et al. (2002) are more optimistic and suggest that some drugs in fact rein in epileptogenesis. Accepting Gowers' dictum that "seizures beget seizures" (see Chapter 6: "The mirror focus"), it may be hoped that suppressing fits at an early stage might at the least retard the progression of the disease. In any case, compared to the total helplessness of the physicians of old, today's neurologists have an impressive array of tools, and many patients are well helped. The adoption of bromides was an advance from having nothing whatsoever, barbiturates were a great advance over bromides, and phenytoin marked a leap from barbiturates. Developments are accelerating. The report of a conference held in 2000 listed 10 antiepileptic drugs (AEDs) licensed recently and 11 others then undergoing various prelicense clinical trials (Bialer et al., 2001).

This chapter provides a brief summary of the mode of action, if known, of the main classes of drugs that suppress seizures. It is emphatically not a catalog of what is on the market and even less a formulary for prescriptions. For reviews from a more practical point of view, see Bialer et al. (2001), McNamara (2001), Voskuyl (2000), and Volume 2 of the textbook edited by Engel and Pedley (1998a).

Classification of anticonvulsant drugs

Anticonvulsants can be classified according to their known or suspected principal mode of action:

1. Ion channel modulators, which can further be subdivided: (a) Na^+ channel inhibitors, (b) Ca^{2+} channel inhibitors, and (c) K^+ channel enhancers.
2. Enhancers of inhibition: (a) GABA agonists, (b) GABA uptake inhibitors, and (c) adenosine-like agonists.
3. Depressants of excitatory synapses: antagonists of (a) non-NMDA glutamatergic synapses, (b) antagonists of NMDA receptor controlled synapses, and (c) of cholinergic synapses.
4. Inducers of cerebral acidosis.
5. Unknown mode of action.

Many of the drugs have *multiple actions*. This should not be too surprising. If a man-made compound successfully attaches to or insinuates itself into a channel, it might disrupt more than one aspect of that channel's functions—for example, its activation as well as its inactivation. Also, systemically administered compounds act on the entire CNS, not just at the sites responsible for initiating seizures. Moreover, selectivity is relative; a drug targeted for one type of channel might also interfere with similar sites on other types of channels. After all, ion channels are members of a superfamily of giant proteins. Multiple actions can sometimes be beneficial, provided that they add up synergistically, allowing (one hopes) low dosage and fewer side effects.

Identifying the mechanism by which a drug relieves a clinical disorder in a patient is not straightforward. An experimentally demonstrated drug effect need not be the one that works in the clinical case, because laboratory tests rarely represent the disease condition realistically. Most of the currently available anticonvulsants were originally identified by screening a number of promising compounds in easily reproducible test models, such as the electroconvulsive threshold in mice. More detailed testing of the mode of action, safety, and efficacy followed. For the most technically advanced investigations of the mode of action, the test object is usually a cell culture or a brain tissue slice. In all such trials the key question is, does a given effect occur at concentrations that are achieved by a therapeutic dosage in patients and is it therefore deemed clinically relevant? Even if it is so, in vitro experiments yield only prima facie evidence, not definitive proof of the mode of action of the drug in patients. Mutated animals suffering from a condition that may be analogous to a human disease are more realistic models, but the most revealing experimental techniques cannot be carried out in intact animals. These reservations apply to most if not all of the interpretations presented in the paragraphs that follow.

Drugs acting on voltage-gated ion channels

Antagonists of Voltage-Gated Na⁺ Currents

Antagonists of voltage-gated Na$^+$ currents include *phenytoin, lamotrigine, valproic acid, carbamazepine, topiramate,* and, weakly, *benzodiazepines.* Also included, but in a different manner, is *ethosuximide.* Several of these agents have multiple actions and will appear again below.

An antiepileptic drug's ability to limit sustained high-frequency firing by neurons has become a screening test for a likely effect on Na$^+$ channels (MacDonald, 1988). The usual test objects are cultured spinal or cortical neurons that, when depolarized, normally fire a steady series of action potentials. A number of antiepileptic drugs drastically reduce such high-frequency firing without affecting the threshold (*rheobase*) of single action potentials. Typically, when the neuron is stimulated while under the influence of such a drug, the first action potential is normal, but then the rate of depolarization of subsequent spikes becomes progressively slower, and the interval between impulses becomes longer, until firing stops completely. This type of drug action is said to be **use-dependent** (McLean and MacDonald, 1983). Further analysis has revealed that the effect is also voltage-dependent. The primary target appears to be the inactivation of the transient Na$^+$ current, $I_{Na,T}$. The steady-state inactivation (h∞) shifts to a more negative voltage, and recovery from inactivation is slowed (MacDonald, 1998). The activation of $I_{Na,T}$ may also be affected, but only at higher concentrations. The usefulness of these agents lies in the fact that at the therapeutic dose level, excitability as such is almost normal, yet excessively high frequency firing, as it occurs during tonic-clonic seizures, is prevented.

Phenytoin (synonyms: *diphenylhydantoin, dilantin*) was introduced in 1938 (Merritt and Putnam, 1938), and it is still among the routinely used antiepileptics. It has the use-dependent action described above (McLean and MacDonald, 1983), and it is not supposed to cause generalized depression of the CNS. Compared to bromide and the barbiturates, this is true, but it cannot be claimed that phenytoin has no side effects. In a toxic overdose it can cause excitation and muscle rigidity of central origin. Phenytoin also depressed veratridine-induced burst firing (Otoom and Alkadhi, 2000). Veratridine enhances Na$^+$ channel activation by hindering inactivation (see Chapter 6: "Drugs that boost sodium current" and Chapter 7: "Somatic bursts . . ."). In addition to its effect on $I_{Na,T}$, phenytoin inhibits the persistent Na$^+$ currents ($I_{Na,P}$) (Chao and Alzheimer, 1995b; Segal and Douglas, 1997). In view of the likely importance of $I_{Na,P}$ in the generation of tonic-clonic seizures (Chapter 9), the selectivity of phenytoin doubtless enhances its usefulness. Finally, phenytoin also suppresses low-voltage activated calcium currents in cultured neuroblastoma cells (Twombly et al., 1988), which could reduce not only neuron excitability but also the release of transmitters from presynaptic terminals.

Several of the newer drugs limit high-frequency firing and are therefore assumed to have actions analogous to, though not necessarily identical to, those of phenytoin. Among these are *valproic acid, carbamazepine, lamotrigine*, and *zonisamide* (MacDonald, 1998; McLean and MacDonald, 1986; Rock et al., 2002; Vreugdenhil and Wadman, 1999). Lamotrigine's block of transient Na$^+$ current is use-dependent and voltage-dependent, and is based on shifting the steady-state inactivation (h∞) (Xie et al., 1995a). Valproic acid also suppresses veratridine-induced spontaneous discharges (Otoom and Alkadhi, 2000).

In the treatment of SW absence seizures lamotrigine is an exception to the rule, because it is effective even though it leaves low-threshold (LVA) Ca^{2+} currents unaffected (Bialer et al., 2001; Gibbs et al., 2002). *Ethosuximide* is the preferred drug for the treatment of absence seizures. It depresses persistent Na$^+$ current ($I_{Na,P}$) (Leresche et al., 1998) but has no effect on transient Na$^+$ currents, and it does not limit high-frequency firing of cultured neurons (McLean and MacDonald, 1986) or the spontaneous bursts induced by veratridine (Otoom and Alkadhi, 2000).

In addition, lamotrigine and carbamazepine depress the **calcium-sensing nonselective cation channel (csNSC)** (see Chapter 15: "Not one spreading depression channel but the cooperation of several . . .") (Xiong et al., 2001).

Antagonists of Ca^{2+} Channels

Antagonists of Ca^{2+} channels include ethosuximide, the methadiones, and, more weakly, valproic acid.

Ethosuximide, trimethadione, and *dimethadione* inhibit low voltage activated LVA Ca^{2+} currents in neurons, and this is believed to be the key to their success in treating SW absence seizures (see Chapter 7: "The pharmacology of spike-wave absence epilepsy . . .") (Bromfield, 1997; Coulter et al., 1989). Dimethadione is the active metabolite of trimethadione (Browne and Ascanape, 1997). These · three compounds inhibited "simple thalamocortical burst complexes" induced by withdrawing Mg^{2+} from the bathing solution of mouse brain slices in which cortex and thalamus remained connected (Zhang et al., 1996a). This discharge pattern was considered an in vitro model of SW seizures. The same preparation also generated very prolonged "compound thalamocortical bursts" that resemble tonic-clonic seizures. Ethosuximide and trimethadione suppressed the compound discharges only at very high concentrations, while phenytoin and carbamazepine were selectively effective against the compound discharges (Zhang and Coulter, 1996).

In addition to inhibiting Na^+ channels, *valproate* and the new wide-spectrum antiepileptic drug *zonisamide* suppress LVA Ca^{2+} currents (Bialer et al., 2001; Kelly et al., 1990). The effect of valproate on Ca^{2+} current is said to be relatively weak (MacDonald, 1998), but in line with its broad spectrum clinical efficacy, valproic acid suppressed both the simple and compound bursts in Mg^{2+}-deprived mouse thalamocortical slices (Zhang et al., 1996b) and it is useful in absence epilepsy (Holmes and Riviello, 2001).

The organic calcium channel antagonists, *verapamil* and *flunarizine,* suppressed some but not all types of experimental seizures (Bingmann et al., 1988; Cereghino, 1997). The anticonvulsant action probably depends on reducing transmitter output due to limitation of presynaptic calcium influx. These compounds found no clinical use in treating epilepsy (Cereghino, 1998).

Not long ago, *levetiracetam* was classified among the compounds whose mode of action was unknown (Bialer et al., 2001), with no demonstrable effect on Na^+ or LVA Ca^{2+} currents or on GABA- or glutamate-controlled currents. It now appears that it selectively inhibits the high-voltage activated (HVA) N-type Ca^{2+} current, albeit only partially (Lukyanetz et al., 2002). Whether the maximal 18% reduction of $I_{Ca,N}$ explains the drug's clinical efficacy remains to be seen.

Drugs That Act by Augmenting K^+ Currents

Retigabine, a relatively new drug, with a novel mode of action, reduces neuronal excitability by hyperpolarizing neurons as it augments K^+ conductance (Armand et al., 2000; Rundfeldt, 1999). This K^+ conductance is nearly ohmic, that is, not voltage sensitive. It may be the channel of the M-current, which is active at resting potential and is suppressed by ACh acting on muscarinic receptors.

Drugs that modify synaptic transmission

Augmenting GABAergic Inhibition

Several of the often used therapeutic agents boost synaptic inhibition. Among them are *phenobarbital, benzodiazepines, gabapentin, felbamate, topiramate,* and *valproic acid*—each by targeting different aspects of either the $GABA_A$ receptor itself or GABA metabolism. Baclofen, originally synthesized as a GABA agonist, turned out to be useless as an anticonvulsant and to be a selective activator of $GABA_B$ receptors, with no effect on $GABA_A$ channels.

The *generally depressant barbiturates* such as *pentobarbital* and *thiopental* depress excitatory synaptic transmission (Barker and Ransom, 1978; Somjen and

Gill, 1963), in part by blocking glutamate receptor–operated channels (Barker and Ransom, 1978) and in part by inhibiting presynaptic voltage-gated Ca^{2+} currents (ffrench-Mullen et al., 1993). Suppression of excitation explains their general anesthetic action, and it makes them less suitable anticonvulsants. *Phenobarbital* is a (sometimes) useful antiepileptic drug because it augments $GABA_A$-mediated inhibition more, and depresses glutamate-mediated excitation less, than the anesthetics (Barker and McBurney, 1979).

Benzodiazepines also augment $GABA_A$ receptor–mediated inhibition, but they attach to a binding site different from that of phenobarbital. While barbiturates increase the GABA channel open time, benzodiazepines increase the opening frequency (Barker and McBurney, 1979; MacDonald, 1998; Study and Barker, 1981). At high concentrations, not reached in clinical practice except possibly when arresting status epilepticus, they also inhibit Na^+ currents (Ko et al., 1997).

Unlike barbiturates and benzodiazepines, *gabapentin* and *tiagabine* have no direct effect on GABA receptors, but they inhibit the reuptake of GABA into neurons, and therefore prolong and increase the presence of GABA at synapses (Bialer et al., 2001; Fink-Jensen et al., 1992; Treiman, 2001).

Drugs That Reduce Glutamatergic Transmission

Felbamate, a drug now withdrawn from practice (McNamara, 2001), depresses NMDA receptor–controlled current, and augments $GABA_A$-controlled inhibition. Several new compounds in various stages of preclinical trials are also NMDA antagonists, among them *harkoseride*, which attaches to the glycine recognition site of NMDA receptors (Bialer et al., 2001).

Therapeutic induction of cerebral acidosis

Acetazolamide is used mainly as a diuretic. By inhibiting carbonic anhydrase, it limits the renal tubular reabsorption of bicarbonate and therefore tends to cause systemic acidosis. In brain tissue, the inhibition of carbonic anhydrase causes accumulation of CO_2, and both intra- and extracellular tissue acidosis. Both inhaled CO_2 and acetazolamide are anticonvulsants (Ramsay and DeToledo, 1997; Woodbury, 1980), as is *sulthiame*, another carbonic anhydrase inhibitor (Leniger et al., 2002). As we have seen (Chapter 4: "Protons inhibit . . ."), acidosis depresses most ion channels, but it augments GABA-mediated inhibition, the net effect being depression of cerebral excitability, which probably accounts for its anticonvulsant effect (Somjen and Tombaugh, 1998; Tombaugh and Somjen, 1998; Traynelis, 1998). Leniger et al. (2002) emphasize the importance of intracellular acidification for seizure control. There is some indication that molecular CO_2 itself has a depressant effect, independently of the acidification (Balestrino and Somjen, 1988).

The practical usefulness of acetazolamide is limited because of the rapid development of tolerance (McNamara, 2001). Besides their other actions, *topiramate* and *zonisamide* are also weak carbonic anhydrase inhibitors (Bialer et al., 2001).

Intracellular acidification can also be brought about by blocking transmembrane acid extrusion by *DIDS* or *amiloride*, both of which also suppress spontaneous burst activity induced by 4-AP or bicuculline in hippocampal slices (Bonnet et al., 2000). Among epilepsy therapies, a *ketogenic diet* also causes cerebral acidosis (Withrow, 1980), although that need not be its only action (Janigro, 1999; Schwartzkroin, 1999). A ketogenic diet imitates diabetic acidosis.

General depressants

As mentioned above, barbiturates are also general depressant drugs that interfere with excitatory synaptic transmission. However, the use of selected members of this drug class in epilepsy therapy is based on the fact that, in a dosage that does not cause sleep or general anesthesia, they augment GABA-mediated inhibition.

Bromide and *paraldehyde* were used in years gone by in sleeping drafts. Their mode of action is ill defined. Br⁻ is believed to enter neurons through Cl⁻ channels, but this does not clearly explain its effect (Browne and Ascanape, 1997). It is mainly of historic interest, because it was the first drug that had a demonstrable anticonvulsant action. It also has many untoward side effects. Paraldehyde is also in disfavor, except as a remedy of last resort in status epilepticus (Browne and Ascanape, 1997).

The body's own anticonvulsants?

Adenosine is a normal ingredient in CNS ECF and is believed to act as a neuromodulator (Sebastião and Ribeiro, 2000). It has both pre- and postsynaptic actions (Haas and Selbach, 2000). It is produced, among other pathways, by the breakdown of ATP. The administration of exogenous adenosine to hippocampal tissue slices suppressed both penicillin-induced and low-calcium-induced spontaneous burst firing (Lee et al., 1984). Conversely, pharmacological blockade of adenosine receptors A_1 and A_{2A} caused burst firing that persisted even after the blocking drugs were washed out (Thümmler and Dunwiddie, 2000). It seems likely that the normally present adenosine has a calming effect on the healthy brain.

Galanin is a neuroactive peptide that appears to have an amazing variety of functions (Mazarati et al., 2001; Wynick et al., 2001). It is found, among other places, in nerve fibers and nerve endings, which it shares with better-known "ordinary" neurotransmitters. In the dorsal horn of the spinal cord, galanin is released when sensory nerves are stimulated (Blakeman et al., 2001), and it supposedly modulates the transmission of nociceptive signals. In the forebrain it coexists most conspicuously with and is coreleased with the transmitters of cholinergic fibers from the septum, noradrenergic fibers from locus coeruleus, and histaminergic fibers of the tuberomammillary nucleus. Cholinergic and noradrenergic systems have abundant connections to hippocampus and to neocortex. Galanin in the bathing fluid limits the release of glutamate from hippocampal tissue slices stimulated by high K^+ or exposed to hypoxia and glucose deprivation (Zini et al., 1993). This effect is due to the augmentation of ATP-dependent K^+ channels by galanin. Presumably, the hyperpolarization achieved by the increased K^+ conductance limited the release of glutamate.

From these data, it has been inferred that galanin, coreleased with ACh and/or noradrenaline, activates ATP-dependent K^+ channels in nearby glutamatergic nerve terminals, limiting excitatory transmission. The reasoning is plausible, but a flaw lies in the fact that both high K^+- and hypoxia-induced glutamate release in the Zini et al. (1993) study were shown to be Ca^{2+}-independent, therefore not vesicular, and not related to normal synaptic transmission. Be that is it may, galanin microinjected into hippocampus or n. accumbens exerts anticonvulsant action against several types of seizures (Mazarati et al., 2001). Even more strikingly, mice become resistant to kindled and other seizures when galanin is produced in excess by genetic manipulation. Conversely, galanin knockouts are excessively seizure-prone (Kokaia et al., 2001 ; Mazarati et al., 1998). There is also some indication that status epilepticus becomes self-sustaining when stored galanin in the dentate hilus becomes exhausted (Mazarati et al., 1998).

Another multifunction endogenous compound with suspected antiepileptic properties is *neuropeptide Y* (Vezzani et al., 1999b). Like galanin, neuropeptide Y is also colocalized with classical transmitters (Hökfelt et al., 2000). It is released when the fibers are strongly stimulated. When released, it limits glutamate excitatory transmission. It is abundant in hippocampus, and it is rapidly overexpressed after acute seizures. Neuropeptide Y added to the bathing solution stopped low Mg^{2+}-induced spontaneous burst activity in hippocampal and neocortical slices. In slices taken from mutant mice deficient in the Y5 receptor, this protective effect was absent. Moreover, kainite status epilepticus killed many more of the Y5 knockout mutants than wild-type controls (Marsh et al., 1999). The antiseizure effect may be related to inhibition of high voltage activated Ca^{2+} currents and the resulting limitation of transmitter release (Wiley et al., 1990).

Galanin and neuropeptide Y are also present in glial cells and are upregulated in certain pathological conditions. The significance of glial neuropeptides is not yet clear (Hökfelt et al., 2000).

Kynurenic acid, derived from kynurenine, a metabolite of tryptophane (Coomes, 2002), is yet another candidate auto-anticonvulsant compound. In the laboratory, kynurenate is widely used to block glutamate synapses. In low concentration it is selective for the glycine site of the NMDA receptor. Normally there is very little kynurenic acid in brain tissue, but there are three reasons why it could perhaps restrain epileptic fits somewhat. First, it appears that very little—less than is needed to block synapses—reduces seizures in tissue slices. This was shown by exposing hippocampal slices to the precursor, l-kynurenine, which induced the endogenous production of kynurenic acid, presumably by glial cells. When magnesium was withdrawn from slices so treated, some failed to develop the customary seizure activity, even though excitatory synaptic transmission remained normal (Scharfman et al., 2000). Second, some kynurenic acid produced outside the brain might perhaps seep through the BBB, if and when seizures render the BBB more permeable (Scharfman et al., 2000). Finally, its production in brain may be increased when seizures threaten. This occurs during kindling, at least in n. accumbens, where kynurenic acid might limit the spread of the seizure from limbic to motor systems, thus restraining overt convulsions (Löscher et al., 1996).

Key points

The majority of clinically useful anticonvulsant drugs acts by modifying ion channel function. Many have multiple effects.

Several drugs limit high-frequency firing without altering the threshold of single action potentials. They do so by shifting the voltage dependence of steady-state activation and slowing the recovery from inactivation of voltage-gated Na^+ current ($I_{Na,T}$). Among them are phenytoin, lamotrigine, and valproic acid.

The drugs that are effective against absence seizures, ethosuximide and dimethadione, inhibit LVA Ca^{2+} current.

Phenobarbital and the benzodiazepines augment $GABA_A$-mediated inhibition.

Acetazolamide inhibits carbonic anhydrase, causing cerebral acidosis, which depresses CNS excitability. A ketogenic diet can sometimes be useful for the same reason.

A number of compounds that are normally present in brain tissue antagonize seizures. Among them are adenosine, galanine, neuropeptide Y, and kynurenic acid.

III

SPREADING DEPRESSION
OF LEÃO

12

Introduction to Spreading Depression:
Extracellular Electric Signs

Spreading depression (*SD*) is perhaps not the best choice of a name, because this peculiar, transient, but profound disorder has nothing to do with mood or affect or with the state of the economy. It is a striking and highly reproducible response of the gray matter of the CNS. Its place in and significance for the functioning of the brain, and its biophysical mechanism have long intrigued yet eluded researchers. Recent developments have moved us closer to solution of the puzzle, and in this part of the book I attempt to put the pieces together. Spreading depression is important for at least two reasons. *First*, it may underlie certain clinical neurological conditions. But, *second*, apart from practical considerations, understanding its mechanism is essential for a complete picture of cerebral function.

What is spreading depression?

At the core of SD is a rapid and nearly complete depolarization of a sizable population of brain cells, associated with a massive redistribution of ions between intracellular and extracellular compartments. The main event in SD lasts for about a 1 min, and it propagates as a wave in gray matter at a slow velocity of 2.5–7 mm/min. Synapses are not required for its spread. A very similar phenomenon occurs a few minutes after interruption of the blood flow or of the oxygen supply, except that the hypoxic event does not recover unless oxygen is restored to the tissue (Chapter 19). Leão, who discovered both phenomena, and several other investigators suspected that the same cellular process underlies the potential shifts and ion fluxes seen in severe acute hypoxia/ischemia and in SD (Hansen and Zeuthen, 1981; Leão, 1947; Marshall, 1959; Van Harreveld and Stamm, 1953a), but others have disputed this (Tegtmeier, 1993). Other names have been used to distinguish the hypoxic event, including *Terminaldepolarisation* (Bureš and Burešová, 1957); Speckmann and Caspers, 1966), *anoxic depolarization (AD)* (Bureš et al., 1974; Tanaka, 1997), and *rapid depolarization*. It could be argued that hypoxia-induced depolarization should not be called *spreading* depression because it starts at once in a wide area and does not propagate. Marshall (1959) had already emphasized that propagation is not the essential feature of the process. More recently we have found that hypoxic SD-like depolarization actually does start in small foci and it spreads at about the same rate as does normoxic SD (Aitken et al., 1998b) (see also Jarvis et al., 2001). Our team favors the term (even if somewhat cumbersome) *SD-like hypoxic depolarization* or *hypoxic SD (HSD)*. It is agreed that the sequence of events that precede and prepare the ground for the depolarization are not the same in SD and in HSD, but no difference has been detected in the biophysics of the depolarization itself. Therefore, the mechanism of both SD and HSD will be discussed here in Part III, while more will be said about the pathophysiological role of HSD in the context of hypoxia and ischemia in Part IV.

Spreading depression is hardly a new phenomenon; in fact, it was described six decades ago (Leão, 1944). Early attempts to explain it failed for two reasons. One was ignorance of the biophysical properties of the membranes of neurons in the mammalian brain; the other was the lack of computational power required to test the feasibility of hypothetical proposals. Both of these handicaps have been overcome, and believable theoretical treatments based on reliable laboratory data have recently emerged.

The early studies have repeatedly been reviewed (Bureš et al., 1974; Marshall, 1959; Ochs, 1962). Recent reviews include Martins-Ferreira et al. (2000) and Somjen (2001).

Discovery

The first seminal paper on SD, titled "Spreading depression of activity in the cerebral cortex" (Leão, 1944), was written by a young, as yet unknown Brazilian investigator, Aristides Leão, working at the Harvard laboratory of R.S. Morison. He originally meant to record the propagation of focally induced experimental seizures, but he became distracted when, instead of the expected seizure, he saw an unexpected silencing of the ongoing normal electrical activity (Fig. 12–1). The flattening of the ECoG trace crept slowly over the cortex, from one recording

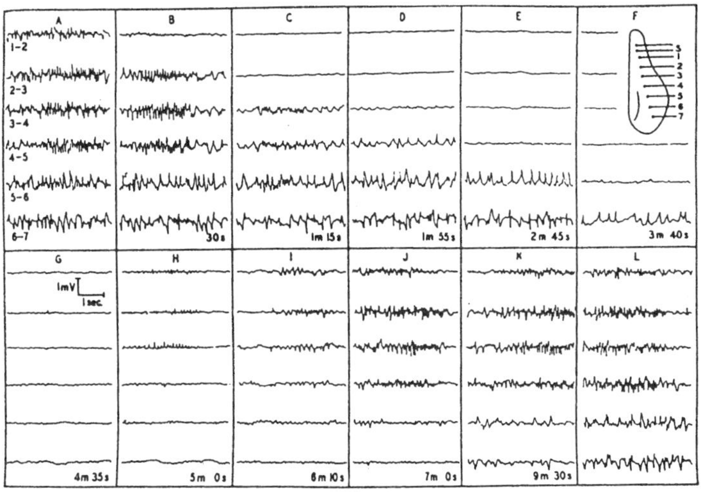

FIGURE 12–1. Leão's historical illustration of spreading depression activity in the cerebral cortex. Bipolar recordings from pairs of electrodes in a row on the exposed cortex of an anesthetized rabbit. The inset shows the electrode placements; "s" marks the site of stimulation. A: Control recordings. B–K: Various times after a brief train of "tetanic" stimulation. Times after the stimulation are shown below the records. L was 9 min after K. The flattening of the electrocorticogram moved from electrode pair to electrode pair. Recovery followed the same sequence. (Reproduced from Leão, 1944.)

electrode pair resting on the cortical surface to the one beside it. According to Leão, SD and propagating focal seizures were related phenomena, forwarded by the same cellular elements, an inference later supported by others (Van Harreveld and Stamm, 1953b). But, as we have seen (Chapter 5: "Seizure propagation"), the propagation of Jacksonian fits has not yet been solved, so we still do not know whether SD and focal seizures "march" by the same means.

After returning to Rio de Janeiro, Leão recorded from the cortical surface the "negative slow voltage variation" (SP or ΔV_o) associated with SD and the similar voltage shift that occurs after a few minutes' delay when the cortex is deprived of blood flow (Leão, 1947), which we now call HSD. Reaching a maximal amplitude of –15 mV, this surface potential shift was astonishingly large compared to those of other brain waves.

Spreading depression can be provoked by many stimuli in most brains

Spreading depression can be triggered by high-frequency electrical pulses or DC (*galvanic*) current, mechanical stimuli such as pressure on or puncture of the cortex, alkaline pH, low osmolarity, and a variety of chemical stimuli (Balestrino et al., 1999b; Bureš et al., 1974; Chebabo et al., 1995a; Lauritzen et al., 1988; Ochs,

1962; Reid et al., 1988; Roitbak and Bobrov, 1975; Somjen, 2001). Among the chemical stimuli potassium ions, glutamate, and, in some areas, ACh, are noteworthy because these compounds are normally present in the brain. In general, similar stimuli can induce SD or provoke seizure discharge, and there are no simple rules by which to predict which of the two will occur. Also, seizures can sometimes terminate in an episode of SD (Chapter 7: "How do seizures stop?"). Waves of SD often emanate from the border of ischemic brain foci and propagate into the surrounding *penumbra* region, where blood flow is only moderately compromised (see also Chapter 19: "The ischemic penumbra . . .") (Hansen and Nedergaard, 1993; Hossmann, 1996; Strong et al., 1996; Walz, 1997). *Endothelin* applied to the exposed neocortex in very low concentration triggered SD, but it had no such effect on isolated cortical tissue slices (Dreier et al., 2002). The onset of SD was preceded by moderate vasoconstriction and elevation of $[K^+]_o$, and the authors suggest that the endothelin may have induced a penumbra-like condition.

Some contended at first that SD can occur only in cortex that is either diseased or ill treated (Marshall, 1959). While it is true that drying, hypoperfusion, and trauma facilitate SD, the condition can be provoked in perfectly healthy, well-nourished, oxygenated brain even when it is protected by its normal coverings, as well as in the brains of unanesthetized, freely moving animals (Bureš et al., 1974; Burešová and Bureš, 1960; Koroleva and Bureš, 1993; Ochs, 1962; Van Harreveld et al., 1956). The same is true, of course, of epileptiform seizures. Moreover, SD has been demonstrated in virtually all the gray matter regions of the CNS, but it is provoked more readily in some areas than in others. The CA1 sector of the hippocampal formation is perhaps the most prone to SD, closely followed by the neocortex. In the cerebellar cortex and olfactory bulb, SD is difficult to produce unless the tissue is suitably "primed" by raising the extracellular potassium concentration or substituting acetate or proprionate for Cl^- (Amemori et al., 1987; Nicholson, 1984; Young, 1980) or low osmolarity (Amemori et al., 1987; Nicholson, 1984). The spinal cord seemed quite "immune" for a long time but, under special conditions, its gray matter can also produce SD-like events (Czéh and Somjen, 1990; Streit et al., 1995). In very young animals, SD cannot be provoked (Bureš et al., 1974; Néverlée and Laget, 1965). The most likely reason is the wide interstitial spaces in the brains of newborns (Lehmenkühler et al., 1993b), which effectively dilute K^+ released from neurons (for the role of $[K^+]_o$ in SD, see Chapter 15).

It has been debated whether SD can occur in the highly convoluted cortex of primates, especially in humans. Indeed, the smooth cortex of rats and rabbits produces SD more readily than that of cats, while the monkey brain is relatively resistant, though by no means immune (Bureš et al., 1974; Van Harreveld et al., 1956).

As pointed out by Strong and Dardis (in press), the species differences may have more to do with neuron density than with cortical convolutions. Tower (1967) and Tower and Young (1973) plotted the log of the glia/neuron ratio against the log of brain weight of numerous mammals, from mouse to elephant and whale. While glial density was about the same in all the brains examined, neuron density decreased steeply with increasing brain size. There are, of course, more neurons in large brains than in small ones; they are just more dispersed. Also, the relative size of the neuropil increases as the synaptic connections become more complex in the larger brains. The relative preponderance of glial elements in larger brains is likely to confer relative protection (but not immunity) against SD in larger animals. Also, the scarcity of glia in hippocampal formation can be the reason for its propensity not only for seizures but also for SD.

Šramka et al. (1977) recorded SD-like potential shifts caudate nucleus and in the hippocampal formation of human patients during stereotactic surgery. By contrast, McLachlan and Girvin (1994) failed to evoke SD in the exposed cortex of patients, using electrode configurations and current intensities similar to those that consistently provoked SD in rat cortex. This failure may have been due to the anesthesia of the patients (Piper and Lambert, 1996) or else the threshold requirements may differ in human compared to rat brain. Mayevsky et al. (1996) saw the unmistakable signs of recurrent SD in at least one patient with a severe head injury whose cortex was monitored with an implanted multiple probe. During surgery, Strong et al. (2002) recorded propagating waves of EEG suppression in the vicinity of cortex injured by trauma or hemorrhage. There is no doubt that in vitro hippocampal and cortical tissue slices prepared from human brain fragments removed during neurosurgery do generate both SD and HSD (Fig. 12–3) (Aitken et al., 1991a; Avoli et al., 1991; Köhling et al., 1996; Somjen et al., 1993a).

Extracellular sustained potential shift (ΔV_o) and extracellular current flow related to spreading depression

The potential shift recorded through DC-coupled amplification from the exposed cerebral cortex of cats, rats, or rabbits during SD has a maximal amplitude of –5 to –15 mV (Leão, 1947, 1951). The initial surface-negative wave is followed by a smaller but more prolonged positive phase. When recorded by extracellular microelectrodes inserted into the gray matter of the neocortex or hippocampus, the ΔV_o can be biphasic or triphasic, with the main component again negative relative to a distant ground and reaching –15 to –30 mV, sometimes preceded and followed by smaller positive shifts. The white matter beneath the cortical gray becomes positive when the cortex itself undergoes the negative wave (Leão, 1951).

From the distribution of voltage shifts in neocortex, Ochs (1962) inferred that apical dendrites of pyramidal neurons were the primary generators. Current source density analysis in hippocampal formation in situ in the brains of anesthetized rats and in organotypic slice cultures confirmed that during SD the main sink of the

ΔV_o—that is, current flow inward—is located in layers containing the dendritic trees of pyramidal neurons, while neuron somas seem to be sources—that is, regions of outward current (Fig. 7–10) (Kraig et al., 1999; Wadman et al., 1992). This is the sink-source distribution of excitatory synaptic currents as well but, as we saw in Chapter 7 ("Hippocampal tonic seizures . . .") and in Figure 7–10, during tonic seizure the current flows in the opposite direction: inward (sink) into the neuron somas, while the dendrites act as passive sources of outward current. Nonetheless, SD is not generated by synaptic current. In fact, SD can be induced with all synapses blocked and even when action potentials are abolished (Sugaya et al., 1975; Tobiasz and Nicholson, 1982). The generators are intrinsic, slowly inactivating channels in the dendritic membranes (Chapter 15: "The role of ion channels . . ." and Chapter 16). We must also remember that CSD reveals the net current, which, more often than not, is the algebraic sum of several components, some of which may be flowing in opposite directions. Although the dendritic depolarization starts earlier, is larger, and lasts longer, the soma also depolarizes. The soma depolarization is also active, but it trails behind and is ignited by the earlier, primary dendritic process. In the CSD trace the somatic current is not detected because it is overshadowed by the more intensive dendritic current (Figs. 7–10, 12–2, 12–4, 16–2B).

The negative ΔV_o results from the inward flow of positive charges, which leaves en excess of negative charges on the outside of neurons. In terms of equivalent ion concentrations, the imbalance between cations and anions is negligible because the voltage generated by the inward current forces a matching outward current after an almost imperceptible delay. This means that for each cation moving inward (mostly Na^+ with some Ca^{2+}) very soon either another cation is pushed outward (mostly K^+), or else an anion is dragged inward (mostly Cl^- with some HCO_3^-). Inward flux of both, Na^+ and Cl^- results in osmotic water flow and cell swelling.

The onset of the ΔV_o is usually preceded by increased neuronal excitability (Grafstein, 1956b), or "fast activity" in the ECoG trace (Rosenblueth and Garcia Ramos, 1966). In hippocampus the prodromal excitation is manifested in a shower of *population spikes*, representing hypersynchron, phase-locked (lockstep) firing of neurons (Herreras and Somjen, 1993c). Rosenblueth and García Ramos (1966) emphasized that the ΔV_o itself has all-or-none character: once it is started, its ultimate magnitude is independent of the triggering stimulus.

Several investigators emphasized that SD must be a complex phenomenon resulting from the interaction of more than one process (Bureš et al., 1984; Do Carmo and Martins-Ferreira, 1984; Kraig and Nicholson, 1978; Oliveira Castro et al., 1985; Rosenblueth and Garcia Ramos, 1966). As seen in Figures 7–10, 12–2, 12–3A, 12–4, 13–4, and 14–1A, the negative ΔV_o is bimodal; it rapidly attains an early negative peak, followed either by a less negative plateau or, after a brief decline or "notch," by a slow second maximum. We (Herreras and Somjen, 1993a)

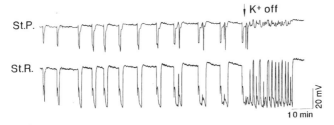

FIGURE 12–2. Extracellular voltage shifts during recurrent spreading depression (SD) waves in hippocampus. Simultaneous recording by microelectrodes in stratum pyramidale (St.P.) and stratum (st.) radiatum (St.R.) of an anesthetized rat. Negative voltage plotted downward. The SD waves were induced by microdialysis of a high K^+ solution into hippocampus about 0.8 mm anterior to the recording electrodes. The voltage shifts were invariably larger and longer in st. radiatum than in st. pyramidale. Note the inverted saddle appearance. The SD episodes increased in duration until, in the end, prolonged unstable SD oscillations occurred in st. radiatum that outlasted high K^+ administration (see arrow marked "K^+ off"). (Modified from Herreras and Somjen, 1993a.)

have called this upside-down peak-and-hump waveform an ***inverted saddle***. It is usually evident in extracellular recordings not only of SD but also of HSD (Figs. 19–1, 19–6a), in retina (Do Carmo and Martins-Ferreira, 1984), neocortex (Hansen and Lauritzen, 1984; Martins-Ferreira, 1954), cerebellar cortex (Nicholson, 1984), and, most prominently, in stratum (st.) radiatum of the CA1 region of the hippocampus (Herreras and Somjen, 1993a, 1993c), in brain in situ, and in tissue slices in vitro, and it is accentuated by CSD analysis (Fig. 7–10) (Wadman et al., 1992). When recordings were made simultaneously from st. pyramidale and st. radiatum of the hippocampal CA1 sector, the ΔV_o invariably started earlier and ended later in the layer of the dendritic trees than among the cell somas (Figs. 12–2, 12–4A). It was the later, slower negative hump at the rear of the saddle that was much more pronounced in st. radiatum (Figs. 12–2, 12–4A). In some of these dual recordings, it seemed as if the somatic current may have subtracted from the dendritic current, and it was this interaction that created the notch between the early peak and the late hump of the dendritic ΔV_o (e.g., Fig. 12–4A). This could not, however, explain the pharmacological dissociation of the early and late components. During microdialysis of the NMDA antagonist drug (3-(2-carboxypiperazin-4-yl))-propyl-1-phophonic acid (CPP), the late phase was suppressed near the dialysis source but the early sharp peak was unaffected and continued to propagate. As the early peak moved away from the source of CPP, the late, slower component reemerged (Herreras and Somjen, 1993a). It seemed that the first peak and the following hump or negative plateau of the ΔV_o were expressions of two distinct ion currents and that NMDA-controlled channels were responsible only for the second current. From computer simulations, it appears that this interpretation is not quite accurate (Chapter 16). Two successive maxima

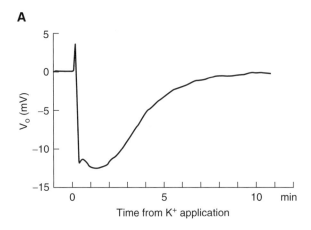

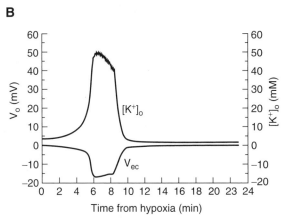

FIGURE 12–3. Spreading depression (SD) and hypoxic spreading depression-like depolarization (HSD) in tissue slices of human hippocampus. Specimens obtained from surgery for intractable temporal lobe epilepsy from two patients. Recordings from CA1 stratum pyramidale. **A:** Spreading depression induced by a small drop of high K^+ solution at a distance from the recording electrode. **B:** Hypoxia induced by switching from 95% O_2, 5% CO_2 to 95% N_2, 5% CO_2. Oxygen was readmitted 6.5 min after N_2 onset. [Recordings made by P.G. Aitken, J. Jing, and J. Young in 1991 (Aitken et al., 1991a). Illustration reproduced from Somjen, 2001.]

need not represent one current being followed by another; instead, the complex interplay of several currents can sum to produce two surges of the net (aggregate) membrane current (I_{mem}), with first one and then the other taking the larger but not the exclusive share (Fig. 16–2B). In the live hippocampus, the first peak is probably dominated by a brief, intense surge of voltage-gated persistent inward currents ($I_{Na,P}$), while during the later phase, the NMDA receptor–controlled I_{NMDA} is the main (but not the only) generator.

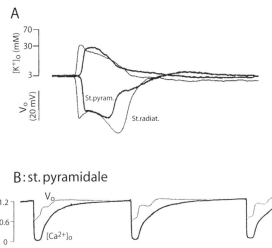

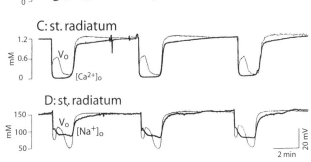

FIGURE 12–4. Extracellular potassium, calcium, and sodium concentration changes associated with spreading depression (SD). Recordings with double-barreled ion-selective microelectrodes from the hippocampal CA1 region in anesthetized rats. Spreading depression induced by high-K^+ microdialysis, as for Figure 12–2. **A:** $[K^+]_o$ in the upper plot, V_o below. The heavy lines trace recordings from stratum pyramidale, the thin lines from stratum (st.) radiatum. Note that the courses of $[K^+]_o$ and of V_o are not mirror images. **B:** Changes in $[Ca^{2+}]_o$ (heavy line) and V_o (thin line) in stratum (st.) pyramidale during SD. The very large fall in $[Ca^{2+}]_o$ outlasts the ΔV_o. The voltage and time calibrations below part D refer to B, C, and D. **C:** Recording as in B, but from st. radiatum. The start and end of $\Delta[Ca^{2+}]_o$ and ΔV_o coincide, but only ΔV_o has the inverted saddle shape. **D:** The decline in $[Na^+]_o$ is marked, but as a fraction of the rest level it is not as drastic as that in $[Ca^{2+}]_o$. (Modified from Herreras and Somjen, 1993.)

A note on negative maxima

To speak of the double wave of the inverted saddle as having two *negative maxima* sounds like a contradiction in terms. It should, however, be remembered that, in electricity, *negative* is arbitrary. It does not mean "less," but rather "opposite in direction to positive." Increasingly negative voltage signifies an increasing electromotive force and it can have a summit, even if conventionally we plot it upside down.

Spreading depression in clinical conditions

The CNS of numerous classes of animals can produce SD. This could mean that SD has been phylogenetically conserved because it is somehow useful (Bureš et al., 1984). Yet it is more plausible that SD, like seizures, is a malfunction, a hazard inherent in the complex biophysics of cerebral neurons. Indeed, there are four clinical conditions in which SD is suspected to play a role: migraine, head trauma, epilepsy (postictal depression), and hypoxia/ischemia (Gorji, 2001; Hansen and Lauritzen, 1984; Somjen, 2001; Strong and Dardis, in press).

Migraine

A link between epilepsy and migraine has been suspected at least since the days of Jackson and Gowers (see the Preface to Andermann et al., 1987). There is statistical evidence for a genetic linkage, albeit not a very strong one (Kullmann, 2002). In a theoretical essay, van Gelder (1987) linked three conditions—migraine, epilepsy, and SD—assuming that an imbalance of glutamate and GABA might be the common factor among them.

Leão and Morison (1945) were the first to suggest that SD may cause the *aural scintillating scotoma* often experienced by patients at the onset of a *classical migraine* attack. This aura, which precedes the headache, consists of an elementary visual hallucination: a dark, blind area surrounded by a bright edge that moves slowly across the visual field. The aural scotoma, as well as other forms of migraine aura, were originally ascribed to localized cerebral vasoconstriction (Biemond, 1961; Walton, 1985). To Leão and Morison, it seemed that the scintillating bright edge corresponds to a brief introductory phase of excitation and the dark field to a subsequent depression of cortical neuron activity, which is also seen during SD. The idea was picked up by Milner (1958), who linked the idea of Leão and Morison to an earlier observation by Lashley (1941). Lashley suffered from migraine and, with the devotion of a true scientist, analyzed his own aura. He correctly assumed that the scintillating border of the scotoma signaled neuron excitation and the subsequent darkness a more enduring depression of neuron populations, and assumed that the site was the cerebral cortex. From the virtual movement of his scotoma and the relationship of the size (visual angles) of the visual field to that of the cortical receiving area, he estimated the velocity of propagation of the postulated brain process. Milner compared the velocity of SD reported by Leão and Morison (1945) to the rate of propagation of the scotoma as estimated by Lashley, and was struck by the congruence of the two data. It would, of course, require direct electrical (or optical) recording from a person's visual cortex while experiencing the aura to remove all doubt concerning the identity of the scotoma and SD, but there are obvious obstacles to this experiment. Conventional EEG is not suited to this purpose. Recent magnetic resonance imaging (MRI) recordings are consistent with but not conclusive for an SD-like process during the migraine aura (Hadjikhani et al., 2001; James et al., 2001). Hadjikhani et al.'s report seeks to link SD to propagating vascular responses associated with the aura.

An aura is typical of classical migraine but not of the more frequent *common migraine*. A question has been raised: could the headache, the visceral symptoms, and the other associated neurological disturbances also be related to SD? Arguments connecting SD with the main complaints of migraine are, however, less compelling than the evidence for the role of SD in the aura. The SD event itself is probably not the direct cause of the pain. From the observations of unanesthetized surgical patients, we know that the handling of the meninges hurts, but handling of brain tissue itself does not. Abnormal CNS activity can nevertheless cause severe pain, for example *thalamic pain* (Walton, 1985) and *ictal pain* (Blume and Young, 1987). Such central pain, however, requires abnormal excitation of nociceptive neurons, whereas during SD, neurons are silenced. Moreover, SD typically lasts only for minutes, and even though it can be repeated and can culminate in a more prolonged oscillating state (Fig. 12–2) (Herreras and Somjen, 1993b), it does not match the time course of migraine attacks, which last for hours or even days. These arguments do not deny a possible indirect link between SD and the clinical syndrome. Several experts, some themselves migraine sufferers, have suggested that cortical SD initiates a long-lasting vascular response that is then the proximate cause of the headache and the other disturbances. Detailed discussion of the various points of view may be found in an anthology of reviews (Lehmenkühler et al., 1993a) and in other papers (Aurora and Welch, 2000; Bolay et al., 2002; Gardner-Medwin and Mutch, 1984; Gorji, 2001; Hansen and Lauritzen, 1984; Shimazawa and Hara, 1996).

The group led by J. Bureš made extensive use of SD in behavioral experiments on conscious rats. They report that SD is not an "aversive" stimulus. (Koroleva and Bureš, 1993). This could be taken to mean that rats do not get a headache while undergoing SD, but, of course, no one has actually asked the rats' opinion. Moreover, Bureš et al. (1984) call attention to the trials by Šramka et al. (1977) who provoked SD in the caudate nucleus and hippocampus (but not neocortex) during surgery of human patients, without causing neurological symptoms. On the contrary, taking the affirmative position, in a recent paper, Bolay et al. (2002) report long-lasting vasodilatation and plasma protein leakage from the middle meningeal artery of rats in response to a stimulus that is assumed to provoke SD. This comes closest to demonstrating a link between SD and a presumably painful vascular response.

Head Trauma and Concussion

In practice, it may be difficult to distinguish concussion from cerebral contusion (Walton, 1985), yet a connection between SD and uncomplicated concussion suggests itself. One of the traditional ways to elicit SD in laboratory experiments is mechanical insult to the exposed brain or isolated tissue. It is easy to imagine that a blow to the head could trigger SD at once in many areas of the brain, perhaps including subcortical nuclei, rendering the victim unconscious (Hansen and Lauritzen, 1984; Irwin et al., 1975; Oka et al., 1977). In the absence of structural damage or bleeding, brain function can return after a knockout in about the same time that it takes for cerebral tissue to recover from SD. Electrophysiological confirmation of this scenario is lacking. As already noted, Strong et al. (2002) recorded signs of SD from the cortex of patients undergoing surgery after brain injury due to trauma or hemorrhage (see above: "Spreading depression can be provoked . . .").

Epilepsy

The brief burst of firing that frequently precedes the depolarization at the leading edge of a wave of propagating SD is not a seizure. Nonetheless, true tonic-clonic seizures can also be followed by SD (Fig. 7–10, 13–6), and this has led to the suggestion that *postictal depression* may be due to SD-like depolarization (Van Harreveld and Stamm, 1955). More often than not, however, neurons become hyperpolarized after termination of tonic-clonic discharges, not depolarized (see Chapter 7: "How do seizures stop?"). Whether a seizure is followed by SD is determined by the behavior of $[K^+]_o$. As long as $[K^+]_o$ respects the ceiling level of about 8–12 mM (Heinemann and Lux, 1977), SD will not occur, but if the regulation of $[K^+]_o$ is overwhelmed and the ceiling is breached, SD can ensue (Fig. 16–6) (Kager et al., 2000, 2002a). We have seen earlier that SD does occasionally follow in the wake of seizures provoked in animal tissues (Fig. 7–10; and Chapter 7: "How do seizures stop?"). Clinically, this is especially plausible in generalized status epilepticus when recurrent intensive convulsions are interrupted by transient relaxation in coma (Biemond, 1961; Walton, 1985). The brief periods of respite may in fact represent episodes of SD. Again, this is a hypothesis, to be tested. Illustrations in a report of an "in vitro model of status epilepticus" show SD-like events, though not so named by the authors (Rafiq et al., 1995).

The pathological conditions in which an SD-like state is almost certainly important are severe acute *hypoxia* and *ischemia/stroke*. These topics will be discussed in detail in part IV.

Key points

Spreading depression was discovered as a slowly propagating wave of flattening of the ECoG activity in the neocortex. In the forebrain of experimental animals and in vitro brain preparations, SD can be provoked by stimuli similar to those triggering seizures.

Spreading depression cannot be elicited in the brains of newborn animals. In cerebellum and spinal cord, SD can be provoked only under special conditions.

Spreading depression is associated with a large negative shift of extracellular potential. The amplitude of this ΔV_o is larger than any other extracellular electrical signal in brain.

In hippocampal formation the ΔV_o is larger, starts earlier, and lasts longer in dendrite layers than among neuron somas. Current source density analysis reveals large, extended, intensive sinks among the dendritic trees. Spreading depression–related ΔV_o and its CSD trace show two successive maxima, forming an inverted saddle pattern.

A process resembling SD in every respect occurs after a short latent period during acute, severe hypoxia and ischemia of brain tissue. It is known as hypoxic SD-like depolarization (HSD) or anoxic depolarization (AD).

In human patients SD is suspected of having a role in migraine, head trauma, and cerebral hypoxia and stroke. Its relationship to epilepsy is uncertain, but it may sometimes occur during post-ictal depression and intermittently during status epilepticus.

13

Ion Fluxes during Spreading Depression

Even before ion changes in live brain tissue could reliably be measured, it was suspected that the unusually large electrical signals recorded during SD may reflect drastic redistribution of ions. Subsequently this has been amply confirmed. Chapter 13 reviews the evidence.

Neuronal and glial ion fluxes

During Spreading Depression K^+ Flows Out, While Na^+, Ca^{2+}, and Cl^- Flow into Neurons

Independently of each other but at about the same time, Brinley and Kandel (Brinley et al., 1960) and Křivánek and Bureš (1960) demonstrated the oozing of potassium from the cortical surface during SD. Using ion-selective microelectrodes, Bureš and colleagues later confirmed the very large increase in interstitial potassium concentration during both SD and the hypoxic SD-like condition (HSD) (Vyskočil et al., 1972) (Figs. 12–3B, 12–4A, 13–1A).

The unparalleled increase in $[K^+]_o$ is accompanied by a drop in $[Cl^-]_o$, in $[Na^+]_o$, and, especially precipitously, in $[Ca^{2+}]_o$ (Figs. 12–3B, 12–4, 13–1, 18–3) (Do Carmo and Martins-Ferreira, 1984; Hansen and Zeuthen, 1981; Kraig and Nicholson, 1978; Nicholson, 1984; Nicholson and Kraig, 1981; Somjen and Aitken,

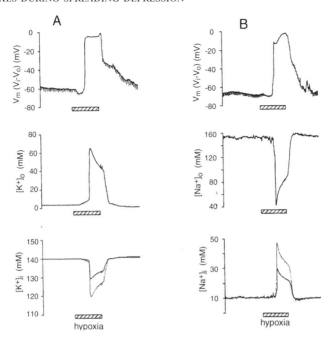

FIGURE 13–1. Neuronal membrane potential, extracellular and calculated intracellular potassium and sodium concentration changes during hypoxic spreading depression–like depolarization (HSD). Recordings from the CA1 region of hippocampal tissue slices. A and B from two preparations. The intracellular voltage of a pyramidal neuron was corrected for the simultaneously recorded extracellular potential shifts to obtain true membrane potential change ($V_m = V_I - V_o$) (V_o not illustrated). $[K^+]_o$ and $[Na^+]_o$ recorded with double-barreled ion-selective microelectrodes in stratum pyramidale near the intracellular recording. Intracellular ion changes ($[K^+]_i$ and $[Na^+]_i$) calculated for two sets of assumptions about volume proportions. True changes probably lie between the calculated extremes. (Modified from Müller and Somjen, 2000a.)

1984). The K^+ ions leaving cells are exchanged for Na^+ that are entering (Nicholson, 1984), but the exchange is not one for one, for the reduction in $[Na^+]_o$ is greater than the increase in $[K^+]_o$ (Fig. 13–1) (Müller and Somjen, 2000a). The concomitant drop in $[Cl^-]_o$ indicates that some of the Na^+ entering the neurons is accompanied by Cl^- (Fig. 16–1), but Cl^- can also accompany K^+ that is taken up by glial cells (Figs. 2–7, 2–8, 16–5). The uptake of NaCl into neurons and of KCl into glial cells draws osmotic water flow and causes cell swelling (Fig. 13–2) (Hansen and Olsen, 1980; Jing et al., 1994). Nicholson (1984) suggested that the deficit in extracellular anions is made up by anions leaving the neuronal cytosol in the company of K^+. Indeed, organic anions, including glutamate, are released during SD (Fabricius et al., 1993; Szerb, 1991; Van Harreveld and Kooiman, 1965)—although some of the glutamate probably comes from glial cells, not neurons (Kimelberg, 2000; Szatkowski et al., 1990). Of all the ions, $[Ca^{2+}]_o$ decreases proportionately the most drastically, from its normal level of 1.2–1.5 mM to less than 0.3 mM. Expressed as a fraction of the resting level, the lowering of $[Na^+]_o$ and $[Cl^-]_o$ is less drastic than that of $[Ca^{2+}]_o$, but in molar terms the influx of Na^+ and Cl^- into cells greatly exceeds that of Ca^{2+}. An accurate and complete balance sheet of all the ingredients displaced during SD is yet to be completed.

The unusual magnitude of the changes in extracellular ion concentrations created the impression that intra- and extracellular ion concentrations equilibrate during SD; this idea was bolstered by the nearly complete depolarization of neurons (Collewijn and Van Harreveld, 1966b; Higashida et al., 1974; Sugaya et al., 1975). The volume of the cytosol is, however, so much larger than that of the ISF that cells need to give up only part of the K^+ they contain in order to achieve the rise in $[K^+]_o$. Calculations based on the recorded levels of $[K^+]_o$ and the known fractional volume of the interstitial space in hippocampus show that a greatly reduced but still substantial transmembrane K^+ concentration gradient remains during SD and HSD (Kager et al., 2002a; Müller and Somjen, 2000a) (Figs. 13–1, 16–5). Unlike K^+, the ratio of $[Na^+]_o/[Na^+]_i$ may reach almost unity at the height of the depolarization. End-stage ratios for Na^+ and K^+ differ because of the unequal availability of the two ions. Per unit tissue volume, there is much more K^+ stored in cells than Na^+ in the restricted interstitial space. During SD, while V_m collapses and Na^+ conductance is (relatively) high, the limited supply of extracellular Na^+ can be depleted to the point where $[Na^+]_o$ becomes nearly equal to $[Na^+]_i$ as it moves from the smaller-capacity interstitium into the larger space inside neurons.

In conclusion

The depolarization to nearly zero V_m is not achieved by the flattening of the K^+ gradient alone, but rather by the combination of a reduced electrochemical gradient and the opening of persistent Na^+ and K^+ (and perhaps Cl^-) conductances.

While Neurons Release K^+, Glial Cells Take Up K^+
During Spreading Depression

Rising $[K^+]_o$ causes the uptake of KCl together with an osmotically equivalent amount of water in cells whose plasma membrane is permeable to Cl^-, such as muscle (Boyle and Conway, 1941) and astrocytes (Bourke et al., 1978). (Fig. 16–5). Insofar as KCl is accompanied by water, $[K^+]_i$ increases only slightly. Intracellular measurement shows, however, that glial $[K^+]_i$ does rise when $[K^+]_o$ increases (Ballanyi, 1995; Walz and Hertz, 1983). Part of the K^+ enters astrocytes unaccompanied by Cl^-, exchanged for Na^+ by the 3Na/2K ATPase ion pump, so that Na^+ is discharged into the extracellular medium. This results in elevation of glial $[K^+]_i$ and decrease of $[Na^+]_i$, changes that are opposite in direction to those in neurons. Both K^+ uptake and Na^+ release serve to buffer extracellular ion changes, but during SD they are apparently overwhelmed by ion tides. Glial membrane resistance decreases only slightly during SD compared to the drastic drop in the neuronal membranes (Fig. 14–2) (Czéh et al., 1992; Müller and Somjen, 2000a), presumably due to the relative scarcity of voltage-gated ion channels (Chapter 2: "Channels in glial membranes"). The exchange of ions across the astrocyte membrane occurs in part by passive flow through ohmic (leaky) conductances. As $[K^+]_o$ increases, it moves the glial E_K to a more positive level, creating an inward-driving force for the ion. The high $[K^+]_o$ depolarizes astrocytes and this is likely to open voltage-gated K^+ channels, accelerating the inflow of K^+ and causing the mild decrease in membrane resistance. At the same time, the glial 3Na/2K ion pump is activated, extruding Na^+ and gathering in additional K^+. As glutamate and other neuroactive substances overflow into interstitial fluid during SD (Fabricius et al., 1993; Szatkowski et al., 1990), they are likely to act on receptors on astrocyte membranes. The degree to which ligand-gated channels contribute to the behavior of glial cells during SD has not yet been assessed.

Tissue electrical resistance and cell swelling

Among the discoveries of Leão was the increase in tissue (extracellular) electrical impedance that accompanies SD, and this was soon confirmed by others (Leão and Martins-Ferreira, 1953; Freygang and Landau, 1955; Hoffman et al., 1973; Van Harreveld and Ochs, 1957). To measure extracellular impedance or resistance, alternating current or DC current pulses are passed between two electrodes in the tissue. The associated voltage drop is measured, usually between two additional electrodes placed between the current delivery electrodes, so that all four electrodes are arranged in a straight line. The increase in impedance during SD represents mainly elevated tissue resistance (R_T), while the reactive components remain less affected. The most likely explanation for the increased R_T is the swelling of cells at the expense of interstitial space. Cell swelling was confirmed in morphological studies (Van Harreveld, 1958; Van Harreveld and Khattab, 1967). Tissue resistance is an exact index of cell volume if and only if cell membrane resistance is so high that (almost) all current is forced through the interstitial spaces and the fraction flowing through cells can neglected, and membrane resistance would be invariant under all conditions. Analyzing impedance and phase angle at several frequencies, Ranck (1964) concluded that, during SD, interstitial space shrinks, neuronal membrane resistance decreases, and, a little later, glial membrane resistance increases (see also Ferreira-Filho and Martins-Ferreira, 1982). This last inference proved false; Ranck's attempt to distinguish glial from neuronal membrane behavior was based on an assumed difference in membrane time constants in excess of 1000 and a very leaky glial membrane (Ranck, 1963). In fact, glial membrane resistance either remains constant or decreases slightly during SD and HSD (Fig. 14–2) (Czéh et al., 1992;

Müller and Somjen, 2000a). More recent measurements confirm that a sizable fraction of current imposed on the brain tissue does flow through cell membranes (Ferreira-Filho and Martins-Ferreira, 1982; Gardner-Medwin, 1983; Gardner-Medwin and Nicholson, 1983; Okada et al., 1994). More importantly, neuronal membrane resistance drops drastically during SD (Fig. 14–1) (Czéh et al., 1993; Müller and Somjen, 2000a ; Snow et al., 1983), so that during SD an increased fraction of the current must take the transcellular route, further degrading the accuracy of estimates of cell swelling based on changes of R_T.

A more reliable measure of the ISVF is obtained from the concentrations of indicator substances that do not penetrate cell membranes. Tried and tested indicators such as inulin, are metabolically and pharmacologically inert and electrically neutral, but these provide only single time point measurements in whole tissue samples. To follow changes in real time and to resolve spatial distributions, indicators that can be measured with ion-selective microelectrodes are preferred. Among them are TMA^+ and TEA^+ and certain anions (Dietzel et al., 1980; Nicholson and Rice, 1988; Phillips and Nicholson, 1979). From the increase in the concentration of such indicators the collapse of the interstitial spaces during SD and HSD could accurately be gauged (Fig. 13–2) (Do Carmo and Martins-Ferreira, 1984; Hansen and Olsen, 1980; Jing et al., 1994; Lundbaek and Hansen, 1992; Pérez-Pinzón et al., 1995). In interpreting the drastic decrease in ISVF, it should be remembered that only moderate cell swelling is needed to compress most of the interstitial space. For example, where the normal ISVF occupies 13% of the tissue volume (McBain et al., 1990), there a 70% decrease in ISVF during SD (Jing et al., 1994) corresponds to only about a 10.5% expansion of the average intracellular volume.

The ISVF also shrinks during neuronal excitation and seizures (Dietzel et al., 1980) (Chapter 8: "Na^+, Cl^-, and cell volume"), but much less than during SD or HSD (Fig. 13–2) (Jing et al., 1994). Neurons, especially dendrites, swell because NaCl uptake exceeds the discharge of K^+ and organic anions (see above), while glial cell swelling is driven by KCl uptake stimulated by the rising $[K^+]_o$ (Kimelberg, 2000; Kimelberg et al., 1995; Mori et al., 1976c).

Spreading depression–related intrinsic optical signals

Osmotic Cell Swelling Is Associated with Decreased Light Scattering

Optical signals recorded from live tissues are called *intrinsic* if they do not require staining of the tissue, only an appropriate light source and a detector, which could be a camera or an array of photodiodes. Scattering of light in cell suspensions has long been used to measure cell volume changes (Lucké and Parpart, 1954; Ørskov, 1935; and see the review by Aitken et al., 1999). Cell swelling is accompanied by reduced scattering, cell shrinkage by the opposite change. Scattering

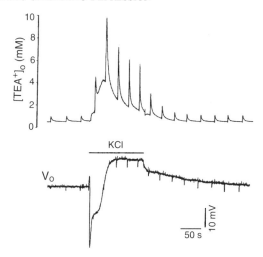

FIGURE 13–2. Interstitial volume fraction shrinkage during spreading depression (SD). Recording in stratum pyramidale of the CA1 region in a hippocampal tissue slice. Tetraethyl ammonium (TEA^+) was the indicator, recorded with a double-barreled ion-selective microelectrode. A total of 0.2 mM TEA^+ was dissolved in the bath, and at regular intervals a brief pulse of constant magnitude was delivered by micro-iontophoresis close to the recording electrode. Spreading depression was induced by applying a high K^+ solution to the surface of the slice. Spreading depression was accompanied by elevation of baseline $[TEA^+]_o$ and a severalfold increase in iontophoresis-evoked transient responses. V_o was recorded from the reference barrel of the ion-selective electrode. On average, the interstitial volume fraction decreased to about 25% of its resting size during SD. (Modified from Jing et al., 1994.)

makes cells and tissues less transparent (decreases light transmittance), but it brightens the surface (increases reflectance). The best explanation of the diminished scattering associated with cell swelling is the dilution of intracellular scattering particles as water enters the cell. Scattering particles include macromolecules and organelles (Barer et al., 1953). Light is not only scattered but also absorbed in tissues, and tissues can also be sources of autofluorescence. Absorption and fluorescence spectra provide information about biochemical events. Scattering changes have a broad spectrum, and they can be recorded independently of absorption and fluorescence changes, because the latter are limited in wavelength band. Besides, absorption diminishes both transmitted and reflected light, fluorescence increases both, while scattering decreases the former and increases the latter. When organs in situ are illuminated, absorption by hemoglobin dominates the changes in reflected light, but in isolated tissue preparations absorption is weak compared to scattering.

Neuron excitation is accompanied by scattering changes, which produce intrinsic optical signals (IOSs). With a charge-coupled digital (CCD) camera attached to a microscope, IOSs produced by brain cells can be recorded and mapped in real time, and their extension and movements followed. This is an advantage over electrodes that register voltages from only a limited number of points (reviewed by Aitken et al., 1999; Andrew et al., 1999). Also, when light is the recorded variable, the puncture wound made by microelectrodes is avoided. As in cell suspensions, light scattering changes in brain tissue are caused in part by water moving into and out of cells. Raising osmolarity causes an increase in light scattering and lowering osmolarity causes a decrease, as expected from the shrinkage of cells in the former case and swelling in the latter (Aitken et al., 1999; Fayuk et al., 2002; Holthoff and Witte, 1996; Kreisman et al., 1995). In hippocampal slices these optical changes are much more marked in dendritic layers than cell body layers, as expected from the relative resistance of neuron somas to volume change (Aitken et al., 1998a) (see chapter 3: "Volume Regulation of Cells . . ."). Cell volume changes are, however, by no means the only source of optical signals in brain tissue (Aitken et al., 1999; Cohen et al., 1972; Fayuk et al., 2002; Syková et al., 2003; Tao et al., 2002).

Spreading Depression Is Associated with an Increase in Light Scattering

Gouras (1958) noticed the "milky area" that expanded over an excised frog retina together with the electrical signs of SD. This was the first report of an IOS coupled to a functional neuronal change in a vertebrate nervous system. Subsequently Martins-Ferreira and de Oliveira Castro (1966; Oliveira Castro et al., 1985) recorded four successive phases of the optical response accompanying SD in isolated retina and identified their cause as changing light scattering. Snow et al. (1983) reported the SD-related IOSs in hippocampal tissue slices. These were less obvious than those in retina, probably because the retina is more translucent than are hippocampal slices. In the retina, the SD-related optical signals are maximal in the inner plexiform layer (Martins-Ferreira and de Oliveira Castro, 1966), corresponding to the region of maximal ΔV_o (Mori et al., 1976a). In hippocampal tissue slices, IOSs associated with SD are most marked in the dendritic layers, while cell body layers are relatively inert (Figs. 13–3, 19–5) (Aitken et al., 1998b; Andrew et al., 1995; Müller and Somjen, 1999), as expected from electrical recordings (Herreras and Somjen, 1993a) and CSD analysis (Wadman et al., 1992). In neocortical tissue slices the SD-related optical signals start in layers II and III (Andrew et al., 2002).

As already stated, the cell volume increase is associated with a decrease in light scattering not only in cell suspensions and cell cultures but also in tissue slices (Aitken et al., 1999; Andrew and MacVicar, 1994; Fayuk et al., 2002; Holthoff and Witte, 1998; but see Syková et al., 2003). This presents a problem, for even though cells undoubtedly swell rapidly and strongly during SD, the main optical change associated with SD is a large, sudden increase, not a decrease, in light scattering (Aitken et al., 1998b; Andrew et al., 1995; Fayuk et al., 2002; Kreisman

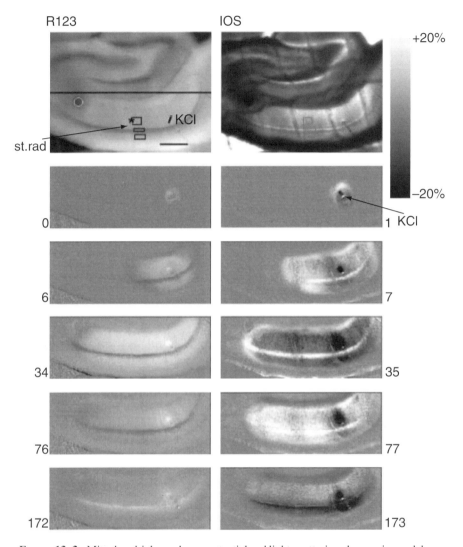

Figure 13–3. Mitochondrial membrane potential and light-scattering changes imaged during spreading depression. Optical recording from a transilluminated hippocampal tissue slice. Spreading depression was provoked by microinjection of KCl solution. Mitochondrial membrane potential assayed by fluorescence of the rhodamine derivative R123; increased fluorescence indicates mitochondrial depolarization. The increase in the intrinsic optical signal (IOS; transmitted light) indicates diminished light scattering. The top two frames show resting reference images; the other frames are difference images: resting reference subtracted from recorded intensities. The horizontal line bisecting the top left image shows the boundary of the imaged area in the frames below. The "regions of interest" for time plots (e.g., Figs. 13–4 and 13–5) and site of KCl microinjection are shown in the top left frame. Scale bar represents 0.5 mm. Note the spreading brightening of the R123 signal in the dendritic zones of the CA1 region and alternation of the light-dark-light sequence of IOS. (Compare with Fig. 19–5.) (From Bahar et al., 2000.)

and LaManna, 1999; Kreisman et al., 2000; Martins-Ferreira and de Oliveira Castro, 1966; Snow et al., 1983; Tao, 2000; Tao et al., 2002; Yoon et al., 1996). The exception seems to be submerged neocortical tissue slices, where SD can apparently be induced without a light scattering increase, while hypoxic SD-like depolarization is associated with a scattering increase in this preparation as well (Andrew et al., 2002).

Kreisman et al. (1995) found a possible artifact that could explain the paradox of an apparent light scattering increase coinciding with cell swelling. When tissue slices are at a liquid–gas interface and the slice takes on extra water, the surface of the slice bulges, the angles of incidence and reflection of light change, and so does the recorded signal, independently of scattering within the tissue. This, however, is not the whole explanation.

In a detailed series of experiments, we (Aitken et al., 1999; Bahar et al., 2000; Fayuk et al., 1999, 2002; Müller and Somjen, 1999) compared the IOSs of hippocampal tissue slices during SD, HSD, and osmotically induced cell volume changes (Figs. 13–3, 13–4, 13–5, 19–5, 19–6). Two kinds of optical signals are generated in these slices, and neither is caused by the artifact described by Kreisman et al. (1995). As expected, mild to moderate hypotonic cell swelling was correlated with

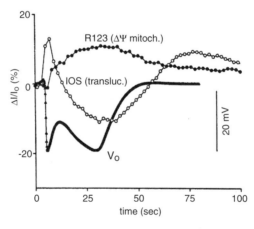

FIGURE 13–4. Light scattering shows triphasic change while mitochondria depolarize during spreading depression. Plots of rhodamine-123 (R123) fluorescence, intrinsic optical signal (IOS) and V_o from stratum radiatum from the experiment of Figure 13–3. R123 fluorescence increase means depolarization of mitochondria ($\Delta\psi_m$). Initiallly, increased IOS (translucence) indicates decreased light scattering, corresponding to cell swelling. Coincident with the onset of the R123 fluorescence increase the IOS turned down, indicating light-scattering increase, probably due to swelling of mitochondria. Extracellular potential, V_o, was recorded from the margin of the area of optical recording, marked by the asterisk in the top left frame of Figure 13–3. Zero time is the moment of KCl injection, which was at some distance from the area of recording. (From Bahar et al., 2000.)

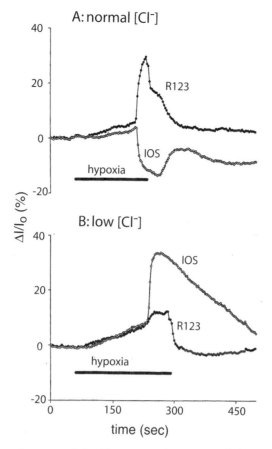

FIGURE 13–5. Lowering extracellular Cl-concentration prevents light-scattering increase and limits mitochondrial depolarization during HSD. Recording of optical signals similar to Figures 3–3 and 3–4. A: In normal artificial cerebrospinal fluid bathing solution. B: With most of the Cl⁻ substituted for by methyl sulfate, which is impermeant to plasma membrane. When oxygen was replaced by nitrogen in the gas space of the chamber, initially both rhodamine-123 (R123) and the intrinsic optical signal (IOS; transmitted light intensity) increased gradually, indicating mild depolarization of mitochondria and moderate decrease of light scattering due to slow cell swelling. In normal $[Cl^-]_o$ (A) the sharp upturn of the R123 fluorescence and the coincident downturn of the IOS signal onset of hypoxic SD-like depolarization (HSD) (cf. Fig. 13–4). In low $[Cl^-]_o$ (B) the HSD-related R123 increase is greatly reduced, and the IOS decrease is replaced by a sharp IOS increase (decreased light scattering). In low $[Cl^-]_o$ the light scattering decrease caused by HSD-related cell swelling is unmasked, probably because the mitochondrial swelling, which in normal ACSF causes the scattering increase, is curtailed. (From Bahar et al., 2000.)

a decrease in light scattering and hypertonic shrinkage with its increase. Spreading depression and especially HSD are preceded by a brief decrease in scattering, but when the SD-related ΔV_o begins, the IOS abruptly reverses polarity. The intense increase in scattering returns to baseline more slowly than does V_o. The IOS changes were qualitatively similar in interfaced and submerged slices, and therefore could not be due to the change in curvature of the surface (bulging or *lensing*) of the tissue slice. The reversal from scattering decrease to scattering increase at the onset of ΔV_o during SD was also confirmed by Tao and associates (Tao, 2000; Tao et al., 2002), who used optical fibers in contact with the tissue to exclude surface artifacts.

Spreading Depression–Related Increase in Light Scattering May Be Caused by Swelling of Mitochondria and of Other Intracellular Organelles

When Cl^- in the bathing solution is replaced by an anion that does not penetrate cell membranes, the scattering increase is abolished (Martins-Ferreira et al., 1971), and in its place the swelling-induced scattering decrease continues during and after the ΔVo (Fig. 13–5) (Aitken et al., 1999; Fayuk et al., 2002; Müller, 2000; Müller and Somjen, 1999). The cell swelling, measured as the shrinkage of the TMA^+ space, was not diminished by deleting Cl^- (Müller, 2000; Müller and Somjen, 1999). In the absence of NaCl, cell swelling was probably due to the influx of $NaHCO_3$. In the absence of extracellular Cl^-, the swelling-related scattering decrease was unmasked, while in the presence of Cl^- the SD-induced scattering increase obscured it. Tao et al. (2002) confirmed that the scattering increase can be converted into a scattering decrease if Cl^- is replaced by methyl sulfate. They also found that proprionate can substitute for Cl^- without abolishing the light-scattering increase. This they attribute to the ability of proprionate to penetrate the neuron membrane, while methyl sulfate is impermeant.

The source of the chloride-dependent scattering increase is not definitely determined, but it probably is related to swelling of mitochondria and other organelles. Using the fluorescence of rhodamine-123 to gauge mitochondrial membrane potential ($\Delta\psi_m$), Bahar et al. (2000) found that during SD and HSD mitochondria are powerfully depolarized, but lowering of $[Cl^-]_o$ suppresses the SD-related mitochondrial depolarization together with the SD-induced increase in light scattering (Figs. 13–3, 13–5). The correlation of the two effects, chloride-dependent mitochondrial depolarization and chloride-dependent light scattering increase, does not prove identity of their source, but at the least, it is very suggestive. We suggest that Cl^--dependent swelling of mitochondria and possibly of other organelles causes the increase in light scattering during SD. This is supported by the observation that in extreme hypotonicity as well, the initial decrease in scattering inverts and turns into an increase (Fayuk et al., 2002).

Unlike low Cl⁻, depriving the preparation of external Ca^{2+} did not prevent SD-induced mitochondrial depolarization (Bahar et al., 1999). This means that it was either initiated by release of Ca^{2+} from ER (Zhang and Lipton, 1999) or that it was not Ca^{2+} dependent. Opening of the ***mitochondrial permeability transition pore (MPTP)*** (Fig. 2–3) is associated with collapse of the mitochondrial membrane potential, and it is said to be usually initiated by rising mitochondrial Ca^{2+} (Zoratti and Szabó, 1995). Opening of the mPTP is associated with lethal events (Duchen, 1999), although some authors suggest that it has reversible physiological functions as well. The SD- and HSD-related mitochondrial depolarization signaled by the rhodamine-123 fluorescence increase was reversible, with return of neuron function, provided that the hypoxic period was not unduly prolonged (Bahar et al., 1999).

Other Proposed Sources of Spreading Depression– and Excitation-related Intrinsic Optical Signals

Andrew and his associates identified another possible source for the light-scattering increase that is caused by combined oxygen-glucose deprivation and also by excitotoxicity (Andrew et al., 1999; Obeidat and Andrew, 1998; Polischuk et al., 1998). They attribute the increased scattering to the *beading of dendrites*, which is a sign of irreversible injury (Andrew et al., 2002; Hori and Carpenter, 1994). Unlike dendritic beading, the scattering increase associated with uncomplicated SD or transient HSD is rapidly and completely reversible and does not lead to loss of neuronal function, provided that oxygenation is restored in time (Aitken et al., 1999; Müller and Somjen, 1999).

Finally, Syková and associates (2003) report that in spinal cord tissue slices of very young rats, IOSs correlate in time and magnitude better with neuronal activity than with cell swelling as measured by interstitial volume changes, reminding us of earlier findings by Cohen (1973) and Cohen et al. (1972) relating scattering changes by squid axon membranes to membrane potential.

In Conclusion: Several Mechanisms Can Alter Light Scattering

Light scattering is a general physical property of living tissue that is not linked to any single specific biophysical variable. It should therefore not be surprising that light scattering can be changed by a variety of conditions. The following explanations have been proposed for the (nonmetabolic) IOSs of brain slices, and these are not mutually exclusive: (*1*) Cell swelling is associated with a light-scattering decrease. (*2*) Spreading depression and (reversible) HSD are associated with a Cl⁻-dependent scattering increase that is probably due to swelling of intracellular organelles. (*3*) Excitation of neurons alters refraction at the plasma membrane, perhaps due to conformation change in channel proteins. (*4*) Strong swelling of tissue slices at liquid–gas interfaces can alter reflected light when the radius of curvature of the slice surface changes. (5) Irreversible beading of dendritic processes can also increase light scattering.

Tissue and cell pH in spreading depression

During SD, extracellular pH (pH$_o$) first becomes alkaline and then acid (Fig. 13–6) (Kraig and Cooper, 1987; Kraig et al., 1983; Lehmenkühler et al., 1982b; Nicholson, 1984; Somjen, 1984). During hypoxia or ischemia strong tissue acidosis begins well before HSD, but the onset of HSD is marked by a brief but strong alkaline transient that interrupts the acid shift (Fig. 19–10A) (Hansen and Lauritzen, 1984; Kraig et al., 1983; Tombaugh, 1994). The acute alkaline transient is related to the membrane change that brings about the depolarization in both SD and HSD. The slower tissue acidosis is generated by metabolic processes.

The local acidosis which outlasts the ΔV_o is due mainly to the production of excess CO_2 and other acid metabolites, especially lactic acid (Cruz et al., 1999; Křivánek, 1961; Scheller et al., 1992b), by-products of the increased metabolic activity required for restoration of the ion distributions (Bureš et al., 1984). The origins of the alkaline shift are less clear, and several factors may contribute to it. The production of ammonium ions appears to be one factor (Kraig and Cooper, 1987). The more moderate increase in pH induced by electrical stimulation (without SD) has been attributed to the extrusion of HCO_3^- at $GABA_A$ receptor–controlled channels (Kaila, 1994), plus uptake of H^+ in response to glutamate-induced depolarization. The latter mechanism is calcium dependent, and it is believed to be caused by countertransport exchanging Ca^{2+} for protons, which compensates

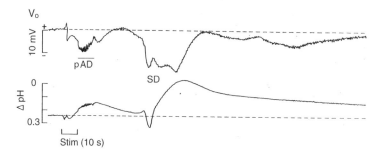

FIGURE 13–6. Seizures and spreading depression are accompanied by transient alkalinization followed by greatly prolonged acidification of interstitial fluid. Recording from dentate gyrus of an anesthetized rat with a double-barreled ion-selective electrode: 10 s 20 Hz stimulation of the angular bundle (similar to Figs. 7–8, 8–1, and 8–2). Increase of pH (decrease of [H^+]) is plotted downward. pAD: paroxysmal afterdischarge. The records were low-pass filtered. (Modified from Somjen, 1984)

for depolarization-induced calcium influx (Grichtchenko and Chesler, 1996; Smith and Chesler, 1999; Smith et al., 1994). This, however, does not completely account for the alkaline shift associated with SD, which does occur even in Ca^{2+}-free medium (Menna et al., 2000). The extracellular alkaline transient is accompanied by alkalinization of glial cytoplasm followed by delayed intracellular acidification, while neurons become acid from the start (Chesler, 1990; Chesler and Kraig, 1987). Glial alkalinization is in part a function of membrane potential and may be caused by transmembrane proton flux (Chesler, 1990; Grichtchenko and Chesler, 1994; Kraig, 1993) but, again, more than one mechanism may be at work (Amos and Chesler, 1998; Lascola and Kraig, 1997).

Key points

During SD $[K^+]_o$ rises to levels unequaled by any other brain condition except the SD-like condition in severe hypoxia and stroke (HSD). $[Na^+]_o$, $[Cl^-]_o$, and $[Ca^{2+}]_o$ decrease drastically.

K$^+$ is released from neurons but taken up by glial cells. Glial K$^+$ uptake is in part in exchange for Na$^+$ and in part combined with uptake of Cl$^-$, causing glial swelling. Neurons, or at least their dendrites, also swell.

Cell swelling is associated with reduced light scattering of the tissue, but at the

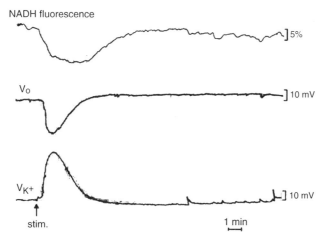

FIGURE 13–7. Reduced nicotinamide adenine dinucleotide (NADH) oxidation, extracellular voltage shift, and potassium concentration during spreading depression. Recording from cat neocortex, with conditions similar to those in Figure 8–4. Spreading depression was provoked by strong electrical stimulation of the cortical surface. Diminished corrected NADH fluorescence indicates oxidation. V_{K^+} is the voltage of the potassium-selective microelectrode. (Modified from Lothman et al., 1975)

onset of SD and HSD light scattering increases suddenly and markedly. Similarly to the SD-related shifts in V_o and $[K^+]_o$, optical responses were much more marked in dendritic layers than in cell body layers. Mitochondria depolarize at the onset of SD. Substituting an impermeant anion for Cl^- prevents the light-scattering increase and the mitochondrial depolarization. The rapid, reversible, Cl-dependent light-scattering increase is probably the result of organelle swelling. Additional sources of light-scattering changes are discussed.

At the onset of SD and HSD, pH_o undergoes a marked but brief alkaline transient, followed by prolonged acidification that outlasts the V_o and ion shifts. The alkaline transient is related to a membrane flux of ions that is not completely understood. The acidification is caused by metabolic production of acid. However in normoxic SD, the tissue is not short of oxygen (Fig. 13–7 and Chapter 15: "Neurons are not short of oxygen . . .")

14

Membrane Potential and Input Resistance during Spreading Depression

Ever since its discovery, there has been a debate about the source and the mechanism of the electric signs that accompany SD—chiefly, whether the primary generator is neuronal or glial. This chapter reviews the electrophysiology of the cells involved in the SD process.

Membrane changes in neurons

Neuron Membrane Potential

Brožek (1966) sampled membrane potentials by advancing a microelectrode through cortex and registering the voltage deflections as the electrode tip penetrated cells before, during, and after the passage of a wave of SD. Average membrane voltages were less negative during SD than before it, suggesting depolarization, and more negative thereafter, indicating transient hyperpolarization following SD. Collewijn and Van Harreveld (1966b) were the first to record the intracellular potential (V_i) of neurons long enough to follow its course through SD. They recognized that the intracellular electrode records the sum of intra- and extracellular voltage shifts and, in the case of SD, ΔV_o is too large to be ignored. After correcting ΔV_i for ΔV_o ($\Delta V_m = \Delta V_I - \Delta V_o$), they concluded that, during SD, the membrane potential of neurons can briefly approach but not reach zero. Their findings have been repeatedly confirmed (Czéh et al., 1993; Higashida et al., 1974; Müller and Somjen, 2000a; Snow et al., 1983; Somjen and Aitken, 1984; Tomita, 1984) (Figs. 13–1, 19–1), but some investigators neglected to correct for ΔV_o. Since V_o shifts in the negative direction while V_i shifts in the positive direction, the two approach one another. If only the movement of V_i is taken into account and that of V_o is neglected, then the depolarization (ΔV_m), will be underestimated (e.g., Goldensohn, 1969; Tanaka et al., 1997). In most cases, neither the trajectory of ΔV_m nor that of $\Delta[K^+]_o$ has the inverted saddle shape, with two maxima, that is typical of the trajectory of ΔV_o. Rather, there is typically an early single peak followed by a lower, prolonged plateau or else a slowly declining late phase (Figs. 12–4A, 13–1, 19–1). If, however, ΔV_i is not corrected for ΔV_o, then ΔV_i can show an artifactual drift in a positive direction.

Neuronal Input Resistance

Neuron R_{in} was measured during SD and HSD by a number of teams using "sharp" intracellular electrodes (Mody et al., 1987; Müller and Somjen, 1998, 2000a; Snow et al., 1983) or using patch-clamp electrodes in a whole-cell configuration (Czéh et al., 1993). Snow et al. (1983) reported the collapse of R_{in} to a degree where it was too small to measure. The apparent elimination of membrane resistance, together with the nearly complete depolarization and the drastic ion fluxes, have led to a concept of *membrane breakdown*, assuming sieve-like transparency of neuronal membranes at the height of SD. This has turned out to be an exaggeration.

    Czéh et al. (1993) patch-clamped CA1 hippocampal neurons in a whole-cell configuration and obtained current-voltage (I-V) plots by subjecting the cells to depolarizing voltage ramps. In control recordings the I-V plot had a linear part in the passive range of voltages negative in relation to the firing threshold. A technical limitation of whole-cell voltage-clamping of large neurons is that the voltage clamp controls only the cell soma. The axon, which is outside the clamped region, can fire action potentials, and the apical dendrites can generate calcium spikes. These out-of-control spikes create current surges (Fig. 14–1B). Input resistance can be determined from the slope of the subthreshold, linear portion of the I-V plot. During SD and HSD the current surges representing active responses disappeared. The I-V plot became entirely linear and quite steep, indicating increased conductance (Figs. 14–1, 19–2). The average R_{in} was reduced to 34% of its control value during SD and to 21% during HSD when cesium-gluconate pipettes were used and to 52% with potassium-gluconate pipettes. The Cs^+ in the pipette blocked most K^+ currents but had no effect on Na^+ and Ca^{2+} currents. This average conceals the wide variability among neurons. R_{in} dropped below 10% in some cells, while others seemed not to participate at all in the SD, even though the extracellular ΔV_o confirmed the SD of their neighbors. Nonparticipating neurons were found earlier by Sugaya et al. (1975). Using sharp electrodes filled with potassium-acetate solution, Müller and Somjen (1998) estimated input resistance

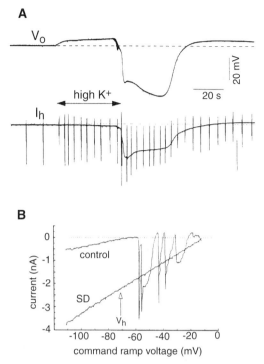

FIGURE 14–1. Neuron membrane current and conductance during spreading depression (SD). Whole-cell patch-clamp recording from a CA1 pyramidal neuron in a rat hippocampal tissue slice. The voltage of the patch pipette was referred to a nearby extracellular micro-electrode (instead of ground) to control membrane voltage without interference by extra-cellular voltage shifts. V_o was recorded from this reference electrode, against ground. Spreading depression was provoked by a small drop of high-K^+ solution at some distance. **A:** I_h is the current holding the membrane at a –71 mV holding potential (V_h). I_h increases greatly during SD, but its trajectory is not congruent with that of V_o. The vertical deflections intersecting the I_h trace are caused by test ramp voltage commands, two of which are illustrated in the current-voltage (I-V) plots of **B**. The ramp was preceded by a 20 ms hyperpolarizing step to -111 mV; then it moved the membrane to –11 mV over 300 ms and then stepped back to V_h. In the control I-V record, the ramp triggered inward current surges caused by impulses and Ca^{2+} spikes generated outside the clamp-controlled region. During SD the I-V plot becomes straight and its steep slope indicates increased membrane conductance. The zero current intercept of the I-V plot indicates the membrane potential that would occur in the absence of voltage clamp (about –12 mV during SD). (Modified from Czéh et al., 1993.)

in *current-clamp* mode, using small hyperpolarizing current pulses. With this method R_{in} was reduced to 11.5% (17.1% for interneurons) of its resting value during HSD. The two methods register different aspects of the membrane response. The whole-cell voltage ramp moves the membrane potential over a wide range, and even within the seemingly linear portion, some conductances are perhaps activated. The small hyperpolarizing pulses delivered by sharp electrodes probably do not significantly activate currents. Although the averages found with the two methods differed, the ranges of the two data sets overlapped.

The main conclusion

Neither method indicated complete breakdown of membrane resistance or ionic transparency of the membrane.

In spreading depression, neurons lead and glial cells follow

In the normal central nervous system the V_m of glial cells (usually astrocytes) is, on average, more negative and more stable than that of neurons, while their input resistance (R_{in}) is lower. Low glial membrane resistance is due in part to the high resting conductance for K^+ and for Cl^-, while input resistance is further lowered by the electrical coupling between cells by gap junctions (see Chapter 2: "Voltage-gated channels, *but* voltage-independent membrane resistance?"). Excitation of neurons causes $[K^+]_o$ to rise. This depolarizes glial cells and, in the spinal gray matter and neocortex K^+-induced glial depolarization contributes a large part of the extracellular sustained potential shifts that accompany prolonged neuron excitation (Figs. 2–10 and 2–11, and Chapter 7: "How much do glial cells contribute . . . ?") (Somjen, 1973). The prominent ΔV_o that is typical of SD has also been assumed to be generated in large part by glia, and this was one of the early reasons for suggesting that glial cells play a leading role in SD (Leibowitz, 1992; Marshall, 1959). In the hippocampal formation the glial contribution to ΔV_o is, however, minor (Somjen, 1987, 1993), yet the glial cells in hippocampus are depolarized just as profoundly as those in neocortex. This is just one of many examples showing that extracellular signals do not reliably reflect membrane potential changes.

The membrane potential of *idle cells*, later proven to be neuroglia, was recorded during SD for the first time by Karahashi and Goldring (1966), followed by Higashida et al. (1971). The depolarization of glial cells more or less mirrored the ΔV_o of the cortical surface. Later, Higashida et al. (1974) and Sugaya et al. (1975) compared neuronal and glial recordings and came to contrasting conclusions. Higashida et al. (1974) found that neurons were more strongly depolarized than glial cells. By contrast, according to Sugaya et al. (1975), depolarization started earlier and was more profound in cortical glial cells than in neurons. They also reported that not all neurons depolarized during SD, while the response of glial cells was uniform. These observations and the lack of effect of TTX on SD led them to believe that glial cells produce SD and that neurons merely follow their lead. This was contradicted by Mori et al. (1976b, 1976c), who reported that Müller (glial) cells in retina take up K^+ during SD. Therefore, they cannot be the source of the rise of $[K^+]_o$; rather, their membrane behaves passively, as a potassium electrode. The sources of the elevated K^+ must have been neurons, and neuronal depolarization had to be the primary event.

We obtained recordings from glial cells in hippocampal slices during SD and HSD. As in the retina (Mori et al., 1976b), the membrane of hippocampal glial cells depolarized with the rise of $[K^+]_o$, as expected for a passive K^+-permeable membrane. R_{in} decreased only slightly and sometimes not at all. This was the case using either the whole-cell patch-clamp method (Fig. 14–2) (Czéh et al., 1992; Somjen et al., 1993a) or sharp electrodes in current-clamp mode (Müller and Somjen, 2000a). Also, at the height of HSD, glial cells still retained a membrane potential of about –20 mV, when neurons were depolarized to near zero. A flaw in the whole-cell recordings was the use of cesium-gluconate-filled patch pipettes in the majority of the recordings. This presumably blocked K^+ currents, but not

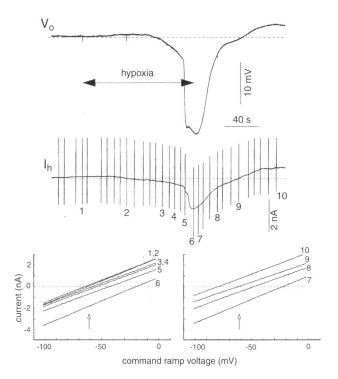

Figure 14–2. Passive behavior of a glial cell during hypoxic spreading depression–like depolarization (HSD). Recording conditions similar to those in Figure 14–1, but from a glial cell. The holding current increased during hypoxia, first gradually and then abruptly during HSD. The current-voltage (I-V) plots below were generated as in Figure 14–1B; the arrow shows the holding potential. 1: Before hypoxia; 2, 3: during hypoxia, before HSD; 4–6: during HSD; 7–10: during recovery. Note that the I-V plot is linear in the control condition and remains so during hypoxia. The I-V lines are shifted along the voltage axis, while the slope barely changes, indicating that the membrane conductance was minimally affected. (Unpublished experiment by G. Czéh. See also Czéh et al., 1992; Somjen, 1995.)

Na$^+$ and Ca^{2+} currents. Using similar electrodes, input resistance of neurons did decrease, however, many times more than that of glial cells. Besides, the sharp electrodes used in the current-clamp trials contained no Cs$^+$. Our data thus agree with those of Higashida et al. (1974).

Interest in the role of neuroglia in SD was rekindled with the discovery of *cal-cium waves* in glial cell cultures (Cornell-Bell et al., 1990; Finkbeiner, 1992; Glaum et al., 1990). When a local stimulus, for example glutamate or NMDA, raises [Ca^{2+}]$_i$ in a cluster of glial cells, other cells that are linked through gap junctions follow suit, and the wave of [Ca^{2+}]$_i$ increase spreads at a slow velocity reminiscent of the propagation of SD. Similarly spreading calcium waves have also been recorded in hippocampal slices (Dani et al., 1992; Dani and Smith, 1995), retina (Fernandes de Lima et al., 1994), and organ cultures (Kunkler and Kraig, 1998). Nedergaard (Martins-Ferreira et al., 2000) has proposed a primary role for the calcium waves in the generation of SD. The Ca^{2+} is thought to diffuse from cell to cell by way of gap junctions, and in each next cell to trigger calcium-induced calcium release from intracellular storage. In line with this scheme, a number of agents that block gap junctions also prevent SD spread (Nedergaard et al., 1995). The notion of SD mediation by calcium waves was refuted, however, by observations of Basarsky et al. (1998), who showed that calcium waves cease when calcium is deleted from the bathing medium, yet SD is not prevented by removing Ca^{2+}. It follows that Ca^{2+} influx from the medium is required for calcium waves but not for SD generation or propagation. In addition, unlike heptanol and halothane, the more selective gap junction blocking agent carbenoxolone failed to stop SD (Világi et al., 2001). (Gap junctions are discussed further in Chapter 16: "Mechanisms of spreading depression propagation").

Do Astrocytes Promote Spreading Depression, or Protect Against It?

Two diametrically opposed interpretations can be found in the literature concerning the significance of glial elements for SD. On the one hand, it is suggested that the glial "functional syncytium" promotes SD either by "broadcasting" K$^+$ ions (see Chapter 2: "Can spatial buffering have unintended consequences?") or by spreading "calcium waves" (see above). On the other hand, it is asserted that the glial spatial buffer and the siphoning system inhibit SD. Reports by Largo, Herreras, and colleagues (Largo et al., 1996, 1997a, 1997b) and, more recently, by Theis et al. (2003) show that poisoning glial cells or selectively interrupting gap junctions among them (leaving neuronal gap junctions intact) enhances SD instead of limiting it. This tips the balance in favor of a protective, inhibitory role for astrocytes.

Glial protection against SD is achieved in part by stabilization of extracellular ion levels, especially [K$^+$]$_o$ (Chapter 2: "Glial cells regulate ion levels . . ."). Computer simulation makes this contention plausible (Fig. 16–6). Ion regulation is a joint function of neuroglia and the capillary endothelium that forms the BBB (Bradbury, 1979; Cancilla et al., 1993; Newman, 1995). Additionally, astrocytes prevent overflow of transmitters into interstitial fluid (Barbour et al., 1988; Schousboe and Westergaard, 1995), although when things go wrong, the glial glutamate transporter can turn around and cause more harm than good (Hansson et al., 2000; Szatkowski et al., 1990).

In conclusion

Glial cells play a passive role in the total SD response (Walz, 1997). They depolarize because their membrane potential is determined by the rise of $[K^+]_o$, and they swell because they take up KCl. Glial membrane conductance changes little, but glial cells depolarize uniformly. The time courses of glial ΔV_m and of the ΔV_o are similar because both voltages are governed by the aggregate behavior of the neuron population. By contrast, in neurons the timing of the depolarization and the magnitude of the underlying membrane conductance increase can vary greatly among members of the population, because they are determined by the activation of specific membrane conductances, which differ among neurons. As we shall see, the SD process is ignited when neuron dendritic persistent inward currents begin to exceed persistent outward currents (Chapter 16: "Spreading depression is ignited . . ."), and for some neurons this moment may precede while in others it may lag behind the group average. In spite of individual variability, neurons initiate and govern the SD process.

Key points

Neurons depolarize to near zero V_m during SD, with input resistance decreasing to a fraction of normal. Glial cells also depolarize, but with input resistance only slightly decreased. Glial depolarization is mainly passive, caused by the rising $[K^+]_o$.

Glial cells take up K^+ during SD, while neurons release it.

Glial calcium waves run with propagating SD but are not required for SD.

Healthy glial tissue inhibits SD.

Changes in neuronal membrane potential and input resistance during HSD are indistinguishable from those in normoxic SD.

15

The Mechanism of Spreading Depression

In preceding chapters we have seen that during SD and HSD neurons, as well as glial cells, undergo profound depolarization, but neurons are the primary agents in the SD process. Chapter 15 examines the various possible ways in which the neuron membrane potential can be brought to near zero volts. The data indicate that several membrane ion channels cooperate in causing SD-related depolarization.

Neurons are not short of oxygen during spreading depression, only during hypoxic spreading depression–like depolarization

Based on the similarities between SD and HSD, and on inspection of pial blood vessels, Van Harreveld and Stamm (1952) proposed that SD resulted from a spreading wave of local ischemia due to vasoconstriction. Localized hypoperfusion would cause the failure of ion transport and hence the collapse of membrane potentials. Referred to as the *asphyxial hypothesis*, this idea was the first attempt to explain SD. It was, however, discarded as evidence mounted.

As it turned out, the vascular responses associated with SD are not simple. Just prior to ΔV_o vessels may constrict, but this is not always observed. The depolarization itself is associated with a marked increase in local blood flow, followed after repolarization by prolonged but moderate hypoperfusion (Gjedde et al., 1981; Hansen and Lauritzen, 1984; Lauritzen, 1987; Lauritzen et al., 1982; Mies and

292

Paschen, 1984; Piper et al., 1991). During uncomplicated SD in otherwise healthy brain tissue, local blood flow is so abundant that hemoglobin oxygenation increases in spite of the increased metabolic demand (Kohl et al., 1999; Wolf et al., 1996). Extracellular tissue oxygen tension (P_{O_2}) is also elevated, especially at the onset of SD, though it may decrease later (Lehmenkühler, 1990; Wolf et al., 1996).

Most importantly, as assayed by their autofluorescence, mitochondrial oxidative enzymes, NADH as well as cytochrome a,a$_3$, become oxidized during SD (Fig. 13–7), (Jöbsis et al., 1977; Lothman et al., 1975; Mayevsky and Chance, 1974, 1975; Mayevsky et al., 1993; Raffin et al., 1991; Rex et al., 1999; Rosenthal and Somjen, 1973) (see also Chapter 2: "Keeping ions in their place . . ."). Unlike cats and rats, in gerbils the local CBF starts to increase only after the passage of the SD wave. Presumably for this reason, NADH/NAD$^+$ ratio briefly shifts in the reduced direction during the early phase of the SD and reverts to oxidation thereafter (Hashimoto et al., 2000).

In contrast to the oxidation during SD, in hypoxia and ischemia mitochondrial enzymes become reduced (Mayevsky and Chance, 1975; Rosenthal et al., 1976; Sick and Perez-Pinzon, 1999). Massive reduction is the true asphyxial response of the NADH/NAD$^+$ and the cytochromes. The SD waves emanating from the penumbra area of an experimental cortical infarct (***peri-infarct depolarizations, PIDs***) (see Chapter 19: "*The ischemic penumbra . . .*") are accompanied by NADH reduction within the area of compromised blood flow but by oxidation when they emerge into the well-perfused zone of the surround (Strong et al., 1996, 2000).

Unlike in intact brain with normal blood flow, in brain tissue slices SD is associated with a predominant reduction of NADH and NADPH as well as FAD (D. Fayuk and D.A. Turner, personal communication). In the absence of a circulation that is governed by tissue energy demand, the supply of oxygen cannot increase and apparently it falls short in the face of the massive load represented by SD-like depolarization.

In conclusion

Convergent evidence of the oversupply of oxygen and the oxidation of mitochondrial enzymes refutes the idea that the profound cellular depolarization during SD is the result of a shortfall in energy and consequent failure of ion homeostasis.

Grafstein's potassium hypothesis

The second and still most influential explanation of SD was Grafstein's (1956b) potassium hypothesis. According to Grafstein, K$^+$ released during intense neuron firing accumulates in the restricted interstitial spaces of brain tissue, and the excess [K$^+$]$_o$ further depolarizes the very cells that released it, resulting in a vicious circle that leads first to increasing firing and eventually to inactivation of neuronal excitability. In the meantime, some of the accumulated K$^+$ diffuses through the interstitial spaces to neighboring cells, which then also depolarize, fire, and go through the same cycle, thus producing the slowly propagating wave of SD. At Grafstein's request, Hodgkin derived a mathematical expression for this process (Grafstein, 1963).

The core of Grafstein's idea survives today. There is little doubt that the huge rise of $[K^+]_o$ is a link in the chain of events causing SD. There were, however, problems with the details of the theory as originally formulated. To the surprise of most, TTX did not prevent SD, even though it suppressed action potential firing (García Ramos and de la Cerda, 1974; Kow and Van Harreveld, 1972; Olsen and Miller, 1977; Tobiasz and Nicholson, 1982). Today we know that K^+ can be released from cells without the firing of action potentials. Yet another problem is that in normoxic SD, at a given point in the tissue, $[K^+]_o$ usually does not start to increase before the arrival of the ΔV_o wave, as it should if K^+ were the agent of its propagation (Herreras and Somjen, 1993a; Lehmenkühler, 1990). As we shall see (Chapter 16), the increase in $[K^+]_o$ is probably a key to the evolution of the SD process (Kager et al., 2000, 2002a) but not necessarily to its propagation. By contrast, during hypoxia there always is a slow, gradual increase in $[K^+]_o$ well before the start of the ΔV_o (Hansen, 1978, 1985), which may be important in the spread of HSD (Aitken et al., 1998b).

Van Harreveld's glutamate hypothesis

The third major proposal was van Harreveld's glutamate hypothesis (Van Harreveld and Fifková, 1970; Van Harreveld and Kooiman, 1965). In a landmark paper, Van Harreveld (1959) proposed, before anyone else thought of it, that glutamate may be a physiologically important excitatory compound. He based this hypothesis on three observations: it was present in extracts of normal brain, it caused the contraction of crustacean muscle, and it induced SD when applied to the cortical surface. As far as SD was concerned, circumstantial evidence seemed to favor glutamate over potassium as its mediator. Neither the release of glutamate nor its excitatory action was antagonized by TTX. Glutamate causes the uptake of NaCl and water into cells (Ames, 1964). Finally, glutamate is released during SD, albeit not in the massive amounts seen during HSD (Fabricius et al., 1993; Iijima et al., 1999; Scheller et al., 1993; Van Harreveld and Fifková, 1970; Van Harreveld and Kooiman, 1965). Nonetheless, doubts about the role of glutamate were and are still voiced (Curatolo et al., 1967; Do Carmo and Leão, 1972; Obrenovitch and Zilkha, 1995; Obrenovitch et al., 1996).

The arguments in favor of glutamate can be extended to any or all excitatory transmitters (Nicholson and Kraig, 1981; Rodrigues et al., 1988; Somjen, 1973). Indeed, there have been reports implicating ACh, at least in the retina (Rodrigues and Martins-Ferreira, 1980; Rodrigues et al., 1988) but not in neocortex (Leão and Morison, 1945).

The Need for More Than One Mediator

There have been flaws with both the K^+ and glutamate hypotheses of SD propagation. While $[K^+]_o$ begins to increase during hypoxia long before the onset of HSD (Hansen and Olsen, 1980; Müller and Somjen, 2000a), no such prodromal rise is observed ahead of an advancing wave of normoxic SD (Herreras and Somjen, 1993a; Lehmenkühler, 1990). Extracellular glutamate concentration increases to a far higher level during HSD than during SD (Fabricius et al., 1993), yet SD and HSD propagate at about the same velocity (Aitken et al., 1998b). Neither dialyzed glutamate nor the inhibition of glutamate uptake facilitates the initiation or propagation of SD (Obrenovitch and Zilkha, 1995; Obrenovitch et al., 1996). Scheller et al., (1993) detected glutamate at the site of SD initiation but not at some distance in the path in which SD was spreading. They attributed this failure to the insensitivity of the assay.

Obrenovitch and Zilkha (1995) and Obrenovitch et al. (1996) reported that neither glutamate nor glutamate uptake inhibitor administered through microdialysis influenced propagating SD waves, but elevated $[K^+]$ facilitated SD. To reconcile this failure with the inhibition of SD by the NMDA antagonist MK 801 and by the blockade of the glycine-binding site of the NMDA receptor (Obrenovitch and Zilkha, 1996a), Obrenovitch and Zilkha (1995) proposed that K^+ ions are the agents of SD propagation, yet high $[K^+]_o$ achieves its effect by depolarizing NMDA receptors and thus relieving the Mg^{2+} block of the NMDA receptor. The NMDA receptor channels can thus be opened without need for a huge overflow of glutamate.

Van Harreveld's dual hypothesis

Transmitters and high $[K^+]_o$ may both play a role. Van Harreveld (1978) himself had modified his views, allowing for two types of SD, one mediated by K^+, the other by glutamate. There is much evidence in favor of this dual hypothesis (Kager et al., 2000, 2002a; see also Chapter 16).

The role of ion channels in spreading depression generation

Sodium Channels and Glutamate-Controlled Channels

As already mentioned ("Grafstein's potassium hypothesis"), TTX in amounts sufficient to abolish action potentials postpones or reduces but does not prevent SD or HSD (Kow and Van Harreveld, 1972; Mori et al., 1976a; Müller and Somjen, 1998; Sugaya et al., 1975; Tobiasz and Nicholson, 1982). Inhibition by TTX is stronger against HSD than against normoxic SD, and in a minority of identically treated slices TTX actually prevented HSD (Aitken et al., 1991b; Müller and Somjen, 2000a; Xie et al., 1994). Other drugs that act on voltage-gated Na^+ channels, such as diphenylhydantoin (phenytoin) and local anesthetics, slow the propagation of SD in retina, raise its threshold, and sometimes block it completely (Chebabo et al., 1988, 1993; Kow and Van Harreveld, 1972).

The rapid, large decline of $[Na^+]_o$ (Hansen and Zeuthen, 1981; Kraig and Nicholson, 1978) leaves little doubt that there is an intense inward surge of this ion during SD. Two questions arise. First, is the influx of Na^+ required for the generation of SD? Second, if not through TTX-sensitive Na^+ channels, then how does Na^+ get into cells?

In the isolated retina, if Na^+ is substituted for by choline or TMA^+, SD is slowed in a concentration-dependent manner, and eventually it is stopped entirely (Martins-Ferreira et al., 1974a). Remarkably, the substitution of $TRIS^+$ for Na^+ had no effect on the circling SD in this preparation (Marrocos and Martins-Ferreira, 1990). In isolated hippocampus, substituting N-methyl-D-glucamine ($NMDG^+$) for Na^+ in the presence of normal $[Ca^{2+}]_o$ suppressed the ΔV_o of HSD, also in a concentration-dependent manner (Müller and Somjen, 2000b). It follows that, ordinarily, the depolarization is mediated mainly, if not exclusively, by Na^+ influx, and Ca^{2+} in the amounts in which it is normally present in ECF cannot take its place.

One must then ask, what pathway do Na^+ ions take when voltage-gated Na^+ channels are blocked by TTX? A clue is provided by the fact that in both SD and HSD the depolarization approaches zero voltage without ever moving into the positive range (Collewijn and Van Harreveld, 1966b; Müller and Somjen, 2000a), and the SD-related whole-cell current reverses at a slightly negative level (Czéh et al., 1993). This points to a mixed ion conductance, because conductance that is exclusively selective for Na^+ (or for Ca^{2+}) would reverse at a strongly positive voltage. Nonselective conductance could also explain the intense outflow of K^+. In theory, such a mixed flux of ions could occur through perforations that are not normally present or at least are not normally open. Alternatively, the mixed conductance could be provided by the opening of transmitter-controlled channels. Like the SD-related current, glutamate-controlled current reverses near zero membrane potential (Langmoen and Hablitz, 1981). Finally, it could be the result of the simultaneous activation of inward and outward currents.

The glutamate hypothesis could be tested once selective agonists and antagonists of glutamate receptors became available. Agonists of all three major ionotropic glutamate receptors—quisqualate, kainate, and NMDA—were able to induce SD (Lauritzen et al., 1988). Antagonists of NMDA receptors in high concentrations inhibited SD, but were ineffective against or actually accelerated the onset of HSD (Aitken et al., 1988; Hernandez-Caceres et al., 1987; Kral et al., 1993; Krüger et al., 1999; Lauritzen and Hansen, 1992; Marrannes et al., 1993). Antagonists of quisqualate and kainate receptors had no effect on either SD or HSD (Avoli et al., 1991; Herreras and Somjen, 1993a; Lauritzen and Hansen, 1992; Lauritzen et al.,

1993). To reconcile the seeming discrepancy between the universal effectiveness of glutamate agonists in triggering SD and the exclusive selectivity of NMDA antagonists in opposing SD, it has been suggested that quisqualate and kainate provoke SD indirectly by stimulating glutamate release, and the released glutamate then activates NMDA receptors (Scheller et al., 1993; Sheardown, 1993).

These observations suggested that activation of NMDA receptors is required for the generation of SD but not of HSD. There are, however, problems with this proposition. The amount of aspartate and glutamate spilled into interstitial space during normoxic SD is quite small compared to the huge amounts released during HSD (Benveniste et al., 1984, 1989; Fabricius et al., 1993; Scheller et al., 1993). Moreover, not all trials with NMDA antagonists were equally successful. A dose of an antagonist that successfully blocked the propagation of SD did not necessarily suppress SD at the site of stimulation (Marrannes et al., 1988b). Also, the selectivity of higher doses of antagonists such as ketamine, kynurenate, or MK-801 is suspect (Collingridge and Lester, 1989; Schurr et al., 1995a). For example, the dose of kynurenate that blocked glutamate-evoked SD failed to prevent SD provoked by high K^+ except when the dose was raised to very high levels (Lauritzen et al., 1988). Lauritzen et al., (1993) pointed out that this difference between glutamate-evoked and K^+-evoked SD supports van Harreveld's (1978) advocacy of two kinds of SD, only one of which is dependent on glutamate. In urethane-anesthetized rats, the highly selective competitive NMDA antagonist CPP blocked only the late component of the SD-related ΔV_o and it did not prevent the propagation of the SD wave (Herreras and Somjen, 1993a).

In conclusion

Neither neuron firing nor synaptic transmission is required for SD generation. Nor is the activation of NMDA receptors an absolute requirement for the generation of SD and even less for HSD. Nonetheless, glutamate and aspartate, as well as some TTX-sensitive Na^+ channels, do play a role.

The Role of Calcium Channels

$[Ca^{2+}]_o$ sinks to very low levels during both SD and HSD. The decrease of $[Ca^{2+}]_o$ starts perhaps a little later than the rise of $[K^+]_o$, (Hansen and Lauritzen, 1984; Lehmenkühler, 1990), and the duration of its decline is considerably longer among apical dendrites than in cell body layers (Fig. 12–4) (Herreras and Somjen, 1993a). The onset and the end of $\Delta[Ca^{2+}]_o$ in st. radiatum coincide with ΔV_o, raising the question of whether the Ca^{2+} current contributes to the depolarization. Adding Ni^{2+} or Co^{2+} to the bathing fluid inhibited SD and, to a lesser degree, HSD without completely suppressing either but, at the concentrations used, these divalent cations are not selective antagonists of Ca^{2+} channels but have other effects, such as strengthening surface charge screening, which makes the interpretation of the results difficult (Jing et al., 1993). More to the point, removing calcium from the ECF does not prevent SD or HSD and may even favor their onset (Balestrino and Somjen, 1986; Basarsky et al., 1998; Garcia Ramos, 1975; Menna et al., 1999; Young and Somjen, 1992). By contrast, substituting Na^+ by a membrane-impermeant cation in the presence of normal $[Ca^{2+}]$ does suppress SD as well as HSD (Martins-Ferreira et al., 1974a; Müller and Somjen, 2000b).

While $[Ca^{2+}]_o$ drops by 0.8–1.1 mM during SD (Figs. 12–4, 18–3) (Hablitz and Heinemann, 1989; Hansen and Lauritzen, 1984; Kraig and Nicholson, 1978; Lehmenkühler, 1990; Nicholson and Kraig, 1981) and HSD (Jing et al., 1993; Young and Somjen, 1992), $[Ca^{2+}]_i$ increases by less than 0.2 μM (Silver and Erecinska, 1990; Wang et al., 2000). Simple arithmetic indicates that, even taking account of the different volume fractions of interstitium and cytosol, the bulk of the Ca^{2+} that enters must be buffered and/or sequestered. Yet, according to Zhang and Lipton (1999), about half of the $[Ca^{2+}]_i$ increase comes from release from intracellular stores. This suggests that when the cytosol is flooded by influx of huge amounts of Ca^{2+}, buffers take up most of it; but, in the absence of an external supply, under the influence of HSD some stores release their content into the cytosol. Increased mitochondrial permeability could cause such release (Bahar et al., 2000). ·

In conclusion

Extracellular Ca^{2+} is neither necessary nor sufficient for SD. This does not mean that the flow of Ca^{2+} into cells during SD does not have important consequences, only that Na^+ ions carry the bulk of the charge necessary for the depolarization.

The Behavior of Anions

Cl^- also disappears from interstitial fluid during SD. Some Cl^- accompanies Na^+ into neurons, and Cl^- also flows into glial cells with K^+, as glia removes some of the excess K^+ from interstitial fluid. Phillips and Nicholson (1979) compared the movements of a series of anions of varying ion radius during SD and concluded that the limit for the size of the channel or "pore" that admits anions during SD lies between 6 and 11.2 Å (see also Martins-Ferreira et al., 2000).

Until recently, it was believed that cell swelling was dependent on Cl^- influx (Van Harreveld and Khattab, 1967; Van Harreveld and Schadé, 1960). Müller (2000) examined the effects of the chloride transport inhibitors furosemide, 4,4-diisothiocyanatostilbene-2,2'-disulfanic acid (DIDS), and 4,4'-dinitrostilbene-2,2' disulfonic acid (DNDS) on HSD and found only minor changes in the magnitude of the ΔV_o and in the onset time of the depolarization. More surprisingly, substituting methyl sulfate or gluconate for Cl^- in the bath did not prevent cell swelling during HSD (measured as the shrinkage of the TMA^+ space) (Müller, 2000; Müller and Somjen, 1999). As discussed in Chapter 13 ("Spreading depression–related intrinsic optical signals"), removal of extracellular chloride suppressed the HSD-related light-scattering increase (Martins-Ferreira et al., 1971) and un-masked the decrease in light scattering, that is caused by cell swelling (Fig. 13–5) (Bahar et al., 2000; Fayuk et al., 2002; Müller and Somjen, 1999). There is little doubt that normally, with Cl⁻ being the most abundant anion in ECF, it is indeed the main anion accompanying cations into cells, causing cell swelling (Van Harreveld and Schadé, 1959, 1960). Which anions take the place of Cl⁻ when Cl⁻ is absent is less clear. Bicarbonate is the most likely candidate because it is the second highest in concentration, and its molecular size is smaller than the limit estimated by Phillips and Nicholson for the SD-induced anion flux (Martins-Ferreira et al., 2000; Müller, 2000; Phillips and Nicholson, 1979).

The Role of Potassium Channels

Last but by no means least, we must ask, what is the role of voltage-gated K^+ channels? In the first place, what causes the massive increase in $[K^+]_o$? It would seem that no matter what initiates SD, the depolarization, the presence of glutamate in the ISF, and the increase in $[Ca^{2+}]_i$ will open wide several K^+-channels, as well as K^+-permeable nonselective channels. The question is, can we differentiate and find the specific role of each of these channels? Data on this issue are still scarce.

In the isolated retina, the broad-spectrum K-channel blocker TEA⁺ slowed the propagation of SD (Garcia Ramos, 1975; Martins-Ferreira et al., 1974a; Scheller et al., 1998).We (Aitken et al., 1991b) tested the effect of TEA as well as that of 4-AP on HSD. 4-Aminopyridine inhibits only the inward rectifier and A-type channels ($I_{K,DR}$ and $I_{K,A}$) (Hille, 2001). Both TEA and 4-AP shortened the delay from oxygen withdrawal to the onset of HSD, probably because blocking K^+ chan-nels enhances the excitability of neurons. Yet even though HSD started earlier, the amplitude of the ΔV_o and of the increase of $[K^+]_o$ were consistently and sub-stantially depressed by TEA, but not by 4-AP. We concluded that some but not all of the K^+ leaving cells flows through TEA-sensitive, 4-AP-insensitive chan-nels (Aitken et al., 1991b). *ATP-dependent K^+ channels* probably carry some of the K^+ released during HSD (Xie et al., 1995b).

Not one spreading depression channel, but the cooperation of several channels, generates spreading depression-like depolarization

Trials with channel-blocking drugs have been inspired by the search for a spe-cific ion current that could explain the precipitous decrease of membrane resis-tance and depolarization of neurons. Diverse selective antagonists partially depressed or delayed SD or HSD, but none completely prevented them. One might conjecture, therefore, that during SD, pathological pathways open that normally are absent or dormant. We rejected this conclusion after finding that simultaneously blocking all known major inward currents with a cocktail of CPP, DNQX, TTX, and Ni^{2+} reliably prevented HSD (Müller and Somjen, 1998). Administered separately, each ingredient in this cocktail delayed the onset of SD or HSD, but even three of the four combined could not reliably prevent it (Jing et al., 1993; Müller and Somjen, 2000b); it takes all four inhibitors to achieve consistent protection. It seems that, normally, several ion channels cooperate in generating HSD or SD, but if some are incapacitated, one of the channels alone is sufficient to mediate a slowed version of the process. Even if delayed, once SD has been initiated, the depolarization progresses to ultimately reach the usual near-zero V_m level (Müller and Somjen, 1998, 2000a, 2000b).

In this context, it is important to remember that the *extracellular voltage shift*, ΔV_o, is a biased *sum* of the signals from many cells. ΔV_o can appear depressed not only when the signal from all participating neurons diminishes, but also if *fewer than the usual number* of neurons are responding. In the latter case, those cells that do take part in the response could depolarize fully. Only intracellular recording, corrected for the simultaneously recorded ΔV_o, can decide the issue.

We missed one piece of the puzzle as we tried to solve it (Müller and Somjen, 1998, 2000a, 2000b). Here was the problem. Reducing $[Na^+]_o$ (by substituting an impermeant cation) suppressed HSD-related depolarization in a dose-dependent manner. Na^+ was evidently the charge carrier for the inward current. Yet blocking voltage-gated as well as glutamate-controlled currents by TTX, CPP, and DNQX did not completely abolish HSD. To completely prevent it, Ni^{2+} had to be added to the cocktail. At first sight, this would suggest a contribution by Ca^{2+} currents, which are known to be blocked by Ni^{2+}. But that explanation did not work because, in the absence of any channel-blocking drugs while $[Na^+]_o$ was drastically reduced but $[Ca^{2+}]_o$ was normal, HSD was effectively suppressed. Ca^{2+} currents were evidently not sufficient to cause the massive depolarization of neurons. The delayed but eventually complete depolarization, seen when voltage-gated and glutamate-controlled avenues were barred, was still due to influx of Na^+, and the question then was, what residual route did Na^+ take? At the time we wrote our paper, we could only vaguely guess (Müller and Somjen, 2000b), but it now seems that the most likely candidate for the missing current is the calcium-sensing non-selective cation channel (csNSC) of Xiong and MacDonald (1999), which is activated by the decrease in $[Ca^{2+}]_o$ and is indeed blocked by divalent cations, including Ni^{2+}. (See also Chapter 16: "Critique of the model.")

In conclusion

The voltage to which the membrane is moved during SD is not determined by the number or type of channels available, but by the feedback that governs the process (Müller and Somjen, 2000b). This is another way of stating that SD is an all-or-none event.

Key points

In otherwise healthy brains with normally regulated blood flow and oxygen supply, SD does not cause a cellular energy shortage.

The application of a high-K^+ solution or glutamate to brain tissue can provoke SD. Both $[K^+]_o$ and extracellular glutamate increase during SD, regardless of the triggering stimulus. Probably both K^+ and glutamate are involved, to varying degrees, in various situations in the evolution and propagation of SD.

Spreading depression can be provoked with synapses and action potentials blocked.

The principal charge carrier of SD- or HSD-related depolarization is Na^+.

The SD-related neuron membrane change is brought about by the cooperative activation of several voltage-, glutamate-, K^+-, and Ca^{2+}-dependent slow inward currents. If one or more of these is blocked, the remaining ones can still produce full-size SD or HSD, albeit more slowly. Only a drug cocktail that blocks all known slowly inactivating inward currents can reliably prevent HSD.

16

Solving the Puzzle of Spreading Depression by Computer Simulation

Several mathematical models of SD have been published (Grafstein, 1963; Nicholson, 1993; Reggia and Montgomery, 1996; Revett et al., 1998; Shapiro, 2001; Tuckwell, 1981; Tuckwell and Miura, 1978). These computations were more concerned with the propagation of SD than with its initiation and its biophysical membrane mechanism. This chapter first presents the results of our simulation of the membrane events producing SD-like depolarization in a single model neuron. Propagation of SD is the topic of a later section ("Mechanisms of spreading depression propagation").

A computer model representing one neuron and its milieu can generate spreading depression-like depolarization

Voltages and Currents of Simulated Spreading Depression

The model described earlier (Fig. 9–1) (Chapter 9), which generated seizure-like afterdischarges, could also produce SD-like depolarization (Kager et al., 2000, 2002a). As we have seen, as long as the $[K^+]_o/[K^+]_i$ ratio of the model neuron was maintained within normal limits, depolarizing stimulation evoked repetitive firing of life-like action potentials that ceased promptly when the stimulus stopped (Figs. 9–2, 9–3) but if the $[K^+]_o/[K^+]_i$ ratio was allowed to rise, paroxysmal afterdischarges could erupt. The same stimulus could evoke normal firing or seizure-like behavior, depending on parameter settings. After appropriate adjustments, simulated SD-like depolarization was also produced (Figs. 16–1, 16–6).

There was a telling contrast between the trajectories of computed $[K^+]_o$ during seizure and during SD, in life as well as in the computer model. During paroxysmal afterdischarge $[K^+]_o$ increases up to a ceiling level no higher than 8–12 mM (Heinemann and Lux, 1977) (Figs. 8–2, 9–5, 9–6). In sharp contrast to seizures, at the onset of SD the ceiling of $[K^+]_o$ is breached. Moreover, while during seizures $[K^+]_o$ increases more in the region of the soma than among dendrites (Somjen and Giacchino, 1985) (Figs. 8–2, 8–3D), at the onset of SD the dendrites take the lead (Herreras and Somjen, 1993a) (Figs. 12–4A, 16–3). In the simulations of Figures 16–1 and 16–3, during the triggering stimulation $[K^+]_o$ rose highest at the

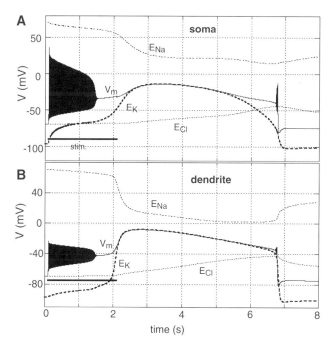

FIGURE 16–1. Simulated spreading depression in a model neuron. The model is illustrated in Figure 9–1. **A:** Membrane potential and Na^+, K^+, and Cl^- equilibrium potentials in the neuron soma. **B:** In the D2 dendrite segment. E_K shifts positively as K^+ is released from the neuron to the interstitial fluid, and E_{Na} shifts negatively as the cell accumulates Na^+. E_{Cl} shifts gradually as Cl^- ions are taken in to make up for charge imbalance due to excess inflow of Na^+ relative to outflow of K^+; Na^+ uptake continues even when E_K begins to recover. Net uptake of NaCl causes neuron swelling at the expense of interstitial space (not illustrated). Note that initial voltage and ion shifts are more abrupt in the dendrite than in the soma. (Modified from Kager et al., 2002a.)

soma, but when SD was ignited, $[K^+]_o$ surged ahead around the dendrites. Spreading depression started in the dendrite segment farthest from the soma (D3); then it approached and eventually ignited in the soma itself (Fig. 16–3). The simulated trajectories of $[K^+]_o$ are very similar to those recorded during SD from st. pyramidale and st. radiatum in hippocampus of anesthetized rats (Fig. 12–4A) (Herreras and Somjen, 1993a). In live hippocampus the SD-related increase of $[K^+]_o$ as well as the voltage shift began in the dendritic tree, whence it was conducted into the soma. Conduction along dendritic processes is faster than propagation among the cells in the neuron population, in simulated as well as real SD (see also Kager et al., 2000).

The currents responsible for the depolarization are examined in Figure 16–2. In this example, the dominant dendritic inward current during SD was I_{NMDA}

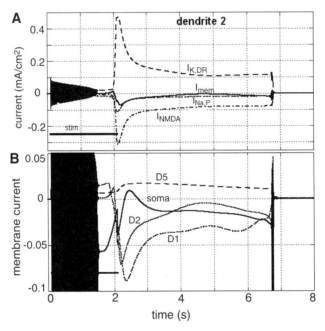

FIGURE 16–2. Membrane currents related to simulated spreading depression (SD). **A:** The main ion currents that generate the depolarization of the D2 dendrite segment during SD. $I_{K,DR}$: delayed rectifier K^+ current. $I_{Na,P}$: persistent Na^+ current. I_{NMDA}: N-methyl-D-aspartate (NMDA) receptor channel–like current (see also the legend to Fig. 9–1). I_{mem} is the net (aggregate) membrane current. **B:** The net membrane current in the soma and in apical dendrite segments D1, D2, and D5. Spreading depression is ignited when the net membrane current in D1 and D2 turns inward. Membrane current in the soma hesitates before joining the sustained inward flow in the dendrites. D5 had no "active" channels (cf. Fig. 9–1) and provides a passive outward current source for the active inward sinks. (Data from the same trial as Fig. 16.1). (Unpublished figure based on data from the study of Kager et al., 2002a.)

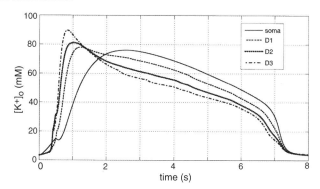

FIGURE 16–3. Simulated extracellular potassium changes demonstrate spreading depression (SD) propagation from distal dendrite toward soma. At the start of SD, $[K^+]_o$ rose fastest and highest around the distalmost active dendrite segment (D3), with D2, D1, and soma following in sequence. (Data from a trial other than Figs. 16–1 and 16–2). (Unpublished study by H. Kager, W.J. Wadman, and G.G. Somjen.)

(Fig. 16–2A). Of the several lesser inward currents, only $I_{Na,P}$ is plotted to avoid crowding the graph. In other simulations, depending on parameter settings, either I_{NMDA} or $I_{Na,P}$ alone was sufficient to generate SD-like depolarization, but when both were operating the SD threshold was lower, its latency shorter, and its duration longer (Kager et al., 2000, 2002a).This confirms the thesis that the ability to generate SD is not specific to any one channel and that it usually involves the cooperation of more than one current (see Chapter 15: "Not one spreading depression channel . . ."). As described above, in hippocampal slices HSD was completely prevented only with a cocktail of blocking drugs that suppressed all known major inward currents (Müller and Somjen, 1998, 2000b).

Tracings of extracellular voltage and of CSD during SD in rat brains show two negative or inward maxima in succession, producing the inverted saddle (or peak-and-hump) shape (Figs. 7–10, 12–2, 12–4) (Herreras and Somjen, 1993a; Wadman et al., 1992). The aggregate (net) membrane current in the model neuron often also has a similar configuration (Kager et al., 2002a; Somjen, 2001). In Figure 16–2A, both I_{NMDA} and $I_{Na,P}$ show an initial inward (negative) surge shortly after SD onset, followed by a sustained plateau for which I_{NMDA} is chiefly responsible. The net (aggregate) membrane current (I_{mem}) shows an early surge, and toward the end a smaller second maximum. More like the inverted saddle is the membrane current of the first dendrite segment, D1, in Figure 16–2B. In rat hippocampus the late component of the extracellular voltage shift appears to be dominated by an NMDA receptor–controlled current (see Chapter 12: "Extracellular sustained potential shifts . . .") (Herreras and Somjen, 1993a), as it also is in the simulation of Figure 16–2.

For the simulations of Figures 16–1 and 16–2 only Na^+, K^+, and Cl^- were represented. Figure 16–4A illustrates the currents carried by Ca^{2+} ions in a simulation when Ca^{2+} and its channels, exchanger, and pump have been added to the model (Fig. 9–1), and Figure 16–4B shows the intracellular concentration of free Ca^{2+} during the simulated SD. $I_{Ca,T}$ was quite small and became rapidly inactivated, and $I_{Ca,L}$ was negligible. Most of the Ca^{2+} entered the cell through the NMDA receptor–controlled conductance. The Ca/3Na exchanger (antiporter), which normally removes Ca^{2+} from cells, worked in reverse (calcium inward) mode throughout much of the late part of the SD. The reversal occurs whenever the membrane potential is positive relative to the reversal potential of the exchanger (Fig. 2–4). The calcium-dependent K^+ channel, through which $I_{K,SK}$ flows, was opened as $[Ca^{2+}]_i$ increased in the neuron (not ilustrated). For each Ca^{2+} ion carried by the Ca/3Na antiporter, three Na^+ ions move in the opposite direction so that excess charge goes where Na^+ goes (not shown here but see Fig. 2–4). This means that in the Ca^{2+} exit mode (cell normally polarized and ion distributions normal), the net Ca/3Na exchanger current aids depolarization (net inward current), but in the Ca^{2+} entry mode, it aids repolarization (net outward current).

Spreading Depression Is Ignited When the Net Dendritic Membrane Current Turns Inward

The critical event igniting SD is the moment when the sum of the slowly inactivating inward currents across the dendritic membrane exceeds the sum of the outward currents so that the total membrane current, I_{mem}, turns inward (Fig. 16–2). Spreading depression ignites in the soma later than in the dendrite; this sequence is the rule, but not an absolute rule. In formal terms:

$$(I_{Na,P} + I_{Na,leak} + I_{NMDA} + I_{Ca,T} + I_{Ca,L}) > (I_{K,DR} + I_{K,SK} + I_{K,leak} + I_{Capump} + I_{Na/Kpump}) \tag{16–1}$$

Note

It is important to remember that every term in Eq. 16–1 is a variable controlled by sets of mostly nonlinear functions.

Also, the NMDA receptor–controlled channel allows the inflow of Na^+ and Ca^{2+} and the outflow of K^+. The aggregate (net) I_{NMDA} is inward (Fig. 16–2A) as long as the membrane potential remains more negative than the reversal potential (E_{NMDA}). During SD this is almost always the case because E_{NMDA} is near zero millivolts. The two ATP-fueled electrogenic pumps, one transporting Ca^{2+} outward and the other moving 3 Na^+ ions out against 2 K^+ ions in, both provide outward currents, aiding re- or hyperpolarization. The Ca/3Na exchanger, which allows 3 Na^+ to be exchanged against 1 Ca^{2+}, has not been entered into Eq. 16–1 because of its ambiguous contribution to the total current (Figs. 2–4, 16–4A). Also not shown, in the cell soma the window current of $I_{Na,T}$ also contributes to the left side of the equation.

There is a striking analogy between the condition for igniting SD and the condition for triggering an action potential. Hodgkin and Huxley (1952; Katz, 1966) defined the threshold of firing as the voltage at which the inward Na+ current begins to exceed the outward K+ current. At the time only one kind of Na+ and one kind of K+ current were recognized. Once this critical state is reached, a positive feedback ensues whereby influx of Na+ depolarizes the membrane, opening more Na+ channels and thus accelerating depolarization (Fig. 9–8). Once the threshold has been reached, the kinetics of the channels take over and the action potential proceeds according to its prescribed course, without regard for the previously delivered stimulus. The action potential begins to subside when inactivation starts to shut down the Na+ channels. Also, the more slowly activated K+ channels initiate

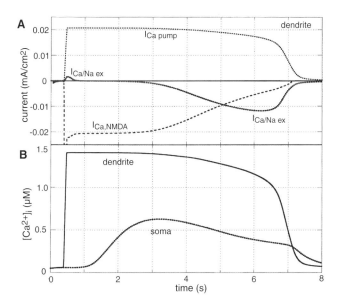

FIGURE 16–4. The main calcium currents responsible for shifts in Ca²⁺ distribution, and the changes in intracellular calcium during simulated spreading depression (SD). **A:** Initially the Ca²⁺ component of the N-methyl-D-aspartate (NMDA) receptor–mediated current ($I_{Ca,NMDA}$) mediated the inflow of Ca²⁺ into the dendrite. The Ca/Na exchanger ($I_{Ca/Na\,ex}$) moved Ca²⁺ out of the neuron at the very beginning of SD, then stalled and later was responsible for the maintained inward flow of Ca²⁺. The turnaround of $I_{Ca/Na\,ex}$ is the result of depolarization (cf. Fig. 2–4). The Ca-ATPase ion pump ($I_{Ca,pump}$) limited the accumulation of Ca²⁺ and eventually restored its distribution. **B:** Intracellular free Ca²⁺ levels in dendrite segment D2 and in the soma during SD. The accumulation of buffered (stored/bound) calcium was much greater (not shown). (Data from the same trial as Fig. 16–3.) (Unpublished study by H. Kager, W.J. Wadman, and G.G. Somjen.)

an outward current in opposition to the (already decaying) Na^+ inward current, accelerating repolarization. The rules that govern SD are quite similar to those producing an action potential, with this amendment. Unlike the fast activation and inactivation of $I_{Na,T}$ mediating the action potential, the inward and outward currents that bring on and terminate SD must be very slowly inactivating. Still, like nerve impulses, SD is an all-or-none event, which means that once it is ignited, its trajectory is controlled by the parameters of the ion currents and not by the antecedent stimulus that had set the process in motion.

Any Slow Inward Current(s) Could Generate Spreading Depression

Any slow inward inward currents could generate spreading depression if the following conditions exist: (*1*) the primary current must flow inward; (*2*) it must be activated by depolarization, elevated $[K^+]_o$, or both; (*3*) the primary current must be inactivated or desensitized slowly or not at all; (*4*) the depolarization achieved by the primary inward current must be able to force the release of K^+ ions into a restricted extracellular space; and (*5*) the removal of K^+ from the interstitium must not keep pace with its release.

The ignition point of SD is not a fixed threshold in one variable. Ignition is reached by the confluence of several processes, reminiscent of the Reynolds number, which defines the transition from laminar to turbulent flow. Pharmacological evidence points to I_{NMDA} and $I_{Na,P}$ as the chief charge carriers in undrugged hippocampus and neocortex (Müller and Somjen, 2000b).

Nor is the dendritic location essential for producing the SD-associated depolarization. This is, however, clearly the site where SD is initiated in hippocampal formation (Herreras and Somjen, 1993a, 1993c). Old and perhaps less compelling evidence suggests the same for neocortex (Ochs, 1962), but data are insufficient to pinpoint the initiating area elsewhere, for example thalamus or cerebellum. Wherever there is a large concentration of slowly inactivating channels carrying inward current, plus the likelihood of interstitial accumulation of K^+, there exists the danger of SD.

In our simulations, the ignition point of SD could be raised or lowered by manipulating the parameters that govern the relevant currents, but the leak conductances of the glia-endothelial ion buffer had an especially powerful effect. High leak conductance of the glial membrane effectively prevented SD, because glial uptake of K^+ restrained the rise of $[K^+]_o$ (Figs. 16–5, 16–6) (Kager et al., 2002a).

In Live Brains Several Factors Can Facilitate Spreading Depression Ignition

$I_{Na,P}$ is augmented by hypoxia (Hammarström and Gage, 1998, 2000) and by elevated $[K^+]_o$ (Somjen and Müller, 2000). Glutamate is released not only by the K^+-induced depolarization of presynaptic terminals (Nicholson and Kraig, 1981;

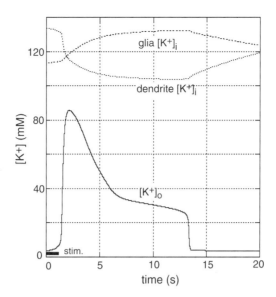

FIGURE 16–5. Changes in intra- and extracellular K+ concentrations during simulated spreading depression (SD). Data from the D2 dendritic segment. The glial compartment accumulated K+, while the neuron dendrite lost K+. [K+]$_o$ reached an early summit and then subsided even as the dendrite was still losing K+ ions, because some of the K+ leaving the dendrite entered the glia. Extracellular change was much larger than intracellular change because the volume of the interstitial space is smaller than that of the neuron and the glial compartment. Extracellular changes were also amplified because interstitial space shrank during SD. (Data from a trial different from Figs. 16–3 and 16–4. Modified from Kager et al., 2002a.)

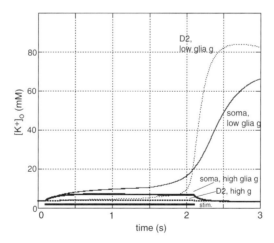

FIGURE 16–6. A change in glial leak conductances and in the glial ion pump can make the difference between spreading depression(SD) and no SD. Simulated extracellular K+ concentrations at the level of the soma and the D2 dendrite segment in two conditions. All neuron parameters and stimulus current were identical, but glial Na and K leak conductances ("glia g") and the glial 3Na/2K pump settings were different. Higher glial leak and higher glial pump current provide more efficient control of [K+]$_o$ and prevent SD. (Unpublished illustration from the database of Kager et al., 2002a.)

Somjen, 1973) and of glia (Billups et al., 1998; Rossi et al., 2000; Szatkowski et al., 1990), but also by the swelling of glial cells (Basarsky et al., 1999; Kimelberg et al., 1990, 1995). Cell swelling restricts the volume into which K^+ is released, amplifying the rise of $[K^+]_o$. Since acidosis hinders and alkalosis favors SD generation while SD itself alters pH, there is yet another possibility for strengthening the feedback. The initial alkalinization produced by the SD process is likely to promote its own regenerative evolution, while the subsequent acidification shortens its trajectory (Tong and Chesler, 1999, 2000).

In conclusion

The following conclusions are derived from these simulations and from the real-life experiments that they imitate: (*1*) Once ignited, SD has an all-or-none trajectory. (*2*) The ignition point of SD is reached when net sustained dendritic currents turn inward. (*3*) Excessive activation of certain physiological membrane ion channels can bring about SD; there is no need to postulate the opening of pathological holes, pores, or a breakdown of the membrane. (*4*) The final level of depolarization is governed by feedback, not by the number of channels that are opened. (*5*) $I_{Na,P}$ dominates HSD while I_{NMDA} is the leader in SD; neither of the two has an exclusive role.

Critique of the Model

Propagation in the tissue could not, of course, be tested in a model consisting of a single neuron. Others have simulated the spread of SD among cells, and these will be the topic of the next section. Our model was deficient in other ways as well—for example, the absence of H^+ and of secondary messengers, as well as of metabolism and other biochemical functions. Still, the purpose of the exercise was to define the minimal *biophysical machinery* capable of generating SD-like depolarization. This, it seems, has been achieved.

We chose to represent $I_{Na,P}$ and I_{NMDA} because when either of these two currents is blocked, SD and HSD onset are slowed and ion fluxes appear to be reduced. Since the combination of TTX, CPP, and DNQX powerfully delayed and sometimes but not always prevented HSD, it seems that in the absence of both $I_{Na,P}$ and I_{NMDA} there are other, still unknown, inward currents that can sometimes produce a delayed SD (Müller and Somjen, 2000b). Among the possible candidates are TTX-resistant Na^+ current (Hoehn et al., 1993) and nonspecific ion currents (Congar et al., 1997; Fraser and MacVicar, 1996; Hoehn-Berlage et al., 1997; Xiong and MacDonald, 1996). Channels activated by cell swelling or membrane stretch have been considered (Somjen et al., 1992), but to date there is no evidence of their presence in central neurons (Aitken et al., 1998a; Somjen et al., 1993c), only in glial cells (Basarsky et al., 1999; Kimelberg and Mongin, 1998).

Mechanisms of spreading depression propagation

Spreading depression spreads in contiguous gray matter as if it were a wave, without recourse to synaptic transmission, at a (more or less) uniform velocity between 2 and 5 mm/min, the exact value depending on the site, the age of the animal, and certain experimental conditions such as temperature (Aitken et al., 1998b; Basarsky et al., 1998; Bureš et al., 1974; Leão and Morison, 1945). The wave stops where white matter begins, and at the edge of glial-fibrous scars left by previous injury or infarction. Cytoarchitecture does matter: some areas are preferentially invaded (Leão and Morison, 1945; Ochs, 1962). Cuts that interrupt some but not all the layers of neocortex do not stop the spread (Grafstein, 1956a). In neocortex as well as in hippocampus, the leading edge of the wave is in the layers containing apical dendrites (Herreras and Somjen, 1993c). Intense excitation conveyed by way of fiber tracts can elicit SD at distant sites (Vinogradova et al., 1991).

The potassium hypothesis (Grafstein, 1956b) and the glutamate hypothesis (Van Harreveld, 1959) had this feature in common: both relied on the release of a substance normally stored in brain cells to explain both the initiation and the propagation of SD. Humoral mediation of SD propagation is supported by two observations. Inspired by the classical experiment of Otto Loewi (1921), Martins-Ferreira et al. (1974b) demonstrated that the fluid in which retinas had been bathed while they were undergoing SD could induce SD in another, otherwise untreated retina. Moreover, Obrenovitch and Zilkha (1996b) reported that intracerebral microdialysis with a drug-free physiological solution inhibits the propagation of SD through the dialyzed area, presumably because the dialysate dilutes the substance that mediates SD propagation. The humoral agent forwarding SD was not identified in these experiments. It could have been glutamate, K^+, or any other excitant compound, singly or in combination.

Several computational models treated SD propagation as a ***diffusion-reaction process*** (Bureš et al. 1974; Davydov and Koroleva, 1993; Grafstein, 1963; Nicholson, 1993; Tuckwell, 1981; Tuckwell and Miura, 1978). Key to these treatments was the calculation of the diffusion of K^+ or of an unspecified humoral agent in the interstitial spaces. Additionally, certain assumptions had to be made about the kinetics of the hypothetical reaction(s) governing the release of the agent. For example, the release of K^+ into the interstitium was assumed to be stimulated by its accumulation in the interstitium, resulting in positive feedback. The membrane mechanism underlying the release was not always specified in explicit biophysical terms. Reasonable velocities of propagation have been computed in this way, even if the waveforms derived from the equations were not always life-like.

Alternative theoretical solutions proposed that the agent mediating SD (or seizures) is spread by way of ***intercellular gap junctions*** instead of by diffusion through interstitial spaces (Amzica et al., 2002; Heinemann et al., 1991, 1995). As a "potassium sponge," glia guards against the eruption of SD (Gardner-Medwin,

1981; Mori et al., 1976c), but once SD erupts, glial tissue could advance its spread by broadcasting K^+ through intercellular gap junctions (see also Chapter 2: "Can spatial buffering have unintended consequences?" and Chapter 14: "In spreading depression neurons lead and glial cells follow"). Observing that the rise of $[K^+]_o$ coincides with ΔV_o but precedes the decrease in $[Na^+]_o$ and $[Ca^{2+}]_o$, Lehmenkühler (1990) agreed that K^+ ions are being propelled by way of the quasi-syncytial network of glial cells. High $[K^+]_o$ and glutamate apparently increase the coupling of astrocytes through gap junctions (Enkvist and McCarthy, 1994), and this effect could facilitate K^+ dispersal. This, then, is a variant of Grafstein's (1956b) hypothesis: K^+ is the mediator of SD propagation but, instead of diffusing through the interstitial spaces, it moves by way of cytoplasmic bridges among glial cells. As we saw earlier, however (Chapter 14: "Do astrocytes promote . . . ?") (Largo et al., 1997a, 1997b; Theis et al., 2003), astrocytes appear to hinder rather than promote SD generation as well as its propagation.

There are, however, other observations that suggest that SD might propagate through intercellular junctions linking neurons rather than astrocytes (Herreras and Somjen, 1993a, 1993c; Herreras et al., 1994; Somjen et al., 1992). In the brains of urethane-anesthetized rats, an oncoming wave of propagating SD is heralded by a brief burst of extracellular *population spikes*. Unlike seizure discharges, which ride on a negative shift of the extracellular potential and are accompanied by a steady elevation of $[K^+]_o$, the pre-SD spike bursts erupt before the onset of the ΔV_o when $[K^+]_o$ is still normal. The large amplitude of these extracellular compound action potentials indicates lockstep firing of many neurons, and the synchronization extends over long distances that could not be spanned by ephaptic interaction. To explain the long-distance synchrony, Herreras proposed that the opening of previously closed interneuronal gap junctions precedes the advancing wave of the depolarization (Herreras and Somjen, 1993a; Herreras et al., 1994). Enkvist and McCarthy (1994) reported improvement of gap junction communication by high $[K^+]_o$ and glutamate among astrocytes, but the same effect, increased coupling, could perhaps operate among neurons as well.

Spreading depression propagation mediated by gap junctions has recently been tested in computer simulation by Shapiro (2001). His model consists of a row of single-compartment *cells* connected by gap junctions and surrounded by an interstitial space. It incorporates a formidable array of ion channels and transporters and provides for the calculation of an equally impressive number of variables. Not only ion concentration changes due to electrodiffusion across cell membranes and through gap junctions, but also osmotic water flow, and hence cell swelling, have been computed. Spreading depression was initiated by raising $[K^+]_o$ to 50 mM, imitating the common laboratory practice of injecting KCl into brain tissue. In this model, SD did not propagate if gap junctions were closed or if cells were not allowed to swell.

Like the K^+ and glutamate hypotheses, the idea of gap junctions has problems. Gap junctions among neurons are more numerous in infant animals than in older ones (Kandler and Katz, 1995; Yuste et al., 1995), yet the inclination for generating SD increases with age. This is not a fatal flaw, because gap junctions are found among pyramidal neurons in hippocampus of mature animals as well (Andrew et al., 1982; Baimbridge et al., 1991; MacVicar and Dudek, 1981). Besides, the postulate is for normally closed junctions to open during SD. The pharmacological evidence is weakened, however, by the fact that agents such as heptanol and halothane, as well as acidity, inhibit not just gap junctions but a wide range of membrane functions (Largo et al., 1997b; Nelson and Makielski, 1991; Pott and Mechmann, 1990; Somjen and Tombaugh, 1998). Besides, in the retina, low concentrations of heptanol and octanol accelerated the propagation of SD; only higher concentrations inhibited it (Martins-Ferreira and Ribeiro, 1995). Finally, recently, Világi et al. (2001) reported that the selective gap junction blocking agent carbenoxolone failed to block SD.

In conclusion

The mechanism of SD propagation could but need not be identical to that of SD initiation. There are four competing hypotheses to explain SD propagation, two of which are based on the interstitial diffusion of a humoral agent, either K^+ or glutamate, and the two others postulating mediation through gap junctions among either glial cells or neurons. There is no conclusive evidence for or against any one of these proposals. Nor are they mutually exclusive. As with SD initiation, there may be more than one path converging toward the same destination.

Key points

The same single-neuron computer model that generated seizures can also produce SD-like depolarization.

Either simulated persistent Na^+ current ($I_{Na,P}$) or imitated NMDA receptor current in the dendritic membrane can produce SD. When both are present, the trigger level is lower and the duration of the depolarization is longer than with either alone.

Spreading depression was ignited when the net (aggregate) dendritic membrane current turned inward.

Once ignited, the membrane changes associated with SD ran along an all-or-none trajectory.

Efficient uptake of interstitial K^+ by the "glia" could prevent SD.

Other published computer models were designed to solve the mechanism of SD propagation in the tissue. Simulations based on a diffusion-reaction process, as well as those assuming dispersal through gap junctions, succeeded in imitating SD propagation. Experimental data are equally ambiguous in this respect.

IV

PATHOLOGICAL BIOPHYSICS OF CEREBRAL HYPOXIA AND STROKE

17

Hypoxia, Asphyxia, and Ischemia

We are acclimated to the partial pressure of oxygen in the atmosphere in which we live. Too much or too little of this gas can cause trouble.

More than other cells, neurons of the forebrain need oxygen for survival. The research reviewed in Part IV shows that maldistribution of ions and malfunction of ion channels have much to do with the selctive vulnerability of cerebral neurons. Chapter 17 introduces the topic, clarifies similarities and differences between cerebral hypoxia and ischemia, and summarizes the chief overt signs in these conditions.

Why do we need oxygen? Boyle, Priestley, Lavoisier

Today it is hard to imagine, but 400 years ago it was not evident that we need something that is in air to live. Robert Boyle proved this around 1660. Boyle (who gave us the first gas laws) and Robert Hooke built a pneumatic engine or gas pump, and with its help they found out that flames are extinguished and small animals die if deprived of air. A few years later, John Mayow determined that only about a fifth of the air is used for breathing and for combustion. He came close to discovering oxygen, but his work was mired in controversy (the story is told by Proctor, 1995 and by Bert, 1943). It took another 100 years to identify the ingredient in air without which we cannot survive.

Depending on whom one believes, oxygen was first obtained as a more or less pure gas either by Joseph Priestley or by Carl Scheele. Priority matters little; the two men worked independently at around the same time (1772–1774). Neither Scheele nor Priestley knew what they had isolated, but Priestly noticed that mice enclosed in a glass jar survived longer when the vessel was filled with his new gas than with air, and when he himself inhaled it, he felt good. Priestley called it *dephlogisticated air* in conformity with the confusion prevailing in the science of his time. During a trip to Paris he showed how to obtain this new gas to Lavoisier, who later named it *oxygen* and figured out its true significance (Lavoisier, 1920). For his discoveries Lavoisier is rightly considered the father of physiological chemistry (Fig. 17–1). Lavoisier was guillotined in 1794 during the Paris Terror— not the first or the last brilliant mind to perish at the hands of crazed mobs. Priestley fared somewhat better: only his house, his laboratory, and the church where he preached were burned by a mob that disliked his religion. He ended up in the United States, probably the first of the many scientists who sought refuge by crossing the Atlantic. The story of the two pioneers, their accomplishments (which were great), and their failures (which, in the long run, were inconsequential) is delightfully and concisely told by Chinard (1995), who also provides references to original sources.

Paul Bert's 1878 volume titled *La Pression Barometrique* established that hypoxemia caused **altitude sickness**, and also that **oxygen is toxic** under high ambi-

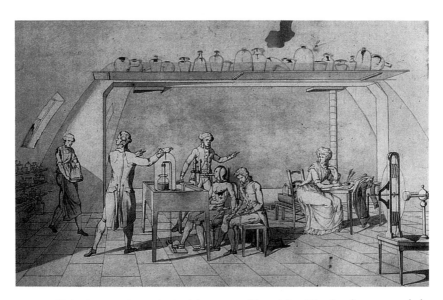

Figure 17–1. An experiment in the laboratory of Lavoisier. The drawing was made by Madame Marie Lavoisier, who is seen seated at the right-hand side of the picture taking notes. [Re-reproduced from a reproduction in Hoffmann (2002). The original is in a private collection.]

ent air pressure. As Fulton recounts in his introduction to the English translation (Bert, 1943), Alberto Mosso opposed Bert's conclusions, attributing mountain sickness to *hypocapnia* (loss of CO_2), induced by hyperventilation. As it turns out, both Bert and Mosso are right. Under normal conditions, meaning the altitude to which a person is acclimated, breathing is controlled by the CO_2 and the pH in the blood, while arterial oxygen has little or no influence. Too much of either CO_2 or H^+ stimulates and too little inhibits respiration. When, however, P_{O_2} falls below a critical level, the low P_{O_2} becomes a more powerful stimulus, overriding the P_{CO_2} signal and causing the increase of alveolar ventilation at the expense of *hypocapnic alkalosis*. The symptoms of altitude sickness result from the combination of hypoxemia and hypocapnia.

Want of oxygen injures cells

The Trouble Is Not Merely "Running Out of Gas"

When an automobile runs out of fuel, it stops, but when the tank is refilled, it can be started again. When cells of an air-breathing animal are deprived of oxygen or of oxidizable substrate, they first stop functioning and then they die. Why can't a living organism be revived when it is "refueled" any time after functional arrest? The limit to resuscitation is a basic problem in pathophysiology. In general, the answer appears to lie in the need for constant renewal. The unabated turnover of membranes and cytoskeleton ensures that the structural elements of living cells are not subject to corrosion, or metal fatigue, or other modes of decay that affect nonliving materials, but the price paid is the incessant need for metabolic energy, required not only to do external work but for survival itself. Because synthesizing structural proteins requires a steady supply of ATP, in its absence cells disintegrate. But this universal rule does not explain why some cells perish so much sooner for want of oxygen than others, certainly much more rapidly than the decay of their structural elements.

When deprived of oxygen, the organs that are arguably most precious to us perish first: brain, heart, kidneys, liver, and intestines, in that order. In the CNS, neurons die of hypoxia long before glial cells do, and among glia, oligodendrocytes before astrocytes (García and Anderson, 1997). The high rate of metabolism has been cited as the reason for the vulnerability of the CNS. The brain is said to consume one-fifth of the oxygen that the body metabolizes. This is true only under *basal conditions*, during relaxed bed rest of a fasting subject. As soon as one gets out of bed or eats a meal, overall metabolic energy demand increases and the (proportional) share of oxygen consumed by the brain decreases. And even at rest, the metabolic rate calculated per unit tissue mass of heart and kidneys exceeds that of brain.

High metabolic rate per se does not explain the unique sensitivity of central neurons to lack of oxygen, but this does not mean that metabolic rate is unimportant. The temperature of the tissue at the time of reduced oxygen makes a big difference for cell survival, and temperature exerts its effect by altering metabolic reaction rates (Busto et al., 1987; Chen et al., 1993; Freund et al., 1990b; Mitani et al., 1991; Wang et al., 2000). Patients undergoing surgery that mandates temporary interruption of blood flow to the brain are routinely cooled before the arrest of cerebral circulation.

Selective Vulnerability Among Neurons

Even among neurons there is wide variability. In hippocampal formation, CA1 pyramidal cells (*Sommer's sector*: see Fig. 17–2) succumb first, followed by CA3 cells and then dentate granule cells. There are also differences in the susceptibility among the different classes of hippocampal interneurons (Schmidt-Kastner and Freund, 1991). Cerebellar Purkinje cells are as vulnerable as CA1 pyramidal cells, and layers III, IV, and V neocortical pyramids and cells in the striatum are also very sensitive to hypoxia (García and Anderson, 1997; Pulsinelli, 1985). Neurons in the brain stem and spinal cord survive longer than most of those in the forebrain, which explains why some patients end up in a functionally decerebrate state when resuscitated after cardiac arrest.

The widely varying sensitivity of neuron populations to ischemic injury intrigued pathologists for many decades (Crain et al., 1988; Kirino et al., 1985; Spielmeyer, 1929; Vogt and Vogt, 1922). For a long time the contended issue was whether the difference lies in variations of the local blood supply or in properties inherent of the vulnerable cells. The latter view carries more weight nowadays but, in times of restricted flow, when the blood supply is marginal but not zero, the distribution of blood flow as determined in large part by the vascular architecture can become the decisive factor for cell survival (Welsh, 1995). The importance of *intrinsic cell properties* is demonstrated in brain tissue slices in vitro, where vascular factors cannot play a role. As in brains in situ, CA1 pyramidal neurons in hippocampal slices succumb to hypoxic injury earlier than do dentate granule cells (Aitken and Schiff, 1986; Balestrino et al., 1989). The specific factors responsible for high sensitivity are gradually being discovered (Haddad and Jiang, 1993; Lipton, 1999; Pulsinelli, 1985; Schmidt-Kastner and Freund, 1991; Somjen et al., 1990; see also Chapter 19: "Selective vulnerability correlates . . .").

Age is also important. Newborns have a much better chance to survive hypoxia than do adults (Cherubini et al., 1989; Kabat, 1940). The very young are protected by the endocrine response (Slotkin and Seidler, 1988), but this is not the whole explanation, because neurons and brain tissue slices harvested from newborn animals and made hypoxic in vitro are also more resistant to hypoxic injury than those from mature brains (Friedman and Haddad, 1993; Luhmann and Kral, 1997).

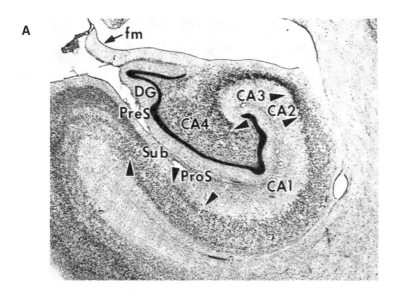

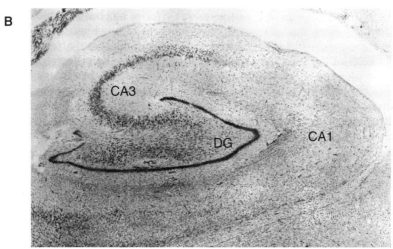

FIGURE 17–2. Selective loss of CA1 pyramidal neurons caused by transient cerebral ischemia (Sommer sector). **A:** Section from the hippocampal formation of a healthy rhesus monkey. PreS: pre-subiculum; ProS: pro-subiculum; Sub: subiculum. **B:** From the hippocampal formation of a 49-year-old man who died 7 months after transient cardiac arrest. Pyramidal cells are depleted in the CA1 region. DG: dentate gyrus. (**A** from Rosene and van Hoesen, 1987; **B** from Brierley and Graham, 1984.)

In Asphyxia and Cerebral Ischemia Lack of Oxygen Dominates the Picture,
but It Is Modified Compared to Pure Hypoxia

Suffocation, or **asphyxia**, may be caused by drowning, airway obstruction, lung disease, or being enclosed in a limited air space. In the asphyxic condition excess CO_2 builds up and complicates the hypoxia, in contrast to altitude sickness, in which low P_{O_2} is combined with low P_{CO_2}. Remarkably, while suffocation causes great distress, hypoxia with hypocapnia does not. Mountain sickness may be unpleasant, but it is not frightening or painful. Fulton in his introduction and Bert in his historical chapter (Bert, 1943) quote from the accounts of several pioneer balloonists, who at great height were overtaken first by a pleasant excitement not unlike drunkenness and then by torpor, quietly subsiding into paralysis and fainting. Because of the euphoric state of mind, miscalculations cost the lives of several early balloonists and aviators. Mistakes in judgment are a hazard for inexperienced mountain climbers as well. All of this points to the fact that hypoxia impairs brain function.

Hypoxia uncomplicated by deviation in CO_2 levels can be achieved only under laboratory conditions. In intact animals, even if blood CO_2 is controlled, cardiovascular and endocrine responses interfere with the direct CNS effects of a reduced oxygen supply. To study truly pure hypoxia, in vitro systems must be used.

Interrupting the blood flow (**ischemia**) deprives the brain not only of oxygen but also of glucose and other metabolic substrates. It also interdicts the clearing of waste products, of which acids are most relevant for their acute effects on brain function. Nonetheless, the immediate effect of ischemia is similar to that of anoxia, except that the former evolves faster than the latter (Graham, 1992). The consequences of depressed oxidative metabolism dominate the syndromes of acute cerebral ischemia and acute anoxia as well as hypoglycemia (Duchen, L.W., 1992a).

The sequence of functional changes in brains deprived of oxygen

Hans Berger wrote a vivid account of his one and only recording of the EEG of a human subject rendered hypoxic by what Berger called the "American method." This consisted of rebreathing in and out of an airtight bag through a trap that absorbed expired CO_2 (Berger, 1934; see also, Gloor, 1969). The subject was his assistant, a certain Dr. W. After 6 min of this treatment the subject started to tremble. Alarmed, Berger ripped off the face mask and found his assistant unconscious. Dr. W recovered, but Berger vowed never to repeat this experiment. He did publish the EEG and ECG recordings taken during the drama. The EEG trace changed quite abruptly from alpha pattern to large amplitude slow waves with interspersed "group formations" (*Gruppenbildung*, in today's terminology spindles?). Berger (1934) commented that the EEG pattern that accompanied loss of consciousness is the opposite of the expected electrical silence, and it represents "unambiguous disinhibition" (*unzweideutige Enthemmung*). Further, he compared the hypoxic EEG to that seen when consciousness is lost in general anesthesia and during an epileptic attack, both also being forms of disinhibition, in his view.

When the blood supply to the brain is suddenly and completely interrupted, it takes much less than 6 min before the patient faints. Loss of various functions were accurately timed first in dogs and then in people by Kabat and colleagues (1941; Rossen et al., 1943). They used a pneumatic cuff in the shape of a collar around the neck, with protuberant inserts the purpose of which was to compress, when inflated, not only the common carotid artery but also the subclavian arteries so that all circulation to the brain would be cut off at once. A picture of this fiendish device, worn by its inventor, was published by Hansen (1988). In dogs the corneal reflex was extinguished in 10 s, and respiration ceased in 20–30 s. The dogs eventually recovered completely, provided that the cerebral circulation was restored in 6 min, but some remained in coma for up to 24 hr. In the postischemic coma involuntary running movements were sometimes seen, but no epileptiform convulsions. Lasting neurological deficits were severe if cerebral circulatory arrest lasted for 8 min or more. Human subjects included the investigators (Rossen et al., 1943). In humans, a tingling sensation and a constriction of the visual field occurred before consciousness was extinguished, on average 6.8 s after inflation of the cuff. The EEG showed large-amplitude slow waves, as in Berger's experiment. The pressure in the collar was released after 100 s, and 25 s after restoration of the circulation some of the subjects underwent mild tonic-clonic convulsion. Reportedly, all recovered completely.

It is important to add here that the "complete" recovery of dogs after 6 min of global cerebral ischemia reported by Kabat et al. (1941) may have been assessed by somewhat crude criteria, and mild malfunction could have gone undetected. At the other extreme, Jung (1953) gives 2 min of total anoxia as the limit for complete reversibility, which is probably a bit short for pure anoxia but may be accurate for the most vulnerable neuron types in case of the withdrawal of both oxygen and glucose (as in ischemia). Many factors influence the chances of survival and of recovery, among them temperature and the age of the patient. There have been medically documented reports of the revival of children pulled out of icy lakes after prolonged submersion who subsequently appeared to do quite well.

Early experiments on animals established the sequence in which function is extinguished in hypoxic mammalian brains (Baumgartner et al., 1961; Hirsch et al., 1957; Jung, 1953; Naquet and Fernandes-Guardiola, 1961; Opitz and Schneider, 1950; see reviews by Hansen, 1985; Somjen, 1990; Somjen et al., 1993b). If oxygen is replaced by nitrogen, with CO_2 kept constant in the inspired air of an experimental animal, the functional disturbances follow a predictable pattern in several distinct phases:

1. Initially there is a short delay before signs of malfunction appear (called the *free interval* by Baumgartner et al. (1961).
2. Next comes the period of ***activation***, during which the EEG shows signs of arousal, that is, fast, irregular, low-voltage activity. (This is Phase 2 according to Baumgartner et al., 1961, and Stage I. according to Naquet and Fernandes-Guardiola, 1961.) Arousal was absent or weak in forebrains disconnected from the midbrain (*cerveau isolé*) (Baumgartner et al., 1961), and it has been attributed to input arriving in the brain stem from stimulated arterial chemoreceptors (Dell et al., 1961). There can be, however, genuine neuronal *hyperexcitability* in the earliest stages due to *disinhibition* (see below).
3. Next there may be brief, generalized α activity of unusually low frequency; alternatively, ***EEG spindles*** may appear (Jung, 1953; Stage II of Naquet and Fernandes-Guardiola, 1961).
4. Alpha activity and spindles are then converted into slower, larger, *δ* ***waves*** (Stage III or the *delta phase*).
5. Then spontaneous oscillations as well as spontaneous neuron impulse discharges cease and the ***EEG*** becomes ***isoelectric*** (stage IV of Naquet and Fernandes-Guardiola, 1961, or the *null phase* of Baumgartner et al., 1961). In rabbits this occurred on average after 36 s of nitrogen breathing. Partial depression of synaptic transmission probably underlies the changing EEG pattern of the earlier phases, but even at the time when the EEG becomes flat, synapses still transmit, albeit weakly (Baumgartner et al., 1961). The EEG activity is first extinguished in the higher regions of the cerebral cortex, later in the subcortical forebrain gray matter, and last in the lower brain stem (Sugar and Gerard, 1938). When the forebrain is inactive, *convulsions* may still emanate from the brain stem or spinal cord (Jung, 1953).
6. Soon thereafter, ***synaptic transmission fails*** altogether (Fig. 17–3, 17–4).
7. ***Hypoxic SD-like depolarization*** of the gray matter of the forebrain always starts after complete synaptic failure. The sequence is important for considerations of mechanisms. Mild, gradual depolarization of forebrain neurons begins well before HSD. Axons in white matter and the neurons in spinal gray depolarize slowly, without ever undergoing the SD-like event. There is an important difference between the gradual loss of membrane potential of axons and neurons in the lower regions of the CNS and the precipitous, nearly complete depolarization of cell bodies and dendrites of forebrain neurons typical of HSD (Somjen, 2001). Timely reoxygenation can restore normal function even after the onset of HSD.
8. If, however, oxygen is not readmitted, neuron injury becomes irreversible and ***hypoxic neuronal damage*** sets in (Duchen, 1992a; Lipton, 1999; Somjen et al., 1993b).

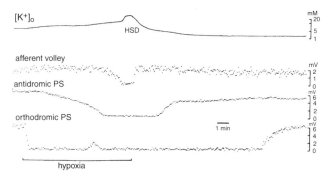

FIGURE 17–3. Neural function during hypoxia in hippocampus. Recording from the CA1 region of a hippocampal tissue slice. $[K^+]_o$ and the antidromic and orthodromic population spikes (PS) from stratum (st.) pyramidale and afferent volley from st. radiatum. Stimulation of the Schaffer collateral-commissural fiber bundle. Synaptic transmission (orthodromic PS) fails first and recovers last but, paradoxically, was slightly restored before the onset of hypoxic spreading depression–like depolarization (HSD). (Modified from Sick et al., 1987.)

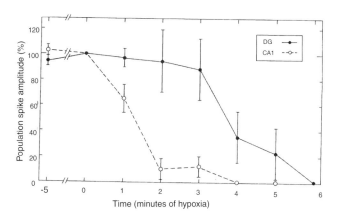

FIGURE 17–4. Selective loss of function during hypoxia. Amplitudes of population spikes evoked by Schaffer collateral bundle stimulation in CA1 stratum pyramidale and by perforant path stimulation in the granule cell layer of the dentate gyrus (DG) recorded simultaneously in hippocampal tissue slices. Mean ±S.E.M. of 19 slices. During hypoxia, synaptic transmission was obliterated earlier (and was less likely to recover after reoxygenation) in CA1 than in DG. (Modified from Balestrino et al., 1989.)

9. Even if the supply of oxygen or of blood is restored and neurons seem to regain some function and look normal in histological sections, certain cells can succumb days after a transient hypoxic or ischemic episode—***delayed neuron degeneration*** (Kirino, 1982).

Key points

Hypoxia of brain tissue, hypoxia combined with glucose deprivation, and ischemia involve similar but increasingly severe pathophysiology.

Certain populations of forebrain neurons are more susceptible to hypoxic/ischemic injury than any other cell type. Selective vulnerability cannot be explained by unequal distribution of cerebral blood vessels, because the different susceptibility is present in brain tissue slices in vitro.

When crebral circulation is interrupted, consciousness is lost before EEG silence, the EEG is flattened before complete failure of synapses, and HSD sets in after synaptic failure.

Hypoxic SD-like depolarization is initially reversible, but in the long run in the absence of re-oxygenation it causes irreversible cell injury.

18

Mechanism of Early, Reversible Hypoxic Synaptic Failure

The most common manifestation of impaired blood flow to the brain is fainting, which can be caused by strong emotions, orthostatic hypotension, or a variety of other conditions, some benign, some not. Fortunately, in most cases it is readily reversible. Consciousness is lost in these cases by impairment of synaptic transmission in critical neuron circuits.

Chapter 18 explores the mechanism of the rapid arrest of brain function during hypoxia and ischemia.

Brain function is arrested before brain cells are injured

Arrest of function in times of energy shortage is believed to aid ultimate recovery, because economizing on metabolic activity during times of want might save reserves and forestall irreversible injury. Plausible as it sounds, to my knowledge this frequently voiced opinion has no rigorous experimental underpinning, although it has been reported that suppressing brain function before clamping a cerebral artery prevents stroke (Maynard et al., 1998). To quote a review by Guillemin and Krasnow: "Hypoxic cells sense diminishing oxygen levels well before their ATP pools are depleted, and respond with a self-imposed austerity program to curb their energy usage by shutting down non-essential cell function" (Guillemin and Krasnow, 1997; Hochachka et al., 1996). In any event, it is a fact that brain function stops when either oxygen or glucose runs low, and it does so long before hope for recovery vanishes. It has also been clear for several decades that synaptic transmission is interrupted well before axonal conduction (see Chapter 17: "The sequence of functional changes . . ." and Somjen, 1990), at a time when energy reserves are not yet exhausted. It has been argued that arrest of function is a coordinated response to a stimulus, the stimulus being low partial pressure of oxygen (Jiang and Haddad, 1994; Opitz and Schneider, 1950). It is a corollary that cells must sense oxygen level, and the hunt is on for the biophysical *oxygen sensor*, to be found perhaps in mitochondria, perhaps in membrane channels, or perhaps in the redox status of cytosolic compounds (Duchen, 1999; Jiang and Haddad, 1994; Müller et al., 2002; O'Kelly et al., 1999).

The absence of molecular oxygen arrests mitochondrial oxidative metabolism, but even under anoxia ATP is produced for a while by anaerobic glycolysis, albeit at a much too low level of efficiency (Harris, 2002). Both neurons and glial cells are equipped for glycolysis, but glia more so than neurons; glia also have more of the necessary glycogen (Fillenz et al., 1997).

During hypoxia synaptic inhibition seems to fail before synaptic excitation, creating a period of hyperexcitability (Krnjević et al., 1991). The disinhibition is, however, not due to selective blockade of GABAergic synapses, but rather to the silencing of inhibitory interneurons. It is the excitatory input to the inhibitory interneurons that is rapidly blocked and puts the interneurons out of action (Khazipov et al., 1995; Zhu and Krnjević, 1994).

Several changes, both pre- and postsynaptic, contribute to synaptic failure. These will now be discussed.

Presynaptic factors in hypoxic transmission failure

In a pioneering study, Rose Eccles et al. (1966b) found that, in the hypoxic spinal cord, EPSPs are initially boosted and then depressed. They concluded that the trouble lay in hypoxic depolarization of presynaptic axon terminals, causing first elevated release of transmitter substance and then blockade of impulse conduction into the terminal. The postsynaptic target cells, the ventral horn motoneurons, gradually depolarized. Initially, the depolarization increased motoneuron excitability, as measured by injected stimulating current (i.e., lowered rheobase); then it suppressed excitability.

Rapid depression of excitatory synaptic transmission was confirmed for other regions of the CNS (Collewijn and Van Harreveld, 1966a; Speckmann and Caspers, 1974). Synaptic transmission can be blocked for many reasons. Transmitter output can fall short or the postsynaptic target cells can fail to respond to the transmitter. Both pre- and postsynaptic failure can have multiple causes.

A number of observations placed the blame on the presynaptic side of synapses. Most importantly, neuron responses to exogenous glutamate, quisqualate, or

NMDA were not depressed or were barely depressed when the transmission of synaptic potentials (or synaptic currents) evoked by afferent fiber volleys was blocked, indicating that hypoxia curtailed the output of transmitter from presynaptic terminals (Crépel et al., 1993; Frenguelli, 1997; Khazipov et al., 1995; Rosen and Morris, 1993).

Four possible causes of hypoxia-induced curtailment of transmitter release

Granted that hypoxia impairs the release of transmitter, the question remained, what prevents the release? In 1987 we listed the following four possibilities (Somjen et al., 1987b):

1. *Depletion of available transmitter* due to the inability to produce fresh supplies. This seemed unlikely, because adding glutamine to the bathing medium of hypoxic hippocampal slices did not alleviate the synaptic block, even though the same treatment did counteract the "fatigue" of transmission caused by intense overstimulation (Schiff et al., 1985).

2. *Branch point failure.* Krnjević and Miledi (1959) found that hypoxia blocked transmission across the neuromuscular junction, because impulses failed to propagate from the myelinated axon into the unmyelinated terminal branches that innervate the endplate. R. Eccles et al. (1966b) came to a similar conclusion concerning spinal cord synapses (see above). In general, conduction is more easily arrested at points with a *low safety factor of propagation*, where large-caliber axons divide into finer branches. Impulse propagation was also arrested at the axon bifurcation in hypoxic mammalian DRG cells (Urbán and Somjen, 1990). Hypoxia inhibits Na^+ currents in neurons (Fig. 18–1) (Cummins et al., 1993 ; O'Reilly et al., 1997). If this also occurs in axons, even if the inhibition is partial, it would reduce action potential amplitude and make impulse propagation less secure. In hippocampal slices, the presynaptic volley amplitude remained unchanged when synaptic transmission was completely blocked, suggesting normal conduction in afferent axons (Fig. 17–3) (Schiff and Somjen, 1985; Sick et al., 1987), but it could be reasoned that conduction into the terminal *boutons* could have been impaired even if the main axon conducted normally.

3. *Depolarization of presynaptic boutons.* In early studies, the loss of membrane potential due to weakening of the 3Na/2K ATPase ion pump was thought to be the early consequence of energy failure (e.g., Collewijn and Van Harreveld, 1966a). Even if impulses do arrive at the terminal, depolarization would reduce the amplitude of the presynaptic spike and partially inactivate Ca^{2+} channels, limiting the release of transmitter. The constancy of the presynaptic volley amplitude, mentioned above, does not support this alternative explanation but, as also mentioned above, it cannot rule it out

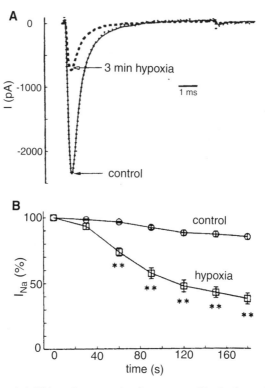

FIGURE 18–1. Hypoxia inhibits voltage-gated sodium current. Single-electrode voltage clamp of isolated CA1 hippocampal pyramidal neurons. K^+ and Ca^{2+} currents were blocked. Na^+ current ($I_{Na,T}$) was evoked by stepping from a holding potential of -70 mV to -10 mV. **A:** Current response from one cell in control condition and in hypoxia. **B:** Mean $\pm$S.E.M. amplitude of $I_{Na,T}$ in 10 cells each in control and hypoxia. The suppression of $I_{Na,T}$ was attributed to activation of protein kinase C by hypoxia. (Modified from O'Reilly et al., 1997.)

either, because the extracellular record might not register a change in impulse amplitude at the terminal.

4. *Failure of presynaptic voltage-gated calcium channels.* In the 1980s it became clear that ATP is required for the operation of calcium channels (Kostyuk, 1984). Lipton and Whittingham (1982) demonstrated early reduction in ATP content in the region of synapses in brain tissue slices. Combining these findings, we proposed hypothetically that hypoxic depletion of ATP in presynaptic terminals could incapacitate presynaptic Ca^{2+} channels and thereby depress the release of transmitter substance (Somjen et al., 1987b). Besides depletion of ATP, calcium current could also be inactivated by an increase of intracellular free Ca^{2+} concentration (Adams et al., 1985; Hille, 2001). Experimental tests support this mechanism.

Hypoxia Inhibits Presynaptic Calcium Channels

Measurements in voltage-clamped neurons confirmed that interference with mitochondrial oxidative metabolism, whether by lack of oxygen, glucose deprivation, or cyanide poisoning, depresses voltage-controlled calcium currents (Figs. 18–2, 18–3, 19–2B–D) (Duchen, 1990; Duchen and Somjen, 1988; Krnjević and Leblond, 1987, 1989). The depression of Ca^{2+} currents recorded from the neuron soma does not necessarily mean, however, a similar effect at presynaptic terminals, because different membranes contain different sets of Ca^{2+} channels. To decide whether presynaptic Ca^{2+} channels respond similarly, we adopted a method invented by Konnerth and Heinemann (1983). In hippocampal tissue slices, Ca^{2+} influx into presynaptic terminals can be assayed from the stimulus-induced decrease of $[Ca^{2+}]_o$, provided that postsynaptic responses are first blocked. With synaptic transmission blocked by glutamate antagonist drugs, stimulus-induced presynaptic Ca^{2+} uptake was depressed early during hypoxia. $[Ca^{2+}]_o$ responses were depressed well before the onset of HSD, at about the time when synapses

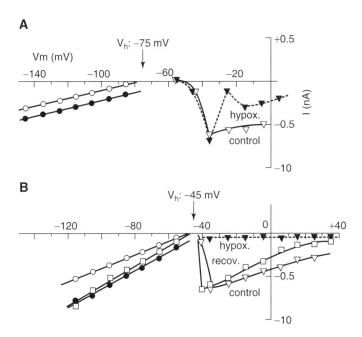

FIGURE 18–2. Hypoxia reversibly suppresses calcium currents in hippocampal neurons. Current-voltage (I-V) plots obtained by single-electrode voltage clamp from one CA1 pyramidal neuron in a hippocaampal slice. Na^+ and K^+ currents were pharmacologically blocked. Open triangles: control; filled triangles: during hypoxia; open squares: during reoxygenation. **A** and **B** taken in sequence so that "control" in **B** corresponds to "recovery" of **A**. **A:** Holding potential –75 mV. **B:** Holding potential –45 mV, which inactivated T-type low-voltage activated (LVA) transient current. (Modified from Krnjević et al., 1989.)

would have started to fail, had they not been blocked in the first place (Fig. 18–3) (Young and Somjen, 1992). It was also evident that baseline $[Ca^{2+}]_o$ began to decline slowly shortly before the stimulus-induced $[Ca^{2+}]_o$ responses, suggesting gradual, stimulus-independent Ca^{2+} uptake into cells. An increase in the resting cytosolic Ca^{2+} level can inactivate voltage-gated Ca^{2+} channels (see the next paragraph and Hille, 2001). After the disappearance of the stimulus-induced $[Ca^{2+}]_o$ responses, there was a very large decrease in $[Ca^{2+}]_o$ caused by HSD. Resupplying the tissue with oxygen allowed recovery of baseline $[Ca^{2+}]_o$, which took place in two phases, and only as the baseline returned toward normal did the stimulus-induced transient $[Ca^{2+}]_o$ responses recover (Fig. 18–3e) (Young and Somjen, 1992).

If insufficiency of Ca^{2+} channels causes hypoxic failure of synapses, then it is to be expected that raising $[Ca^{2+}]_o$ would delay the synaptic block. Increased driving force should overcome incomplete opening of the channel. This indeed proved to be the case in isolated mouse spinal cords (Fig. 18–4) (Czéh and Somjen, 1990).

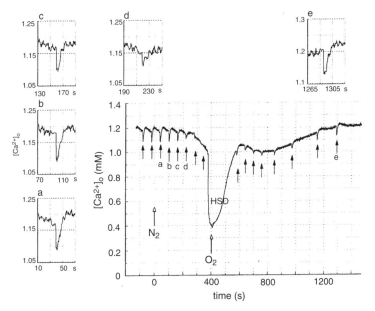

FIGURE 18–3. Suppression of presynaptic calcium current in hypoxia and subsequent $[Ca^{2+}]_o$ decrease during hypoxic spreading depression–like depolarization (HSD). Recording of $[Ca^{2+}]_o$ in stratum radiatum of the CA1 region in a hippocampal tissue slice, with postsynaptic responses pharmacologically blocked. Oxygen was withheld between the arrows marked "N_2" and "O_2." The solid arrows mark $[Ca^{2+}]_o$ responses evoked by 5 s 20 Hz afferent stimulus trains; the transient dips in $[Ca^{2+}]_o$ correspond to Ca^{2+} influx into presynaptic fibers. Small frames (a–e) are expanded segments illustrating selected presynaptic responses; note the time scales. Hypoxic spreading depression caused the large drop in $[Ca^{2+}]_o$. Presynaptic Ca^{2+} currents became depressed before the onset of HSD, and HSD was not prevented by the blockade of glutamate receptors. (From Young and Somjen, 1992.)

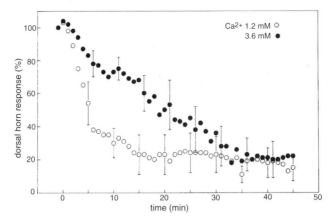

FIGURE 18–4. Elevated calcium level postpones hypoxic failure of synaptic transmission. Recordings of synaptically transmitted dorsal horn response in mouse spinal cord in vitro. Oxygen was withdrawn at zero time. Mean ±S.E.M. from seven preparations, each subjected to hypoxia in control (1.2 mM) as well as elevated (3.6 mM) bath [Ca^{2+}] (the sequence was varied). (From Czéh and Somjen, 1990.)

Failure of presynaptic calcium channels

There are three possible explanations for the failure of presynaptic calcium channels:

1. *High-voltage activated calcium currents are inactivated by elevated* [Ca^{2+}]$_i$. The decline of the [Ca^{2+}]$_o$ baseline in hypoxic hippocampus (Fig. 18–3) indicated uptake into cells. Elevation of [Ca^{2+}]$_i$ inactivates voltage-gated Ca^{2+} channels, and this can impede transmitter release (Adams et al., 1985; Hille, 2001). In some preparations the early, slow [Ca^{2+}]$_o$ decrease may be masked by the swelling of cells that restrict the interstitial volume and concentrate the ion (Hansen, 1985). Indeed, intracellular recording by Silver and Erecińska (1990) did show an early, moderate increase of [Ca^{2+}]$_i$ before the later, much larger increase coincident with the rapid SD-like depolarization of the neuron. The inflow could begin through low-threshold voltage-gated Ca^{2+} channels before they become plugged by inactivation. As the extracellular glutamate level starts to increase, NMDA receptor–operated channels could add to the inflow (see Chapter 19: "Glutamate is released . . ."). [Ca^{2+}]$_i$ may be raised not only by entry from the outside but also by release from internal stores. In addition, its removal from the cell by the calcium pump may be in jeopardy due to the decreased ATP level.

2. *Decreased ATP content.* Besides calcium-induced inactivation, calcium currents could be depressed due to a decline of ATP (see above and Kostyuk, 1984). Reduction ATP has yet another effect: it allows the opening of ATP-

inhibited K channels. Enhanced K+ conductance could counteract depolarization, and therefore the activation of Ca^{2+} channels, and reduce transmitter release (Krnjević, 1990). Data reported by Alici and Heinemann (1995) appear to refute, however, the role of ATP depletion. They found that withdrawal of glucose (with normal oxygenation) augmented presynaptic calcium currents in hippocampal slices instead of blocking them. The augmentation persisted for more than 1 hr, at which time the ATP supply must have been severely curtailed. The hypoxic failure of presynaptic Ca^{2+} appears to be caused by factors other than depletion of ATP.

3. *Adenosine.* Adenosine concentration increases in ISF during hypoxia (Van Wylen et al., 1986). It has both pre- and postsynaptic receptors and generally inhibitory effects (Haas and Selbach, 2000). Adenosine *antagonist drugs* retard the failure of excitatory but not of inhibitory synapses during hypoxia (Fowler, 1989; Katchman and Hershkowitz, 1993; Khazipov et al., 1995). On the other hand, Doherty and Dingledine (1997) contend that the hypoxic depression of the EPSP of inhibitory interneurons is caused by presynaptic metabotropic glutamate receptors, not by adenosine receptors.

In conclusion

The three proposed mechanisms that interfere with presynaptic function are not mutually exclusive. One or the other might dominate, or several could cooperate, at different synapses. Whatever the mechanism, it seems clear that transmitter release fails in all hypoxic synapses that have been studied.

Postsynaptic hyperpolarization mediated by enhanced K+ conductance

In early studies, mostly on nerve or nerve-muscle preparations, oxygen lack was seen to initially increase excitation, followed by suppression of function. This was linked to a decrease of the *demarcation current* (DC current flowing between the intact surface and the cut or crushed end of a nerve or muscle), indicating depolarization (Gerard, 1930; Jung, 1953). When the ATP dependence of the 3Na/2K ion pump was discovered, it was easy to conclude that hypoxic depolarization was due to shortage of ATP. The first direct recordings from central neurons during hypoxia showed depolarization, reinforcing the concept (Collewijn and Van Harreveld, 1966a, 1966b).

Against this background, it was quite surprising when Glötzner (1967) reported that cortical neurons of hypoxic cats undergo hyperpolarization before they depolarize. It took 15 years before Hansen et al. (1982) showed that the same happens in pyramidal cells in hippocampal slices and attributed the hyperpolarization to enhanced K+ conductance (Fig. 18–5). Subsequently, hyperpolarization of neu-

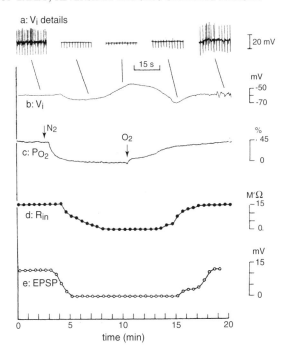

Figure 18–5. Hypoxic hyperpolarization, reduced input resistance, and synaptic failure in a neuron. Recording from a CA1 neuron in a guinea pig hippocampal tissue slice. a: Intracellular recordings before, during, and after a hypoxic period. Downward deflections represent pulses used to measure input resistance. Upward deflections are truncated action potentials. Firing was abolished during hypoxia and returned only several minutes after reoxygenation. b: Low-pass filtered continuous record of V_i. Hypoxic hyperpolarization changed to mild depolarization before reoxygenation. A second wave of hyperpolarization was seen during recovery. Hypoxic hyperpolarization was attributed to K^+ conductance and posthypoxic hyperpolarization (in part?) to activation of the 3Na/2K ion pump. c: Tissue partial pressure of oxygen measured polarographically, expressed as a percentage of P_{O_2} in a solution saturated with 100% oxygen. Arrows mark the onset of hypoxia and reoxygenation. d: Input resistance. e: Excitatory postsynaptic potential (EPSP) amplitude. Note early failure and late recovery. (Modified from Hansen et al., 1982.)

rons due to increased K^+ conductance received much attention (Fujimura et al., 1997; Krnjević and Xu, 1990; Leblond and Krnjević, 1989; Mercuri et al., 1994). However, not all neurons hyperpolarize, yet all synapses, both excitatory and inhibitory, become rapidly blocked during hypoxia, (Krnjević and Ben-Ari, 1989; Luhmann and Heinemann, 1992; Morris et al., 1995; Rosen and Morris, 1991, 1993). The method used for the recording sometimes influences the outcome. Cells that hyperpolarized when "sharp" recording electrodes were used usually depolarized under whole-cell conditions created with patch-clamp electrodes filled with potassium-gluconate, cesium-gluconate, or KCl (Czéh et al., 1993; Hershkowitz et al., 1993; Zhang and Krnjević, 1993). With potassium-methylsulfate in the patch pipette, the hyperpolarization was again revealed (Erdemli et al., 1998). A small, short-lived depolarization sometimes precedes the hyperpolarization. Subsequent analysis of membrane currents suggested that inward and outward currents compete in the early phases of hypoxia (Haddad and Jiang, 1993; Hershkowitz et al., 1993). Depending on which of the two is in ascendance, the membrane might depolarize or hyperpolarize.

It should be emphasized that the early, gradual, and mild depolarization is not related to the dramatic SD-like event (HSD) that follows later. The full course of early hypoxic membrane changes consists of (*1*) an initial, small depolarization, (*2*) then the somewhat longer-lasting hyperpolarization, and (*3*) then gradual depolarization, which leads to (*4*) major, rapid depolarization of the HSD. These four phases have been reported in various situations, but all four are rarely seen as a sequence in one cell.

The mechanism of the hyperpolarization was investigated in detail by Krnjević and associates (Belousov et al., 1995; Erdemli et al., 1998; Krnjević and Xu, 1990). The likely candidate K^+ currents included the ATP-sensitive $I_{K,ATP}$ and several calcium-dependent K^+ currents. The latest conclusions of the Krnjević team identify it, at least for hippocampal neurons, as a G-protein–dependent outward K^+ current initiated by Ca^{2+} released from internal stores. It is apparently independent of ATP (Erdemli et al., 1998). However, Müller et al. (2002) report that under hypoxic condition $I_{K,ATP}$ can open, independently of any change in ATP level. There are also other advocates for $I_{K,ATP}$ mediation of hypoxic hyperpolarization (Ben-Ari, 1989; Fujimura et al., 1997; Jiang et al., 1994; Murphy and Greenfield, 1991).

In conclusion

In light of accumulating evidence, decreased output of synaptic transmitter from axon terminals appears to be the most important reason for hypoxic failure of synaptic transmission. Decreased postsynaptic excitability caused by enhanced K^+ conductance is an added factor in many neurons. Elevation of $[Ca^{2+}]_i$ may be important for both presynaptic and postsynaptic failure of hypoxic synapses. In presynaptic terminals, high $[Ca^{2+}]_i$ inactivates voltage-gated Ca^{2+} current and therefore reduces transmitter output. In postsynaptic target cells it activates $I_{K,(Ca)}$ and therefore raises the threshold of firing.

Key points

The function of hypoxic brain tissue is suppressed before high-energy phosphates are depleted. This suggests a protective function of conserving the energy reserve. It also suggests the existence of a cellular oxygen sensor that acts as a sentinel of hypoxic threat.

Synaptic transmission is interrupted chiefly by failure of transmitter release.

The most likely explanation of hypoxic synaptic failure is impaired calcium channel function. Reduced Na^+ current and consequent failure of impulse propagation into terminal axon branches may contribute. Ca^{2+} channel failure may be the result of Ca^{2+}-dependent inactivation or inhibition by adenosine.

Inhibitory synaptic transmission fails before EPSPs, causing transient hyperexcitation. The cause is failure of excitation of inhibitory interneurons, not selective block of GABA synapses.

Transient hyperpolarization of postsynaptic neurons caused by enhanced K^+ conductance occurs in many but not all hypoxic neurons and contributes to the failure of excitatory synaptic transmission. Hyperpolarization is transformed into depolarization during continued hypoxia.

19

Irreversible Hypoxic (Ischemic) Neuron Injury

Cerebral stroke is a devasting condition. The distinguished neuroanatomist Alf Brodal (1973) wrote a restrained yet gripping first-hand account of a stroke he suffered. He self-diagnosed the anatomical extent of the lesion, and recounted the struggle to re-learn with the remaining parts of his brain the skills that were lost in the affected parts. As he wrote, "even if the patient seems to be as he was . . . he is painfully aware himself that this is not so."

Brain cells can't do without oxygen even for a relatively short time. This last chapter examines the reasons for their low tolerance of hypoxia.

Oxygen-starved cells can die in three ways

When CNS tissue is deprived of oxygen or of oxidizable substrate, there comes a time when resupply no longer achieves recovery even though the cell structure still seems intact. This limit has been called *Wiederbelebungszeit* (Hirsch et al., 1957), meaning *resuscitation time* or revivability time, or, more recently, the **commitment point**. Irreversible hypoxic or ischemic neuron injury can be one of three kinds: *acute rapid*, *acute slow*, or *delayed*. (*1*) The most vulnerable neurons fall victim most rapidly, within a few minutes of oxygen lack (Chapter 17: "The sequence of functional changes . . ."). (*2*) The *acute but slow* process requires 45 min or more of severe hypoxia or anoxia before recovery becomes impossible. The immature brain is relatively resistant to anoxia, and acute rapid cell death does not occur in the newborn. If this were not so, none of us would have made safely the journey through the birth canal. In mature nervous systems, death comes slowly to neurons in the lower brain stem and even later to the spinal cord. It should be noted that within each of these major divisions there are differences among neuron populations. Axons perish more slowly than the cells from which they issue: it takes an extended period of oxygen and glucose deprivation to injure an optic nerve in vitro (Garthwaite et al., 1999; Stys et al., 1992a). Hypoxia slowly kills the neurons in cell cultures, which are customarily grown from cells harvested from newborn animals. This must be kept in mind when interpreting data from cultures. (*3*) *Delayed* neuron injury can follow an episode of hypoxia/anoxia, and it can damage certain selectively vulnerable cells that look healthy at first and may even regain function but subsequently succumb over 2–5 days (Kirino, 1982; Kirino et al., 1985; Pulsinelli et al., 1982a).

In each of these three modes, cells are damaged by a different pathophysiological process. We shall examine the mechanism of each.

Selectively vulnerable neuron populations are the ones first shut down by reversible synaptic failure. They are also the ones most prone to acute and delayed irreversible injury.

Hypoxic spreading depression–like depolarization hastens irreversible injury, but only in the presence of calcium

Hypoxic Spreading Depression–Like Depolarization Is Not Immediately Lethal, but It Turns into Terminal Depolarization with Time

The most easily recognizable predictor of the threat of a rapid demise of selectively vulnerable neurons is the occurrence of HSD, also known as *anoxic depolarization (AD)* or *rapid depolarization* (Figs. 19–1, 19–2). If oxygen is returned in time, HSD can be reversed, and it is then followed by full recovery of function, but if it persists, the depolarized neurons become committed to cell death in a matter of minutes. All cells of the mammalian CNS depolarize in the absence of oxygen, but those that are relatively resistant to hypoxic injury do so slowly and gradually. For example, the relative resistance of neonatal brain tissue is explained, at least in part, by the absence of the HSD response (Hansen, 1977) (Chapter 12: "Spreading depression can be provoked . . ."). Gradual depolarization is not SD-like.

Leão (1947) discovered the negative shift of the extracellular voltage of the cortical gray matter that is typical of sudden ischemia of the cerebral cortex. He

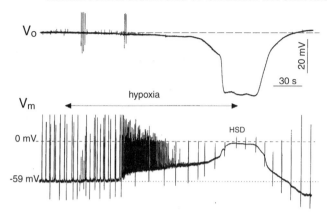

Figure 19–1. Extracellular and membrane potential changes during hypoxia of a neuron. Whole-cell patch clamp recording in the current clamp configuration from a CA1 pyramidal neuron in a rat hippocampal tissue slice. V_o is the extracellular potential near the neuron. V_m is the membrane potential referenced to V_o. The cell was firing spontaneously in the control state. Hypoxia caused an early depolarization and a storm of impulses that were stopped by depolarization-induced inactivation. Hypoxic spreading depression–like depolarization (HSD) is followed by hyperpolarization. The vertical up-down deflections intersecting the V_m trace are caused by injected current pulses used to test input impedance and excitability; these became small but not zero during HSD. (Modified from (Czéh et al., 1993.)

correctly assumed that it represented profound depolarization of cortical cells, and he suspected that the depolarization of normoxic SD and the one caused by ischemia resulted from the same biophysical change. This position was supported by some investigators and disputed by others (see below: "Comparing spreading depression and hypoxic spreading depression–like depolarization"). Intracellular recordings confirmed that neurons undergo depolarization in much the same way during normoxic SD as they do during ischemia or hypoxia (Collewijn and Van Harreveld, 1966b), and changes in other membrane properties are also alike. The processes that precede and trigger the depolarization are, however, different (Somjen, 2001).

Bureš and Burešová (1957) recorded a very large negative voltage shift from the cortex of animals dying of anoxia or ischemia and labeled it *anoxische Terminaldepolarisation*, assuming that it was the hallmark of the dying brain. They also noted that cooling the brain postponed the depolarization. As discussed below, HSD can indeed become terminal if it is permitted to persist, but this need not be so if the flow of oxygen (or of blood) is restored soon enough. And depolarization per se does not kill cells unless calcium enters in large amounts through open ion channels.

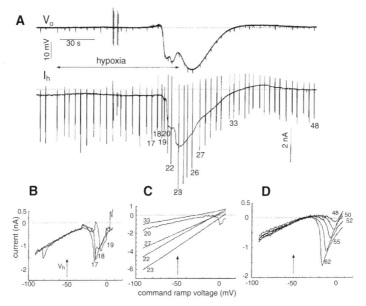

FIGURE 19–2. Neuron membrane currents and input resistance during hypoxia. Whole-cell patch-clamp recording in the voltage clamp configuration from a CA1 pyramidal neuron in a rat hippocampal slice. Conditions are similar to those in Figure 14–1, except that the pipette contained the local anesthetic QX-314, which blocked Na^+ action potentials but not dendritic Ca^{2+} spikes. **A:** Continuous record of extracellular potential (V_o) and holding current (I_h). The clamped pipette voltage was referred to V_o to obtain true transmembrane current and voltage. **B:** Three current-voltage (I-V) plots generated by ramp voltage commands during hypoxia just before the onset of hypoxic spreading depression–depolarization (HSD). The numbers next to the current-voltage (I-V) plots match those of the I_h trace in A. Note the progressively delayed onset of the Ca^{2+} spike. The slope of the linear portion of the I-V plot did not yet change, indicating the constancy of passive input resistance (Na^+ and K^+ conductances were blocked by QX-314). **C:** Current-voltage plots during and immediately after HSD. Steep slopes fo the lines signify reduced input resistance. **D:** Recovery of the Ca^{2+} spike. The I-V plots labeled 50–62 were taken after the end of the recording shown in A. The early depression and late recovery of the Ca^{2+} spike are related to the hypoxic suppression of voltage-gated Ca^{2+} current, as also seen in Figure 18–2. (Unpublished recordings of G. Czéh from the study reported in Czéh et al., 1993.)

Delaying Hypoxic Spreading Depression–Like Depolorization Favors Posthypoxic Recovery

During the 1970s, attention began to focus on cell injury caused by the accumulation of excess calcium in cytoplasm (Schanne et al., 1979; Wrogemann and Pena, 1976; see also the review by Kristián and Siesjö, (1998). Schanne, Farber, and colleagues (Farber et al., 1981; Schanne et al., 1979) showed that ischemic liver cells lived longer if they were perfused with calcium-free solution and also that ischemic necrosis of isolated, perfused livers was delayed by pretreatment with *chlorpromazine*. Earlier, Benešová et al. (1957) had reported that chlorpromazine, administered to rats before subjecting them to hypoxia or cerebral ischemia, postponed the onset of *Terminaldepolarisation*, that is, HSD.

Taking these hints, Balestrino and Somjen (1986) applied chlorpromazine to hippocampal tissue slices. They made four interrelated observations. *First*, chlorpromazine protected brain slices against hypoxic injury, defined as irreversibly impaired synaptic transmission. *Second*, the protection was correlated with postponement of SD-like depolarization. *Third*, if the slice was superfused with low-calcium medium for 30 min before oxygen deprivation, it was protected against hypoxia even in the absence of chlorpromazine (see also Young et al., 1991, and Fig. 19–3). *Fourth*, low calcium did not prevent or postpone HSD; on the contrary, it hastened its onset. The last two points proved to be most important. Together they strongly suggested that Ca^{2+} admitted into neurons by SD-like depolarization starts the process that causes irreversible neuron injury. Roberts

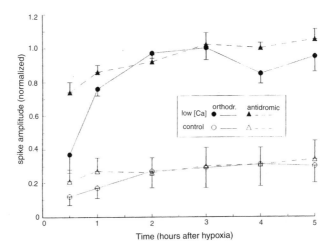

FIGURE 19–3. Withdrawing calcium during hypoxia aids posthypoxic recovery of neuron function. Pairs of slices cut from the same hippocampus were exposed simultaneously to 9 min of severe hypoxia in two wells of a double tissue slice chamber. Calcium concentration was reduced from 1.2 to 0.12 mM in one of the two chambers 30 min before hypoxia; $[Ca^{2+}]$ and O_2 were restored at the same time. Orthodromic (synaptically transmitted) and antidromic population spikes were recorded in CA1 stratum pyramidale. Synaptic transmission recovered more slowly than antidromic conduction because Ca^{2+} takes longer to diffuse into the tissue than does oxygen, but both recovered almost completely in Ca^{2+}-deprived slices, even though hypoxic spreading depression–like depolarization started earlier in low Ca^{2+} than in normal artificial cerebrospinal fluid. (The points show mean ±SEM in six pairs of slices.) (From Young et al., 1991.)

and Sick (1988) confirmed this point and also showed that too high $[Ca^{2+}]_o$ promotes irreversible hypoxic failure of synapses.

A similar relationship was found for other compounds: those that delayed the onset of HSD offered protection (Aitken et al., 1988; Balestrino et al., 1988, 1992, 1999a; Jarvis et al., 2001; Obeidat et al., 2000). Exposing hippocampal slices to a moderately acidic bath also greatly improved the chances of functional recovery from transient hypoxia (Fig. 19–10; Tombaugh, 1994; and see below: "Hyperglycemia and acidosis"). There appeared to be two components to the protection by acidosis. One was that acidity markedly delayed the onset of HSD, but even when the length of the hypoxic period was adjusted to make HSD equal for acidified and control slices, the slices maintained at the lower pH still recovered somewhat better than those at a bath pH of 7.4 (Tombaugh, 1994). The protective effect of low temperature can also be attributed, in large part, to the suppression or delay of HSD (Joshi and Andrew, 2001; Obeidat and Andrew, 1998; Taylor and Weber, 1993).

Selective Vulnerability Correlates with Rapid Onset of Hypoxic Spreading Depression–Like Depolarization

The selective vulnerability of the pyramidal cell population of the CA1 region of the hippocampus contrasts with the relative resistance of the granule cells of the dentate gyrus. Originally this was discovered by postmortem examination of histopathological brain tissue (*Sommer sector*, Fig. 17–2) (Graham, 1992). The difference in vulnerability is present in hippocampal tissue slices exposed to hypoxia in vitro. Synaptic transmission fails first and also becomes irreversible, first in CA1 and later in dentate gyrus (Fig. 17–4) (Aitken and Schiff, 1986; Balestrino et al., 1989). Simultaneous recording from CA1 and dentate gyrus demonstrated that HSD always began earlier in CA1. Moreover, in comparing individual slices exposed to equal lengths of hypoxia, it was evident that in both regions the chances of functional recovery after reoxygenation worsened the longer the time spent in the depolarized state (Balestrino et al., 1989). As already mentioned, the protective effect of chlorpromazine and other treatments appeared to be linked to the postponement of HSD (see the previous paragraph).

Prolonged Hypoxic Spreading Depression–Like Depolarization–Induced Calcium Influx Impairs not only Synaptic Transmission but also Action Potential Generation

These observations suggested a relationship between prolonged HSD and irreversible neuron injury but left lingering doubts. It could be argued that synapses failed to recover in the hour or so of observation following hypoxia, but the cells may have survived and perhaps more prolonged reoxygenation could eventually have restored neuron function. Young et al. (1991) addressed these two points (Fig. 19–3). Not only synaptic transmission but also antidromically conducted action potentials were abolished by 9 min of hypoxia of the slices. While still not proving cell necrosis, this did demonstrate abolition of all physiological responses of the pyramidal neurons. Furthermore, neuron responses remained absent for 5 hr after reoxygenation, which is longer than the usual period of observation in this type of experiment. Yet, if calcium was withdrawn from the slice before hypoxia and then readmitted together with oxygen, then both synaptic transmission and antidromic conduction were restored and remained stable for 5 hr (Fig. 19–3).

Prolonged Calcium Overload Kills Well-Oxygenated Neurons

This still left one puzzle. Just as much Ca^{2+} is taken up during normoxic SD as during HSD, yet function returns to normal even after many bouts of SD (Herreras and Somjen, 1993a; Nedergaard and Hansen, 1988). The answer seems to lie, at least in large part, in the *duration of the calcium overload*. The depolarizing phase of typical normoxic SD is over in about 1 min. When, however, cells are forced to remain depolarized by the continued elevation of $[K^+]_o$ for an extended period of time, recovery is jeopardized and eventually fails altogether, even if abundant oxygen was available during the whole time. As with HSD, the damage caused by prolonged K^+-induced normoxic depolarization can be prevented by depleting Ca^{2+} before raising $[K^+]_o$ (Fig. 19–4) (Jing et al., 1991; Kawasaki et al., 1988).

But the evidence, though strong, could still be considered circumstantial. It might be hard to believe that an innocuous and ubiquitous element such as calcium could do so much harm. To test this point, Jones et al. (1986) iontophoresed Ca^{2+} into some *Aplysia* neurons and Mg^{2+} into others. The cells receiving Ca^{2+} depolarized and disintegrated; those that received Mg^{2+} did not. More recently, Gwag et al. (1999) exposed cultured cortical neurons to calcium ionophores in the presence of normal Ca^{2+} in the medium. The ionophore made the plasma membrane permeable to calcium and raised $[Ca^{2+}]_i$. With a low ionophore concentration the neurons underwent *apoptosis*; with a higher concentration, *necrosis* (Figs. 19–8, 19–9) (see below: "Apoptosis and necrosis"). Thus is calcium judged guilty as charged.

Comparing spreading depression and hypoxic spreading depression–like depolarization

Differences between SD and HSD have been emphasized from time to time (Bureš et al., 1974; Scheller et al., 1992a; Tegtmeier, 1993). No doubt the total syndromes of cerebral hypoxia and ischemia include changes that are absent in uncomplicated normoxic SD. Depolarization in SD is self-limiting, but V_m and excitability recover

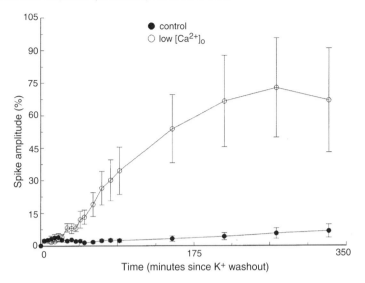

FIGURE 19–4. Prolonged high potassium-induced depolarization causes calcium-dependent neuron injury. Pairs of rat hippocampal tissue slices were irrigated by elevated K+ solution (130 mM K+ replacing Na+) for 40 min in both wells of a double tissue slice chamber. In one chamber the bath calcium was reduced from 1.2 mM to 0.12 30 min before the high K+ treatment, and the $[Ca^{2+}]$ and $[K^+]$ were restored to normal at the same time. Orthodromic population spikes were recorded in the CA1 region. The graph shows mean ±S.E.M. for five pairs of slices. Synaptic transmission recovered only in the slices that were Ca^{2+} deprived during high K+ exposure. (From Jing et al., 1991.)

from HSD only if oxygen is restored soon after the onset of depolarization. Oxidative energy is required for the restoration of ion gradients (Hansen and Lauritzen, 1984; Lipton, 1999). As we have already seen, during normoxic SD mitochondria produce an oxidation response, but in hypoxic brain tissue mitochondrial enzymes become reduced (Fig. 13–7 and Chapter 15: "Neurons are not short of oxygen . . .") (Rosenthal and Somjen, 1973; Rosenthal et al., 1976). It has also been pointed out that cells release inorganic phosphate during HSD but not during SD (Scheller et al., 1992a, 1996). This is the result of the shortfall in oxidative energy and the consequent breakdown of high-energy phosphates (Nioka et al., 1990; Scheller et al., 1996). Tissue becomes acidotic in the course of both SD and HSD, but during hypoxia pH begins to fall well before the onset of the SD-like depolarization due to the accumulation of lactic acid, produced in anaerobic glycolysis (Hansen and Lauritzen, 1984; Hanwehr et al., 1986; Siesjö et al., 1990), while during normoxic SD the acid shift evolves slowly, following the initial transient alkaline shift (Figs. 13–6, 19–10). It is important to remember that, similarly to normoxic SD, during hypoxia the onset of the SD-like depolarization is marked by a sharp, transient alkaline shift superimposed on the already acidotic baseline (Fig. 19–10A) (Hansen and Lauritzen, 1984; Kraig et al., 1983; Tombaugh, 1994).

Experimental withdrawal from brain slices of both oxygen and glucose has sometimes been called *oxygen-glucose deprivation* (*OGD*) and sometimes *ischemia in vitro*. With this treatment HSD starts earlier than during hypoxia with normal glucose, and the depolarization can become almost immediately irreversible (terminal), especially if the tissue slice is submerged under flowing bath fluid (Rader and Lanthorn, 1989; Tanaka et al., 1997). There are two reasons why OGD of submerged slices is more lethal than uncomplicated hypoxia of interface slices. First, glucose diffuses slowly, and after it has been first depleted and then returned to the bath, it takes a while before it again becomes available to the cells. Besides, even at high P_{O_2}, aqueous media contain little dissolved oxygen, and therefore the tissue oxygen level is restored slowly. Unlike submerged slices, slices maintained at the gas–liquid interface can be rapidly flooded with abundant oxygen after the termination of a period of hypoxia, favoring recovery. In intact brain, the distance for diffusion from capillaries to cells in much shorter than it is in brain slices in vitro, and the limit of revivability after experimental transient ischemia is longer for brain in situ than for submerged brain slices subjected to OGD.

Another difference between normoxic SD and HSD is the timing of synaptic failure. Synapses fail to transmit minutes before the onset of HSD, whereas in normoxic SD synapses continue to function until depolarization inactivates ion channels. Both presynaptic and postsynaptic malfunction contribute to the early synaptic block during hypoxia, and these have nothing to do with the HSD that follows later (Chapter 18).

Finally, there is a difference in the pharmacology of the two conditions. N-methyl-D-aspartate antagonist drugs are more effective against SD than against HSD, while TTX postpones HSD more powerfully than SD (Aitken et al., 1988; Lauritzen et al., 1993; Scheller et al., 1993; Tegtmeier, 1993).

Every one of these differences concerns events that precede or lead up to the depolarization, but none speaks to the biophysical mechanism of the depolarization itself. In this respect the similarities are overwhelming. The waveform of the ΔV_o is essentially identical in SD and HSD, provided that oxygenation is restored shortly after the onset of HSD (reviewed in Somjen, 2001). Holding current and input resistance change in identical fashion in patch-clamped neurons during SD and HSD (Figs. 14–1 and 19–2). So do the IOSs that accompany the voltage shift (Figs. 13–3, 13–4, 19–5, 19–6) (Aitken et al., 1998b; Bahar et al., 2000). Both the ΔV_o and the IOS propagate at similar velocities in the tissue during SD and HSD (Aitken et al., 1998b; Andrew et al., 2000). Ion concentrations change in identical fashion (Hansen and Zeuthen, 1981). The interstitial space shrinks to the same degree (Jing et al., 1994). The reduction in membrane potential and input resistance of neurons and glial cells are indistinguishable in the two processes (Czéh et al., 1993).

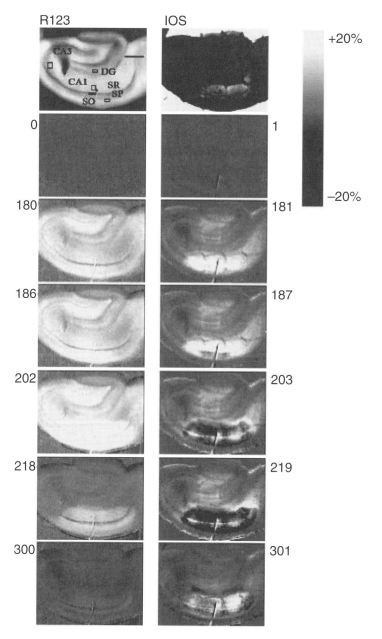

FIGURE 19–5. Mitochondrial depolarization and light scattering increase associated with hypoxic spreading depression–like depolarization. Images of rhodamine-123 (R123) fluorescence and transmitted light intensity (intrinsic optical signal, IOS) of a rat hippocampal slice. Conditions are similar to those in Figure 13–3. The top two frames are unsubtracted; the others show difference images. Areas of interest used for intensity plots of Figure 19–6 are defined in the top left image. The numbers next to the frames show times in seconds after oxygen withdrawal; oxygen was restored after 210 s. (From Bahar et al., 2000.)

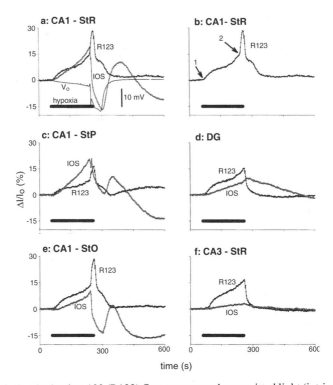

FIGURE 19–6. Rhodamine-123 (R123) fluorescence and transmitted light (intrinsic optical signal [IOS]) intensity changes in different hippocampal regions caused by hypoxia. Data from the same trial as Figure 19–5. The intensity scales show changes as a percentage of control ($\Delta I/I_o$ %). **a:** R123 fluorescence, IOS, and extracellular potential (V_o) in stratum radiatum of the CA1 region. Early during hypoxia, mitochondria start to depolarize (R123 fluorescence increase), cells swell (IOS increase indicating light-scattering decrease), and V_o shifts in negatively. Later during hypoxia V_o turns abruptly negative, signaling the onset of hypoxic spreading depression–like depolarization (HSD). Coincident with HSD, R123 fluorescence shoots up and the IOS suddenly decreases (light scattering increases). R123 begins to recover before IOS and V_o. **b:** The R123 trace of part a is repeated. The arrows show the onset of the two main phases of R123 fluorescence increase, where rates of change have been calculated (see Bahar et al., 2000). **c:** Light signals from CA1 stratum (st.) pyramidale. **d:** Same from dentate gyrus. **e:** Same from CA1 st. oriens. **f:** Same from CA3 st. radiatum. Note that spreading depression–related R123 and IOS responses occur only in CA1 and are much milder in st. pyramidale than in the two dendritic layers (radiatum and oriens). Dentate gyrus and CA3 apparently did not undergo HSD. In CA1, HSD is related to selective vulnerability of CA1 neurons. (Modified from Bahar et al., 2000.)

What ignites hypoxic spreading depression–like depolarization?

Glutamate Is Released by Both Calcium-Dependent
and Calcium-Independent Processes

Glutamate and aspartate overflow into ISF during hypoxia and ischemia (Fig. 19–7) (Benveniste et al., 1984; Mitani et al., 1992; Torp et al., 1993). It is a fair guess that such a surge of glutamate might initiate HSD. The excess is discharged by both calcium-dependent and calcium-independent processes (Drejer et al., 1985). Calcium-dependent release probably comes from synaptic terminals, while glial cells were initially suspected to be the source that does not require calcium (Drejer et al., 1985; Kimelberg et al., 1990; Szatkowski et al., 1990). Gebhardt et al. (2002) suggest that glutamate is released from hypoxic presynaptic terminals by both a vesicular (normal) and a nonvesicular (pathological) process, while glial cells take it up and do not release it. They compared the onset of HSD in brain slices prepared from mice made deficient in neuronal **glutamate membrane transporter excitatory amino acid carrier 1** (**EAAC1**) with normal wild-type controls. The onset of HSD was greatly delayed in the slices from the mutant mice but not abolished. By contrast, the glial uptake inhibitor DL-threo-β-benzyloxyaspartate (TBOA) dramatically shortened the latent period before HSD onset. Gebhardt et al. (2002) concluded that in depolarized terminals the EAAC1

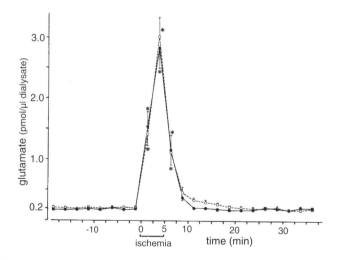

FIGURE 19–7. Dramatic but transient increase in glutamate overflow during ischemia of gerbil hippocampus. Glutamate levels were assayed in microdialysate. Five minutes of global cerebral ischemia was caused by clamping both carotid arteries. In gerbils but not in rats, carotid obstruction interrupts almost all blood flow to the cerebral hemispheres. Filled circles show data from CA1, open circles from CA3. Points are mean ±S.E.M. (From Mitani et al., 1992.)

transporter works in the reverse direction, mediating nonvesicular release. This nonvesicular component was absent in the knockout mice. Since inhibiting the glial glutamate transporter hastened HSD onset, Gebhardt et al. (2002) suggested that glial cells normally continue to remove glutamate from the synaptic cleft even during hypoxia, at least right up to the onset of HSD. This is at variance with the suggestion that glutamate is released from astrocytes by a reversal of glutamate transport (Szatkowski et al., 1990). In their latest contribution, Attwells' group report that knocking out the glial glutamate transporter, GLT-1, had no effect on the membrane current associated with HSD and is therefore presumably of minor importance in ischemia (Hamann et al., 2002), a conclusion in agreement with that of Gebhardt et al. (2002).

Release of glutamate in the selectively vulnerable CA1 region is not different from that in the less sensitive CA3 area (Fig. 19–7) (Mitani et al., 1992). It is the defense of the target neuron—or the lack of it—that determines selective vulnerability, not the attack by the excitotoxin.

Glutamate Receptor–Controlled and Voltage-Gated Currents Cooperate in Generating Hypoxic Spreading Depression–Like Depolarization

Selective blockade of NMDA receptors has little effect on HSD (Aitken et al., 1988; Kral et al., 1993; Marrannes et al., 1988a), but blocking all three ionotropic glutamate receptors postpones it (Müller and Somjen, 2000b). Yet, even though it starts later, once it is ignited, HSD runs its full course even if glutamate receptors are fully suppressed. Inhibition of voltage-gated Na^+ channels with TTX also delays the onset of HSD but, even in the presence of both TTX and glutamate antagonists, HSD occurred in about half of the hypoxic trials. Only when Ni^{2+} was added to the cocktail could HSD be reliably prevented (Müller and Somjen, 1998) (see Chapter 12: "Not one spreading depression channel . . ."). Rossi et al. (2000) recorded the HSD-related huge neuronal membrane current in patch-clamped neurons and found that they could prevent this current when glutamate receptors were blocked. In their trials, however, the patch pipettes contained Cs^+ and the local anesthetic drug QX-314, effectively suppressing voltage-dependent currents.

We are led to the same conclusion that we have already reached concerning the mechanism of normoxic SD (Chapter 15: "Not one spreading depression channel . . ."). Several slowly inactivating dendritic inward currents cooperate in initiating and generating HSD. Before the onset of HSD, $[K^+]_o$ in hypoxic brain tissue starts to increase slowly, $[Ca^{2+}]_o$ decreases slightly, and neurons briefly hyperpolarize and then start to depolarize slowly and gradually. The most likely reason for the early, mild depolarization and mild, gradual ion shifts is the slowing of the ATP-dependent ion transport by both the 3Na/2K ion pump and the calcium pump. Whether the pumps slow down because ATP is in short supply, or whether they are inhibited by "sensing" low P_{O_2} or by some other chemical signal, is not clear. For the moderate ion shifts seen at this stage, ion pumps need not be arrested, only somewhat inhibited. Eventually these ion shifts and the resulting depolarization reach a critical stage, and then set into motion the self-reinforcing processes that lead to HSD. Entry of Ca^{2+} into presynaptic terminals causes the release of glutamate (and other excitatory transmitters). Whether or not glutamate is also released from astrocytes is uncertain (see above). Elevated $[K^+]_o$ also depolarizes neuron dendrites, activating voltage-dependent calcium and sodium channels. Persistent Na^+ current $I_{Na,P}$ is potentiated by both high $[K^+]_o$ and low P_{O_2} (Hammarström and Gage, 2000; Somjen and Müller, 2000). Reduced $[Ca^{2+}]_o$ activates the calcium-sensitive nonspecific cation current (Xiong and MacDonald, 1997). When the sum of the inward currents through all these dendritic channels exceeds the opposing outward currents, HSD is ignited (Chapter 16). When any one of these channels is blocked, HSD is delayed, but only blockade of all channels can reliably prevent it.

Computer simulation of hypoxic arrest of ion pump function supports this scenario (Kager et al., 2002a).

Zinc: The guardian of neurons or the new villain?

Millions of persons take zinc in dietary supplements. It is universally accepted as an essential trace metal, indispensable for good health. There is about 15 μM of zinc in normal human blood plasma, most of it bound to protein and complexed to small molecule ligands. Only between 10^{-9} and 10^{-10} M exists as the free ion (Takeda, 2001). Thus $[Zn^{2+}]_{plasma}$ is at least two orders of magnitude less than the concentration in protons (pZn $\geq$ 9 compared to pH 7.4), but not all the bonds that hold zinc are tight. The fractions bound to albumin and to small molecules, even though not active, is *exchangeable*, that is, available as needed. The concentration in CSF is about 0.15 μM, which is lower than the total plasma concentration but much higher than the free ion concentration in plasma, suggesting active transport across the BBB (Davson and Segal, 1996; Takeda, 2001). The estimated average concentration in brain cells is 150 μM but, again, only a small fraction is present in cytosol as the free ion, most of it being bound as metalloprotein. Zinc is, however, also present in synaptic vesicles of some nerve terminals, where the level is said to be as high as 350 μM, much or all of it probably as the free ion. More Zn^{2+} has been found in the mossy fibers of dentate gyrus granule cells than anywhere else, but zinc-containing synaptic vesicles are also present in the amygdala and neocortex. The Zn^{2+} is packaged together with the glutamate of glutamatergic nerve endings, but not all glutamate fibers contain Zn^{2+}. When a zinc-containing synapse transmits a signal and the vesicles are emptied, free Zn^{2+} is released together with glutamate. Once released, glutamate and Zn^{2+} part company, each being bound at different receptor sites. While glutamate activates its ligand-operated channels, Zn^{2+} can modulate the NMDA receptor channel (Molnár and Nadler, 2001; Vogt et al., 2000), enhance AMPA receptor–mediated current (Lin et al., 2001), or dampen glutamate transmission and reduce seizure activity (reviewed by (Frederickson and Bush, 2001). After glutamate does its job, it is removed for the most part by perisynaptic glial cells (Billups et al., 1998; Hansson et al., 2000). Of the synaptically released Zn^{2+}, some is taken back by the presynaptic nerve ending that released it, but about half is admitted into the target cell, where presumably it then performs useful functions that are yet to be completely defined (Frederickson and Bush, 2001; Frederickson et al., 2000).

Among its functions, zinc is said to regulate apoptosis (Truong-Tran et al., 2001), reduce oxidative stress, and scavenge free radicals (Takeda, 2001). Accordingly, elevation of free Zn^{2+} saves neurons from untimely death. On the other hand, we are also told that under pathological conditions, an excess of zinc delivered to the wrong address can cause havoc (Weiss et al., 2000). In cell cultures, elevating the $[Zn^{2+}]_o$ level caused death of neurons (Kim et al., 1998) and enhanced the lethality of excitotoxic or hypoxic neuron injury. Conversely, if Zn^{2+} was removed by chelating compounds, neurons were spared from damage (Aizenman et al., 2000). Moreover, zinc accumulates in excitotoxically injured cells in CNS regions where normally no intracellular zinc is found (reviewed by Frederickson and Bush, 2001). Ports of entry for Zn^{2+}, beside specific zinc transporters, include the same voltage-gated and ligand operated ion channels that admit Ca^{2+} (Colvin et al., 2000).

The Jekyll-and-Hyde character of Zn^{2+} is, of course, not unique. Ca^{2+} also serves as a normal cell signal but, in excess, it can also initiate lethal processes. It has also been suggested that a moderate increase of neuron $[Ca^{2+}]_i$, similarly to $[Zn^{2+}]_i$, modulates apoptosis and protects neurons (Yu et al., 2001). Pathological depolarization opens ion channels that admit both Ca^{2+} and Zn^{2+} in abnormally large amounts. Which of the two is more of a menace in real clinical conditions may vary according to the specific circumstances. In either case, preventing HSD or interdicting divalent cation entry could mitigate acute hypoxic/ischemic neuron injury.

Apoptosis and necrosis: Two paths leading to the demise of neurons

Cells are shed on purpose in organisms in good health, or they can succumb to disease or injury. The two routes to cell death, apoptosis and necrosis, can be visualized conceptually as running in parallel and converging toward the same endpoint. Siesjö and collaborators (1999) called this dual-lane, one-way road the *cell death pathway*. Both paths can be triggered by excess $[Ca^{2+}]_i$ (Figs. 19–8, 19–9).

Apoptosis is also called *programmed* or *controlled* or *gene-directed cell death* to distinguish it from the accidental nature of cell necrosis. In good health, apoptosis

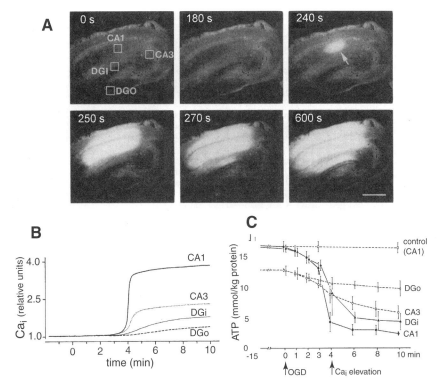

FIGURE 19–8. Intracellular calcium and adenosine triphosphate (ATP) levels during oxygen-glucose deprivation (OGD). Gerbil hippocampal tissue slices. For $[Ca^{2+}]_i$ determination slices were loaded with the fluorescent indicator dye rhod-2. For ATP determination, slices were rapidly frozen at various times before, during, and after OGD. **A:** Rhod-2 images at increasing times after OGD. The regions of interest for the plots in B are shown in the first frame. DGi and DGo are the inner and outer leaves of the dentate gyrus. Fluorescence increase starts in CA1 stratum (st.) radiatum, then spreads over CA1 but (relatively) spares the st. pyramidale. **B:** Time course of the increase in $[Ca^{2+}]_i$ from the regions of interest in images of A. **C:** Adenosine triphosphate levels in various regions of groups of slices. Zero time shows OGD onset. The second arrow marks the time of the abrupt $[Ca^{2+}]_i$ increase, presumably caused by hypoxic spreading depression–like depolarization (HSD). Adenosine triphosphate levels begin to decrease before HSD but dive steeply with HSD onset. Data show mean ±S.D. (Modified from Mitani et al., 1994.)

is a normal method of eliminating superfluous tissue. It occurs on a spectacular scale during metamorphosis, for example when tadpoles discard the tail as they become frogs, but it is also essential in shaping mammalian organs during development. Inappropriate apoptosis is, however, pathological. Too little fosters tumor growth; too much destroys cells that are needed. Physiological apoptosis is governed by gene products. The pathological varieties can be caused by pathological genes or they are initiated by some noxious agent. In neuropathology, apoptosis

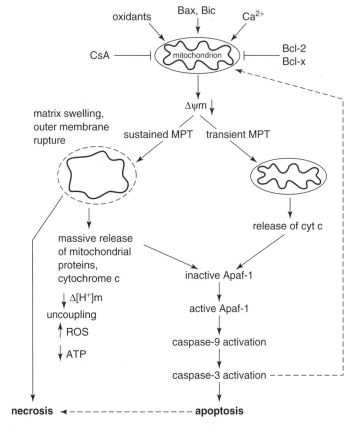

FIGURE 19–9. Injury to mitochondria commits cells to eventual death. Pathways to necrosis and apoptosis. Mitochondria may be injured by oxidants, shortage of oxygen or of fuel, the pro-apoptotic factors Bax and Bic, or a greatly elevated $[Ca^{2+}]_i$ level (primarily in cytosol, secondarily in the mitochondria). The anti-apoptotic factors Bcl-2 and Bcl-x$_l$ have a natural protective function; the drug cyclosporin-A (CsA) can prevent the opening of mitochondrial permeability transition (MPT) pores. Injury of the mitochondria depolarizes the inner membrane (diminished $\Delta\psi$). Low $\Delta\psi_m$ initiates MPT, which makes the mitochondrial membrane indiscriminately permeable. If MPT is sustained, the mitochondria swell, the outer membrane ruptures, and mitochondrial contents are released. With the collapse of the proton gradient ($\Delta[H^+]_m$), oxidative metabolism is uncoupled, reactive oxygen species (ROS) are produced, and adenosine triphosphate (ATP) production stops. The result is necrosis. If MPT is short-lived, a smaller amount of cytochrome c is released, which activates the cytoplasmic protein Apaf-1, which activates caspase-9, which activates caspase-3, which feeds back to further impair mitochondrial function, and the cycle leads to apoptosis. The end stage of apoptosis is indistinguishable from that of necrosis. (Modified from Siesjö et al., 1999.)

is blamed for cell loss in a number of progressive diseases, including Alzheimer's, Parkinson's and Huntington's diseases. It is also one of the paths, though not the only one, leading to the demise of neurons in excitotoxic insults and in the slow and delayed forms of hypoxic/ischemic neuron death.

John Kerr, a foremost pioneer of apoptosis research, recounts in a short memoir (Kerr, 1999) that the term *apoptosis* was suggested to him by James Cormack, professor of Greek at the University of Aberdeen. The word, a composite of *apo* and *ptosis*, means "shedding of tree leaves in the fall" in classical Greek.

Before it has been named apoptosis, Kerr (1999) called the process **shrinkage necrosis** to distinguish it from the then better-known form of necrotic cell death that begins with cell swelling. Besides the compacting of cell volume and the condensation of intracellular organelles, its diagnostic signs include a characteristic fragmentation of DNA that creates a "ladder" pattern; staining of DNA in the nucleus by a procedure dubbed terminal deoxynucleotidyltransferase-mediated nick-end labeling (*TUNEL*); and activation of a group of proteolytic enzymes called *caspases*. The hallmarks of normal and pathological apoptosis are the same, as if certain noxae could switch on the program at times when it is not at all desirable. The supposed uniformity of apoptosis in so many different normal as well as pathological processes is not universally accepted. Sloviter (2002) argued that it is a "created concept and not a real entity," and he preferred to abolish the term. It may be too late for that.

In spite of the overwhelming amount of research output of the past decade or two, not all the details have been clarified. There is, however, agreement about the broad outlines of the process, illustrated in Figure 19–9. Apoptosis can be induced in a variety of cell cultures by a variety of interventions, but it is not completely clear which of these models realistically represents which situations encountered by living organisms. The main features that are common to all models are as follows. An (unspecified) insult causes a change in the plasma membrane, permitting the influx of calcium or zinc and the efflux of potassium plus chloride. **Apoptotic volume decrease (AVD)** is perhaps a perverted form of *regulatory volume decrease (RVD)*, and it occurs early in the process (Maeno et al., 2000; Yu and Choi, 2000). The changed ion composition inside the cell then triggers a change in the mitochondrial membrane, the **mitochondrial permeability transition (MPT)**, causing the release of **cytochrome 3** and other compounds from the mitochondria into the cytoplasm, which then activate a cytoplasmic protein, **Apaf-1**, which in turn activates various **caspases**, which then mediate the eventual dissolution of the cell structure (Fig 19–9) (Siesjö et al., 1999). **Cyclosporin A (CsA)**, which inhibits the mitochondrial permeability transition, also improves the survival of neurons after transient cerebral ischemia (Li et al., 2000a). Beneath this relatively simple story there is a dizzying array of subplots, which fall outside the scope of this book. For detailed reviews, see Kumar (1999), Lipton (1999), Ravagnan et al. (2002), Siesjö et al. (1999), and Yu et al. (2001).

Necrosis (from *necroun*, Greek, "to kill") formerly meant all forms of cell or tissue death in a live organism, but since the separate identification of apoptosis, it has come to mean cell death by means other than apoptosis. Unlike apoptosis, necrosis never is a normal process. Like apoptosis, it can (but need not) be initiated by elevated $[Ca^{2+}]_i$. When localized ischemia kills all cells in a contiguous but restricted volume of tissue, it is called an *infarct*. Cell necrosis can be caused by a wide variety of pathologies, including infectious agents and poisons, in addition to energy shortfall. High $[Ca^{2+}]_i$ initiates neuron necrosis after hypoxia of ischemia, or during excitotoxicity, by the excessive and persistent activation of proteolytic and lipolytic enzymes. Calcium-induced destructive processes have been studied in great detail by Siesjö and associates (Deshpande et al., 1987; Kristián and Siesjö, 1998; Siesjö, 1993).

The necrotic version of acute, irreversible hypoxic neuron injury is morphologically quite different from the apoptotic form. While apoptosis begins with cell shrinkage, ordinary acute hypoxic cell change begins with cell swelling. Electron microscopy reveals swelling of mitochondria and the appearance of cytoplasmic vacuoles. The plasma membrane disintegrates during necrosis much earlier than in apoptosis. On stained sections chromatin appears to dissolve. In the final stage, neurons become compact and are then eaten by phagocytes (Duchen, 1992a; Graham, 1992; Lipton, 1999).

Generally, apoptosis takes longer than necrosis, and it would be easy to suggest that the acute hypoxic injury is the result of necrosis, while the delayed injurious process is mediated by apoptosis. Indeed, several investigators reported that a mild insult leads to slow apoptosis and more severe injury to more rapid necrosis (Gwag et al., 1999; Nicotera et al., 1999; Walton et al., 1999). When cortical cell cultures were deprived of oxygen and glucose for 45–55 min, neurons died by a necrotic process, imitating the acute slow process. When such cultures were protected by blocking glutamate receptors and then deprived for 90–100 min, an apoptotic process killed neurons over the following 24–48 hr (Gwag et al., 1995). The trouble is that most of these model experiments concerned cell cultures. In whole brains that have undergone focal or global ischemia, the findings are less clear-cut. In gerbils subjected to transient global cerebral ischemia, Colbourne et al. (1999) found only necrotic neurons, no matter how hard they tried to create conditions that favor apoptosis. Yet signs of apoptosis were evident in some studies of delayed neuron death after transient global cerebral ischemia of rats (Ouyang et al., 1999; Siesjö et al., 1999), but again, in others, the signs of DNA fragmentation were seen only after cell death (Petito et al., 1997). In mutant mice lacking the pro-apoptotic protein BID, following transient focal ischemia cytochrome release was partially inhibited and the infarct was smaller than that in control animals (Plesnila et al., 2001). It seems that apoptosis, necrosis, or a mixture of both can occur after either mild or severe bouts of ischemia. Petito et al. (1997) argue for the importance of mixed forms, defined as *type II programmed cell death*.

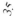

It will take more work to define precisely the conditions that decid'
by which cells die during and after cerebral hypoxia and ischem'
et al., 2001).

Two mechanisms cause the acute swelling of energy-starved neurons

Uptake of Ions Exceeds Their Release During Excitation and Spreading Depression

Excited neurons swell. This was first demonstrated unequivocally by Dietzel et al.
(1980; Dietzel and Heinemann, 1986). They used the method invented by
Nicholson et al. (1979) to measure changes in the size of the interstitial space by
the indicator dilution method, using the membrane-impermeant cations TMA^+ and
choline. During intense, repeated electrical stimulation and during seizure activity the interstitial volume fraction shrank, usually by 10%–20% of its resting size,
sometimes by more. Keep in mind that electrical stimulation resembles seizures
more than it does normal neuronal activity. The interstitium was evidently squeezed
by the increase of cell volume. Both neurons and glial cells can swell, but in neurons swelling occurs mainly in the dendritic tree (Aitken et al., 1998a). Neurons
swell because they gain more Na^+ than they lose K^+ as they fire, and the excess
Na^+ is presumably accompanied by Cl^- and to a lesser degree by HCO_3^- and other
anions, with osmotically driven water following the ions. Glial cells take up K^+
with Cl^- in response to rising $[K^+]_o$ by two routes, actively because their Na/K
exchange pump is stimulated and passively by the Boyle-Conway mechanism
(Chapter 2: "Net uptake of K^+") (Boyle and Conway, 1941).

Excitation, even during seizures, causes moderate swelling of neurons, but
during SD and HSD the interstitium collapses to a bare 4% of the total tissue volume (Jing et al., 1994). This is the same ISVF size found on electron micrographs
of conventionally fixed specimens; in other words, it corresponds in magnitude
to the maximal swelling of dying brain cells (see Chapter 1: "The discovery of
the blood–brain barrier" and Van Harreveld and Schadé, 1959). It is therefore likely
that the rapid swelling of neurons destined for hypoxic acute necrosis is related to
HSD. But the swelling happens before reaching the "point of commitment," and
rapid reoxygenation can still save the cells, followed by undershooting (posthypoxic shrinkage) of the cell volume.

Gibbs-Donnan Forces Take Over When Active Transport Stops

Even in the absence of HSD, neuronal as well as nonneuronal cells *swell if they
run short of metabolic energy*, albeit more slowly than during HSD. In these cases
the cells gain water driven by Gibbs-Donnan forces (see Chapter 3: "Volume regu-

ıation of cells . . ."). The cytoplasm of all cells contains *membrane-impermeant anions*, besides permeant cations (mainly K^+) and a smaller amount of permeant anions (mainly Cl^- and HCO_3^-). The bulk of the ions in the ECF (Na^+, Cl^-, HCO_3^-, and a few others) can penetrate cell membranes to varying degrees. As shown both theoretically and experimentally, in nonliving system, such a distribution of ions forces excess ions and water from the outside to the inside. Equilibrium is obtained only if elevated hydrostatic pressure "inside," that is, on the side of the impermeant anions, prevents further inward movement. This pressure is, by definition, the osmotic pressure (Chapter 3). In normal living cells, however, there is little if any pressure difference between cytosol and ECF. Maintaining equal pressures is possible only because of the steady work of ion pumps that remove excess osmotically active ions almost as rapidly as they enter the cell. This is mainly the work of the ATP-fueled sodium pump, which extrudes 3 Na^+ ions in exchange for 2 K^+. If, however, oxygen or glucose is insufficient, the pumps falter. The ions drawn into the cell by the Gibbs-Donnan force are no longer removed fast enough, and the excess causes the cell to swell.

Following swelling, RVD (Chapter 3: "Osmotic volume changes . . .") can sometimes achieve partial recovery of the cell volume. Eventually, when the necrotic process is more advanced, the integrity of the cytoskeleton and of the cell membrane is destroyed and the membrane becomes permeable to the larger, originally impermeant anions and osmotic and electrochemical gradients dissipate. As its contents are shed, the cell shrinks before final disintegration and removal by phagocytosis.

Hypotonic Swelling Is Relatively Well Tolerated by Otherwise Healthy and Well-Nourished Central Nervous System Neurons

Based on experiments with neuron cultures, it once seemed that excitotoxic and hypoxic neuron injury were caused by the swelling of the cells. It was assumed that the stretched membrane was rendered incontinent for ions and that this was the primary initiator of the necrotic process (Rothman, 1985). But cell swelling in the presence of sufficient oxygen and glucose is not a cause of irreversible neuron injury. When brain tissue slices are exposed to hypotonic bathing solution, excitatory synaptic transmission is greatly enhanced (Chapter 4: "Sodium, chloride and osmotic effects . . .") (Chebabo et al., 1995a; Huang et al., 1997; Rosen and Andrew, 1990). In severely hypotonic solution, recurrent spontaneous SD episodes can occur (Chebabo et al., 1995a). When bath osmolarity is restored, the synapses first undergo rebound depression, but eventually, normal function recovers. Only if the osmolarity of the medium is kept very low for a very long time does the tissue suffer irreversible injury (Huang et al., 1995). At least in hippocampus, the swelling alone cannot be blamed for hypoxic loss of function. Conversely, in cultured neurons, preventing cell swelling does not protect against irreversible injury caused by simulated ischemia (Goldberg and Choi, 1993). Still, while hypotonic cell swelling is relatively harmless for cells in normal energy status, it does worsen the outlook for recovery after hypoxia (Payne et al., 1996).

Is excitotoxicity causing the slow death of neurons?

Less than 10 min of oxygen deprivation and even shorter combined OGD is enough to kill the most vulnerable neurons in mature brains. Such rapid injury is related to HSD. In the brains of newborns and in cell cultures, the limit of revivability is much longer for the same types of neurons. Even in the adult, many neurons survive much longer periods of anoxia, especially in the brain stem and spinal cord. The resistance of immature neurons, and of those in the gray matter in the lower brain stem and spinal cord, may be explained in part by the fact that they do not undergo HSD (Hansen, 1977). Immunity to HSD is not the whole explanation, however, because single neurons dissociated from the CA1 region of immature brains also tolerate energy shortage better than similarly isolated cells from adult animals, even though HSD does not occur under these experimental conditions (Cummins et al., 1991; Friedman and Haddad, 1993). The slower death of the (relatively) resistant neurons may also be caused by the slower buildup of $[Ca^{2+}]_i$ in the resistant cells compared to the vulnerable cells. Much has been written about the role of *excitotoxicity* in causing hypoxic and ischemic injury. Central to these discussions was the role of the NMDA receptor channel in admitting Ca^{2+} during energy shortage.

Seminal papers by Lucas and Newhouse (1957) and Olney (1969) called attention to the toxicity of monosodium glutamate. Olney's paper appeared not long after glutamate has been recognized as an excitatory synaptic transmitter (Eccles, 1964). Not much later, Van Harreveld and Fifková (1970) discovered the release of glutamate from retinal tissue during SD. The next development was Sloviter's demonstration of cell injury caused by intense electrical stimulation (Olney et al., 1983; Sloviter and Damiano, 1981). Benveniste and colleagues (1984, 1989; Drejer et al., 1985) then collected excess glutamate in microdialysate from ischemic brains and linked the excessive overflow to neuron injury. Supporting the concept of excitotoxicity, glutamate or aspartate added to the bathing medium irreversibly injures neurons in cell cultures or brain tissue slices (Choi and Rothman, 1990). Other transmitters can also become harmful in excess. For example, in regions rich in dopamine, it too is released during ischemia and could mediate cell injury (Baker et al., 1991; Sarna et al., 1990).

The toxicity of glutamate and aspartate has been attributed specifically to the excessive activation of NMDA receptors (Rothman and Olney, 1987), but activation of AMPA and kainate receptors can also cause harm (Carriedo et al., 1998;

Diemer et al., 1990; McDonald et al., 1998). The greater toxic potential of NMDA receptors is attributed to the calcium permeability of the channel. Ischemia might make AMPA receptors permeable to calcium (Pellegrini-Giampietro et al., 1992), but even if the non-NMDA receptor–operated channels themselves reject Ca^{2+}, persistent and profound depolarization will open voltage-gated calcium channels and produce the same end result. We have already seen that blockade of NMDA receptors by the selective competitive antagonist APV, which does not block the other glutamate receptors, had little or no effect on HSD or on the accelerated neuron injury related to HSD (Aitken et al., 1988; Diemer et al., 1990). Against the more insidious slow neuron injury seen in cell cultures, blockade of NMDA receptors is apparently quite effective (Choi and Rothman, 1990; Marcoux et al., 1990; Rothman et al., 1987). Similar success was reported for hippocampal tissue slices, but only under conditions in which HSD was precluded even in the drug-free control slices. When slices are kept submerged under bath fluid at a slightly cool (34°C) temperature, and oxygen is withheld but glucose is available, no HSD occurs (Schiff and Somjen, 1987) and synaptic failure becomes irreversible only after 40 min. Under such conditions, NMDA antagonists augment the recovery of function following long periods of hypoxia (Clark and Rothman, 1987; Rothman et al., 1987; Zhu and Krnjević, 1999). However, after comparing interaction between the L-type calcium-channel antagonist diltiazem with APV and with dizocilpine maleate (MK-801), Schurr et al. (1995b) concluded that the success of MK-801 may be due, in part or in whole, to blockade of voltage-dependent calcium channels rather than NMDA receptors. From a different set of data on hippocampal slices, Brooks and Kaupinnen (1993) came to the conclusion that NMDA did not aggravate and NMDA antagonists did not ameliorate hypoxic injury, and that the damage was mediated by the opening of L-type voltage-gated calcium channels. In cerebral ischemia in experimental animals, protection by glutamate antagonist drugs was variable, depending on the specifics of the model (Block and Pulsinelli, 1988; Diemer et al., 1990; Nellgard et al., 1991; Simon et al., 1984), and in clinical trials on stroke, their efficacy was disappointing (DeGraba and Pettigrew, 2000; Dirnagl et al., 1999).

In parentheses we should recall that glutamate receptors are not the only receptors the excessive excitation of which can injure the very cells that have them. Pilocarpine acting on muscarinic receptors can also cause neuron injury (Chapter 6: "Pilocarpine"). This too could be called excitotoxicity, although it usually is not.

Besides glutamate and aspartate, GABA is also released into ISF during hypoxia. This could be considered a protective mechanism, as GABA-mediated inhibition counteracts the depolarization by excitatory amino acids. Indeed, in experimental models, GABA agonist drugs provided some protection against hypoxic neuron injury (reviewed by Schwartz-Bloom and Sah, 2001). On the other hand, if neurons become increasingly loaded with Cl⁻ due to failure of ion pump activity and the continued activation of GABA receptor channels plus other Cl⁻ transporters, the inhibition can gradually lose its power and the GABA-controlled conductance could eventually add to the damage.

In conclusion

Excitotoxicity is certainly not the only killer of hypoxic neurons. Its contribution to hypoxic/ischemic neuron injury varies in different models. It is least important in the rapid, HSD-augmented form of hypoxic injury and more so in the slow and delayed forms. When glutamate and aspartate do cause damage, they may do so through NMDA as well as non-NMDA receptor channels (see also the reviews by Haddad and Jiang, 1993; Lipton, 1999).

Sodium channels and hypoxic-ischemic neuron injury

The likely participation of voltage-gated Na^+ channels in the depolarization and the chain of events that kills neurons has led to testing of the effect of this ion and of channel-blocking drugs. Friedman and Haddad (1994) found that removing Na^+ from the bathing solution protected dissociated neurons against injury caused by anoxia. Tetrodotoxin postpones HSD (Müller and Somjen, 2000a), and in part for this reason, it also protects to some degree against hypoxic damage (Ames et al., 1995; Boening et al., 1989). Indiscriminately interdicting Na^+ channel function is, of course, not useful in clinical practice. More promisingly, Carter et al. (2000) tested a selective use- and depolarization-dependent channel blocker that appears to act by binding to the same site in the channel pore as local anesthetic drugs. This compound reportedly reduced infarct size after permanent local cerebral ischemia without impairing motor coordination of rats.

Reperfusion, delayed neuron injury, and the role of reactive oxygen species

Delayed neuron damage was first clearly defined in gerbils by Kirino (1982) and in rats by Pulsinelli et al. (1982a), based on histological examination of brain tissue at varying times following transient global cerebral ischemia. Immediately after such an ischemic episode, cells destined for delayed injury look intact. As we shall see shortly, the normal morphology is misleading; functional abnormality is detectable early. Signs of degeneration become obvious on electron micrographs of selectively vulnerable cell populations after 1 day, and the cells are dead after 4 days (Kirino and Sano, 1984). Even though rigorous testing would be almost impossible in human cases, careful postmortem examination of the brains of patients who died after varying intervals following transient cardiac arrest and resuscitation indicated that delayed neuron injury occurs in people as well (Petito et al., 1987).

Reperfusion Injury of Myocardium

Reports on *cardiac reperfusion injury* preceded those on delayed brain damage. There are similarities between the two processes. In hearts of experimental animals, much of the damage seems to take place in the moments after blood is allowed to flow through a previously ischemic myocardium (Opie, 1997; Shen and Jennings, 1972). Two factors received special attention in this context: calcium and reactive oxygen species. The previously ischemic heart muscle cells are defenseless when suddenly confronted by the Ca^{2+} in the returning blood, because voltage-gated channels are wide open and ion pumps are temporarily out of service. Moreover, with the membrane depolarized, the 3Na/Ca exchanger works in reverse mode, favoring Ca^{2+} influx, and calcium-activated calcium release becomes operative (Figs. 2–3, 2–4 and Chapter 2: "Intracellular calcium ion activity . . ."). Much of the Ca^{2+} flooding the cytoplasm is taken up by mitochondria, hindering oxidative metabolism even after oxygen is returned (for review see Carmeliet, 1999). Ca^{2+} also triggers the mitochondrial permeability transition, liberating cytochrome C and other apoptosis-activating factors (Fig. 19–9). Moreover, the mitochondria that have become incapacitated cannot detoxify the sudden surge of oxygen, resulting in the formation of large amounts of ***reactive oxygen species (ROS)*** (Fridovich, 1979). Reactive oxygen species include free radicals, H_2O_2, and nitric oxide (NO). Like Ca^{2+} and Zn^{2+}, NO has many useful functions in healthy tissue, but it can become a menace when produced in large, uncontrolled quantities. Many of the discussions of myocardial reperfusion injury are echoed in the proposed mechanisms of delayed neuron death.

Persistent Vascular Insufficiency (No reflow) Plays a Subsidiary Role

The first plausible explanation of delayed damage concerned inadequate reperfusion of previously ischemic areas: the *no-reflow* phenomenon (Ames et al., 1968; Hossman, 1983; LaManna et al., 1985; Liu et al., 2001). Ischemic damage to vessel walls can plug the vessel and hinder the return of local circulation. While poor blood flow may aggravate the process, it is not the only culprit. Tissue slices taken after transient ischemia and maintained in vitro also show signs of progressive deterioration of function (Jensen et al., 1991; Urbán et al., 1989).

Neither Postischemic Seizures nor Spreading Depression Explains
Delayed Neuron Injury

Since prolonged, continuous, or oft-repeated seizure activity can also cause neuron injury (Sloviter, 1983), and since patients sometimes suffer convulsions after cardiac arrest and resuscitation (Bladin and Norris, 1998; Rossen et al., 1943), it seemed logical to suppose that delayed neuron injury could be caused by postischemic seizures. Yet continuous monitoring of gerbils for 4 days after transient global cerebral ischemia revealed no sign of electrical seizures or behavioral convulsions, or for that matter SD-like events (Armstrong et al., 1989; Buzsáki et al., 1989). Instead, there was progressive depression of EEG wave amplitude in hippocampal CA1 and the striatum, beginning after 24 hr and reaching a minimum in 3 days. In the clinical study of Petito et al. (1987) mentioned above, in which postmortem brain pathology suggested delayed injury, those patients who had seizures after the initial stroke were excluded from the data.

Therefore, data from animal and human studies alike suggest that delayed injury can occur without seizures. This does not mean that if seizures do happen, they could not contribute to the damage.

Calcium Accumulates in Two Waves in the Mitochondria of Doomed Cells

Global cerebral ischemia induces HSD throughout the forebrain, and calcium enters in large quantities into neurons, where much of it is bound to calmodulin and absorbed into ER and mitochondria (Dux et al., 1987; Picone et al., 1989). If the ischemia is of short duration, the excess calcium is pumped out of the surviving neurons. Even the cells committed to delayed injury can at first clear their mitochondria of the excess during the first hour or two after the ischemic insult. But then, as the delayed degenerative process takes hold, beginning after about 6 hr, a second wave of calcium invades the damaged mitochondria (Dux et al., 1987).

Not Too Much Transmitter, but Upregulation of Receptors May Play a Role in Delayed Neuron Injury

Even though overt seizures have not been seen, excessive synaptic excitation has been suspected to be the main factor in delayed neuron loss. Early reports of increased spontaneous activity of hippocampal neurons in the days after transient ischemia (Chang et al., 1989; Suzuki et al., 1983b) were contradicted by others (Buzsáki et al., 1989; Imon et al., 1991). Increased spontaneous firing, if it occurred, could not have been due to overflow of glutamate or aspartate, for their level returns to normal soon after ischemia (Fig. 19–7) (Benveniste et al., 1984; Torp et al., 1993). More detailed examination of postischemic changes showed that excitatory synaptic potentials were enhanced but postsynaptic excitability was depressed. These changes were evident in hippocampal tissue slices taken from gerbils after an ischemic episode (Urbán et al., 1989) as well as in hippocampus in situ (Miyazaki et al., 1993; Xu and Pulsinelli, 1996). The raised threshold of firing explains the absence of detectable increased spontaneous activity, while the exaggerated synaptic current still allows for the possibility of excitotoxic damage, especially since the EPSP was enhanced mainly by upregulated NMDA-controlled current (Hori and Carpenter, 1994; Mittmann et al., 1998; Urbán et al., 1990b, 1990c).

In a remarkable study, Gao et al. (1998b, 1999) related the demise or survival of individual CA1 neurons to specific changes in their synaptic responses, revealed in intracellular recordings. Ischemia was induced in rats by a modification of the so-called four-vessel occlusion method of Pulsinelli and Brierley (1979). As an unusual refinement, the extracellular DC potential was recorded during ischemia, and the insult was standardized by maintaining HSD (called *ischemic depolarization* [*ID*], by the authors) for 14 min before the obstructed arteries were opened. Intracellular recordings were then made from CA1 pyramidal cells at varying intervals, up to 48 hr after the ischemic episode. In normal rats, stimulating the contralateral commissural pathway evoked an EPSP followed by a prolonged and profound hyperpolarizing IPSP. In many cells in postischemic animals the IPSP was replaced by a late, long depolarizing potential. Confirming Urban et al.'s (1990c) recordings in hippocampal slices, this late EPSP was found to be mediated by NMDA receptors. The first cells producing the late EPSP were found 4 hr after ischemia; the largest proportion, some 70% of the ones encountered, at around 19 hr; and a few were still present after 48 hr. A certain, more or less invariant, number of the cells produced EPSPs that were smaller than control responses but otherwise normal, and these were followed by IPSPs. At around 31 hours, cells appeared that produced only quite small EPSPs with no late component. MK-801, which is known to ameliorate delayed neuron injury (Miyazaki et al., 1993), also suppressed the late EPSP. For this and other reasons, the authors concluded that the cells producing late NMDA-operated EPSPs, as well as the ones with severely depressed EPSPs, were the ones committed to die, whereas the cells with relatively normal if somewhat subdued synaptic responses were the survivors. Gao et al. (1999) also confirmed the reduced excitability of CA1 pyramidal neurons reported by Urbán et al. (1989), which was most marked in the cells showing the late NMDA dependent EPSPs.

Besides enhanced excitation, decreased inhibition probably aggravates postischemic delayed neuron injury. This has two aspects. If neurons accumulate Cl^-, the driving force enabling $GABA_A$- or glycine receptor–controlled, Cl^--mediated IPSPs diminishes or, in the extreme case, it might even reverse, causing IPSPs to become excitatory. In addition, there is evidence for downregulation of $GABA_A$ receptors (reviewed by Schwartz-Bloom and Sah, 2001). The importance of reduced inhibition in delayed neuron injury is emphasized by the protection afforded by benzodiazepines administered after ischemic insult (Galeffi et al., 2000; Schwartz-Bloom et al., 2000). Benzodiazepines positively modulate $GABA_A$ receptor function.

In conclusion

These data make delayed neuron injury seem like an ultraslow, insidious form of excitotoxicity. Unlike the situation during acute hypoxic injury, there is no excess transmitter overflowing into the ISF during postischemic reperfusion. Instead, the postsynaptic receptors are overperforming. One might say that *it is not the broadcast signal, but the amplifier in the receiver that is turned to a damagingly high volume.* In agreement with this concept, glutamate antagonist drugs, specifically NMDA receptor–blocking drugs, appear to be more effective against delayed injury than they are against acute, rapid, HSD-dependent ischemic injury (Simon et al., 1984; Urbán et al., 1990c).

Adenosine-Mediated Depression of Excitatory Synapses Protects Some Neurons Against Delayed Postischemic Injury

In the hippocampal formation, CA3 pyramidal neurons and dentate granule cells have a much better chance to survive transient episodes of ischemia than the selectively vulnerable CA1 pyramidal neurons. While EPSPs of CA1 pyramidal cells are exaggerated after transient ischemia (see above), in CA3 pyramidal and dentate granule cells EPSPs are depressed (Gao et al., 1998a). This could be a factor protecting these cells against delayed neuron injury. A similar situation prevails in striatum, where spiny neurons are selectively vulnerable but large, aspiny cells are resistant to transient ischemic damage. In the immediate postischemic period, EPSPs of the large, aspiny cells are depressed (Pang et al., 2002). This depression affects both AMPA- and NMDA receptor–mediated transmission, and it appears to be caused by *adenosine* acting on *presynaptic terminals.* A protective role of endogenous adenosine has been suspected for some time in ischemia, as well as in epilepsy (Rudolphi et al., 1992).

Postischemic Calcium Overload Explained

During a transient ischemic episode, HSD drives $[Ca^{2+}]_o$ to very low levels as Ca^{2+} flows into cells. When the flow of blood is restored, $[Ca^{2+}]_o$ recovers, albeit not immediately to its normal level . Even as $[Ca^{2+}]_o$ remains lower than normal, the total tissue calcium *content* in the reperfused area can greatly increase, indicating *transfer from blood into brain* and continued accumulation in cells (Kristián et al., 1998). As Ca^{2+} is transported into the brain, it is taken up into cells so rapidly that the interstitial concentration remains low. Too much of the excess calcium entering neurons ends up in mitochondria (Dux et al., 1987; see also the next paragraph). Abnormally functioning NMDA-controlled and non-NMDA channels reportedly cooperate in admitting excess Ca^{2+} into neurons (Gorter et al., 1997; Hori et al., 1991; Mitani et al., 1993; Tsubokawa et al., 1994).

Mitochondrial Permeability Transition and the Role of Reactive Oxygen Species

As in reperfused heart muscle, in postischemic brain tissue the delayed damage is said to be mediated by a calcium-induced *mitochondrial permeability transition* and the release of cytochrome C from impaired mitochondria (Fig. 19–9)

(Sugawara et al., 1999) (but see Ouyang et al., 1999). According to Matsumoto et al. (1999), a derivative of cyclosporin A, which prevents the mitochondrial permeability transition, could limit infarct size when the drug is administered during postischemic reperfusion.

Mitochondrial dysfunction promotes the formation of reactive oxygen species. A role for reactive oxygen species in delayed neuron damage was formerly controversial but is increasingly being accepted (Kogure et al., 1985; Siesjö, 1993). Pérez-Pinzón et al. (1997a, 1998) used NADH fluorescence to assay the mitochondrial redox status (Jöbsis et al., 1971) during and after hypoxia of hippocampal slices. Oxygen withdrawal caused a reduction, as expected, but reoxygenation induced hyperoxidation. Administration of ascorbate and glutathione, both antioxidants, blunted the posthypoxic hyperoxidation and greatly improved functional recovery in the slices. Lowering $[Ca^{2+}]_o$ had a similar protective effect. Nitric oxide has an ambiguous status; it may be protective in low amounts and injurious in higher amounts (Shen and Gundlach, 1999).

Form and Function of Surviving Neurons

As already discussed, signs of both apoptosis and necrosis have been found in neurons undergoing delayed injury (Li et al., 2000a; Ouyang et al., 1999). Inhibition of caspases saved neurons from delayed death, as judged by histology supporting apoptosis as the main process of delayed injury (Gillardon et al., 1999). The neurons that were saved, however, lost their ability to produce LTP. This disquieting dissociation of histological appearance and normal function raises a cautionary note for studies in which the mere survival of the cells is used as an endpoint to evaluate the efficacy of therapeutic interventions, without testing function.

The ischemic penumbra and peri-infarct spreading depression waves

When one of the main cerebral arteries becomes obstructed, the area that it exclusively supplies becomes infarcted. Surrounding the infarct is a region supplied by branches of the obstructed artery plus collaterals from adjacent vessels. This is called the ***penumbra***, the shadowed surround, where blood flow is insufficient but not zero. In the hours and days following ischemic stroke, the patient's condition can deteriorate or improve, the outcome depending, among other things, on the evolving condition of the penumbral cells.

In experimental animals, focal ischemia is frequently created by temporary clamping or permanent ligation of the middle cerebral artery. From the border of an infarct so created, waves of spreading depression-like depolarization invade the penumbral region (Hossmann, 1996; Strong et al., 2000). These have been called *peri-infarct depolarizations* (*PIDs*). They arise just outside the border of the dead core and propagate into the penumbra, and they may or may not invade the healthy tissue. Over time the infarct can grow, and the frequency of the SD waves correlates with the expansion of the dead zone (Mies et al., 1993; Nedergaard, 1996). According to Dijkhuizen et al. (1999), the critical variable is not the number of SD episodes but the time spent in the depolarized state, echoing our earlier conclusion about acute HSD in hippocampal slices (see above: "Hypoxic spreading depression–like depolarization is not immediately lethal . . ."). Treatment with NMDA antagonist drugs (Hossmann, 1994; Iijima et al., 1992) or blockade of nonselective cation channels (Hoehn-Berlage et al., 1997) inhibits both the SD waves and the growth of the damage.

All these data point to the conclusion that the peri-infarct SD waves are instrumental in expanding the infarct. Normal brain tissue tolerates many repeated SD episodes without suffering lasting damage (Herreras and Somjen, 1993a; Nedergaard and Hansen, 1988), but apparently the metabolic stress of recurrent SD is too much when the blood supply is marginal (Gidö et al., 1994; Hossmann, 1994). The role of metabolic sufficiency is underscored by the fact that hyperglycemia limits while hypoglycemia augments both SD waves and the damage they do in the penumbra (Els et al., 1997; Strong et al., 2000).

Blood glucose leads us to our next topic.

Hyperglycemia and acidosis: good or bad?

Moderate Acidosis Protects Neurons In Vitro but Aggravates Damage in Ischemic Brain

The clinical outcome of stroke is worse for diabetics than for other persons (Pulsinelli et al., 1983). The main reason for the bad prognosis is believed to be the lactic acidosis that is secondary to hyperglycemia (Kagansky et al., 2001). The clinical experience is duplicated in animal experiments (Kalimo et al., 1981; Li et al., 2000b; Pulsinelli et al., 1982b; Smith and Siesjö, 1994). The poor outlook for diabetics has been known for decades, and when Schurr et al. (1987) first reported that raising the glucose concentration protected hippocampal tissue slices against hypoxic injury, the news understandably raised some eyebrows. Yet the protective effect was amply confirmed, not only for high glucose but also for *tissue acidosis* that can be induced without raising glucose (Fig. 19–10) (Ebine et al., 1994; Ou-Yang et al., 1994; Roberts and Sick, 1992; Roberts et al., 1998; Takadera et al., 1992; Tombaugh, 1994; Tombaugh and Sapolsky, 1993).

Schurr et al. (1999) called the seemingly contradictory data the *glucose paradox.* Here are some of the theoretical considerations that need to be taken into account in trying to interpret the facts. When oxygen is in short supply, anaerobic glycolysis

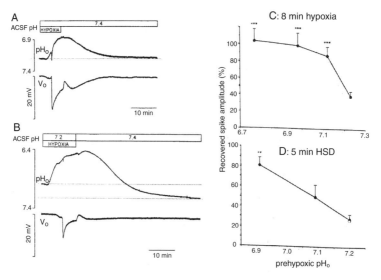

FIGURE 19–10. Moderate acidosis delays hypoxic spreading depression–like depolarization (HSD) and protects brain tissue in vitro against hypoxic injury. Recordings from the CA1 region of rat hippocampal tissue slices. Bath artificial cerebrospinal fluid (ACSF) pH was adjusted by titration with hydrochloric acid or sodium hydroxide. A: pH_o and extracellular potential (V_o) during and after hypoxia, with bath pH at 7.4 (normal). Low pH (high [H^+]) is plotted upward. The slice interstitial fluid is always more acid than the bath, even in control condition. During oxygen withdrawal, tissue pH_o begins to acidify early. At HSD onset there is a brief, sharp alkaline transient (cf. Fig. 13–6) followed by more acid shift, which outlasts the hypoxic period. B: In a slightly more acid bath HSD was postponed and the amplitude of the V_o shift was smaller. C: Recovery of synaptic transmission 2 hr after 8 min of hypoxia as a function of prehypoxic tissue pH_o (note: a pH_o of 7.23 corresponds to a bath pH of 7.4). D: Acidosis provides protection, even if HSD duration is kept constant. To achieve equal HSD, the total hypoxia period had to increase when acidosis postpones HSD onset. (Modified from Tombaugh, 1994.)

can still produce some high-energy phosphates, albeit less efficiently than by mitochondrial oxidative metabolism. Astrocytes are especially well endowed with glycolytic enzymes, and they also contain glycogen (Fillenz et al., 1997). Astrocytes could perhaps supply extra glucose, and perhaps even ATP or creatine phosphate to oxygen-starved neurons. In any event, at first glance it would seem that stocking up on glucose in advance of a scarcity of oxygen could bolster energy reserves and hence neuron survival. On the other hand, glycolysis produces lactic acid and lowers tissue pH. Until recently, acidosis was considered an unmitigated bane and lactic acid useless as a metabolic substrate for CNS neurons. But it now appears that, while severe acidosis undoubtedly kills cells (Kraig et al., 1987; Nedergaard et al., 1991), mild acidosis actually protects them. There are two components to this process. Acidosis postpones SD and HSD, but some additional protection works independently of and in spite of HSD (Roberts and Sick, 1992; Tombaugh, 1994). Moreover, it appears that lactate can be utilized by brain cells as a metabolic substrate, substituting for glucose (Ames, 2000; Cassady et al., 2001; Fillenz et al., 1997; Schurr et al., 1997, 2001b; but see Chih et al., 2001).

Hyperglycemia and acidosis curtail HSD and the associated massive influx of Ca^{2+} into neurons, while low glucose levels prolong HSD in hypoxic and ischemic brain tissue, not only in vitro but also in brains in situ (Hansen, 1978). This was confirmed by Kristián and Siesjö (1998), who found, however, that brain damage was worse in hyperglycemic animals even though HSD was curtailed. Other recent observations on brains in situ have, however, also challenged the concept that hyperglycemia aggravates hypoxic/ischemic brain damage (Phillis et al., 1999, 2001). In squirrel monkeys, hypoglycemia boosted peri-infarct SD-like depolarizations and expanded the infarct volume (Strong et al., 2000), while in another study hyperglycemia improved the outcome (Els et al., 1997).

In conclusion

There are two aspects to the protection afforded by high glucose levels. One is the provision of extra substrate for energy metabolism: not just the extra glucose, but also the lactate that is produced in glycolysis can be utilized by brain cells. The other effect is the acidosis caused by high glucose, which reduces excitation and inhibits the onset of SD-like depolarization.

This leaves open the question, why is the clinical outcome so much worse for diabetics? This is addressed next.

Extracerebral Effects Can Influence the Clinical Outcome

Schurr et al. (1999) attributed the deleterious effect of high glucose on ischemic brain in situ to secondary systemic effects, possibly hormonal and specifically related to corticosterone release (Schurr et al., 2001a). There is also the possibility that the *no-reflow* phenomenon plays a part: failure of the circulation due to plugging of capillaries, due to damage to the endothelium caused by acidosis (see above: "Persistent vascular insufficiency . . .") (Liu et al., 2001). Yet Siesjö's group reported that hyperglycemia aggravates ischemic injury without damaging capillaries (Li et al., 1998). It should be noted, however, that besides obstructing the flow of blood, mild injury to the endothelium could make the BBB abnormally permeable. Breaching of the BBB and cerebral edema have indeed been blamed for the unfavorable prognosis in diabetic acidosis (Kagansky et al., 2001).

The Paradox Solved?

The apparent contradiction could be reconciled by considering the criteria by which damage has been assessed in different experimental paradigms. Those who found that high glucose and mild acidosis are beneficial gauged the outcome based on the acute effects, such as recovery of synaptic transmission, or of depolarization, or of ion levels, or respiratory enzyme status shortly after oxygen withdrawal. Those who found that hyperglycemia and acidosis aggravate hypoxic/ischemic injury counted cells (intact or in the process of dying) some time after the insult. It could be that *high glucose and mild acidosis ameliorate acute hypoxic neuron injury but aggravate delayed neuron damage.* This proposal is in line with the known facts. It has occurred to others (see also Hammerman and Kaplan, 1998; Kristián et al., 2001).

Natural defenses

Preconditioning and Adaptation

After moving to a high altitude, people adapt to the low P_{O_2}. Acquired tolerance of low oxygen levels involves adjustments in the renal regulation of pH and in the responsiveness of arterial chemoreceptors, as well as a host of other general physiological adjustments such as production of more erythrocytes, all of which are outside the scope of this book. Besides responses of systemic homeostatic regulation, the tolerance of oxygen insufficiency of cells, including central neurons, can also improve. Cellular adaptation has been linked to gene induction, mediated by the **hypoxia-inducible factor (HIF)** (Chavez and LaManna, 2002).

A condition that calls such adaptation to mind can be achieved in hippocampal tissue slices. Schurr and colleagues (Schurr and Rigor, 1987; Schurr et al., 1986) withheld oxygen from hippocampal tissue slices for 5 min and then, in some cases a half hour later, and in others 2 hours later, exposed them to hypoxia for a much longer period. The pretreated slices survived 13 or 16 min of anoxic condition well, while untreated controls perished after anoxic periods of this length. Other investigators confirmed this observations (Pérez-Pinzón et al., 1996). There appears to be three-way cross-tolerance among hypoxia, excitotoxicity, and SD in vitro and brain in situ (Kawahara et al., 1995; Kobayashi et al., 1995). Preconditioning with brief exposure to high glutamate protects against later, longer, normally lethal glutamate administration and, importantly, 5 min hypoxic pretreatment also protects brain slices against a subsequent glutamate insult (Schurr et al., 2001c). Moreover, an antecedent episode of SD protects against subsequent hypoxia (Pérez-Pinzón et al., 1999). In neuron cultures sublethal oxygen-glucose deprivation, high $[K^+]_o$, glutamate, or NMDA administration protected the cells against subsequent prolonged, usually lethal, oxygen-glucose withdrawal (Grabb and Choi, 1999). Brief transient ischemia of brain in situ affords some degree of tolerance against subsequent ischemia already after 30 min (Stagliano et al., 1999) that lasts for 3 days but not for 7 days (Pérez-Pinzón et al., 1997b). A more recent report by Chavez and LaManna (2002) confirms the similarity between changes following brief, severe oxygen deprivation and prolonged, moderate hypoxia.

These authors demonstrated powerful upregulation of hypoxia-inducible factor and insulin-like growth factor that persisted for several days following 7 min cardiac arrest.

Even though the brief anoxia or ischemia preconditioning trials do not replicate adaptation to high altitudes where oxygen want is constant and tolerance builds up gradually over days and weeks, the underlying mechanisms may be related. Addressing the question of mechanism, Pérez-Pinzón et al. (1999) found that calcium had to be available to the hippocampal slice during preconditioning for effective protection. This team also emphasized the role of adenosine (Pérez-Pinzón et al., 1996). Adenosine is produced as ATP is hydrolyzed, and it accumulates when ATP cannot be reconstituted due to energy shortage. Schurr and colleagues (2001c) proposed that preconditioning depends on long-term enhancement of lactate production by glial cells and the transfer of lactate from glia to neurons. This is in line with their view that lactic acid is the preferred metabolic substrate favoring recovery from hypoxia (Schurr et al., 1997; but see also Chih et al., 2001). Kawahara et al. (1999) concluded that SD induces tolerance against subsequent ischemia because it causes long-lasting upregulation of protein and growth factor synthesis. Clearly, elucidation of the mechanism of preconditioning is continuing, and the relative importance of the several proposed mechanisms has not yet been clarified.

Ischemia-Induced Neurogenesis

A number of recent papers have reported increased formation of newborn neurons in adult rodent brains in the days and weeks following transient focal or global cerebral ischemia (Jin et al., 2001; Zhu et al., 2003; and other reports quoted in these papers). The phenomenon is reminiscent of neuron proliferation after cell loss following status epilepticus (Chapter 6: "Neuron loss, neuron proliferation . . ."). Typically, the mitotic cells appear in regions at some distance from the infarct. Whether or not they could become incorporated into the brain circuits in a way that helps to restore function instead of disturbing it is not yet clear. Nor is it clear whether similar ischemia-stimulated neurogenesis occurs in the brains of animals other than rodents. Nonetheless, it must be the optimists' credo that it might be possible to stimulate and steer the birth of new neurons or of grafts, in a way that could achieve a cure after stroke (Shetty and Turner, 1999; Turner and Shetty, 2003).

Key points

Cerebral neurons can be killed by hypoxia in three distinct processes: acute fast, acute slow, and delayed. Delayed neuron injury is similar to reperfusion damage of myocardium.

Acute fast neuron injury occurs in selectively vulnerable neurons, and it is hastened by HSD. If Ca^{2+} is withdrawn from brain slices before oxygen, then hypoxia is better tolerated even though HSD occurs even earlier than in the presence of normal Ca^{2+}. Prolonged depolarization-induced Ca^{2+} overload kills well-oxygenated brain cells as well.

It is probable that HSD is ignited by overflowing glutamate and aspartate and it is generated by the cooperation of ligand-controlled and voltage-gated slowly inactivating inward currents. The biophysical mechanism of the neuron depolarization during HSD is indistinguishable from that of normoxic SD, but the events that precede the depolarization are different in the two conditions.

Besides Ca^{2+}, excess cytosolic Zn^{2+} is suspected to be partly responsible for hypoxic/ischemic neuron injury.

The swelling of energy-starved cells is caused by failure of the active transport-regulating cell volume and the resulting dominance of Gibbs-Donnan forces.

Acute, fast hypoxic neuron injury is a necrotic process. In acute, slow and delayed (reperfusion) neuron injury, apoptosis may be the usual path to cell death, but the issue is controversial. Calcium uptake, mitochondrial permeability transition, release of cytochromes from mitochondria, and the unbridled formation of reactive oxygen species are stages in the apoptotic pathway.

During reperfusion following transient cerebral ischemia there is no evidence for glutamate overflow, overt excessive neuron excitation, seizures, or SD. Nonetheless, EPSPs, especially the NMDA-mediated component, are enhanced, but postsynaptic excitability is depressed. Upregulation of NMDA receptors may be the critical factor in initiating the delayed neuronal apoptotic process.

Peri-infarct SD waves invade the ischemic penumbra adjacent to the infarcted core of focal ischemia. These SD waves cause expansion of brain damage.

Hyperglycemic acidosis aggravates clinical strokes but ameliorates hypoxic damage in brain slices in vitro. Systemic rather than cerebral factors are the likely reason for the bad prognosis in diabetics.

Exposure to a sublethal hypoxic episode improves the outcome of a subsequent more severe hypoxia in brain tissue in vitro as well as in situ. Similar preconditioning can be achieved by inducing SD prior to hypoxia.

Postscript

After all the data reviewed in the foregoing pages, some generalization and a bit of speculation may be permitted.

As remarked in the preface, we don't really know how the brain normally works. Yet, without understanding the normal operation of the brain, we have seen how its function can be interrupted or destroyed.

We do know that the CNS uses signals received from the senses to construct a representation of the outside world, and it uses similar signals to govern muscles. Such signals also appear to be essential for the processing of information within the brain. Although we cannot read the code, it seems a priori that the information flows through many channels in parallel, and processed-to-generate patterns that are dynamic, multidimensional, subtly shaded and, in the words of Charles Sherrington, never abiding. This exquisite living pattern is overrun and submerged by seizures and SD.

Nerve impulses and synaptic potentials are the neural signals with which we are familiar, and ions are the elementary particles that generate such nerve signals. The well controlled distribution of ions in brain tissue forms an electrochemical landscape of microscopic and submicroscopic dimensions. This landscape is not static, but constantly in motion. Steep energy gradients are created by the work of ion pumps, and the stored energy is dissipated when neurons emit signals.

It is a peculiarity of the system that the ebb and flow of ions can feed back and influence the pathways through which the ions have surged. In some cases one can surmise a useful function of the feedback. For example, the entry of Ca^{2+} through NMDA controlled channels into neurons mediates LTP, and LTP is achieved by the augmentation of ion currents. Many believe that LTP is a stage in memory formation. Ionic feedback may be important in other normal functions, not yet discovered. Intense localized neuron excitation can raise $[K^+]_o$ and moderate elevation of $[K^+]_o$ could perhaps facilitate transmission in key synaptic systems, when haste, or great mental effort and concentrated attention are important. Mild changes in global ion levels could cooperate with transmitters and neuromodulator substances in changing moods, fatigue level, and attention. One could conjecture other examples.

The significance of the feedback between ions and their channels for pathological processes is, on the other hand, no longer a matter of conjecture but of well-founded inference. We have examined in some detail the evidence that major shifts in the distribution of K^+, Ca^{2+}, H^+, Cl^-, HCO_3^- are instrumental in the evolution of seizures, SD, and HSD. High $[K^+]_o$, low $[Ca^{2+}]$, alkalinization, and perhaps intracellular accumulation of Cl^- appear to sustain tonic-clonic seizures, but ion shifts probably do not start seizures. The initial trigger must come from misdirected synaptic activity or faulty ion channel function. Once the seizure is initiated, excessive ion shifts keep it going. The rise of $[K^+]_o$ during the seizure is limited by a ceiling, ensured by a large mobilization of extra metabolic energy, perhaps reflecting the sudden engagement of the glial ATP-fueled 3Na/2K pump. If the ceiling is breached, SD is ignited and ion shifts reach unprecedented levels.

Astonishing is the ability of mammalian brains to rapidly process a great deal of information, to carry out a multitude of tasks at once, to store large quantities of data, and to anticipate future events based on past experience. No less amazing is the way in which the CNS is constructed during development. Without an explicit blueprint, cells find their place and make the right connections. Here again, the governance of cell proliferation and the guidance of cell migration and axon growth are only very partially understood. It is clear, nevertheless that, in many cases, the sprouting of aberrant connections, unbridled cell proliferation, or uncalled-for programmed cell death can underlie chronic pathologic conditions.

To end on a hopeful note: whenever pathological conditions result from normal functions gone awry, it should be possible to set them right again. Not easy, but possible.

References

Abbott, N.J. Comparative physiology of the blood–brain barrier. In M.W.B. Bradbury (ed.), *Physiology and pharmacology of the blood–brain barrier*. Springer: Berlin, 371–396 (1992).

Abbott, N.J. Astrocyte-endothelial interactions and blood-brain barrier permeability. *J. Anat.* 200, 629–638 (2002).

Adams, D.J., Takeda, K., and Umbach, J.A. Inhibitors of calcium buffering depress evoked transmitter release at the squid giant synapse. *J. Physiol.* 369, 145–159 (1985).

Adrian, E.D. and Matthews, B.H.C. Berger rhythm: potential changes from the occipital lobes in man. *Brain* 57, 355–385 (1934).

Agopyan, N. and Avoli, M. Synaptic and non-synaptic mechanisms underlying low calcium bursts in the in vitro hippocampal slice. *Exp. Brain Res.* 73, 533–540 (1988).

Aitken, P.G., Balestrino, M., and Somjen, G.G. NMDA antagonists: lack of protective effect against hypoxic damage in CA1 region of hippocampal slices. *Neurosci. Lett.* 89, 187–192 (1988).

Aitken, P.G., Borgdorff, A.J., Juta, A.J.A., Kiehart, D.P., Somjen, G.G., and Wadman, W.J. Volume changes induced by osmotic stress in freshly isolated rat hippocampal neurons. *Pflügers Arch.* 436, 991–998 (1998a).

Aitken, P.G., Fayuk, D., Somjen, G.G., and Turner, D.A. Use of intrinsic optical signals to monitor physiological changes in brain tissue slieces. *Methods* 18, 91–103 (1999).

Aitken, P.G., Jing, J., Young, J., Friedman, A., and Somjen, G.G. Spreading depression in human hippocampal tissue in vitro. *Third IBRO Congr. Montreal Abstr.* 329 (1991a).

Aitken, P.G., Jing, J., Young, J., and Somjen, G.G. Ion channel involvement in hypoxia-induced spreading depression in hippocampal slices. *Brain Res.* 541, 7–11 (1991b).

Aitken, P.G. and Schiff, S.J. Selective neuronal vulnerability to hypoxia in vitro. *Neuroscie. Lett.* 67, 92–96 (1986).

Aitken, P.G., Tombaugh, G.C., Turner, D.A., and Somjen, G.G. Similar propagation of SD and hypoxic SD-like depolarization in rat hippocampus recorded optically and electrically. *J. Neurophysiol.* 80, 1514–1521 (1998b).

Aizenman, E., Stout, A.K., Hartnett, K.A., Dineley, K.E., McLaughlin, B., and Reynolds, I.J. Induction of neuronal apoptosis by thiol oxidation: putative role of intracellular zinc oxidase. *J. Neurochem.* 75, 1878–1888 (2000).

Ajmone-Marsan, C. Pentylenetetrazol: historical notes and comments on its electroencephalographic activation properties. In H.O. Lüders and S. Noachtar (eds.), *Epileptic seizures: pathophysiology and clnical semiology.* Churchill Livingstone: New York, 563–569 (2000).

Albrecht, D. and Heinemann, U. Low calcium-induced epileptiform activity in hippocampal slices from infant rats. *Dev. Brain Res.* 48, 316–320 (1989).

Alici, K. and Heinemann, U. Effects of low glucose levels on changes in $[Ca^{2+}]_o$ induced by stimulation of Schaffer collaterals under conditions of blocked chemical synaptic transmission in rat hippocampal slices. *Neurosci. Lett.* 185, 5–8 (1995).

Alkadhi, K.A. and Tian, L.-M. Veratridine-enhanced persistent sodium current induces bursting in CA1 pyramidal neurons. *Neuroscience* 71, 625–631 (1996).

Allen, B.W., Somjen, G.G., and Sanders, D.B. Effect of hypocalcemia on neuromuscular function. In M. Kessler, D.K. Harrison, and J. Höper (eds.), *Ion measurements in physiology and medicine.* Springer: Berlin, 243–248 (1985).

Amemori, T., Gorelova, N.A., and Bureš, J. Spreading depression in the olfactory bulb of rats: reliable initiation and boundaries of propagation. *Neuroscience* 22, 29–36 (1987).

Ames, A. Effect of glutamate and glutamine on the intracellular electrolytes of nervous tissue. *Neurology* 8, Suppl. 1, 64–66 (1964).

Ames, A., Maynard, K.I., and Kaplan, S. Protection against CNS ischemia by temporary interruption of function-related processes of neurons. *J. Cereb. Blood Flow Metab.* 15, 433–439 (1995).

Ames, A., Wright, R.L., Kowada, M., Thurston, J.M., and Majno, G. Cerebral ischemia: II. The no-reflow phenomenon. *Am. J. Pathol.* 52, 437–453 (1968).

Ames, A.I. CNS energy metabolism as related to function. *Brain Res. Rev.* 34, 42–68 (2000).

Amitai, Y., Gibson, J.R., Beierlein, M., Patrick, S.L., Ho, A.M., Connors, B.W., and Golomb, D. The spatial dimensions of electrically coupled networks of interneurons in the neocortex. *J. Neurosci.* 22, 4142–4152 (2002).

Amos, B.J. and Chesler, M. Characterization of an intracellular alkaline shift in rat astrocytes triggered by metabotropic glutamate receptors. *J. Neurophysiol.* 79, 695–703 (1998).

Amzica, F., Massimini, M., and Manfridi, A. Spatial buffering during slow and paroxysmal sleep oscillations in cortical networks of glial cells *in vivo. J. Neurosci.* 22, 1042–1053 (2002).

Amzica, F. and Neckelmann, D. Membrane capacitance of cortical neurons and glia during sleep oscillations and spike-wave seizures. *J. Neurophysiol.* 82, 2731–2746 (1999).

Amzica, F. and Steriade, M. Electrophysiological correlates of sleep delta waves. *Electroencephalogr. Clin. Neurophysiol.* 107, 69–83 (1998).

Amzica, F. and Steriade, M. Spontaneous and artifical activation of neocortical seizures. *J. Neurophysiol.* 82, 3123–3138 (1999).

Amzica, F. and Steriade, M. Neuronal and glial membrane potentials during sleep and paroxysmal oscillations in the neocortex. *J. Neurosci.* 20, 6648–6665 (2000).

Andermann, F. and Lugaresi, E. (eds.). *Migraine and epilepsy.* Butterworth: Boston (1987).

Andersen, P. and Andersson, S.A. *Physiological basis of the alpha rhythm.* Appleton-Century-Crofts: New York (1968).

Andersen, P., Blackstad, T.W., and Lømo, T. Location and identification of excitatory synapses on hippocampal pyramidal cells. *Exp. Brain Res.* 1, 236–248 (1966).

Andersen, P., Dingledine, R., Gjerstad, L., Langmoen, I.A., and Mosfeldt-Larsen, A. Two different responses of hippocampal pyramidal cells to application of gamma-aminobutyric acid. *J. Physiol.* 305, 279–296 (1980).

Andersen, P., Eccles, J.C., and Løyning, Y. Location of postsynaptic inhibitory synapses on hippocampal pyramids. *J. Neurophysiol.* 27, 592–607 (1964).

Anderson, J.M. and Van Itallie, C.M. Tight junctions and the molecular basis for regulation of paracellular permeability. *Am. J. Physiol.* 269, G467–G475 (1995).

Anderson, W.W., Lewis, D.V., Swartzwelder, H.S., and Wilson, W.A. Magnesium-free medium activates seizure-like events in the rat hippocampal slice. *Brain Res.* 398, 215–219 (1986).

Anderson, W.W., Swartzwelder, H.S., and Wilson, W.A. The NMDA receptor antagonist 2-amino-5-phosphonovalerate blocks stimulus-induced epileptogenesis but not epileptiform bursting in the rat hippocampal slice. *J. Neurophysiol.* 57, 1–21 (1987).

Andrew, R.D. Seizure and acute osmotic change: clinical and neurophysiological aspects. *J. Neurol. Sci.* 101, 7–18 (1991).

Andrew, R.D., Anderson, T.R., Biedermann, A.J., and Jarvis, C.R. Imaging and preventing spreading depression independent of cerebral blood flow. *Int.Congr. Ser.* 1235, 421–437 (2002).

Andrew, R.D., Anderson, T.R., Biedermann, A.J., Joshi, I., and Jarvis, C.R. Imaging the anoxic depolarization, a multifocal and propagating event. In J. Krieglstein and S. Klumpp (eds.), *Pharmacology of cerebral ischema.* Medpharm: Stuttgart, 75–94 (2000).

Andrew, R.D., Duffy, S., and MacVicar, B.A. Imaging spreading depression in the rat hippocampal slice using intrinsic optical signals. *Soc. Neurosci. Abstr.* 21, 982 (1995).

Andrew, R.D., Fagan, M., Ballyk, B.A., and Rosen, A.S. Seizure susceptibility and the osmotic state. *Brain Res.* 498, 175–180 (1989).

Andrew, R.D., Jarvis, C.R., and Obeidat, A.S. Potential sources of intrinsic optical signals imaged in live brain slices. *Methods*, 18, 185–196 (1999).

Andrew, R.D., Lobinowich, M.E., and Osehobo, E.P. Evidence against volume regulation by cortical brain cells during acute osmotic stress. *Exp. Neurol.* 143, 300–312 (1997).

Andrew, R.D. and MacVicar, B.A. Imaging cell volume changes and neuronal excitation in the hippocampal slice. *Neuroscience* 62, 371–383 (1994).

Andrew, R.D., Taylor, C.P., Snow, R.W., and Dudek, F.E. Coupling in rat hippocampal slices: dye transfer between CA1 pyramidal cells. *Brain Res. Bull.* 8, 211–222 (1982).

Armand, V., Rundfeldt, C., and Heinemann, U. Effects of retigabine (D-23129). on different patterns of epileptiform activity induced by low magnesium in rat entorhinal cortex hippocampal slices. *Epilepsia* 41, 28–33 (2000).

Armstrong, D.R., Neill, K.H., Crain, B.J., and Nadler, J.V. Absence of electrographic seizures after transient forebrain ischemia in the mongolian gerbil. *Brain Res.* 476, 174–178 (1989).

Ashcroft, F.M. *Ion channels and disease.* Academic Press: San Diego, CA (2000).

Augustine, G.J. How does calcium trigger neurotransmiter release? *Curr. Opin. Neurobiol.* 11, 320–326 (2001).

Aurora, S.K. and Welch, K.M. Migraine: imaging the aura. *Curr. Opin. Neurol.* 13, 273–276 (2000).

Avanzini, G., de Curtis, M., Franceschetti, S., Sancini, G., and Spreafico, R. Cortical versus thalamic mechanisms underlying spike and wave discharges in GAERS. *Epilepsy Res.* 26, 37–44 (1996).

Avanzini, G., Moshé, S.L., Schwartzkroin, P.A., and Engel, J., Jr. Animal models of localization-related epilepsy. In J. Engel, Jr., and T.A. Pedley (eds.), *Epilepsy: a comprehensive textbook*, Vol. 1. Lippincott-Raven: Philadelphia, 427–442 (1998).

Avoli, M. Penicillin induced hyperexcitability in the in vitro hippocampal slice can be unrelated to impairment of somatic inhibition. *Brain Res.* 323, 154–158 (1984).

Avoli, M. Do interictal discharges promote or control seizure? Experimental evidence from an in vitro model of epileptiform discharge. *Epilepsia* 42 Suppl. 3, 2–4 (2001).

Avoli, M., Drapeau, C., Louvel, J., Pumain, R., Olivier, A., and Villemure, J.-G. Epileptiform activity induced by low extracellular magnesium in the human cortex in vitro. *Ann. Neurol.* 30, 589–596 (1991).

Avoli, M., Drapeau, C., Perreault, P., Louvel, J., and Pumain, R. Epileptiform activity induced by low chloride medium in the CA1 subfield of the hippocampal slice. *J. Neurophysiol.* 64, 1747–1757 (1990).

Avoli, M. and Gloor, P. Epilepsy. In G. Adelman (ed.), *Encyclopedia of neuroscience*. Birkhäuser: Boston, 400–403 (1987).

Avoli, M., Gloor, P., Kostopoulos, G , and Gotman, J. An analysis of penicillin-induced generalized spike and wave discharges using simultaneous recordings of cortical and thalamic neurons. *J. Neurophysiol.* 50, 819–837 (1983).

Avoli, M. and Kostopoulos, G. Participation of corticothalamic cells in penicillin-induced generalized spike and wave discharges. *Brain Res.* 247, 159–163 (1982).

Avoli, M., Nagao, T., Köhling, R., Lücke, A., and Mattia, D. Synchronization of rat hippocampal neurons in the absence of excitatory amino acid-mediated transmission. *Brain Res.* 735, 188–196 (1996).

Avoli, M. and Olivier, A. Electrophysiological properties and synaptic responses in the deep layers of the human epileptogenic neocortex in vitro. *J. Neurophysiol.* 61, 589–606 (1989).

Ayala, G.F., Dichter, M., Gumnit, R.J., Matsumoto, H., and Spencer, W.A. Genesis of epileptic interictal spikes: new knowledge of cortical feedback systems suggests a neurophysiological explanation of brief paroxysms. *Brain Res.* 52, 1–17 (1973).

Babb, T.L. Axonal growth and neosynaptogenesis in human and experimental hippocampal epilepsy. *Adv. Neurol.* 72, 45–51 (1997).

Babb, T.L. Synaptic reorganization in human and rat hippocampal epilepsy. *Adv. Neurol.* 79, 763–779 (1999).

Babcock, D.F. and Hille, B. Mitochondrial oversight of cellular Ca^{2+} signaling. *Curr. Opin. Neurobiol.* 8, 398–404 (1998).

Bahar, S., Fayuk, D., Somjen, G.G., Aitken, P.G., and Turner, D.A. Mitochondrial depolarization and intrinsic optical signal imaged during hypoxia and spreading depression in rat hippocampal slices. *J. Neurophysiol.* 84, 311–324 (2000).

Bahar, S., Turner, D.A., and Aitken, P.G. Mitochondrial depolarization precedes hypoxic spreading depression in rat hippocampal slices. *Soc. Neurosci. Abstr.* 25, 1847 (1999).

Baimbridge, K.G., McLennan, P.M.J., and Church, J. Bursting response to current-evoked depolarization in rat CA1 pyramidal neurons is correlated with Lucifer Yellow dye coupling but not with the presence of calbindin-D28k. *Synapse* 7, 269–277 (1991).

Baker, A.J., Zornow, M.H., Scheller, M.S., Yaksh, T.L., Skilling, S.R., Smullin, D.H., Larson, A.A., and Kuczenski, R. Changes in extracellular concentrations of glutamate, aspartate, glycine, dopamine, serotonin and dopamine metabolites after transient global ischemia in the rabbit brain. *J. Neurochem.* 57, 1370–1379 (1991).

Balestrino, M., Aitken, P.G., Jones, L.S., and Somjen, G.G. The role of spreading depression-like hypoxic depolarization in irreversible neuron damage, and its prevention. In G.G. Somjen, (ed.), *Mechanisms of cerebral hypoxia and stroke*. Plenum: New York, 291–301 (1988).

Balestrino, M., Aitken, P.G., and Somjen, G.G. The effects of moderate changes of extracellular K^+ and $Ca2^+$ on synaptic and neural function in the CA1 region of the hippocampal slice. *Brain Res.* 377, 229–239 (1986).

Balestrino, M., Aitken, P.G., and Somjen, G.G. Spreading depression-like hypoxic depolarization in CA1 and fascia dentata of hippocampal slices: relationship to selective vulnerability. *Brain Res.* 497, 102–107 (1989).

Balestrino, M., Cogliolo, I., Lunardi, G., Leon, A., and Mazzari, S. Delay of anoxic depolarization by creatine, sphingosine derivatives or mannitol. *Soc. Neurosci. Abstr.* 18, 1256 (1992).

Balestrino, M., Rebaudo, R., and Lunardi, G. Exogenous creatine delays anoxic depolarization and protects from hypoxic damage: dose-effect relationship. *Brain Res.* 816, 124–130 (1999a).

Balestrino, M. and Somjen, G.G. Chlorpromazine protects brain tissue in hypoxia by delaying spreading depression-mediated calcium influx. *Brain Res.* 385, 219–226 (1986).

Balestrino, M. and Somjen, G.G. Concentration of carbon dioxide, interstitial pH and synaptic transmission in hippocampal formation of the rat. *J. Physiol.* 396, 247–266 (1988).

Balestrino, M., Young, J., and Aitken, P.G. Block of (Na^+, K^+).ATPase with ouabain induced spreading depression-like depolarization in hippocampal slices. *Brain Res.* 838, 37–44 (1999b).

Ballanyi, K. Modulation of glial potassium, sodium and chloride activities by the extracellular milieu. In H. Kettenmann and B.R. Ransom (eds.), *Neuroglia*. Oxford University Press: New York, 289–298 (1995).

Ballanyi, K., Grafe, P., and Ten Bruggencate, G. Ion activities and potassium uptake mechanisms of glial cells in guinea-pig olfactory cortex slices. *J. Physiol.* 382, 159–174 (1987).

Ballyk, B.A., Quackenbush, S.J., and Andrew, R.D. Osmotic effects on the CA1 neuronal population in hippocampal slices with special reference to glucose. *J. Neurophysiol.* 65, 1055–1066 (1991).

Barbour, B., Brew, H., and Attwell, D. Electrogenic glutamate uptake in glial cells is activated by intracellular potassium. *Nature* 335, 433–435 (1988).

Barchi, R.L. Molecular pathology of the skeletal muscle sodium channel. *Annu. Rev. Physiol.* 57, 355–385 (1995).

Barer, R., Ross, K.F.A., and Tkaczyk, S. Refractometry of living cells. *Nature* 171, 720–724 (1953).

Barker, J.L. and McBurney, R.N. Phenobarbitone modulation of postsynaptic GABA receptor function on cultured mammalian neurons. *Proc. R. Soc. B.* 206, 319–327 (1979).

Barker, J.L. and Ransom, B.R. Pentobarbitone pharmacology of mammalian central neurones grown in tissue culture. *J. Physiol.* 280, 355–372 (1978).

Barres, B.A. Five electrophysiological properties of glial cells. *Ann. N.Y. Acad. Sci.* 633, 248–254 (1991).

Barres, B.A., Chun, L.Y., and Corey, D.P. Ion channels in vertebrate glia. *Annu. Rev. Neurosci.* 13, 441–474 (1990).

Basarsky, T.A., Duffy, S.N., Andrew, R.D., and MacVicar, B.A. Imaging spreading depression and associated intracellular calcium waves in brain slices. *J. Neurosci.* 18, 7189–7199 (1998).

Basarsky, T.A., Feighan, D., and MacVicar, B.A. Glutamate release through volume-activated channels during spreading depression. *J. Neurosci.* 19, 6439–6445 (1999).

Baudry, M. and Lynch, G. Remembrance of arguments past: how well is the glutamate receptor hypothesis of LTP holding up after 20 years? *Neurobiol. Learning Memory* 76, 284–297 (2001).

Baumgartner, G., Creutzfeldt, O., and Jung, R. Microphysiology of cortical neurones in acute anoxia and in retinal ischemia. In H. Gastaut and J.S. Meyer (eds.), *Cerebral anoxia and the electroencephalogram.* Charles C. Thomas: Springfield, Ill., 5–34 (1961).

Beattie, D.S. Bioenergetics and oxidative metabolism. In T.M. Devlin (ed.), *Textbook of biochemistry with clinical correlations.* Wiley-Liss: New York, 537–595 (2002).

Beck, H., Steffens, R., Elger, C.E., and Heinemann, U. Voltage-dependent Ca^{2+} currents in epilepsy. *Epilepsy Res.* 32, 321–332 (1998).

Behr, J., Heinemann, U., and Mody, I. Glutamate receptor activation in the kindled dentate gyrus. *Epilepsia* 42 Suppl. 6, S100–S103 (2000).

Behr, J., Heinemann, U., and Mody, I. Kindling induces transient NMDA receptor-mediated facilitation of high-frequency input in the rat dentate gyrus. *J. Neurophysiol.* 85, 2195–2202 (2001).

Bekenstein, J.W. and Lothman, E.W. Dormancy of inhibitory interneurons in a model of temporal lobe epilepsy. *Science* 259, 97–100 (1993).

Belousov, A.B., Godfraind, J.-M., and Krnjević, K. Internal Ca^{2+} stores involved in anoxic responses of rat hippocampal neurons. *J. Physiol.* 486, 547–556 (1995).

Ben-Ari, Y. Effect of glibenclamide, a selective blocker of an ATP-K^+ channel, on the anoxic response of hippocampal neurones. *Pflügers Arch.* 414 (Suppl. 1), S111–S114 (1989).

Ben-Ari, Y., Khazipov, R., Leinekugel, X., Caillard, O., and Gaiarsa, J.-L. $GABA_A$, NMDA and AMPA receptors: a developmentally regulated "ménage à trois." *Trends Neurosci.* 20, 523–529 (1997).

Ben-Ari, Y. and Krnjević, K. Actions of GABA on hippocampal neurons with special reference to the aetiology of epilepsy. In P.L. Morselli (ed.), *Neurotransmitters, seizures and epilepsy.* Raven Press: New York, 63–73 (1981).

Benešová, O., Burešová, O., and Bureš, J. Die Wirkung des Chlorpromazins un der Glykämie auf das elektrophysiologisch kontrollierte Überleben der Hirnrinde bei verschiedenen Körpertemperaturen. *Arch. Exper. Pathol. Pharmacol.* 231, 550–561 (1957).

Bengzon, J., Kokaia, Z., Elmér, E., Nanobashvili, A., Kokaia, M., and Lindvall, O. Apoptosis and proliferation of dentate gyrus neurons after single and intermittent limbic seizures. *Proc. Natl. Acad. Sci. USA* 94, 10432–10437 (1997).

Benninger, C., Kadis, J., and Prince, D.A. Extracellular calcium and potassium changes in hippocampal slices. *Brain Res.* 187, 165–182 (1980).

Benveniste, H., Drejer, J., Schousboe, A., and Diemer, N.H. Elevations of the extracellular concentrations of glutamate and aspartate in rat hippocampus during transient cerebral ischemia monitored by intracerebral microdialysis. *J. Neurochem.* 43, 1369–1374 (1984).

Benveniste, H., Jorgensen, M.B., Sandberg, M., Christensen, T., Hagberg, H., and Diemer, N.H. Ischemic damage in hippocampal CA1 is dependent on glutamate release and intact innervation of CA3. *J. Cereb. Blood Flow Metab.* 9, 629–645 (1989).

Berger, H. Über das Elektrenkephalogram des Menschen. *Arch. Psychiatr. Nervenkr.* 87, 527–570 (1929).

Berger, H. Über das Elektrenkephalogramm des menschen. Zweite Mitteilung. *J. Psychol. Neurol.* 40, 160–179 (1930).

Berger, H. Über das Elektrenkephalogram des Menschen. Neunte Mitteilung. *Arch. Psychiatr. Nervenkr.* 102, 538–557 (1934).

Berkovic, S.F. and Scheffer, I.E. Genetics of the epilepsies. *Epilepsia* 42 (Suppl. 5), 16–23 (2001).

Bernard, C., Cossart, R., Hirsch, J.C., Esclapez, M., and Ben-Ari, Y. What is GABAergic inhibition? How is it modified in epilepsy? *Epilepsia* 41 (Suppl. 6), S90–S95 (2000).

Bernard, C., Esclapez, M., Hirsch, J.C., and Ben-Ari, Y. Interneurons are not so dormant in temporal lobe epilepsy: a critical reappraisal of the dormant basket cell hypothesis. *Epilepsy Res.* 32, 93–103 (1998).

Berridge, M.J. Neuronal calcium signaling. *Neuron* 21, 13–26 (1998).

Bert, P. *Barometric pressure.* (Original title: *La pression barometrique*, 1878). Columbus, Ohio: College Book Co. (1943).

Bertram, E.H. and Lothman, E.W. Morphometric effects of intermittent kindled seizures and limbic status epilepticus. *Brain Res.* 603, 25–31 (1993).

Bertram, E.H., Zhang, D.X., Mangan, P., Fountain, N., and Rempe, D. Functional anatomy of limbic epilepsy: a proposal for central synchronization of a diffusely hyperexcitable network. *Epilepsy Res.* 32, 194–205 (1998).

Besson, J.M., Woody, C.D., and Marshall, W.H. Influences of respiratory acidosis and of cerebral blood flow variations on the DC potential. In B.K. Siesjö and S.C. Sørensen (eds.), *Ion homeostasis of the brain.* Munksgaard: Copenhagen, 97–118 (1971).

Betz, A.L. Epithelial properties of brain capillary endothelium. *Fed. Proc.* 44, 2614–2615 (1985).

Bevensee, M.O. and Boron, W.F. pH regulation in mammalian neurons. In K. Kaila and B.R. Ransom (eds.), *pH and brain function.* Wiley-Liss: New York, 253–276 (1998).

Biagini, G., Avoli, M., Marcinkiewicz, J., and Marcinkiewicz, M. Brain-derived neurotrophic factor superinduction parallels anti-epileptic–neuroprotective treatment in the pilocarpine epilepsy model. *J. Neurochem.* 76, 1814–1822 (2001).

Bialer, M., Johanessen, S.I., Kupferberg, H.J., Levy, R.H., Loiseau, P., and Perucca, E. Progress report on new antiepileptic drugs: a summary of the Fifth Eilat Conference (Eilat V). *Epilepsy Res.* 43, 11–58 (2001).

Biemond, A. *Hersenziekten.* De Erven Bohn: Haarlem, the Netherlands (1961).

Bikson, M., Baraban, S.C., and Durand, D.M. Conditions sufficient for nonsynaptic epileptogenesis in the CA1 region of hippocampal slices. *J. Neurophysiol.* 87, 62–71 (2002).

Bikson, M., Ghai, R.S., Baraban, S.C., and Durand, D.M. Modulation of burst frequency, duration and amplitude in the zero-Ca^{2+} model of epileptiform activity. *J. Neurophysiol.* 82, 2262–2270 (1999).

Billups, B., Rossi, D., Oshima, T., Warr, O., Takahashi, M., Sarantis, M., Szatkowski, M., and Attwell, D. Physiological and pathological operation of glutamate transporters. *Prog. Brain Res.* 116, 45–57 (1998).

Binder, D.K., Croll, S.D., Gall, C.M., and Scharfman, H.E. BDNF and epilepsy: too much of a good thing? *Trends Neurosci.* 24, 47–53 (2001a).

Binder, D.K. and McNamara, J.O. Kindling: a pathologic activity-driven structural and functional plasticity in mature brain. In M.E. Corcoran and S.L. Moshé (eds.), *Kindling 5.* Plenum Press: New York, 245–253 (1998).

Binder, D.K., Oshio, K., Verkman, A.S., and Manley, G.T. Altered seizure susceptibility in mice deficient in the aquaporin-4 membrane water channel. *Soc. Neurosci. Abstr.* 27, Program No.350.2 (2001b).

Binder, D.K., Routbort, M.J., Ryan, T.E., Yancopoulos, G.D., and McNamara, J.O. Selective inhibition of kindling development by intraventricular administration of trkB receptor body. *J. Neurosci.* 19, 1424–1436 (1999).

Bingmann, D., Speckmann, E.-J., Baker, R.E., Ruijter, J., and de Jong, B.M. Differential antiepileptic effects of the organic calcium antagonists verapamil and flunarizine in neurons of organotypic neocortical explants from newborn rats. *Exp. Brain Res.* 72, 439–442 (1988).

Binnie, C.D. Electroencephalography and epilepsy. In A. Hopkins (ed.), *Epilepsy.* Demos: New York, 169–199 (1987).

Bladin, C.E. and Norris, J.W. Epilepsy and stroke. In M.D. Ginsberg and J. Bogousslavsky (eds.), *Cerebrovascular disease: pathophysiology, diagnosis and management*, Volume 2. Blackwell Science: Malden, Mass., 1119–1125 (1998).

Blakeman, K.H., Wiesenfeld-Hallin, Z., and Alster, P. Microdialysis of galanin in rat spinal cord: in vitro and in vivo studies. *Exp. Brain Res.* 139, 354–358 (2001).

Blaustein, M.P. and Golovina, V.A. Structural complexity and functional diversity of endoplasmic reticulum Ca^{2+} stores. *Trends Neurosci.* 24, 602–608 (2001).

Blaustein, M.P. and Lederer, W.J. Sodium/calcium exchange: its physiological implications. *Physiol. Rev.* 79, 763–854 (1999).

Bliss, T.V.P. and Collingridge, G.L. A synaptic model of memory: long-term potentiation in the hippocampus. *Nature* 361, 31–39 (1993).

Bliss, T.V.P. and Gardner-Medwin, A.R. Long-lasting potentiation of synaptic transmission in the dentate area of the unanaesthetized rabbit following stimulation of the perforant path. *J. Physiol.* 232, 357–374 (1973).

Block, G.A. and Pulsinelli, W.A. Excitatory amino acid and purinergic transmitter involvement in ischemia-induced selective neuronal death. In G. Somjen (ed.), *Mechanisms of cerebral hypoxia and stroke.* Plenum: New York, 359–365 (1988).

Blümcke, I., Beck, H., Lie, A.A., and Wiestler, O.D. Molecular neuropathology of human mesial temporal lobe epilepsy. *Epilepsy Res.* 36, 205–223 (1999).

Blume, W.T. and Young, G.B. Ictal paIn unilateral, cephalic and abdominal. In F. Andermann and E. Lugaresi, (eds.), *Migraine and epilepsy.* Boston: Butterworth, 235–247 (1987).

Bock, G. and Goode, J.A. (eds.), *Sodium Channels and Neuronal Hyperexcitability*, Novartis Foundation Symposium 241, Chichester, New York, Wiley (2002).

Boening, J.A., Kass, I.S., Cottrell, J.E., and Chambers, G. The effect of blocking sodium influx on anoxic change in the rat hippocampal slice. *Neuroscience* 33, 253–268 (1989).

Bolay, H., Reuter, U., Dunn, A.K., Huang, Z., Boas, D.A., and Moskowitz, M.A. Intrinsic brain activity triggers trigeminal meningeal afferents in a migraine model. *Nature Med.* 8, 136–142 (2002).

Bollmann, J.H., Helmchen, F., Borst, J.G.G., and Sakmann, B. Postsynaptic Ca^{2+} influx mediated by three different pathways during synaptic transmission at a calyx-type synapse. *J. Neurosci.* 18, 10409–10419 (1998).

Bonnet, U., Leniger, T., and Wiemann, M. Alteration of intracellular pH and activity of CA3-pyramidal cells in guinea pig hippocampal slices by inhibition of transmembrane acid extrusion. *Brain Res.* 872, 116–124 (2000).

Bootman, M.D., Lipp, P., and Berridge, M.J. The organisation and functions of local Ca^{2+} signals. *J. Cell Sci.* 114, 2213–2222 (2001).

Borck, C. and Jefferys, J.G.R. Seizure-like events in disinhibited ventral slices of adult rat hippocampus. *J. Neurophysiol.* 82, 2130–2142 (1999).

Bordey, A. and Sontheimer, H. Passive glial cells, fact or artifact? *J. Memb. Biol.* 166, 213–222 (1998).

Bouffard, G. Injection des couleurs de benzidine aux animaux normaux. Etude expérimentale et histologique. *Ann. Inst. Pateur* 20, 539–550 (1906).

Bouilleret, V., Schwaller, B., Schurmans, S., Celio, M.R., and Fritschy, J.M. Neurodegenerative and morphologic changes in a mouse model of temporal lobe epilepsy do not depend on the expression of calcium-binding proteins parvalbumin, calbindin or calretinin. *Neuroscience* 97, 47–58 (2000).

Bourke, R.S., Dazé, R.S., and Kimelberg, H.K. Chloride transport in mammalian astroglia. In E. Schoffeniels, G. Franck, D.B. Tower, and L. Hertz (eds.), *Dynamic properties of glia cells*. Pergamon: Oxford, 337–346 (1978).

Boyle, P.J. and Conway, E.J. Potassium accumulation in muscle and associated changes. *J. Physiol.* 100, 1–63 (1941).

Bracci, E., Vreugdenhil, M., Hack, S.P., and Jefferys, J.G.R. On the synchronizing mechanisms of tetanically induced hippocampal oscillations. *J. Neurosci.* 19, 8104–8113 (1999).

Bracci, E., Vreugdenhil, M., Hack, S.P., and Jefferys, J.G.R. Dynamic modulation of excitation and inhibition during stimulation at gamma and beta frequencies in the CA1 hippocampal region. *J. Neurophysiol.* 85, 2412–2422 (2001).

Bradbury, M.W.B. *The concept of the blood-brain barrier*. Wiley: Chichester, UK: (1979).

Bradbury, M.W.B., Cserr, H., and Westrop, R.J. Drainage of cerebral interstitial fluid into deep cervical lymph of the rabbit. *Am. J. Physiol.* 240, F329–F336 (1981).

Bradbury, M.W.B. and Stulcova, B. Efflux mechanism contributing to the stability of the potassium concentration in cerebrospinal fluid. *J.Physiol.* 208, 415–430 (1970).

Bragdon, A.C., Kojima, H., and Wilson, W.A. Suppression of interictal bursting in hippocampus unleashes seizures in entorhinal cortex: a proepileptic effect of lowering [K$^+$]$_o$ and raising [Ca^{2+}]$_o$. *Brain Res.* 590, 128–135 (1992).

Bragin, A., Jando, G., Nádasdy, Z., Hetke, J., Wise, K., and Buzsáki, G. Gamma (40–100 Hz). oscillation in the hippocampus of the behaving rat. *J. Neurosci.* 15, 47–60 (1995).

Bragin, A., Penttonen, M., and Buzsáki, G. Termination of epileptic afterdischarge in the hippocampus. *J. Neurosci.* 17, 2567–2579 (1997).

Brailowsky, S., Menini, C., Silva-Barrat, C., and Naquet, R. Epileptogenic gamma-aminobutyric acid-withdrawal syndrome after chronic intracortical infusion in baboons. *Neurosci. Lett.* 74, 75–80 (1987).

Brazier, M.A.B. *A history of neurophysiology in the 19th century*. Raven Press: New York (1988).

Bremer, F. Action de la strychnine en application locale sur l'activité électrique du cortex cérébral. *Comp. Rend. Soc. Biol.* 123, 90–95 (1936).

Brew, H., Gray, P.T., Mobbs, P., and Attwell, D. Endfeet of glial cells have higher densities of ion channels that mediate K$^+$ buffering. *Nature* 324, 466–468 (1986).

Brierley, J.B. and Graham, D.I. Hypoxia and vascular disorders of the nervous system. In H.J. Adams, J.A.N. Corsellis, and L.W. Duchen (eds.), *Greenfield's neuropathology*. Wiley: New York, 125–207 (1984).

Brightman, M.W. Ultrastructure of brain endothelium. In M.W.B. Bradbury (ed.), *Physiology and pharmacology of the blood-brain barrier*. Springer: Berlin, 1–22 (1992).

Brightman, M.W. and Reese, T.S. Junctions between intimately apposed cell membranes in the vertebrate brain. *J. Cell Biol.* 40, 648–677 (1969).

Brinley, F.J., Kandel, E.R., and Marshall, W.H. Potassium outflux from rabbit cortex during spreading depression. *J. Neurophysiol.* 23, 246–256 (1960).

Brodal, A. Self-observation and neuro-anatomical consideration after a stroke. *Brain* 96, 675–694 (1973).

Bromfield, E.B. Ethosuximide and other siccinimides. In J. Engel, Jr., and T.A. Pedley (eds.), *Epilepsy: a comprehensive textbook*. Vol. 2. Lippincott-Raven: Philadelphia, 1503–1508 (1997).

Brooks, K.J. and Kauppinen, R.A. Calcium-mediated damage following hypoxia in cerebral cortex ex vivo studied by NMR spectroscopy. Evidence for direct involvement of voltage gated Ca^{2+} channels. *Neurochem. Int.* 23, 441–450 (1993).

Brown, D.A. and Adams, P. Muscarinic suppression of a novel voltage sensitive K^+ current in a vertebrate neurone. *Nature* 283, 673–676 (1980).

Browne, T.R. and Ascanape, J.S. Diones, paraldehyde, phenacemide, bromides and sulthiame. In J. Engel, Jr., and T.A. Pedley (eds.), *Epilepsy: a comprehensive textbook*, Vol. 2. Lippincott-Raven: Philadelphia, 1627–1644 (1997).

Brozek, G. Changes in the membrane potential of cortical cells during spreading depression. *Physiol. Bohemoslov.* 15, 98–103 (1966).

Bryant, S.H. Cable properties of external intercostal muscle fibres from myotonic and nonmyotonic goats. *J. Physiol.* 204, 539–550 (1969).

Buckmaster, P.S. and Dudek, F.E. In vivo intracellular analysis of granule cell axon reorganization in epileptic rats. *J. Neurophysiol.* 81, 712–721 (1999).

Bureš, J. and Burešová, O. Die anoxische Terminaldepolarisation als Indicator der Vulnerabilität des Grosshirnrinde bei Anoxie un Ischämie. *Pflügers Arch.* 264, 325–334 (1957).

Bureš, J., Burešová, O., and Krivánek, J. *The mechanism and applications of Leão's spreading depression of electroencephalographic activity.* Academia: Prague (1974).

Bureš, J., Burešová, O., and Krivánek, O. The meaning and significance of Leão's spreading depression. *An. Acad. Bras. Cienc.* 56, 385–400 (1984).

Burešová, O. and Bureš, J. The use of partial functional decortication in the study of the localization of conditioned reflexes. *Physiologia Bohemoslovenica* 9, 210–218 (1960).

Burgess, D.L. and Noebels, J.L. Single gene defects in mice: the role of voltage-dependent calcium channels in absence models. *Epilepsy Res.* 36, 111–122 (1999).

Burns, B.D. *The mammalian cerebral cortex.* Arnold: London (1958).

Busto, R., Dietrich, W.D., Globus, M.Y.T., Valdés, I., Scheinberg, P., and Ginsberg, M.D. Small differences in intraischemic brain temperature critically determine the extent of ischemic neuronal injury. *J. Cereb. Blood Flow Metab.* 7, 729–738 (1987).

Buzsáki, G., Freund, T.F., Bayardo, F., and Somogyi, P. Ischemia-induced changes in the electrical activity of the hippocampus. *Exp. Brain Res.* 78, 268–278 (1989).

Buzsáki, G. and Traub, R.D. Physiological basis of EEG activity. In J. Engel, Jr., and T.A. Pedley (eds.), *Epilepsy. a comprehensive textbook*, Vol. 1. Lippincott-Raven: Philadelphia, 819–830 (1998).

Cain, D.P., Desborough, K.A., and McKitrick, D.J. Retardation of amygdala kindling by antagonism of NMDA-aspartate and muscarinic cholinergic receptors: evidence for summation of excitatory mechanisms in kindling. *Exp. Neurol.* 100, 179–187 (1988).

Calcagnotto, M.E., Barbarosie, M., and Avoli, M. Hippocampus-entorhinal cortex loop and seizure generation in the young rodent limbic system. *J. Neurophysiol.* 83, 3183–3187 (2000).

Calvin, W.H. Comments on human epileptic neurons. In G.G. Somjen (ed.), *Neurophysiology studies in man.* Excerpta Medica: Amsterdam, 110–111 (1972).

Calvin, W.H., Ojemann, G.A., and Ward, A.A. Human cortical neurons in epileptogenic foci: comparison of interictal firing patterns to those of "epileptic" neurons in animals. *Electroencephalogr. Clin. Neurophysiol.* 34, 337–351 (1973).

Calvin, W.H., Sypert, G.W., and Ward, A.A. Structured timing patterns within bursts from epileptic neurons in undrugged monkey cortex. *Exp. Neurol.* 21, 535–549 (1968).

Cancilla, P.A., Bready, J., and Berliner, J. Astrocyte-endothelial cell interactions. In S. Murphy (ed.), *Astrocytes*. Academic Press: San Diego, Calif., 383–397 (1993).

Cannon, W.B.A. A law of denervation. *Am. J. Med. Sci.* 198, 737 (1939).

Carmeliet, E. Cardiac ionic currents and acute ischemia: from channels to arrhythmias. *Physiol. Rev.* 79, 917–1017 (1999).

Carpenter, D.O., Hubbard, J.H., Humphrey, D.R., Thompson, H.K., and Marshall, W. Carbon dioxide effects on nerve cell function. In G. Nahas and K.E. Schaefer (eds.), *Carbon dioxide and metabolic regulation.* Springer: New York, 49–62 (1974).

Carpenter, M.B. and Sutin, J. *Human neuroanatomy.* Williams & Wilkins: Baltimore (1983).

Carriedo, S.G., Yin, H.Z., Sensi, S.L., and Weiss, J.H. Rapid Ca^{2+} entry through Ca^{2+}-permeable AMPA/kainate channels triggers marked intracellular Ca^{2+} rises and consequent oxygen radical production. *J. Neurosci.* 18, 7727–7738 (1998).

Carter, A.J., Grauert, M., Pschorn, U., Bechtel, W.D., Bartmann-Lindholm, C., Qu, Y., Scheuer, T., Catterall, W.A., and Weiser, T. Potent blockade of sodium channels and protection of brain tissue from ischemia by BIII 890 CL. *Proc. Natl. Acad. Sci. USA* 97, 4944–4949 (2000).

Casasola, C., Bargas, J., Arias-Montaño, J.-A., Calixto, E., Montiel, T., Galarraga, E., and Brailowsky, S. Hippocampal hyperexcitability induced by GABA withdrawal is due to down-regulation of $GABA_A$ receptors. *Epilepsy Res.* 47, 257–271 (2002).

Cassady, C.J., Phillis, J.W., and O'Regan, M.H. Further studies on the effects of topical lactate on amino acid efflux from the ischemic rat cortex. *Brain Res.* 901, 30–37 (2001).

Castellucci, V.F. and Goldring, S. Contribution to steady potential shifts of slow depolarization in cells presumed to be glia. *Electroencephalogr. Clin. Neurophysiol.* 28, 109–118 (1970).

Castro-Alamancos, M.A. and Connors, B.W. Short-term synaptic enhancement and long-term potentiation in neocortex. *Proc. Natl. Acad. Sci. USA* 93, 1335–1339 (1996).

Casullo, J. and Krnjević, K. Glial potentials in hippocampus. *Can. J. Physiol. Pharmacol.* 65, 847–855 (1987).

Cavazos, J.E., Das, J., and Sutula, T.P. Neuronal loss induced in limbic pathways by kindling: evidence for induction of hippocampal sclerosis by repeated brief seizures. *J. Neurosci.* 14, 3106–3121 (1994).

Cereghino, J.J. Flunarizine. In J. Engel, Jr., and T.A. Pedley (eds.), *Epilepsy: a comprehensive textbook*, Vol. 2. Lippincott-Raven: Philadelphia, 1515–1519 (1997).

Chamberlin, N.L. and Dingledine, R. GABAergic inhibition and the induction of spontaneous epileptiform activity by low chloride and high potassium in the hippocampal slice. *Brain Res.* 445, 12–18 (1988).

Chance, B., Cohen, P., Jöbsis, F., and Schoener, B. Intracellular oxidation-reduction states in vivo. *Science* 137, 499–508 (1962).

Chang, H.S., Sasaki, T., and Kassell, N.F. Hippocampal unit activity after transient cerebral ischemia in rats. *Stroke* 20, 1051–1058 (1989).

Chao, T.I. and Alzheimer, C. Do neurons from rat neostriatum express both a TTX-sensitive and a TTX-insensitive slow Na^+ current? *J. Neurophysiol.* 74, 934–941 (1995a).

Chao, T.I. and Alzheimer, C. Effects of phenytoin on the persistent Na current of mammalian CNS neurons. *NeuroReport* 6, 1778–1780 (1995b).

Chavez, J.C. and LaManna, J.C. Activation of hypoxia-inducible factor-1 in the rat cerebral cortex after transient global ischemia: potential role of insulin-like growth factor-1. *J. Neurosci.* 22, 8922–8931 (2002).

Chebabo, S.R., Do Carmo, R.J., and Martins-Ferreira, H. The effect of diphenylhydantoin on spreading depression. *Braz. J. Med. Biol. Res.* 21, 603–605 (1988).

Chebabo, S.R., Do Carmo, R.J., and Martins-Ferreira, H. Effects of local anaesthetics on retinal spreading depression. *Exp. Brain Res.* 96, 363–364 (1993).

Chebabo, S.R., Hester, M.A., Aitken, P.G., and Somjen, G.G. Hypotonic exposure enhances synaptic transmission and triggers spreading depression in hippocampal tissue slices. *Brain Res.* 695, 203–216 (1995a).

Chebabo, S.R., Hester, M.A., Jing, J., Aitken, P.G., and Somjen, G.G. Interstitial space, electrical resistance and ion concentrations during hypotonia of hippocampal slices of rats. *J. Physiol.* 487, 685–697 (1995b).

Chen, K.C. and Nicholson, C. Spatial buffering of potassium ions in brain extracellular space. *Biophys. J.* 78, 2776–2797 (2000).

Chen, Q., Chopp, M., Bodzin, G., and Chen, H. Temperature modulation of cerebral depolarization during focal cerebral ischemia in rats: correlation with ischemic injury. *J. Cereb. Blood Flow Metab.* 13, 389–394 (1993).

Cherubini, E., Ben-Ari, Y., and Krnjević, K. Anoxia produces smaller changes in synaptic transmission, membrane potential and input resistance in immature rat hippocampus. *J. Neurophysiol.* 62, 882–895 (1989).

Chesler, M. The regulation and modulation of the pH in the nervous system. *Progr. Neurobiol.* 34, 401–427 (1990).

Chesler, M. and Kraig, R.P. Intracellular pH of astrocytes increases rapidly with cortical stimulation. *Am. J. Physiol.* 253, R666–R670 (1987).

Chih, C.-P., Lipton, P., and Roberts, E.L. Do active cerebral neurons really use lactate rather than glucose? *Trends Neurosci.* 24, 573–578 (2001).

Chinard, F.P. Priestley and Lavoisier: oxygen and carbon dioxide. In D.F. Proctor (ed.), *A history of breathing.* Marcel Dekker: New York, 203–221 (1995).

Choi, D.W. and Rothman, S.M. The role of glutamate neurotoxicity in hypoxic-ischemic neuronal death. *Annu. Rev. Neurosci.* 13, 171–182 (1990).

Church, J. and Baimbridge, K.G. Exposure to high-pH medium increases the incidence and extent of dye coupling between rat hippocampal neurons in vitro. *J. Neurosci.* 11, 3289–3295 (1991).

Chvátal, A., Andêroivá, M., Ziak, D., Orkand, R.K., and Syková, E. Membrane currents and morphological properties of neurons and glial cells in the spinal cord and filum terminale of the frog. *Neurosci. Res.* 40, 23–35 (2001).

Chvátal, A., Pastor, A., Mauch, M., Syková, E., and Kettenmann, H. Distinct populations of identified glial cells in the developing rat spinal cord slice: ion chanel properties and cell korphology. *Eur. J. Neurosci.* 7, 129–142 (1995).

Clark, G.D. and Rothman, S.M. Blockade of excitatory amino acid receptors protects anoxic hippocampal slices. *Neuroscience* 21, 665–671 (1987).

Coenen, A.M.L., Blezer, E.H.M., and van Luijtelaar, E.L.J.M. Effects of the GABA-uptake inhibitor tiagabine on electroencephalogram, spike-wave discharges and behaviour of rats. *Epilepsy Res.* 21, 89–94 (1995).

Cohen, L.B. Changes in neuron structure during action potential propagation and synaptic transmission. *Physiol. Rev.* 53, 373–418 (1973).

Cohen, L.B., Keynes, R.D., and Landowne, D. Changes in light scattering that accompany the action potential in squid giant axons: potential-dependent component. *J. Physiol.* 224, 701–725 (1972).

Colbourne, F., Sutherland, G.R., and Auer, R.N. Electron microscopic evidence against apoptosis as the mechanism of neuronal death in global ischemia. *J. Neurosci.* 19, 4200–4210 (1999).

Collewijn, H. and Van Harreveld, A. Intracellular recording from cat spinal motoneurones during acute asphyxia. *J. Physiol.* 185, 1–14 (1966a).

Collewijn, H. and Van Harreveld, A. Membrane potential of cerebral cortical cells during spreading depression and asphyxia. *Exp. Neurol.* 15, 425–436 (1966b).

Collingridge, G.L. and Lester, R.A. Excitatory amino acid receptors in the vertebrate central nervous system. *Pharmacol. Rev.* 41, 143–210 (1989).

Colvin, R.A., Davis, N., Nipper, R.W., and Carter, P.A. Zinc transport in the brain: routes of zinc influx and efflux in neurons. *J. Nutr.* 130, 1484S–1487S (2000).

Congar, P., Leinekugel, X., Ben-Ari, Y., and Crépel, V. A long-lasting calcium-activated nonselective cationic current is generated by synaptic stimulation or exogenous activation of group I metabotropic glutamate receptors in CA1 pyramidal neurons. *J. Neurosci. Meth.* 17, 5366–5379 (1997).

Connors, B., Dray, A., Fox, P., Hilmy, M., and Somjen, G. LSD's effect on neuron populations in visual cortex gauged by transient responses of extracellular potassium evoked by optical stimuli. *Neurosci. Lett.* 13, 147–150 (1979).

Connors, B.W. *Physiological and pharmacological studies of the membrane properties of mammalian dorsal root ganglion cells.* Doctoral dissertation, Duke University, Durham, North Carolina (1979).

Connors, B.W. Initiation of synchronized bursting in neocortex. *Science* 310, 685–687 (1984).

Connors, B.W., Benardo, L.S., and Prince, D.A. Coupling between neurons of the developing rat neocortex. *J. Neurosci.* 3, 773–782 (1983).

Connors, B.W. and Gutnick, M.J. Cellular mechanisms of neocortical epileptogenesis in an acute experimental model. In P.A. Schwartzkroin and H.V. Wheal (eds.), *Electrophysiology of epilepsy.* Academic Press: London, 79–105 (1984).

Connors, B.W. and Gutnick, M.J. Intrinsic firing patterns of diverse neocortical neurons. *Trends Neurosci.* 13, 99–104 (1990).

Connors, B.W. and Telfeian, A.E. Dynamic properties of cells, synapses, circuits and seizures in neocortex. *Adv. Neurol.* 84, 141–152 (2002).

Contreras, D. and Steriade, M. Cellular basis of EEG slow rhythms: a study of dynamic corticothalamic relationships. *J. Neurosci.* 15, 504–622 (1995).

Coomes, M.W. Amino acid metabolism. In T.M. Devlin (ed.), *Textbook of biochemistry.* Wiley-Liss: New York, 779–823 (2002).

Cooper, E.C., Harrington, E., Jan, Y.N., and Jan, L.Y. M channel KCNQ2 subunits are localized to key sites for control of neuronal network oscillations and synchronization in mouse brain. *J. Neurosci.* 15, 9529–9540 (2001).

Corcoran, M.E., Armitage, L.L., Hannesson, D.K., Jenkins, E.M., and Mohapel, P. Dissociation between kindling and mossy fiber sprouting. In M.E. Corcoran and S.L. Moshé (eds.), *Kindling 5.* Plenum Press: New York, 211–222 (1998).

Cordingley, G.E. and Somjen, G.G. The clearing of excess potassium from extracellular space in spinal cord and cerebral cortex. *Brain Res.* 151, 291–306 (1978).

Cornell-Bell, A.H., Finkbeiner, S.M., Cooper, M.S., and Smith, S.J. Glutamate induces calcium waves in cultured astrocytes: long-range glial signalling. *Science* 247, 470–473 (1990).

Coulter, D.A. Thalamocortical anatomy and physiology. In J. Engel, Jr., and T.A. Pedley (eds.), *Epilepsy: a comprehensive textbook*, Vol. 1. Lippincott-Raven: Philadelphia, 341–351 (1998).

Coulter, D.A., Huguenard, J.R., and Prince, D.A. Characterization of ethosuximide reduction of low-threshold calcium current in thalamic neurons. *Ann. Neurol.* 25, 582–593 (1989).

Crain, B.J., Westerkam, W.D., Harrison, A.H., and Nadler, J.V. Selective neuronal death after transient forebrain ischemia in the mongolian gerbil: a silver impregnation study. *Neuroscience* 27, 387–402 (1988).

Crépel, V., Hammond, C., Chinestra, P., Diabira, D., and Ben-Ari, Y. A selective LTP of NMDA receptor-mediated currents induced by hypoxia in CA1 hippocampal neurons. *J. Neurophysiol.* 70, 2045–2055 (1993).

Crill, W.E. Persistent sodium current in mammalian central neurons. *Annu. Rev. Physiol.* 58, 349–362 (1996).

Croucher, M.J., Cotterell, K.L., and Bradford, H.F. Amygdaloid kindling by repeated focal *N*-methyl-D-aspartate administration: comparison with electrical kindling. *Eur. J. Pharmacol.* 286, 265–271 (1995).

Crunelli, V. and Leresche, N. Childhood absence epilepsy: genes, channels, neurons and networks. *Nature Rev. Neurosci.* 3, 371–382 (2002).

Cruz, N.F., Adachi, K., and Dienel, G.A. Rapid efflux of lactate from cerebral cortex during K^+-induced spreading cortical depression. *J. Cereb. Blood Flow Metab.* 19, 380–392 (1999).

Cserr, H.F. Relationship between cerebrospinal fluid and interstitial fluid of brain. *Fed. Proc.* 33, 2075–2078 (1974).

Cserr, H.F., DePasquale, M., Nicholson, C., Patlak, C.S., Pettigrew, K.D., and Rice, M.E. Extracellular volume decreases while cell volume is maintained by ion uptake in rat brain during acute hypernatremia. *J. Physiol.* 442, 277–295 (1991).

Cserr, H.F. and Patlak, C.S. Secretion and bulk flow of interstitial fluid. In M.W.B. Bradbury (ed.), *Physiology and pharmacology of the blood-brain barrier.* Springer: Berlin, 245–261 (1992).

Cummins, T.R., Donelly, D.F., and Haddad, G.G. Effects of metabolic inhibition on the excitability of isolated hippocampal CA1 neurons: developmental aspects. *J. Neurophysiol.* 66, 1471–1482 (1991).

Cummins, T.R., Jiang, C., and Haddad, G.G. Human neocortical excitability is decreased during anoxia via sodium channel modulation. *J. Clin. Invest.* 91, 608–615 (1993).

Curatolo, A., Marchetti, M., Salleo, A., and Brancati, A. Azione degli aminoacidi de-carbossilici sull'attività elettrica spontanea della corteccia cerebrale di gatto. *Arch. Sci. Biol.* 51, 89–97 (1967).

Czéh, G., Aitken, P.G., and Somjen, G.G. Whole cell patch clamp analysis of membrane changes during hypoxic and normoxic spreading depression in hippocampal CA1 pyramidal and glial cells. *Soc. Neurosci. Abstr.* 18, 1579 (1992).

Czéh, G., Aitken, P.G., and Somjen, G.G. Membrane currents in CA1 hippocampal cells during spreading depression (SD). and SD-like hypoxic depolarization. *Brain Res.* 632, 195–208 (1993).

Czéh, G., Obih, J.C., and Somjen, G.G. The effect of changing extracellular potassium concentration on synaptic transmission in isolated spinal cords. *Brain Res.* 446, 50–60 (1988).

Czéh, G. and Somjen, G.G. Changes in extracellular calcium and magnesium and synaptic transmission in isolated mouse spinal cord. *Brain Res.* 486, 274–285 (1989).

Czéh, G. and Somjen, G.G. Hypoxic failure of synaptic transmission in the isolated spinal cord, and the effects of divalent cations. *Brain Res.* 527, 224–233 (1990).

D'Ambrosio, R., Wenzel, J., Schwartzkroin, P.A., McKhann, G.M.I., and Janigro, D. Functional specialization and topographic segregation of hippocampal astrocytes. *J. Neurosci.* 18, 4425–4438 (1998).

Dalby, N.O. and Mody, I. The process of epileptogenesis: a pathophysiological approach. *Curr. Opin. Neurol.* 14, 187–192 (2001).

Dam, A.M. and Meencke, H.-J. Neuropathology of epilepsy. In H. Meinardi (ed.), *The epilepsies, part I.* Elsevier: Amsterdam, 107–121 (1999).

Dani, J.W., Chernjavsky, A., and Smith, S.J. Neuronal activity triggers calcium waves in hippocampal astrocyte networks. *Neuron* 8, 429–440 (1992).

Dani, J.W. and Smith, S.J. The triggering of astrocytic calcium waves by NMDA-induced neuronal activation. *CIBA Foundation Symp.* 188, 195–209 (1995).

Danober, L., Deransart, C., Depaulis, A., Vergnes, M., and Marescaux, C. Pathophysiological mechanisms of genetice absence epilepsy in the rat. *Prog. Neurobiol.* 55, 27–57 (1998).

David, R.J., Wilson, W.A., and Escueta, A.V. Voltage clamp analysis of pentylenetetrazol effects on *Aplysia* neurons. *Brain Res.* 67, 549–554 (1974).

Davies, N.W. Modulation of ATP-sensitive K^+ channels in skeletal muscle by intracellular protons. *Nature* 343, 375–377 (1990).

Davies, S.N., Lester, R.A.J., Reymann, K.G., and Collingridge, G.L. Temporally distinct pre- and postsynaptic mechanisms maintain long-term potentiation. *Nature* 338, 500–503 (1989).

Davson, H. and Segal, M.B. *Physiology of the CSF and blood-brain barriers*. CRC Press: Boca Raton, Fla. (1996).

Davydov, V.I. and Koroleva, V.I. [The modeling of the modes of propagation of SD waves in brain structures taking into account the nonuniform density of the active elements] (in Russian). *Zhurnal Vysshei Nervnoi Deiatelnosti Imani I.P. Pavlova* 43, 695–706 (1993).

de Curtis, M. and Avanzini, G. Interictal spikes in focal epileptogenesis. *Prog. Neurobiol.* 63, 541–567 (2001).

de Curtis, M., Manfridi, A., and Biella, G. Activity-dependent pH shifts and periodic recurrence of spontaneous interictal spikes in a model of focal epileptogenesis. *J. Neurosci.* 18, 7543–7551 (1998).

de Curtis, M., Radici, C., and Forti, M. Cellular mechanisms underlying spontaneous interictal spikes in an acute model of focal cortical epileptogenesis. *Neuroscience* 88, 107–117 (1999).

De Deyn, P.P., Marescau, B., and MacDonald, R.L. Epilepsy and the GABA-hypothesis: a brief review and some examples. *Acta Neurol. Belg.* 90, 65–81 (1990).

de Meduna, L. New methods of medical treatment of schizophrenia. *Arch. Neurol. Psychiatry* 35, 361–363 (1936).

Dean, J.B., Bayliss, D.A., Erickson, J.T., Lawing, W.L., and Millhorn, D.E. Depolarization and stimulation of neurons in nucleus tractus solitarii by carbon dioxide does not require chemical synaptic input. *Neuroscience* 36, 207–216 (1990).

Degen, R. A study of the diagnostic value of waking and sleep EEGs after sleep deprivation in epileptic patients on anticonvulsant therapy. *Electroencephalogr. Clin. Neurophysiol.* 49, 577–584 (1980).

DeGraba, T.J. and Pettigrew, I.C. Why do neuroprotective drugs work in animals but not in humans? *Stroke* 19, 475–493 (2000).

Deisz, R.A. A tetrodotoxin-insensitive sodium current initiates burst firing of neocortical neurons. *Neuroscience* 70, 341–351 (1996).

Deitmer, J.W. pH regulation. In H. Kettenmann and B.R. Ransom (eds.), *Neuroglia*. Oxford University Press: New York, 230–245 (1995).

Del Castillo, J. and Engbaek, L. Nature of the neuromuscular block by magnesium. *J. Physiol.* 124, 370–384 (1954).

Delgado, J.M.R. and Sevillano, M. Evolution of repeated hippocampal seizures in the cat. *Electroencephalogr. Clin. Neurophysiol.* 13, 722–733 (1961).

Dell, P., Hugelin, A., and Bonvallet, M. Effects of hypoxia on the reticular and cortical diffuse systems. In H. Gastaut and J.S. Meyer (eds.), *Cerebral anoxia and the electro-encephalogram.* Charles C. Thomas: Springfield, Ill., 46–58 (1961).

DeLorenzo, R.J. Clinical syndromes and epidemiology of status epilepticus. In H.O. Lüders and S. Noachtar (eds.), *Epileptic seizures: pathophysiology and clincial semiology.* Churchill Livingstone: New York, 697–710 (2000).

DeLorey, T.M. and Olsen, R.W. GABA and epileptogenesis: comparing gabrb3 gene-deficient mice with Angleman syndrome in man. *Epilepsy Res.* 36, 123–132 (1999).

Demir, R., Haberly, L.B., and Jackson, M.B. Voltage imaging of epileptiform activity in slices from rat piriform cortex: onset and propagation. *J. Neurophysiol.* 80, 2727–2742 (1998).

Dempsey, E.W. and Morison, R.S. The production of rhythmically recurrent cortical potentials after localized thalamic stimulation. *Am. J. Physiol.* 135, 293–300 (1942).

Deschenes, M., Feltz, P., and Lamour, Y. A model for an estimate in vivo of the ionic basis of presynaptic inhibition: an intracellular analysis of the GABA-induced depolarization in rat dorsal root ganglia. *Brain Res.* 118, 486–493 (1976).

Deshpande, J.K., Siesjö, B.K., and Wieloch, T. Calcium accumulation and neuronal damage in the rat hippocampus following cerebral ischemia. *J. Cereb. Blood Flow Metab.* 7, 89–95 (1987).

Destexhe, A. Spike-and-wave oscillations based on the properties of $GABA_B$ receptors. *J. Neurosci.* 18, 9099–9111 (1998).

Destexhe, A. Modelling corticothalamic feedback and the gating of the thalamus by the cerebral cortex. *J. Physiol. (Paris)* 94, 391–410 (2000).

Dichter, M. and Spencer, W.A. Penicillin-induced interictal discharges from the cat hippocampus. II. Mechanisms underlying origin and restriction. *J. Neurophysiol.* 32, 663–687 (1969).

Dichter, M.A., Herman, C.J., and Selzer, M. Silent cells during interictal discharges and seizures in hippocampal penicillin foci. Evidence for the role of extracellular K^+ in the transition from the interictal state to seizures. *Brain Res.* 48, 173–183[1](1972).

Diemer, N.H., Johansen, F.F., and Jorgensen, M.B. *N*-methyl-D-aspartate and non-*N*-methyl-D-aspartate antagonists in global cerebral ischemia. *Stroke* 21(Suppl)., III–39–III-42 (1990).

Dietzel, I. and Heinemann, U. Dynamic variations of the brain cell microenvironment in relation to neuronal hyperactivity. *Ann. N.Y. Acad. Sci.* 481, 72–85 (1986).

Dietzel, I., Heinemann, U., Hofmeier, G., and Lux, H.-D. Transient changes in the size of extracellular space in the sensorimotor cortex of cats in relation to stimulus-induced changes in potassium concentration. *Exp. Brain Res.* 40, 432–439 (1980).

Dietzel, I., Heinemann, U., Hofmeier, G., and Lux, H.-D. Stimulus-induced changes in extracellular Na^+ and Cl^- concentration in relation to changes in the size of the extracellular space. *Exp. Brain Res.* 46, 73–84 (1982).

Dietzel, I., Heinemann, U., and Lux, H.D. Relations between slow extracellular potential changes, glial potassium buffering and electrolyte and cellular volume changes during neuronal hyperactivity in cat brain. *Glia* 2, 25–44 (1989).

Dijkhuizen, R.M., Beekwilder, J.P., van der Worp, H.B., Berkelbach van der Sprenkel, J.W., Tulleken, K.A., and Nicolay, K. Correlation between tissue depolarizations and damage in focal ischemic rat brain. *Brain Res.* 840, 194–205 (1999).

Dingledine, R., Borges, K., Bowie, D., and Traynelis, S.F. The glutamate receptor ion channels. *Pharmacol. Rev.* 51, 7–61 (1999).

Dingledine, R., Dodd, J., and Kelly, J.S. The in vitro brain slice as a useful neurophysiological preparation for intracellular recording. *J. Neurosci. Meth.* 2, 323–362 (1980).

Dingledine, R. and Somjen, G.G. Calcium dependence of synaptic transmission in the hippocampal slice. *Brain Res.* 207, 218–222 (1981).

Dinner, D.S. and Lüders, H.O. Electrical stimulation of cortical language areas. In H.O. Lüders and S. Noachtar (eds.), *Epileptic seizures: pathophysiology and clinical semiology.* Churchill Livingstone: New York, 211–217 (1998).

Dirnagl, U., Iadecola, C., and Moskowitz, M.A. Pathobiology of ischaemic stroke: an integrated view. *Trends Neurosci.* 22, 391–397 (1999).

Dittman, J.S. and Regehr, W.G. Calcium dependence and recovery kinetics of presynaptic depression at the climbing fiber to Purkinje cell synapse. *J. Neurosci.* 18, 6147–6162 (1998).

Do Carmo, R.J. and Leão, A.A.P. On the relation of glutamic acid and some allied compounds to cortical spreading depression. *Brain Res.* 39, 515–518 (1972).

Do Carmo, R.J. and Martins-Ferreira, H. Spreading depression of Leão probed with ion-selective microelectrodes in isolated chick retina. *An. Acad. Bras. Cienc.* 56, 401–421 (1984).

Doherty, J. and Dingledine, R. Regulation of excitatory input to inhibitory interneurons of the dentate gyrus during hypoxia. *J. Neurophysiol.* 77, 393–404 (1997).

Dreier, J.P., Kleeberg, J., Petzold, G., Priller, J., Windmüller, O., Orzechowski, H.-D., Lindauer, U., Heinemann, U., Einhäupl, K.M., and Dirnagl, U. Endothelin-1 potently induces Leão's cortical spreading depression *in vivo* in the rat. A model for an endothelial trigger of migrainous aura? *Brain* 125, 102–112 (2002).

Drejer, J., Benveniste, H., Diemer, N.H., and Schousboe, A. Cellular origin of ischemia-induced glutamate release from brain tissue in vivo and in vitro. *J. Neurochem.* 45, 145–151 (1985).

Drouin, H. and The, R. The effect of reducing extracellular pH on the membrane current of the Ranvier node. *Pflügers Arch.* 313, 80–88 (1969).

Duchen, L.W. General pathology of neurons and neuroglia. In J.H. Adams and L.W. Duchen (eds.), *Greenfield's neuropathology.* Oxford University Press: New York, 1–68 (1992a).

Duchen, M.R. Effects of metabolic inhibition on the membrane properties of isolated mouse primary sensory neurones. *J. Physiol.* 424, 387–409 (1990).

Duchen, M.R. Ca^{2+}-dependent changes in the mitochondrial energetics in single dissociated mouse sensory neurons. *Biochem. J.* 283, 41–50 (1992b).

Duchen, M.R. Contributions of mitochondria to animal physiology: from homeostatic sensor to calcium signalling and cell death. *J. Physiol.* 516, 1–17 (1999).

Duchen, M.R. Mitochondria and calcium: from cell signalling to cell death. *J. Physiol.* 529, 57–68 (2000).

Duchen, M. R. and Somjen, G. Effects of cyanide and low glucose on the membrane currents of dissociated mouse primary sensory neurones. *J. Physiol.* 401, 61P (1988).

Dudek, F.E., Andrew, R.D., MacVicar, B.A., Snow, R.W., and Taylor, C.P. Recent evidence for, and possible significance of, gap junctions and electrotonic synapses in the mammalian brain. In H.H. Jasper and N.M van Gelder (eds.), *Basic mechanisms of neuronal hyperexcitability.* Alan R Liss: New York, 31–73 (1983).

Dudek, F.E., Obenaus, A., and Tasker, J.G. Osmolality-induced changes in extracellular volume alter epileptiform bursts independently of chemical synapses in the rat: importance of non-synaptic mechanisms in hippocampal epileptogenesis. *Neurosci. Lett.* 120, 267–270 (1990).

Dudek, F.E., Snow, R.E., and Taylor, C.P. Role of electrical interactions in synchronization of epileptiform bursts. *Adv. Neurol.* 44, 593–617 (1986).

Duffy, S., Fraser, D.D., and MacVicar, B.A. Potassium channels. In H. Kettenmann and B.R. Ransom (eds.), *Neuroglia*. Oxford University Press: New York, 185–201 (1995).

Duffy, S. and MacVicar, B.A. Voltage-dependent ionic channels in astrocytes. In S. Murphy (ed.), *Astrocytes: pharmacology and function*. Academic Press: San Diego, Calif., 137–169 (1993).

During, M.J., Fried, I., Leone, P., Katz, A., and Spencer, D.D. Direct measurement of extracellular lactate in the human hippocampus during spontaneous seizures. *J. Neurochem.* 62, 2356–2361 (1994).

During, M.J. and Spencer, D.D. Extracellular hippocampal glutamate and spontaneous seizure in the conscious human brain. *Lancet* 341, 1607–1610 (1993).

Dürmüller, N., Craggs, M., and Meldrum, B.S. The effecrt of the non-NMDA receptor antagonists GYKI 52466 and NBQX and the competitive NMDA receptor antagonist D-CPPene on the development of amygdala kindling and on amygdala-kindled seizures. *Epilepsy Res.* 17, 167–174 (1994).

Dux, E., Mies, G., Hossmann, K.-A., and Siklós, L. Calcium in the mitochondria following brief ischemia of gerbil brain. *Neurosci. Lett.* 78, 295–300 (1987).

Ebine, Y., Fujiwara, N., and Shimoji, K. Mild acidosis inhibits the rise in intracellular Ca^{2+} concentration in response to oxygen-glucose deprivation in rat hippocampal slices. *Neurosci. Lett.* 168, 155–158 (1994).

Eccles, J.C. *The neurophysiological basis of mind*. Clarendon: Oxford (1953).

Eccles, J.C. *The physiology of synapses*. Springer: New York (1964).

Eccles, J.C., Llinas, R., and Sasaki, K. The excitatory synaptic action of climbing fibers on the Purkinje cells of the cerebellum. *J. Physiol.* 182, 268–296 (1966a).

Eccles, R.M., Löyning, Y., and Oshima, T. Effects of hypoxia on the monosynaptic reflex pathway in the cat spinal cord. *J. Neurophysiol.* 29, 315–332 (1966b).

Ehrlich, P. *Das Sauerstoff-Bedürfniss Des Organismus. Eine Farbenanalytische Studie. Hirschwald.* Reprinted in *Collected papers*, Vol. 1, Pergamon Press: London, 364–342; English translation, 433–496, Berlin (1885).

Els, T., Rother, J., Beaulieu, C., de Crespigny, A., and Moseley, M. Hyperglycemia delays terminal depolarization and enhances repolarization after peri-infarct spreading depression as measured by serial diffusion MR mapping. *J. Cereb. Blood Flow Metab.* 17, 591–595 (1997).

Engel, A.K., Fries, P., König, P., Brecht, M., and Singer, W. Temporal binding, binocular rivalry and consciousness. *Consciousness Cognition* 8, 128–151 (1999).

Engel, A.K., Fries, P., and Singer, W. Dynamic predictions: oscillations and synchrony in top-down processing. *Nature Rev. Neurosci.* 2, 704–716 (2001).

Engel, J., Jr. Research on the human brain in an epilepsy surgery setting. *Epilepsy Res.* 32, 1–11 (1998a).

Engel, J., Jr. The syndrome of mesial temporal lobe epilepsy: A role for kindling. In M.E. Corcoran and S.L. Moshé (eds.), *Kindling 5*. Plenum Press: New York, 469–480 (1998b).

Engel, J., Jr. So what can we conclude—do seizures damage the brain? In T. Sutula and A. Pitkänen (eds.), *Do seizures damage the brain?* Elsevier: Amsterdam, 509–512 (2002).

Engel, J., Jr. and Ackerman, R.F. Interictal EEG spikes correlate with decreased, rather than increased, epileptogenicity in amygdaloid kindled rats. *Brain Res.* 190, 543–548 (1980).

Engel, J., Jr., Driver, M.V., and Falconer, M.A. Electrophysiological correlates of pathology and surgical results in temporal lobe epilepsy. *Brain* 98, 129–156 (1975).

Engel, J., Jr. and Pedley, T.A. Introduction: What is epilepsy? In J. Engel, Jr., and T.A. Pedley (eds.), *Epilepsy: a comprehensive textbook*, Vol. 1. Lippincott-Raven: Philadelphia, 1–7 (1998a).

Engel, J., Jr., and Pedley, T.A. (eds.). *Epilepsy. a comprehensive textbook*. Lippincott-Raven: Philadelphia (1998b).

Engel, J., Jr., Williamson, P.D., and Wieser, H.-G. Mesial temporal lobe epilepsy. In J. Engel, Jr., and T.A. Pedley (eds.), *Epilepsy. a comprehensive textbook*, Vol. 3. Lippincott-Raven: Philadelphia, 2417–2426 (1998c).

Enkvist, M.O. and McCarthy, K.D. Astroglial gap junction communication is increased by treatment with either glutamate or high K^+ concentration. *J. Neurochem.* 62, 489–495 (1994).

Erdemli, G., Xu, Y.Z., and Krnjević, K. Potassium conductance causing hyperpolarization of CA1 hippocampal neurons during hypoxia. *J. Neurophysiol.* 80, 2378–2390 (1998).

Erlanger, J. and Gasser, H.S. *Electrical signs of nervous activity.* University of Pennsylvania Press: Philadelphia (1937).

Erulkar, S.D., Dambach, G.E., and Mender, D. The effect of magnesium at motoneurons of the isolated spinal cord of the frog. *Brain Res.* 66, 413–424 (1974).

Escayg, A., De Waard, M., Lee, D.D., Bichet, D., Wolf, P., Mayer, T., Johnston, J., Baloh, R., Sander, T., and Meisler, M.H. Coding and noncoding variation of the human calcium-channel β_4-subunit gene CACNB4 in patients with idiopathic generalized epilepsy and episodic ataxia. *Am. J. Hum. Genet.* 66, 1531–1539 (2000).

Esclapez, M., Hirsch, J.C., Ben-Ari, Y., and Bernard, C. Newly formed excitatory pathways provide a substrate for hyperexcitability in experimental temporal lobe epilepsy. *J. Comp. Neurol.* 408, 449–460 (1999).

Faber, D.S. and Korn, H. Electrical field effects: their relevance in central neural networks. *Physiol. Rev.* 69, 821–863 (1989).

Fabricius, M., Jensen, L.H., and Lauritzen, M. Microdialysis of interstitial amino acids during spreading depression and anoxic depolarization in rat neocortex. *Brain Res.* 612, 61–69 (1993).

Farber, J.L., Chien, K.R., and Mittnacht, S., Jr. The pathogenesis of irreversible cell injury in ischemia. *Am. J. Pathol.* 102, 271–281 (1981).

Fawcett, W.J., Haxby, E.J., and Male, D.A. Magnesium: physiology and pharmacology. *Br. J. Anaesth.* 83, 302–320 (1999).

Fayuk, D., Aitken, P.G., Somjen, G.G., and Turner, D.A. Dissociation of interstitial volume changes and intrinsic optical signals during normoxic spreading depression in hippocampal slices with low Cl^- and hypertonia. *Soc. Neurosci. Abstr.* 25, 743 (1999).

Fayuk, D., Aitken, P.G., Somjen, G.G., and Turner, D.A. Two different mechanisms underlie reversible intrinsic optical signals in rat hippocampal slices. *J. Neurophysiol.* 87, 1924–1937 (2002).

Fayuk, D., Margraf, R.R., and Turner, D.A. NADH fluorescence and intrinsic optical signal imaging during hypoxic spreading depression in rat hippocampal slices. *Soc. Neurosci. Abstr.* 26, 243 (2000).

Feldberg, W. and Sherwood, S.L. Effects of calcium and potassium injected into the cerebral ventricles of the cat. *J. Physiol.* 139, 408–416 (1957).

Fencl, V. Distribution of H^+ and HCO_3^- in cerebral fluids. In B.K. Siesjö and S.C. Sörensen (eds.), *Ion homeostasis of the brain*. Academic Press: New York, 175–185 (1971).

Fencl, V., Miller, T.B., and Pappenheimer, J.R. The respiratory response to disturbances of acid-base balance, with deductions concerning the ionic composition of cerebral interstitial fluid. In W.F. Caveness and A.E. Walker (eds.), *Head injury*. J.B. Lippincott: Philadelphia, 414–430 (1966).

Feng, Z.-C., Roberts, E.L., Sick, T.J., and Rosenthal, M. Depth profile of local oxygen tension and blood flow in rat cerebral cortex, white matter and hippocampus. *Brain Res.* 445, 280–288 (1988).

Fernandes de Lima, V.M., Goldermann, M., and Hanke, W.R.L. Calcium waves in gray matter are due to voltage-sensitive glial membrane channels. *Brain Res.* 663, 77–83 (1994).

Ferreira-Filho, C.R. and Martins-Ferreira, H. Electrical impedance of isolated retina and its changes during spreading depression. *Neuroscience* 7, 3231–3239 (1982).

Fertziger, A.P. and Ranck, J.B. Potassium accumulation in interstitial space during epi-leptiform seizures. *Exp. Neurol.* 26, 571–585 (1970).

ffrench-Mullen, J.M., Barker, J.L., and Rogawski, M.A. Calcium current block by (−)-pentobarbital, phenobarbital and CHEB but not by (+)-pentobarbital in acutely iso-lated hippocampal CA1 neurons: comparison with effects in GABA-activated Cl⁻ cur-rent. *J. Neurosci.* 13, 3211–3221 (1993).

Fill, M. and Copello, J.A. Ryanodine receptor calcium release channels. *Physiol. Rev.* 82, 893–922 (2002).

Fillenz, M., Demestre, M., Fellows, L.K., Berenrs, M.O.M., and Boutelle, M.G. The source of metabolic substrates for neuronal energy metabolism. In A. Teelken and J. Korf (eds.), *Neurochemistry*. Plenum Press: New York, 561–569 (1997).

Finger, S. *Minds behind the brain*. Oxford University Press: New York (2000).

Fink-Jensen, A., Suzdak, P.D., Swedberg, M.D., Judge, M.E., Hansen, L., and Nielsen, P.G. The gamma-aminobutyric acid (GABA) uptake inhibitor, tiagabine, increases extracel-lular brain levels of GABA in awake rats. *Eur. J. Pharmacol.* 220, 197–201 (1992).

Finkbeiner, S. Calcium waves in astrocytes—filling in the gaps. *Neuron* 8, 1101–1108 (1992).

Flatman, P.W. Mechanisms of magnesium transport. *Annu. Rev. Physiol.* 53, 259–271 (1991).

Flint, A.C. and Connors, B.W. Two types of network oscillations in neocortex mediated by distinct glutamate receptor subtypes and neuronal populations. *J. Neurophysiol.* 75, 951–962 (1996).

Foerster, O. Hyperventilationsepilepsie. *Deut. Z. Nervenheilk.* 83, 347–356 (1924).

Forsythe, I.D. and Redman, S.J. The dependence of motoneurone membrane potential on extracellular ion concentrations studied in isolated rat spinal cord. *J. Physiol.* 404, 83–99 (1988).

Fowler, J.C. Adenosine antagonists delay hypoxia-induced depression of neuronal activ-ity in hippocampal brain slice. *Brain Res.* 490, 378–384 (1989).

Frankenhaeuser, B. and Hodgkin, A.L. The after-effects of impulses in the giant nerve fibers of Loligo. *J. Physiol.* 131, 341–376 (1956).

Fraser, D.D. and MacVicar, B.A. Cholinergic-dependent plateau potential in hippocam-pal CA1 pyramidal neurons. *J. Neurosci.* 16, 4113–4128 (1996).

Frederickson, C.J. and Bush, A.I. Synaptically released zinc: physiological functions and pathological effects. *BioMetals* 14, 353–366 (2001).

Frederickson, C.J., Suh, S.W., Silva, D., Frederickson, C.A.J., and Thompson, R.B. Im-portance of zinc in the central nervous system: the zinc-containing neuron. *J. Nutr.* 130, 1471S–1483S (2000).

French, C.R., Sah, P., Buckett, K.J., and Gage, P.W. A voltage-dependent persistent so-dium current in mammalian hippocampal neurons. *J. Gen. Physiol.* 95, 1139–1157 (1990).

Frenguelli, B.G. The effects of metabolic stress on glutamate receptor-mediated depolarizations in the in vitro rat hippocampal slice. *Neuropharmacology* 36, 981–991 (1997).

Freund, T.F., Buzsáki, G., Leon, A., Baimbridge, K.G., and Somogyi, P. Relationship of neuronal vulnerability and calcium binding protein immunoreactivity in ischemia. *Exp. Brain Res.* 83, 55–66 (1990a).

Freund, T.F., Buzsáki, G., Leon, A., and Somogyi, P. Hippocampal cell death following ischemia: effects of brain temperature and anesthesia. *Exp. Neurol.* 108, 251–260 (1990b).

Freygang, W.H. and Landau, W.M. Some relations between resistivity and electrical activity in the cerebral cortex of the cat. *J. Cell. Comp. Physiol.* 45, 377–392 (1955).

Fridovich, I. Hypoxia and oxygen toxicity. *Adv. Neurol.* 26, 255–259 (1979).

Friedman, J.E. and Haddad, G.G. Major differences in Ca^{2+}_i response to anoxia between neonatal and adult rat CA1 neurons: role of Ca^{2+}_o and Na^+_o. *J. Neurosci.* 13, 63–72 (1993).

Friedman, J.E. and Haddad, G.G. Removal of extracellular sodium prevents anoxia-induced injury in freshly dissociated rat CA1 hippocampal neurons. *Brain Res.* 641, 57–64 (1994).

Fritsch, G. and Hitzig, E. Über die elektrische Erregbarkeit des Grosshirns. *Arch. Anat. Physiol. Wissensch. Med.* 37, 300–332 (1870).

Fujimura, N., Tanaka, E., Yamamoto, S., Shigemori, M., and Higashi, H. Contribution of ATP-sensitive potassium channels to hypoxic hyperpolarization in rat hippocampal CA1 neurons in vitro. *J. Neurophysiol.* 77, 378–385 (1997).

Furshpan, E.J. and Potter, D.D. Seizure-like activity and cellular damage in rat hippocampal neurons in cell culture. *Neuron* 3, 199–207 (1989).

Futamachi, K.J., Mutani, R., and Prince, D.A. Potassium activity in rabbit cortex. *Brain Res.* 75, 5–25 (1974).

Galeffi, F., Sinnar, S., and Schwartz-Bloom, R.D. Diazepam promotes ATP recovery and prevents cytochrome c release in hippocampal slices after in vitro ischemia. *J. Neurochem.* 75, 1242–1249 (2000).

Gao, T.M., Howard, E.M., and Xu, Z.C. Transient neurophysiological changes in CA3 neurons and dentate granule cells after severe forebrain ischemia in vivo. *J. Neurophysiol.* 80, 2860–2869 (1998a).

Gao, T.M., Pulsinelli, W.A., and Xu, Z.C. Prolonged enhancement and depression of synaptic transmission in CA1 pyramidal neurons induced by transient forebrain ischemia *in vivo*. *Neuroscience* 87, 371–383 (1998b).

Gao, T.M., Pulsinelli, W.A., and Xu, Z.C. Changes in membrane properties of CA1 pyramidal neurons after transient forebrain ischemia *in vivo*. *Neuroscience* 90, 771–780 (1999).

García, J.L. and Anderson, M.L. Circulatory disorders and their effects on the brain. In R.L. Davis and D.M. Robertson (eds.), *Textbook of neuropathology*. Williams & Wilkins: Baltimore, 715–822 (1997).

García Ramos, J. Ionic movements in the isolated chicken retina during spreading depression. *Acta Physiol. Latinoam.* 25, 112–119 (1975).

García Ramos, J. and de la Cerda, E. On the ionic nature of the slow potential and impedance changes of spreading depression. *Acta Physiol. Latinoam.* 24, 216–227 (1974).

Gardiner, R.M. Genetic basis of the human epilepsies. *Epilepsy Res.* 36, 91–95 (1999).

Gardner-Medwin, A.R. Possible roles of vertebrate neuroglia in potassium dynamics, spreading depression and migraine. *J. Exp. Biol.* 95, 111–127 (1981).

Gardner-Medwin, A.R. A study of the mechanisms by which potassium moves through brain tissue in the rat. *J. Physiol.* 335, 353–374 (1983).

Gardner-Medwin, A.R. and Mutch, W.A.C. Experiments on spreading depression in relation to migraine and neurosurgery. *An. Acad. Bras. Cienc.* 56, 423–430 (1984).

Gardner-Medwin, A.R. and Nicholson, C. Changes of extracellular potassium activity induced by electric current through brain tissue in the rat. *J. Physiol.* 335, 375–392 (1983).

Garthwaite, G., Brown, G., Batchelor, A.M., Goodwin, D.A., and Garthwaite, J. Mechanisms of ischaemic damage to central white matter axons: a quantitative histological analysis using rat optic nerve. *Neuroscience* 94, 1219–1230 (1999).

Gastaut, H. and Broughton, R. *Epileptic seizures: clinical and electrographic features, diagnosis and treatment.* C.C. Thomas: Springfield, Ill. (1972).

Gebhardt, C., Körner, R., and Heinemann, U. Delayed anoxic depolarization in hippocampal neurons of mice lacking the excitatory amino acid carrier 1. *J. Cereb. Blood Flow Metab.* 22, 569–575 (2002).

Geinisman, Y., Morrell, F., de Toledo-Morrell, L., Persina, I.S., and Van der Zee, E.S. Comparison of synapse remodeling following hippocampal kindling and long-term potentiation. In M.E. Corcoran and S.L. Moshé (eds.), *Kindling 5.* Plenum Press: New York, 179–191 (1998).

Gerard, R.W. The response of nerve to oxygen lack. *Am. J. Physiol.* 92, 498–541 (1930).

Giacchino, J.L., Somjen, G.G., Frush, D.P., and McNamara, J.O. Lateral entorhinal cortical kindling can be established without potentiation of the entorhinal-granule cell synapse. *Exp. Neurol.* 86, 483–492 (1984).

Giaretta, D., Kostopoulos, G., Gloor, P., and Avoli, M. Intracortical inhibitory mechanisms are preserved in feline generalized penicillin epilepsy. *Neurosci. Lett.* 59, 203–208 (1985).

Gibbs, F.A., Davis, H., and Lennox, W.G. Electroencephalogram in epilepsy and in conditions of impaired consciousness. *Arch. Neurol. Psychiatry* 34, 1133–1148 (1935).

Gibbs, F.A. and Gibbs, E.L. The convulsion threshold of various parts of the cat brain. *Arch. Neurol. Psychiatry* 35, 109–116 (1936).

Gibbs, J.W., Zhang, Y.F., Ahmed, H.S., and Coulter, D.A. Anticonvulsant action of lamotrigine on spontaneous thalamocortical rhythms. *Epilepsia* 43, 342–349 (2002).

Gibson, J.R., Beierlein, M., and Connors, B.W. Two networks of electrically coupled inhibitory neurons in neocortex. *Nature* 402, 75–79 (1999).

Gidö, G., Kristián, T., and Siesjö, B.K. Induced spreading depressions in energy-compromised neocortical tissue: calcium transients and histopathological correlates. *Neurobiol. Dis.* 1, 31–41 (1994).

Gillardon, F., Kiprianova, I., Sandkühler, J., Hossman, K.-A., and Spranger, M. Inhibition of caspases prevents cell death of hippocampal CA1 neurons, but not impairment of long-term potentiation following global ischemia. *Neuroscience* 93, 1219–1222 (1999).

Gjedde, A., Hansen, A.J., and Quistorff, B. Blood-brain glucose transfer in spreading depression. *J. Neurochem.* 37, 807–812 (1981).

Glaum, S.R., Holzwarth, J.A., and Miller, R.J. Glutamate receptors activate Ca^{2+} mobilization and Ca^{2+} influx into astrocytes. *Proc. Natl. Acad. Sci. USA* 87, 3454–3458 (1990).

Gloor, P. Generalized cortico-reticular epilepsies. Some considerations on the pathophysiology of generalized bilaterally synchronous spike and wave discharges. *Epilepsia* 9, 249–263 (1968).

Gloor, P. Hans Berger on the electroencephalogram of man. *Electroenceph. Clin. Neurophysiol.* Suppl. 28 (1969).

Gloor, P. Electrophysiology of generalized epilepsy. In P.A. Schwartzkroin and H.V. Wheal (eds.), *Electrophysiology of epilepsy.* Academic Press: London, 107–136 (1984).

Gloor, P. *The temporal lobe and limbic system.* Oxford University Press: New York (1997).

Gloor, P. and Fariello, R.G. Generalized epilepsy: some of its cellular mechanisms differ from those of focal epilepsy. *Trends Neurosci.* 11, 63–68 (1988).

Gloor, P., Sperti, L., and Vera, C.L. A consideration of feedback mechanisms in the genesis and maintenance of hippocampal seizure activity. *Epilepsia* 5, 213–238 (1964).

Gloor, P., Vera, C.L., Sperti, L., and Ray, S.N. Investigation on the mechanism of epileptic discharge in the hippocampus. *Epilepsia* 2, 42–62 (1961).

Gloor, S.M., Wachtel, M., Bolliger, M.F., Ishihara, H., Landmann, R., and Frei, K. Molecular and cellular permeability control at the blood-brain barrier. *Brain Res. Rev.* 36, 258–264 (2001).

Glötzner, F. Intracelluläre Potentiale, EEG und kortikale Gleichspannung an der sensorimotorischen Rinde der Katze bei akuter Hypoxie. *Arch. Psychiatr. Nervenkr.* 210, 274–296 (1967).

Glötzner, F. Membrane properties of neuroglia in epileptogenic gliosis. *Brain Res.* 55, 159–171 (1973).

Glötzner, F. and Grüsser, O.-J. Membranpotential und Entladungsfolgen corticaler Zellen, EEG und corticales DC-Potential bei generalisierten Krampfanfällen. *Arch. Psychiatr. Neurol.* 210, 313–339 (1968).

Gluckman, B.J., Neel, E.J., Netoff, T.I., Ditto, W.L., Spano, M.L., and Schiff, S.J. Electric field suppression of epileptiform activity in hippocampal slices. *J. Neurophysiol.* 76, 4202–4205 (1996).

Goddard, G.V. Development of epileptic seizures through brain stimulation at low intensity. *Nature* 214, 1020–1021 (1967).

Goddard, G.V. The kindling model of epilepsy. *Trends Neurosc.* 6, 275–279 (1983).

Goldberg, M.P. and Choi, D.W. Combined oxygen and glucose deprivation in cortical cell culture: calcium-dependent and calcium-independent mechanisms of neuronal injury. *J. Neurosci.* 13, 3510–3524 (1993).

Goldensohn, E.S. Experimental seizure mechanisms. In H.H. Jasper, A.A. Ward, and A. Pope (eds.), *Basic mechanisms of the epilepsies.* Little, Brown: Boston, 289–298 (1969).

Goldmann, E.E. Die äussere und innere Sekretion des gesunden und kranken Organismus im Lichte der "vitalen Farbung." *Beitr. Klin. Chirurg.* 64, 192–265 (1909).

Goldmann, E.E. Vitalfärbung am Zentralnervensystem. *Abhandl. Preuss. Akad. Wiss. Phys. Math. Kl.* 1, 1–60 (1913).

Gordon, L.M. and Sauerheber, R.D. Calcium and membrane stability. In L.J. Anghileri, and A.M. Tuffet-Anghileri (eds.), *The role of calcium in biological systems.* CRC Press: Boca Raton, Fla., 3–16 (1982).

Gorji, A. Spreading depression: a review of the clinical relevance. *Brain Res. Rev.* 38, 33–60 (2001).

Gorji, A., Madeja, M., Straub, H., Köhling, R., and Speckmann, E.-J. Lowering of the potassium concentration induces epileptiform activity in guinea pig hippocampal slices. *Brain Res.* 908, 130–139 (2001).

Gorter, J.A., Petrozzino, J.J., Aronica, E.M., Rosenbaum, D.M., Opitz, T., Bennett, M.V.L., Connor, J.A., and Zukin, R.S. Global ischemia induces downregulation of Glur2 mRNA and increases AMPA receptor-mediated Ca^{2+} influx in hippocampal CA1 neurons of gerbil. *J. Neurosci.* 17, 6179–6188 (1997).

Gotman, J. Relationship between interictal spiking and seizures: human and experimental evidence. *Can. J. Neurol. Sci.* 18, 573–576 (1991).

Gouras, P. Spreading depression of activity in amphibian retina. *Am. J. Physiol.* 195, 28–32 (1958).

Grabb, M.C. and Choi, D.W. Ischemic tolerance in murine cortical cell culture: critical role for NMDA receptors. *J. Neurosci.* 19, 1657–1662 (1999).

Grafstein, B. Locus of propagation of spreading cortical depression. *J. Neurophysiol.* 19, 308–316 (1956a).

Grafstein, B. Mechanism of spreading cortical depression. *J. Neurophysiol.* 19, 154–171 (1956b).

Grafstein, B. Neuronal release of potassium during spreading depression. In M.A.B. Brazier (eds.), *Brain function: Cortical Excitability and Steady Potentials.* University of California Press: Berkeley, 87–124 (1963).

Graham, D.I. Hypoxia and vascular disorders. In J.H. Adams and L.W. Duchen (eds.), *Greenfield's neuropathology.* Oxford University Press: New York, 153–268 (1992).

Grant, S.B. and Goldman, A. A study of forced respiration: experimental production of tetany. *Am. J. Physiol.* 52, 209–232 (1920).

Green, J.D. The hippocampus. *Physiol. Rev.* 44, 561–608 (1964).

Grichtchenko, I.I. and Chesler, M. Depolarization induced alkalinization of astrocytes in gliotic hippocampal tissue. *Neuroscience* 62, 1071–1078 (1994).

Grichtchenko, I.I. and Chesler, M. Calcium- and barium-dependent extracellular alkaline shifts evoked by electrical activity in rat hippocampal slices. *Neuroscience* 75, 1117–1126 (1996).

Grundfest, H. Electrical inexcitability of synapses and some consequences in the central nervous system. *Physiol. Rev.* 37, 337–361 (1957).

Guillemin, K. and Krasnow, M.A. The hypoxic response: huffing and HIFing. *Cell* 89, 9–12 (1997).

Gullans, S.R. and Verbalis, J.G. Control of brain volume during hyperosmolar and hypoosmolar conditions. *Annu. Rev. Med.* 44, 289–301 (1993).

Gumnit, R.J. and Takahashi, T. Changes in direct current activity during experimental focal seizures. *Electroencephalogr. Clin. Neurophysiol.* 19, 63–74 (1965).

Gunter, T.E., Gunter, K.K., Sheu, S.-S., and Gavin, C.E. Mitochondrial calcium transport: physiological and pathological relevance. *Am. J. Physiol.* 267, C313–C339 (1994).

Gutnick, M.J., Connors, B.W., and Prince, D.A. Mechanisms of neocortical epileptogenesis in vitro. *J. Neurophysiol.* 48, 1321–1335 (1982).

Gutnick, M.J., Connors, B.W., and Ransom, B.R. Dye-coupling between glial cells in the guinea pig neocortical slice. *Brain Res.* 213, 486–492 (1981).

Gutnick, M.J. and Prince, D.A. Thalamocortical relay neurons: antidromic invasion of spikes from a cortical epileptogenic focus. *Science* 176, 424–426 (1972).

Gutschmidt, K.U., Stenkamp, K., Buchheim, K., Heinemann, U., and Meierkord, H. Anticonvulsant actions of furosemide *in vitro. Neuroscience* 91, 1471–1481 (1999).

Gwag, B.J., Canzoniero, L.M.T., Sensi, S.L., Demaro, J.A., Koh, J.-Y., Goldberg, M.P., Jacquin, M., and Choi, D.W. Calcium ionophores can induce either apoptosis or necrosis in cultured cortical neurons. *Neuroscience* 90, 1339–1348 (1999).

Gwag, B.J., Lobner, D., Koh, J.-Y., Wie, M.B., and Choi, D.W. Blockade of glutamate receptors unmasks neuronal apoptosis after oxygen-glucose deprivation *in vitro. Neuroscience* 68, 615–619 (1995).

György, P. and Vollmer, H. Über den Chemismus der Atmungstetanie. *Biochem. Z.* 140, 391–400 (1923).

Haas, H.L. and Jefferys, J.G.R. Low-calcium field burst discharges of CA1 pyramidal neurones in rat hippocampal slices. *J. Physiol.* 354, 185–201 (1984).

Haas, H.L. and Selbach, O. Functions of neuronal adenosine receptors. *Naunyn-Schmiedeberg's Arch. Pharmacol.* 362, 375–381 (2000).

Hablitz, J.J. and Heinemann, U. Extracellular K^+ and Ca^{2+} changes during epileptiform discharges in the immature rat neocortex. *Brain Res.* 433, 299–303 (1987).

Hablitz, J.J. and Heinemann, U. Alterations in the microenvironment during spreading depression associated with epileptiform activity in the immature neocortex. *Dev. Brain Res.* 46, 243–252 (1989).

Hablitz, J.J. and Lundervold, A. Hippocampal excitability and changes in extracellular potassium. *Exp. Neurol.* 71, 410–420 (1981).

Haddad, G.G. and Jiang, C. O_2 deprivation in the central nervous system: on mechanisms of neuronal response, differential sensitivity and injury. *Progr. Neurobiol.* 40, 277–318 (1993).

Hadjikhani, N., Sanchez del Rio, M., Wu, O., Schwartz, D., Bakker, D., Fischl, B., Kwong, K.K., Cutrer, F.M., Rosen, B.R., Tootell, R.B., Sorensen, A.G., and Moskowitz, M.A. Mechanisms of migraine aura revealed by functional MRI in human visual cortex. *Proc. Natl. Acad. Sci. USA* 98, 4687–4692 (2001).

Hallows, K.R. and Knauf, P.A. Principles of cell volume regulation. In K. Strange (eds), *Cellular and molecular physiology of cell volume regulation.* CRC Press: Boca Raton, Fla., 3–29 (1994).

Hamann, M., Rossi, D.J., Marie, H., and Attwell, D. Knocking out the glutamate transporter GLT-1 reduces glutamate uptake but does not affect hippocampal glutamate dynamics in early simulated ischaemia. *Eur. J. Neurosci.* 15, 308–314 (2002).

Hammarström, A.K.M. and Gage, P.W. Inhibition of oxidative metabolism increases persistent sodium current in rat CA1 hippocampal neurons. *J. Physiol.* 510, 735–741 (1998).

Hammarström, A.K.M. and Gage, P.W. Oxygen-sensing persistent sodium channels in rat hippocampus. *J. Physiol.* 529, 107–118 (2000).

Hammerman, C. and Kaplan, M. Ischemia and reperfusion injury. The ultimate pathophysiologic paradox. *Clin. Perinatol.* 25, 757–777 (1998).

Hammond, C., Crépel, V., Gozlan, H., and Ben-Ari, Y. Anoxic LTP sheds light on the multiple facets of NMDA receptors. *Trends Neurosci.* 17, 497–503 (1994).

Hamprecht, B. and Dringen, R. Energy metabolism. In H. Kettenmann and B.R. Ransom (eds.), *Neuroglia.* Oxford University Press: New York, 473–499 (1995).

Hansen, A.J. Extracellular potassium concentration in juvenile and adult rat brain cortex during anoxia. *Acta Physiol. Scand.* 99, 412–420 (1977).

Hansen, A.J. The extracellular potassium concentration in brain cortex following ischemia in hypo- and hyperglycemic rats. *Acta Physiol. Scand.* 102, 324–329 (1978).

Hansen, A.J. Effects of anoxia on ion distribution in the brain. *Physiol. Rev.* 65, 101–148 (1985).

Hansen, A.J. Effects of anoxia on nerve cell function. In G. Somjen (ed.), *Mechanisms of cerebral hypoxia and stroke.* Plenum Press: New York, 165–173 (1988).

Hansen, A.J., Hounsgaard, J., and Jahnsen, H. Anoxia increases potassium conductance in nerve cells. *Acta Physiol. Scand.* 115, 301–310 (1982).

Hansen, A.J. and Lauritzen, M. The role of spreading depression in acute brain disorders. *An. Acad. Bras. Cienc.* 56, 457–480 (1984).

Hansen, A.J. and Nedergaard, M. Spreading depression evoked by focal ischemia. In A Lehmenkühler, K.-H. Grotemeyer, and F. Tegtmeier (eds.), *Migraine: basic mechanisms and treatment*. Urban & Schwarzenberg: München, 319–327 (1993).

Hansen, A.J. and Olsen, C.E. Brain extracellular space during spreading depression and ischemia. *Acta Physiol.Scand.* 108, 355–365 (1980).

Hansen, A.J. and Zeuthen, T. Extracellular ion concentrations during spreading depression and ischemia in the rat brain cortex. *Acta Physiol. Scand.* 113, 437–445 (1981).

Hansson, E., Muyderman, H., Leonova, J., Allanson, L., Sinclair, J., Blomstrand, F., Thorlin, T., Nilsson, M., and Rönnbäck, L. Astroglia and glutamate in physiology and pathology: aspects on glutamate transport, glutamate-induced cell swelling and gap junction communication. *Neurochem. Int.* 37, 317–329 (2000).

Hanwehr, R.v., Smith, M.-L., and Siesjö, B.K. Extra- and intracellular pH during near-complete forebrain ischemia in the rat. *J. Neurochem.* 46, 331–339 (1986).

Harris, R.A. Carbohydrate metabolism I: major metabolic pathways and their control. In T.M. Devlin (ed.), *Textbook of biochemistry with clinical correlations*. Wiley-Liss: New York, 597–664 (2002).

Hartmann, B.K., Swanson, L.W., Raichle, M.E., Preskorn, S.H., and Clark, H.B. Central adrenergic regulation of cerebral microvascular permeability and blood flow; anatomic and physiologic evidence. *Adv. Exp. .Med. Biol.* 131, 113–126 (1980).

Hartmann, H.A., Colom, L.V., Sutherland, M.L., and Noebels, J.L. Selective localization of cardiac SCN5 sodium channels in limbic region of rat brain. *Nature Neurosci.* 2, 593–595 (1999).

Hashimoto, M., Takeda, Y., Sato, T., Kawahara, H., Nagano, O., and Hirakawa, M. Dynamic changes of NADH fluorescence images and NADH content during spreading depression in the cerebral cortex of gerbils. *Brain Res.* 872, 294–300 (2000).

Hauser, W.A. Incidenc and prevalence. In J. Engel, Jr., and T.A. Pedley (eds.), *Epilepsy: a comprehensive textbook*, Vol. 1. Lippincott-Raven: Philadelphia, 47–58 (1998).

Heinemann, U., Albrecht, D., Köhr, G., Rausche, G., Stabel, J., and Wisskirchen, T. Nonsynaptic spread of epileptiform activity in rat hippocampal slices. In M.R. Klee, H.D. Lux, and E.-J. Speckmann (eds.), *Physiology, pharmacology and development of epileptogenic phenomena*. Springer: Experimental Brain Research Series 20, Berlin, 17–21 (1991).

Heinemann, U., Beck, H., Dreier, J.P., Ficker, E., Stabel, J., and Zhang, C.L. The dentate gyrus as a regulated gate for the propagation of epileptiform acitivity. *Epilepsy Res.* (Suppl. 7), 273–280 (1992).

Heinemann, U., Buchheim, K., Gabriel, S., Kann, O., Kovacs, R., and Schuchmann, S. Cell death and metabolic activity during epileptiform discharges and status epilepticus in the hippocampus. In T. Sutula and A. Pitkänen (eds.), *Do seizures damage the brain?* Elsevier: Amsterdam, 197–210 (2002a).

Heinemann, U., Buchheim, K., Gabriel, S., Kann, O., Kovács, R., and Schuchmann, S. Coupling of electrical and metabolic activity during epileptiform discharges. *Epilepsia* 43 (Suppl. 5), 168–173 (2002b).

Heinemann, U. and Dietzel, I. Extracellular potassium concentration in chronic alumina foci of cats. *J. Neurophysiol.* 52, 421–434 (1984).

Heinemann, U., Eder, C., and Laß, A. Epilepsy. In H. Kettenmann and B.R. Ransom (eds.), *Neuroglia*. Oxford University Press: New York, 936–949 (1995).

Heinemann, U., Gabriel, S., Jauch, R., Schulze, K., Kivi, A., Kovács, R., and Lehmann, T.N. Alterations of glial cell function in temporal lobe epilepsy. *Epilepsia* 41 (Suppl. 6), S185–S189 (2000).

Heinemann, U. and Konnerth, A. Changes in extracellular free Ca²⁺ during epileptic activity in chronic alumina cream foci in cats. In R. Canger, F. Angeleri, and J.K. Penry (eds.), *Advances in epileptology: 11th epilepsy international symposiuum*. Raven Press: New York, 371–375 (1980).

Heinemann, U., Konnerth, A., Pumain, R., and Wadman, W.J. Extracellular calcium and potassium concentration changes in chronic epileptic brain tissue. *Adv. Neurol.* 44, 641–661 (1986).

Heinemann, U. and Lux, H.D. Undershoots following stimulus-induced rises of extracellular potassium concentration in cerebral cortex of cat. *Brain Res.* 93, 63–76 (1975).

Heinemann, U. and Lux, H.D. "Ceiling" of stimulus induced rises in extracellular potassium concentration in cerebral cortex of cats. *Brain Res.* 120, 231–250 (1977).

Heinemann, U., Lux, H.D., and Gutnick, M.J. Extracellular free calcium and potassium during paroxysmal activity in the cerebral cortex of the cat. *Exp. Brain Res.* 27, 237–243 (1977).

Heinemann, U., Lux, H.D., and Gutnick, M.J. Changes in extracellular free calcium and potassium activity in the somatosensory cortex of cats. In N. Chalazonitis and M. Boisson (eds.), *Abnormal neuronal discharges*. Raven Press: New York, 329–345 (1978).

Heinemann, U., Schaible, H.G., and Schmidt, R.F. Changes in extracellular potassium concentration in cat spinal cord in response to innocuous and noxious stimulation of legs with healthy and inflamed knee joints. *Exp. Brain Res.* 79, 283–292 (1990a).

Heinemann, U., Stabel, J., and Rausche, G. Activity-dependent ionic changes and neuronal plasticity in rat hippocampus. *Prog. Brain Res.* 83, 197–214 (1990b).

Held, D., Fencl, V., and Pappenheimer, J.R. Electrical potential of cerebrospinal fluid. *J. Neurophysiol.* 27, 942–959 (1964).

Helmchen, F., Svoboda, K., Denk, W., and Tank, D.W. In vivo dendritic calcium dynamics in deep-layer cortical pyramidal neurons. *Nature Neurosci.* 2, 989–996 (1999).

Henn, F.A., Haljamäe, H., and Hamberger, A. Glial cell function: active control of extracellular K⁺ concentration. *Brain Res.* 43, 437–443 (1972).

Hernandez-Caceres, J., Macias-Gonzalez, R., Brozek, G., and Bureš, J. Systemic ketamine blocks cortical spreading depression but does not delay the onset of terminal anoxic depression. *Brain Res.* 437, 360–364 (1987).

Herreras, O. Propagating dendritic action potential mediates synaptic transmission in CA1 pyramidal cells in situ. *J. Neurophysiol.* 64, 1429–1441 (1990).

Herreras, O., Largo, C., Ibarz, J.M., Somjen, G.G., and Martín del Río, R. Role of neuronal synchronizing mechanisms in the propagation of spreading depression in the in vivo hippocampus. *J. Neurosci.* 14, 7087–7098 (1994).

Herreras, O. and Somjen, G.G. Analysis of potential shifts associated with recurrent spreading depression and prolonged unstable SD induced by microdialysis of elevated K⁺ in hippocampus of anesthetized rats. *Brain Res.* 610, 283–294 (1993a).

Herreras, O. and Somjen, G.G. Prolonged unstable depression: a modified manifestation of spreading depression in rat hippocampus. In W. Haschke, E.-J. Speckmann, and A.I. Roitbak (eds.), *Slow potential changes in the brain*. Birkhäuser: Boston, 131–138 (1993b).

Herreras, O. and Somjen, G.G. Propagation of spreading depression among dendrites and somata of the same cell population. *Brain Res.* 610, 276–282 (1993c).

Hershkowitz, N., Katchman, A.N., and Veregge, S. Site of synaptic depression during hypoxia: a patch-clamp analysis. *J. Neurophysiol.* 69, 432–441 (1993).

Hertz, L. An intense potassium uptake into astrocytes, its further enhancement by high concentrations of potassium, and its possible involvement in potassium homeostasis at the cellular level. *Brain Res.* 145, 202–208 (1978).

Higashida, H., Mitarai, G., and Watanabe, S. A comparative study of membrane potential changes in neurons and neuroglial cells during spreading depression in the rabbit. *Brain Res.* 65, 411–425 (1974).

Higashida, H., Miyake, A., Tarao, M., and Watanabe, S. Membrane potential changes of neuroglial cells during spreading depression in the rabbit. *Brain Res.* 32, 207–211 (1971).

Hille, B. Charges and potentials at the nerve surface. Divalent ions and pH. *J. Gen. Physiol.* 51, 221–236 (1968).

Hille, B. *Ionic channels of excitable membranes.* Sinauer: Sunderland, Mass. (2001).

Hille, B., Woodhull, A.M., and Shapiro, B.I. Negative surface charge near sodium channels of nerve: divalent ions, monovalent ions, and pH. *Phil. Trans. R. Soc. Lond. B* 270, 301–318 (1975).

Hilmy, M.I. and Somjen, G.G. Distribution and tissue uptake of magnesium related to its pharmacological effects. *Am. J. Physiol.* 214, 406–413 (1968).

Hines, M. and Carnevale, N.T. The NEURON simulation environment. *Neural Comput.* 9, 1179–1209 (1997).

Hirose, S., Okada, M., Yamakawa, K., Sugawara, T., Fukuma, G., Ito, M., Kaneko, S., and Mitsudome, A. Genetic abnormalities underlying familial epilepsy syndromes. *Brain Dev.* 24, 211–222 (2002).

Hirsch, H., Euler, K.H., and Schneider, M. Über die Erholung und Wiederbelebung des Gehirns nach Ischaemie bei Normothermie. *Pflügers Arch.* 265, 281–313 (1957).

Hochachka, P.W., Buck, L.T., Doll, C.J., and Land, S.C. Unifying theory of hypoxia tolerance: molecular/metabolic defense and rescue mechanisms for surviving oxygen lack. *Proc. Natl. Acad. Sci. USA* 93, 9493–9498 (1996).

Hodgkin, A.L. and Huxley, A.F. A quantitative description of membrane current and its application to conduction and excitation in nerve. *J. Physiol.* 117, 500–544 (1952).

Hoehn, K., Watson, T.W.J., and MacVicar, B.A. A novel tetrodotoxin-insensitive slow sodium current in striatal and hippocampal neurons. *Neuron* 10, 543–552 (1993).

Hoehn-Berlage, M., Hossmann, K.-A., Busch, E., Eis, M., Schmitz, B., and Gyngell, M.L. Inhibition of nonselective cation channels reduces focal ischemic injury of rat brain. *J. Cereb. Blood Flow Metab.* 17, 534–542 (1997).

Hoffman, C.J., Clark, F.J., and Ochs, S. Intracortical impedance changes during spreading depression. *J. Neurobiol.* 4, 471–486 (1973).

Hoffman, E.P., Lehmann-Horn, F., and Rüdel, R. Overexcited or inactive: ion channels in muscle disease. *Cell* 80, 681–686 (1995).

Hoffmann, R. Mme Lavoisier. *Amer. Scientist* 90, 22–24 (2002).

Hoffman, S.N., Salin, P.A., and Prince, D.A. Chronic neocortical epileptogenesis in vitro. *J. Neurophysiol.* 71, 1762–1763 (1994).

Hökfelt, T., Broberger, C., Xu, Z.-Q.D., Sergeyev, V., Ubink, R., and Diez, M. Neuropeptides—an overview. *Neuropharmacology* 39, 1337–1356 (2000).

Holmes, G.L. and Riviello, J.J., Jr. Medical treatment of generalized epilepsy. In H.O. Lüders (ed.), *Epilepsy: comprehensive review and case discussions.* Martin Dunitz: London, 241–260 (2001).

Holmes, K.H., Bilkey, D.K., Laverty, R., and Goddard, G.V. The *N*-methyl-D-aspartate antagonists aminophosphonovalerate and carboxypiperazinephosphonate retard the development and expression of kindled seizures. *Brain Res.* 506, 227–235 (1990).

Holthoff, K. and Witte, O.W. Intrinsic optical signals in rat neocortical slices measured with near-infrared dark-field microscopy reveal changes in extracellular space. *J. Neurosci.* 16, 2740–2749 (1996).

Holthoff, K. and Witte, O.W. Intrinsic optical signals in vitro: a tool to measure alterations in extracellular space with two-dimensional resolution. *Brain Res. Bull.* 47, 649–655 (1998).

Hopkins, A. E. Definitions and epidemiology of epilepsy. In A. Hopkins (ed.), *Epilepsy.* Demos: New York, 1–17 (1987a).

Hopkins, A.E. *Epilepsy.* Demos: New York (1987b).

Hori, N. and Carpenter, D.O. Functional and morphological changes induced by transient in vivo ischemia. *Exp. Neurol.* 129, 279–289 (1994).

Hori, N., Doi, N., Miyahara, S., Shinoda, Y., and Carpenter, D.O. Appearance of NMDA receptors triggered by anoxia indepedent of voltage *in vivo* and *in vitro. Exp. Neurol.* 112, 304–311 (1991).

Horstmann, E. and Meves, H. Die Feinstruktur des molekularen Rindengraues und ihre physiologische Bedeutung. *Z. Zellforsch. Mikrosk. Anat.* 49, 569–604 (1959).

Hossman, K.-A. Neuronal survival and revival during and after cerebral ischemia. *Am. J. Emerg. Med.* 1, 191–197 (1983).

Hossmann, K.-A. Periinfarct depolarizations. *Cerebrovasc. Brain Metab. Rev.* 8, 195–208 (1996).

Hossmann, K.-A. Glutamate-mediated injury in focal cerebral ischemia: the excitotoxin hypothesis revised. *Brain Pathol.* 4, 23–36 (1994).

Hotson, J.R., Sypert, G.W., and Ward, A.A. Extracellular potassium concentration changes during propagated seizures. *Exp. Neurol.* 38, 20–26 (1973).

Howland, B., Lettvin, J.Y., McCulloch, W.S., Pitts, W., and Wall, P.D. Reflex inhibition by dorsal root interaction. *J. Neurophysiol.* 18, 1–17 (1955).

Huang, R., Aitken, P.G., and Somjen, G.G. The extent and mechanism of the loss of function caused by strongly hypotonic solutions in rat hippocampal tissue slices. *Brain Res.* 695, 195–202 (1995).

Huang, R., Bossut, D.F., and Somjen, G.G. Enhancement of whole-cell synaptic current by low osmolarity and by low [NaCl] in rat hippocampal slices. *J. Neurophysiol.* 77, 2349–2359 (1997).

Huang, R. and Somjen, G.G. The effect of graded hypertonia on interstitial volume, tissue resistance and synaptic transmission in rat hippocampal tissue slices. *Brain Res.* 702, 181–187 (1995).

Huang, R. and Somjen, G.G. Effects of hypertonia on voltage-gated ion currents in freshly isolated hippocampal neurons and on synaptic currents in hippocampal slices. *Brain Res.* 748, 157–167 (1997).

Huber, J.D., Egleton, R.D., and Davis, T.P. Molecular physiology and pathophysiology of tight junctions in the blood-brain barrier. *Trends Neurosci.* 24, 719–725 (2001).

Hughes, S.W., Cope, D.W., Toth, T.I., Williams, S.R., and Crunelli, V. All thalamocortical neurones possess a T-type Ca^{2+} "window" current that enables the expression of bistability-mediated activities. *J. Physiol.* 517, 805–815 (1999).

Hwa, G.G. and Avoli, M. Excitatory synaptic transmission mediated by NMDA and non-NMDA receptors in the superficial/middle layers of the epileptogenic human neocortex maintained in vitro. *Neurosci. Lett.* 143, 83–86 (1992).

Hwa, G.G., Avoli, M., Olivier, A., and Villemure, J.-G. Bicuculline-induced epileptogenesis in human neocortex maintained in vitro. *Exp. Brain Res.* 83, 329–339 (1991).

Iijima, T., Iwao, Y., and Sankawa, H. Amino acid release during spreading depression in a flow-compromised cortical area. *Brain Res.* 818, 553–555 (1999).

Iijima, T., Mies, G., and Hossmann, K.A. Repeated negative DC deflections in rat cortex following middle cerebral artery occlusion are abolished by MK-801: effect on volume of ischemic injury. *J. Cereb. Blood Flow Metab.* 12, 727–733 (1992).

Ikeda, A., Lüders, H.O., and Shibasaki, H. Ictal direct-current shifts. In H.O. Lüders and S. Noachtar (eds.), *Epileptic seizures: pathophysiology and clinical semiology.* Churchill Livingstone: New York, 53–62 (2000).

Ikeda, A., Taki, W., Kunieda, T., Terada, K., Mikuni, N., Nagamine, T., Yazawa, S., Ohara, S., Hori, T., Kaji, R., Kimura, J., and Shibasaki, H. Focal ictal direct current shifts in human epilepsy as studied by subdural and scalp recording. *Brain* 122, 827–838 (1999).

Ikeda, A., Terada, K., Mikuni, N., Burgess, R.C., Comair, Y., Taki, W., Hamano, T., Kimura, J., Lüders, H.O., and Shibasaki, H. Subdural recording of ictal DC shifts in neocortical seizures in humans. *Epilepsia* 37, 662–674 (1996).

Imon, H., Mitani, A., Andou, Y., Arai, T., and Kataoka, K. Delayed neuronal death is induced without postischemic hyperexcitability: continuous multiple-unit recording from ischemic CA1 neurons. *J. Cereb. Blood Flow Metab.* 11, 819–823 (1991).

Inagaki, C., Hara, M., and Zeng, X.-T. A Cl⁻ pump in rat brain neurons. *J. Exp. Zool.* 275, 262–268 (1998).

Irwin, D.A., Kakolewski, J.W., Criswell, H.E., and Popov, A. An injury-induced diffuse slow potential from brain. *Electroencephalogr. Clin. Neurophysiol.* 38, 367–377 (1975).

Isokawa, M., Levesque, M.F., Babb, T.L., and Engel, J., Jr. Single mossy fiber axonal systems of human dentate granule cells studied in hippocampal slices from patients with temporal lobe epilepsy. *J. Neurosci.* 13, 1511–1522 (1993).

Izquierdo, I., Nasello, A.G., and Marichich, E.S. Effects of potassium on rat hippocampus: the dependence of hippocampal evoked and seizure activity on extracellular potassium levels. *Arch. Int. Pharmacodyn.* 187, 318–328 (1970).

Jackson, J.H. A study of convulsions, Transactions St. Andrews Medical Graduates Association, volume iii, (1870), Reprinted in: J. Taylor, G. Holmes, F.M.R. Walshe (eds.), *Selected Writings of John Hughlings Jackson*, Volume 1, Basic Books: New York, 8–36 (1958).

Jacobs, K.M., Kharazia, V.N., and Prince, D.A. Mechanisms underlying epileptogenesis in cortical malformations. *Epilepsy Res.* 36, 165–188 (1999).

Jahnsen, H. and Llinas, R. Electrophysiological properties of guinea-pig thalamic neurones: an in vitro study. *J.Physiol.* 349, 205–226 (1984a).

Jahnsen, H. and Llinas, R. Ionic basis for the electro-responsiveness and oscillatory properties of guinea pig thalamic neurones in vitro. *J. Physiol.* 349, 227–247 (1984b).

Jahromi, S.S., Wentlandt, K., Piran, S., and Carlen, P.L. Anticonvulsant actions of gap junctional blockers in an in vitro seizure model. *J. Neurophysiol.* 88, 1893–1902 (2002).

James, M.F., Smith, J.M., Boniface, S.J., Huang, C.L.H., and Leslie, R.A. Cortical spreading depression and migraine: new insights from imaging? *Trends Neurosci.* 24, 266–271 (2001).

Jami, L. Patterns of cortical population discharges during metrazol-induced seizures in cats. *Electroencephalogr. Clin. Neurophysiol.* 32, 641–654 (1972).

Janigro, D. Blood-brain barrier, ion homeostasis and epilepsy: possible implications towards the understanding of ketogenic diet mechanisms. *Epilepsy Res.* 37, 223–232 (1999).

Janzer, R.C. and Raff, M.C. Astrocytes induce blood-brain barrier properties in endothelial cells. *Nature* 325, 253–257 (1987).

Jarvis, C.R., Anderson, T.R., and Andrew, R.D. Anoxic depolarization mediates acute damage independent of glutamate in neocortical brain slices. *Cereb. Cortex* 11, 249–259 (2001).

Jarvis, C.R., Xiong, Z.-G., Plant, J.R., Churchill, D., Lu, W.-Y., and MacVicar, B.A. Neurotrophin modulation of NMDA receptors in cultured murine and isolated rat neurons. *J. Neurophysiol.* 78, 2363–2371 (1997).

Jasper, H.H. Mechanisms of propagation: extracellular studies. In H.H. Jasper, A. Pope, and A.A. Ward (eds.), *Basic mechanisms of the epilepsies.* Little, Brown: Boston, 421–438 (1969).

Jasper, H.H. and Drooglever-Fortuyn, J. Experimental studies on the functional anatomy of petit mal epilepsy. *Res. Publ. Assoc. Res. Nerv. Ment. Dis.* 26, 272–298 (1947).

Jefferys, J.G.R. Influence of electric fields on the excitability of granule cells in guinea-pig hippocampal slices. *J. Physiol.* 319, 143–152 (1981).

Jefferys, J.G.R. Nonsynaptic modulation of neuronal activity in the braIn electric currents and extracellular ions. *Physiol. Rev.* 75, 689–723 (1995).

Jefferys, J.G.R. and Haas, H.L. Synchronized bursting of CA1 hippocampal pyramidal cells in the absence of synaptic transmission. *Nature* 300, 448–450 (1982).

Jefferys, J.G.R. and Roberts, R. The biology of epilepsy. In A.E. Hopkins (ed.), *Epilepsy.* Demos: New York, 19–81 (1987).

Jefferys, J.G.R. and Traub, R.D. "Dormant" inhibitory neurons: do they exist and what is their functional impact? *Epilepsy Res.* 32, 104–113 (1998).

Jefferys, J.G.R., Traub, R.D., and Whittington, M.A. Neuronal networks for induced "40 Hz" rhythms. *Trends Neurosci.* 19, 203–208 (1996).

Jensen, M.S., Lambert, J.D.C., and Johansen, F.F. Electrophysiological recordings from rat hippocampus slices following in vivo brain ischemia. *Brain Res.* 554, 166–175 (1991).

Jensen, M.S. and Yaari, Y. The relationship between interictal and ictal paroxysms in an in vitro model of focal hippocampal epilepsy. *Ann. Neurol.* 24, 591–598 (1988).

Jensen, M.S. and Yaari, Y. Role of intrinsic burst firing, potassium accumulation and electrical coupling in the elevated potassium model of hippocampal epilepsy. *J. Neurophysiol.* 77, 1224–1233 (1997).

Jiang, C. and Haddad, G.G. A direct mechanism for sensing low oxygen levels by central neurons. *Proc. Natl. Acad. Sci. USA* 91, 7198–7201 (1994).

Jiang, C., Sigworth, F.J., and Haddad, G.G. Oxygen deprivation activates an ATP-inhibitable K^+ channel in substantia nigra neurons. *J. Neurosci.* 14, 5590–5602 (1994).

Jin, K., Minami, M., Lan, J.Q., Mao, X.O., Batteur, S., Simon, R.P., and Greenberg, D.A. Neurogenesis in dentate subgranular zone and rostral subventricular zone after focal cerebral ischemia. *Proc. Natl. Acad. Sci. USA* 98, 4710–4715 (2001).

Jing, J., Aitken, P.G., and Somjen, G.G. Lasting neuron depression induced by high potassium and its prevention by low calcium and NMDA receptor blockade. *Brain Res.* 557, 177–183 (1991).

Jing, J., Aitken, P.G., and Somjen, G.G. Role of calcium channels in spreading depression in rat hippocampal slices. *Brain Res.* 604, 251–259 (1993).

Jing, J., Aitken, P.G., and Somjen, G.G. Interstitial volume changes during spreading depression (SD) and SD-like hypoxic depolarization in hippocampal tissue slices. *J. Neurophysiol.* 71, 2548–2551 (1994).

Jöbsis, F.F. Basic processes in cellular respiration. In W. Fenn, H. Rahn, and M.B. Vischer (eds.), *Handbook of physiology: Respiration I.* Amer. Physiological Society: Bethesda, Md., 63–124 (1964).

Jöbsis, F.F., Keizer, J.H., LaManna, J.C., and Rosenthal, M. Reflectance spectrophotometry of cytochrome aa$_3$ in vivo. *J. Appl. Physiol.* 43, 858–872 (1977).

Jöbsis, F.F., O'Connor, M., Vitale, A., and Vreman, H. Intracellular redox changes in functioning cerebral cortex. I. Metabolic effects of epileptiform activity. *J. Neurophysiol.* 34, 735–749 (1971).

Johnston, D. and Brown, T.H. Giant synaptic potential hypothesis for epileptiform activity. *Science* 211, 294–297 (1981).

Joliot, M., Ribary, U., and Llinas, R. Human oscillatory brain activity near 40 Hz coexists with cognitive temporal binding. *Proc. Natl. Acad. Sci. USA* 91, 11748–11751 (1994).

Jones, L.S., Balestrino, M., and Lewis, D.V. Toxicity of intracellular calcium: an invertebrate model. *Soc. Neurosci. Abstr.* 12, 1402 (1986).

Jones, R.S. Epileptiform events induced by GABA-antagonists in entorhinal cortical cells in vitro are partly mediated by *N*-methyl-D-aspartate receptors. *Brain Res.* 457, 113–121 (1988).

Joshi, I. and Andrew, R.D. Imaging anoxic depolarization during ischemia-like conditions in the mouse hemi-brain slice. *J. Neurophysiol.* 85, 414–424 (2001).

Jouvenceau, A., Eunson, L.H., Spauschus, A., Ramesh, V., Zuberi, S.M., Kullmann, D.M., and Hanna, M.G. Human epilepsy associated with dysfunction of the brain P/Q-type calcium channel. *Lancet* 358, 801–807 (2001).

Joyner, R. and Somjen, G.G. A model simulating the hypothetical contribution of glial cells to extracellular potentials. *Progr. Neurobiol.* 1, 227–237 (1973).

Jung, R. Hirnelektrische Befunde bei Kreislaufstörungen und Hypoxieschäden des Gehirns. *Abh. Dtsch. Gesellsch. Kreisl. Forsch.* 19, 170–196 (1953).

Jung, R. and Tönnies, J.F. Hirnelekrrische Untersuchungen über Entstehung und Erhaltung von Krampfenladungen: die Vorgänge am Reizort und die Bremsfähigkeit des Gehirns. *Arch. Psychiatr. Z. Neurol.* 185, 701–735 (1950).

Kabat, H. The greater resistance of very young animals to arrest of brain circulation. *Am. J. Physiol.* 130, 588–599 (1940).

Kabat, H., Dennis, C., and Baker, A.B. Recovery of function following arrest of the brain circulation. *Am. J. Physiol.* 132, 737–747 (1941).

Kagansky, N., Levy, S., and Knobler, H. The role of hyperglycemia in acute stroke. *Arch. Neurol.* 58, 1209–1212 (2001).

Kager, H., Wadman, W.J., and Somjen, G.G. Simulated seizures and spreading depression in a neuron model incorporating interstitial space and ion concentrations. *J. Neurophysiol.* 84, 495–512 (2000).

Kager, H., Wadman, W.J., and Somjen, G.G. Simulation of membrane current and ion concentrations in a neuron predicts epileptiform discharge and spreading depression (SD). *Soc. Neurosci. Abstr.* 27, Prog. No. 559.3 (2001).

Kager, H., Wadman, W.J., and Somjen, G.G. Conditions for the triggering of spreading depression studied with computer simulation. *J. Neurophysiol.* 88, 2700–2712 (2002a).

Kager, H., Wadman, W.J., and Somjen, G.G. Ion currents and ion fluxes responsible for self-sustained and self-limiting tonic seizure-like discharges in a neuron model. *Soc. Neurosci. Abst.* 28, Prog. No. 602.7 (2002b).

Kahana, M.J., Seelig, D., and Madsen, J.R. Theta returns. *Curr. Opin. Neurobiol.* 11, 739–744 (2001).

Kaila, K. Ionic basis of GABA-A receptor channel function in the nervous system. *Prog. Neurobiol.* 42, 489–537 (1994).

Kaila, K. and Chesler, M. Activity-evoked changes in extracellular pH. In K. Kaila and B.R. Ransom (eds.), *pH and brain function*. Wiley-Liss: New York, 309–337 (1998).

Kaila, K., Lamsa, K., Smirnov, S., Taira, T., and Voipio, J. Long-lasting GABA-mediated depolarization evoked by high-frequency stimulation of pyramidal neurons of rat hippocampal slice is attributable to a network-driven, bicarbonate-dependent K^+ transient. *J. Neurosci.* 17, 7662–7672 (1997).

Kalimo, H., Rehncrona, S., and Soderfeldt, B. The role of lactic acidosis in the ischemic nerve cell injury. *Acta Neuropathol.* (Suppl. 7), 20–22 (1981).

Kamphuis, W., Gorter, J.A., and Lopes da Silva, F.H. A long-lasting decrease in the inhibitory effect of GABA on glutamate responses of hippocampal pyramidal neurons induced by kindling epileptogenesis. *Neuroscience* 41, 425–431 (1991).

Kamphuis, W., Wadman, W.J., Buijs, R.M., and Lopes da Silva, F.H. The development of changes in hippocampal GABA immunoreactivity in the rat kindling model of epilepsy: a light microscopic study with GABA antibodies. *Neuroscience* 23, 433–446 (1987).

Kandel, A. and Buzsáki, G. Cellular-synaptic generation of sleep spindles, spike-and-wave discharges and evoked thalamocortical responses in the neocortex of the rat. *J. Neurosci.* 17, 6783–6797 (1997).

Kandel, E.R. and Spencer, W.A. Electrophysiological properties of an archicortical neuron. *Ann. N.Y. Acad. Sci.* 94, 570–603 (1961a).

Kandel, E.R. and Spencer, W.A. Excitation and inhibition of single pyramidal cells during hippocampal seizure. *Exp. Neurol.* 4, 162–178 (1961b).

Kandel, E.R. and Spencer, W.A. The pyramidal cell during hippocampal seizure. *Epilepsia* 2, 63–69 (1961c).

Kandler, K. and Katz, L.C. Neuronal coupling and uncoupling in the developing nervous system. *Curr. Opinion Neurobiol.* 5, 98–105 (1995).

Kann, O., Schuchmann, S., Buchheim, K., and Heinemann, U. Coupling of neuronal activity and mitochondrial metabolism as revealed by NAD(P)H fluorescence signals in organotypic hippocampal slice cultures. *Neuroscience* 119, 87–100 (2003).

Kanner, A.M. and Parra, J. Psychogenic pseudoseizures. In H.O. Lüders and S. Noachtar (eds.), *Epileptic seizures: pathophysiology and clinical semiology*. Churchill Livingstone: New York, 766–773 (1998).

Kapur, J. and Lothman, E.W. Loss of inhibition precedes delayed spontaneous seizures in the hippocampus after tetanic electrical stimulation. *J. Neurophysiol.* 61, 427–434 (1989).

Kapur, J., Stringer, J.L., and Lothman, E.W. Evidence that repetitive seizures in the hippocampus cause a lasting reduction of GABAergic inhibition. *J. Neurophysiol.* 61, 417–426 (1989).

Karahashi, Y. and Goldring, S. Intracellular potentials from "idle" cells in cerebral cortex of cat. *Electroencephalogr. Clin. Neurophysiol.* 20, 600–607 (1966).

Karst, H., Joëls, M., and Wadman, W.J. Low-threshold calcium current in dendrites of the adult rat hippocampus. *Neurosci. Lett.* 164, 154–158 (1993).

Karwoski, C.J., Newman, E.A., Shimazaki, H., and Proenza, L.M. Light-evoked increases in extracellular K^+ in the plexiform layers of amphibian retinas. *J. Gen. Physiol.* 86, 189–213 (1985).

Karwoski, C.J. and Proenza, L.M. Light-evoked changes in extracellular potassium concentration in mudpuppy retina. *Brain Res.* 142, 515–530 (1978).

Kass, I.S., Cottrell, J.E., and Chambers, G. Magnesium and cobalt, not nimodipine, protect neurons against anoxic damage in the rat hippocampal slice. *Anesthesiology* 69, 710–715 (1988).

Katchman, A.N. and Hershkowitz, N. Adenosine antagonists prevent hypoxia-induced depression of excitatory but not inhibitory synaptic currents. *Neurosci. Lett.* 159, 123–126 (1993).

Katz, B. *Nerve, muscle and synapse.* McGraw-Hill: New York (1966).

Katzman, R. and Pappius, H.M. *Brain electrolytes and fluid metabolism.* Williams & Wilkins: Baltimore (1973).

Kaura, S., Bradford, H.F., Young, A.M., Croucher, M.J., and Hughes, P.D. Effect of amygdaloid kindling on the content and release of amino acids from the amygdaloid complex: in vivo and in vitro studies. *J. Neurochem.* 65, 1240–1249 (1995).

Kawahara, N., Ruetzler, C.A., and Klatzo, I. Protective effect of spreading depression against neuronal damage following cardiac arrest cerebral ischemia. *Neurol. Res.* 17, 9–16 (1995).

Kawahara, N., Ruetzler, C.A., Mies, G., and Klatzo, I. Cortical spreading depression increases protein synthesis and upregulates basic fibroblast growth factor. *Exp.Neurol.* 158, 27–36 (1999).

Kawasaki, K., Czéh, G., and Somjen, G.G. Prolonged exposure to high potassium concentration results in irreversible loss of synaptic transmission in hippocampal tissue slices. *Brain Res.* 457, 322–329 (1988).

Kearney, J.A., Plummer, N.W., Smith, M.R., Kapur, J., Cummins, T.R., Waxman, S.G., and Goldin, A.L. A gain-of-function mutation in the sodium channel gene Scn2a results in seizures and behavioral abnormalities. *Neuroscience* 102, 307–317 (2001).

Kelly, J.P. and Van Essen, D.C. Cell structure and function in the visual cortex of the cat. *J. Physiol.* 238, 515–547 (1974).

Kelly, K.M., Gross, R.A., and MacDonald, R.L. Valproic acid selectively reduces the low-threshold (T) calcium current in rat nodose neurons. *Neurosci. Lett.* 116, 233–238 (1990).

Kemény, A., Boldizsár, H., and Pethes, G. The distribution of cations in plasma and cerebrospinal fluid following infusions of solutions of salts of sodium, potassium, magnesium and calcium. *J. Neurochem.* 7, 218–227 (1961).

Kempski, O. Cerebral edema. *Semin. Nephrol.* 21, 303–307 (2001).

Kempski, O., Von Rosen, S., Weigt, H., Staub, F., Peters, J., and Baethmann, A. Glial ion transport and volume control. *Ann. N.Y. Acad. Sci.* 633, 306–317 (1991).

Kerr, J.F.R. A personal account of events leading to the definition of the apoptotic concept. In S. Kumar (ed.), *Apoptosis: biology and mechanisms.* Vol. 23. Springer: Berlin, 1–10 (1999).

Ketelaars, S.O.M., Gorter, J.A., Van Vliet, E.A., Lopes da Silva, F.H., and Wadman, W.J. Sodium currents in isolated rat CA1 pyramidal and dentate granule neurones in the post-status epilepticus model of epilepsy. *Neuroscience* 105, 109–120 (2001).

Kettenmann, H., Sonnhof, U., and Schachner, M. Exclusive potassium dependence of the membrane potential in cultured mouse oligodendrocytes. *J. Neurosci.* 3, 500–505 (1983).

Khazipov, R., Congar, P., and Ben-Ari, Y. Hippocampal CA1 lacunosum-moleculare interneurons: comparison of effects of anoxia on excitatory and inhibitory postsynaptic currents. *J. Neurophysiol.* 74, 2138–2149 (1995).

Kim, D., Song, I., Keum, S., Lee, T., Jeong, M.J., Kim, S.S., McEnery, M.W., and Shin, H.S. Lack of burst firing of thalamocortical relay neurons and resistance to absence seizures in mice lacking α_{1G} T-type Ca^{2+} channels. *Neuron* 31, 35–45 (2001).

Kim, Y.-H., Kim, E.Y., Gwag, B.J., Sohn, S., and Koh, J.-Y. Zinc-induced cortical neuronal death with features of apoptosis and necrosis: mediation by free radicals. *Neuroscience* 89, 175–182 (1998).

Kimelberg, H.K. Chloride transport across glial membranes. In F.J. Alvarez-Leefmans and J.M. Russell (eds.), *Chloride channels and carriers in nerve, muscle and glial cells.* Plenum Press: New York, 159–191 (1990).

Kimelberg, H.K. Cell volume in the CNS: regulation and implications for nervous system function and pathology. *Neuroscientist* 6, 14–25 (2000).

Kimelberg, H.K. and Frangakis, M.V. Volume regulation in primary astrocyte cultures. *Adv. Biosci.* 61, 177–185 (1986).

Kimelberg, H.K. and Goderie, S.K. Volume regulation after swelling in primary astrocyte cultures. In M.D. Norenberg and L. Hertz (eds.), *The biochemical pathology of astrocytes*. Alan R. Liss: New York, 299–311 (1988).

Kimelberg, H.K., Goderie, S.K., Higman, S., Pang, S., and Waniewski, A. Swelling-induced release of glutamate, aspartate and taurine from astrocyte cultures. *J. Neurosci.* 10, 1563–1591 (1990).

Kimelberg, H.K., Jalonen, T., and Walz, W. Regulation of the brain microenvironment: transmitters and ions. In S. Murphy (ed.), *Astrocytes: pharmacology and function.* Academic Press: San Diego, Calif., 193–228 (1993).

Kimelberg, H.K. and Mongin, A.A. Swelling-activated release of excitatory amino acids in the brain: relevance for pathophysiology. In F. Lang (ed.), *Cell volume regulation.* Karger: Basel, 240–257 (1998).

Kimelberg, H.K., Rutledge, E., Goderie, S., and Charniga, C. Astrocytic swelling due to hypotonic or high K^+ medium causes inhibition of glutamate and aspartate uptake and increases their release. *J. Cereb. Blood Flow Metab.* 15, 409–416 (1995).

Kimelberg, H.K., Sankar, P., O'Connor, E.R., Jalonen, T., and Goderie, S.K. Functional consequences of astrocyte swelling. *Prog. Brain Res.* 94, 57–68 (1992).

King, R.D., Wiest, M.C., and Montague, P.R. Extracellular calcium depletion as a mechanism of short-term synaptic depression. *J. Neurophysiol.* 85, 1952–1959 (2001).

Kinnes, C.G., Connors, B.W., and Somjen, G.G. The effects of convulsant doses of penicillin on primary afferents, dorsal root ganglion cells, and on "presynaptic" inhibition in the spinal cord. *Brain Res.* 192, 495–512 (1980).

Kirino, T. Delayed neuronal death in the gerbil hippocampus. *Brain Res.* 239, 57–69 (1982).

Kirino, T. and Sano, K. Fine structural nature of delayed neuronal death following ischemia in the gerbil hippopcampus. *Acta Neuropathol.* 62, 209–218 (1984).

Kirino, T., Tamura, A., and Sano, K. Selective vulnerability of the hippocampus to ischemia—reversible and irreversible types of ischemic damage. *Prog. Brain Res.* 63, 39–58 (1985).

Kivi, A., Lehmann, T.N., Kovacs, R., Eilers, A., Jauch, R., Meencke, H.-J., von Deimling, A., Heinemann, U., and Gabriel, S. Effects of barium on stimulus-induced rises of $[K^+]_o$ in human epileptic non-sclerotic and sclerotic hippocampal area CA1. *Eur. J. Neurosci.* 12, 2039–2048 (2000).

Klapstein, G.J., Meldrum, B.S., and Mody, I. Decreased sensitivity to group III mGluR agonists in the lateral perforant path following kindling. *Neuropharmacology* 38, 927–933 (1999).

Klee, M.R., Faber, D.S., and Heiss, W.-D. Strychnine- and pentyleneterazol-induced changes in excitability in *Aplysia* neurons. *Science* 179, 1133–1136 (1973).

Klink, R. and Alonso, A. muscarinic modulation of the oscillatory and repetitive firing properties of entorhinal cortex layer II neurons. *J. Neurophysiol.* 77, 1813–1828 (1997).

Knowles, W.D., Funch, P.G., and Schwartzkroin, P.A. Electrotonic and dye coupling in hippocampal CA1 pyramidal cells in vitro. *Neuroscience* 7, 1713–1722 (1982).

Ko, D.Y., Rho, J.M., DeGiorgio, C.M., and Sato, S. Benzodiazepines. In J. Engel, Jr., and T.A. Pedley (eds.), *Epilepsy: a comprehensive textbook*, Vol. 2. Lippincott-Raven: Philadelphia, 1475–1489 (1997).

Kobayashi, S., Harris, V.A., and Welsh, F.A. Spreading depression induces tolerance of cortical neurons to ischemia in rat brain. *J. Cereb. Blood Flow Metab.* 15, 721–727 (1995).

Kogure, K., Arai, H., Abe, K., and Nakano, M. Free radical damage of the brain following ischemia. *Prog. Brain Res.* 63, 237–259 (1985).

Kohl, M., Lindauer, U., Dirnagl, U., and Villringer, A. Separation of changes in light scattering and chromophore concentrations during cortical spreading depression in rats. *Optics Lett.* 23, 555–557 (1999).

Köhling, R., Gladwell, S.J., Bracci, E., Vreugdenhil, M., and Jefferys, J.G.R. Prolonged epileptiform bursting induced by 0 Mg^{2+} in rat hippocampal slices depends on gap junctional coupling. *Neuroscience* 105, 579–587 (2001).

Köhling, R., Lücke, A., Straub, H., Speckmann, E.-J., Tuxhorn, I., Wolf, P., Pannek, H., and Oppel, F. Spontaneous sharp waves in human neocortical slices excised from epileptic patients. *Brain* 121, 1073–1087 (1998).

Köhling, R., Qü, M., Zilles, K., and Speckmann, E.-J. Current-source-density profiles associated with sharp waves in human epileptic neocortical tissue. *Neuroscience* 94, 1039–1050 (1999).

Köhling, R., Schmidinger, A., Hülsmann, S., Vanhatalo, S., Lücke, A., Straub, H., Speckmann, E.-J., Tuxhorn, I., Wolf, P., Lahl, R., Pannek, H., Oppel, F., Greiner, C., Moskopp, D., and Wassmann, H. Anoxic terminal negative DC-shift in human neocortical slices in vitro. *Brain Res.* 741, 174–179 (1996).

Köhr, G. and Mody, I. Endogenous intracellular calcium buffering and the activation/inactivation of HVA calcium currents in rat dentate gyrus granule cells. *J. Gen. Physiol.* 98, 941–967 (1991).

Köhr, G. and Mody, I. Kindling increases *N*-methyl-D-aspartate potency at single *N*-methyl-D-aspartate channels in dentate gyrus granule cells. *Neuroscience* 62, 975–981 (1994).

Kokaia, M., Holmberg, K., Nanobashvili, A., Xu, Z.-Q.D., Kokaia, Z., Lendahl, U., Hilke, S., Theodorsson, E., Kahl, U., Bartfai, T., Lindvall, O., and Hökfelt, T. Suppressed kindling epileptogenesis in mice with extopic overexpression of galanin. *Proc. Natl. Acad. Sci. USA* 98, 14006–14011 (2001).

Konnerth, A. and Heinemann; U. Effects of GABA on presumed presynaptic calcium entry in hippocampal slices. *Brain Res.* 270, 185–189 (1983).

Konnerth, A., Heinemann, U., and Yaari, Y. Slow transmission of neural activity in hippocampal area CA1 in absence of active chemical synapses. *Nature* 307, 69–71 (1983).

Konnerth, A., Heinemann, U., and Yaari, Y. Nonsynaptic epileptogenesis in the mammalian hippocampus in vitro. I. Development of seizurelike activity in low extracellular calcium. *J. Neurophysiol.* 56, 409–423 (1986).

Korn, S.J., Giacchino, J.L., Chamberlin, N.L., and Dingledine, R. Epileptiform burst activity induced by potassium in the hippocampus and its regulation by GABA-mediated inhibition. *J. Neurophysiol.* 57, 325–340 (1987).

Koroleva, V.I. and Bureš, J. Rats do not experience cortical or hippocampal spreading depression as aversive. *Neurosci. Lett.* 149, 153–156 (1993).

Korytová, H. Arousal induced increase of cortical [K^+] in unrestrained rats. *Experientia* 33, 242–244 (1977).

Kostopoulos, G.K. Spike-and-wave discharges of absence seizures as a transformation of sleep spindles: the continuing development of a hypothesis. *Clin. Neurophysiol.* 111, (Suppl. 2), S27–S38, (2000).

Kostyuk, P.G. Metabolic control of ionic channels in the neuronal membrane. *Neuroscience* 13, 983–989 (1984).

Kotagal, P. and Lüders, H.O. Simple motor seizures. In J. Engel, Jr., and T.A. Pedley (eds.), *Epilepsy: a comprehensive textbook*, Vol. 1. Lippincott-Raven: Philadelphia, 525–532 (1998).

Kovács, R., Schuchmann, S., Gabriel, S., Kardos, J., and Heinemann, U. Ca^{2+} signalling and changes of mitochondrial function during low-Mg2+- induced epileptiform activity in organotypic hippocampal slice cultures. *Eur. J. Neurosci.* 13, 1311–1319 (2001).

Kovács, R., Szilágyi, N., Barabás, P., Heinemann, U., and Kardos, J. Low-[Mg^{2+}]-induced Ca^{2+} fluctuations in organotypic hippocampal slice cultures. *NeuroReport* 11, 2107–2111 (2000).

Kow, L.-M. and Van Harreveld, A. Ion and water movements in isolated chicken retinas during spreading depression. *Neurobiology* 2, 61–69 (1972).

Kraig, R.P. Interrelationship of astrocytic pH and calcium changes during spreading depression. In A. Lehmenkühler, K.-H. Grotemeyer, and F. Tegtmeier (eds.), *Migraine: basic mechanisms and treatment*. Urban & Schwarzenberg: München, 309–318 (1993).

Kraig, R.P. and Cooper, A.J. Bicarbonate and ammonia changes in brain during spreading depression. *Can. J. Physiol. Pharmacol.* 65, 1099–1104 (1987).

Kraig, R.P., Ferreira-Filho, C.R., and Nicholson, C. Alkaline and acid transients in cerebellar microenvironment. *J. Neurophysiol.* 49, 831–850 (1983).

Kraig, R.P., Hulse, R.E., Kunkler, P.E., and Nicholson, C. Optical current source densities with spreading depression in hippocampal organ cultures. *Soc. Neurosci. Abstr.* 25, 2102 (1999).

Kraig, R.P. and Nicholson, C. Extracellular ionic variations during spreading depression. *Neuroscience* 3, 1045–1059 (1978).

Kraig, R.P., Petito, C.K., Plum, F., and Pulsinelli, W.A. Hydrogen ions kill brain at concentrations reached in ischemia. *J. Cereb. Blood Flow Metab.* 7, 379–386 (1987).

Kral, T., Luhmann, H.J., Mittmann, T., and Heinemann, U. Role of NMDA receptors and voltage-activated calcium channels in an in vitro model of cerebral ischemia. *Brain Res.* 612, 278–288 (1993).

Kraus, J.E. and McNamara, J.O. Measurement of NMDA receptor protein subunits in discrete hippocampal regions of kindled animals. *Mol. Brain Res.* 61, 114–120 (1998).

Kraus, J.E., Yeh, G.C., Bonhaus, D.W., Nadler, J.V., and McNamara, J.O. Kindling induces the long-lasting expression of a novel population of NMDA receptors in hippocampal region CA3. *J. Neurosci.* 14, 4196–4205 (1994).

Kreisman, N.R. and LaManna, J. Rapid and slow swelling during hypoxia in the CA1 region of rat hippocampal slices. *J. Neurophysiol.* 82, 320–329 (1999).

Kreisman, N.R., LaManna, J.C., Liao, S.-C., Yeh, E.R., and Alcala, R. Light transmission as an index of cell volume in hippocampal slices: optical differences of interfaced and submerged positions. *Brain Res.* 693, 179–186 (1995).

Kreisman, N.R., LaManna, J.C., Rosenthal, M., and Sick, T.J. Oxidative metabolic responses with recurrent seizures in rat cerebral cortex: role of systemic factors. *Brain Res.* 218, 175–188 (1981).

Kreisman, N.R., Rosenthal, M., Sick, T.J., and LaManna, J.C. Oxidative metabolic responses during recurrent seizures are indepedent of convulsant, anesthetic or species. *Neurology* 33, 861–867 (1983a).

Kreisman, N.R., Sick, T.J., and Rosenthal, M. Importance of vascular responses in determining cortical oxygenation during recurrent paroxysmal events of varying duration and frequency of repetition. *J. Cereb. Blood Flow Metab.* 3, 330–338 (1983b).

Kreisman, N.R., Soliman, S., and Gozal, D. Regional differences in hypoxic depolarization and swelling in hippocampal slices. *J. Neurophysiol.* 83, 1031–1038 (2000).

Kristián, T., Bernardi, P., and Siesjö, B.K. Acidosis promotes the permeability transition in energized mitochondria: implications for reperfusion injury. *J. Neurotrauma* 18, 1059–1074 (2001).

Kristián, T., Gidö, G., Kuroda, S., Schütz, A., and Siesjö, B.K. Calcium metabolism of focal and penumbral tissues in rats subjected to transient middle cerebral artery occlusion. *Exp. Brain Res.* 120, 503–509 (1998).

Kristián, T. and Siesjö, B.K. Calcium in ischemic cell death. *Stroke* 29, 705–718 (1998).

Krivánek, J. Some metabolic changes accompanying cortical spreading depression. *J. Neurochem.* 6, 183–189 (1961).

Krivánek, J. and Bureš, J. Ion shifts during Leão's spreading cortical depression. *Physiol. Bohemoslov.* 9, 494–503 (1960).

Krnjević, K. Acetylcholine receptors in vertebrate CNS. In L.L. Iversen, S.D. Iversen, and S.H. Snyder (eds.), *Handbook of psychopharmacology*, Vol. 6. Plenum Press: New York, 97–125 (1975).

Krnjević, K. Adenosine triphosphate-sensitive potassium channels in anoxia. *Stroke* 21(Suppl. III), III.190–III.193 (1990).

Krnjević, K. and Ben-Ari, Y. Anoxic changes in dentate granule cells. *Neurosci. Lett.* 107, 89–93 (1989).

Krnjević, K., Cherubini, E., and Ben-Ari, Y. Anoxia on slow inward currents of immature hippocampal neurons. *J. Neurophysiol.* 62, 896–906 (1989).

Krnjević, K. and Leblond, J. Anoxia reversibly suppresses neuronal calcium currents in rat hippocampal slices. *Can. J. Physiol. Pharmacol.* 65, 2157–2161 (1987).

Krnjević, K. and Leblond, J. Changes in membrane currents of hippocampal neurons evoked by brief anoxia. *J. Neurophysiol.* 62, 15–30 (1989).

Krnjević, K. and Miledi, R. Presynaptic failure in neuromuscular propagation in rats. *J. Physiol.* 149, 1–22 (1959).

Krnjević, K. and Xu, Y.Z. Mechanisms underlying anoxic hyperpolarization of hippocampal neurons. *Can. J. Physiol. Pharmacol.* 68, 1609–1613 (1990).

Krnjević, K., Xu, Y.Z., and Zhang, L. Anoxic block of GABAergic IPSPs. *Neurochem. Res.* 16, 279–284 (1991).

Krnjević, K. and Zhao, Y.-T. 2-Deoxyglucose-induced long-term potentiation of monosynaptic IPSPs in CA1 hipocampal neurons. *J. Neurophysiol.* 83, 879–887 (2000).

Krüger, H., Heinemann, U., and Luhmann, H.J. Effects of ionotropic glutamate receptor blockade and 5HT1A receptor activation on spreading depression in rat neocortical slices. *NeuroReport* 10, 2651–2656 (1999).

Kuffler, S.W. Neuroglial cells: physiological properties and a potassium mediated effect of neuronal activity on the glial membrane potential. *Proc. R. Soc. B* 168, 1–21 (1967).

Kuffler, S.W. and Nicholls, J.G. The physiology of neuroglial cells. *Erg. Physiol.* 57, 1–90 (1966).

Kullmann, D.M. The neuronal channelopathies. *Brain* 125, 1177–1195 (2002).

Kumar, S. (ed.). *Apoptosis: biology and mechanisms*. Springer: Berlin (1999).

Kunkler, P.E. and Kraig, R.P. Calcium waves precede electrophysiological changes of spreading depression in hippocampal organ cultures. *J. Neurosci.* 18, 3416–3425 (1998).

Kutchai, H.C. Cellular membranes and transmembrane transport of solutes and water. In R.M. Berne and M.N. Levy (eds.), *Physiology*. Mosby: St. Louis, 3–26 (1993).

LaManna, J., Romeo, S.A., Crumrine, R.C., and McCracken, K.A. Decreased blood volume with hypoperfusion during recovery from total cerebral ischaemia in dogs. *Neurol. Res.* 7, 161–165 (1985).

LaManna, J.C., Sick, T.J., Pikarsky, S.M., and Rosenthal, M. Detection of an oxidizable fraction of cytochrome oxidase in intact rat brain. *Am. J. Physiol.* 253, C477–C483 (1987).

Langmoen, I.A. and Hablitz, J.J. Reversal potential for glutamate receptors in hippocampal pyramidal cells. *Neurosci. Lett.* 23, 61–65 (1981).

Largo, C., Cuevas, P., Somjen, G.G., Martín del Río, R., and Herreras, O. The effect of depressing glial function in rat brain in situ on ion homeostasis, synaptic transmission and neuron survival. *J. Neurosci.* 16, 1219–1229 (1996).

Largo, C., Ibarz, J.M., and Herreras, O. Effects of the gliotoxin fluorocitrate on spreading depression and glial membrane potential in rat brain in situ. *J. Neurophysiol.* 78, 295–307 (1997a).

Largo, C., Tombaugh, G.C., Aitken, P.G., Herreras, O., and Somjen, G.G. Heptanol but not fluoroacetate prevents the propagation of spreading depression in rat hippocampal slices. *J. Neurophysiol.* 77, 9–16 (1997b).

Larkman, A.U. and Jack, J.J.B. Synaptic plasticity: hippocampal LTP. *Curr. Opin. Neurobiol.* 5, 324–334 (1995).

Lascola, C. and Kraig, R.P. Astroglial acid-base dynamics in hyperglycemic and normoglycemic global ischemia. *Neurosci. Biobehav. Rev.* 21, 143–150 (1997).

Lashley, K.S. Patterns of cerebral integration indicated by the scotomas of migraine. *Arch. Neurol. Psychiatry* 46, 331–339 (1941).

Lau, D., de Miera, E.V.S., Contreras, D., Ozaita, A., Harvey, M., Chow, A., Noebels, J.L., Paylor, R., Morgan, J.I., Leonard, C.S., and Rudy, B. Impaired fast-spiking, suppressed cortical inhibition, and increased susceptibility to seizures in mice lacking Kv3.2 K$^+$ channel proteins. *J. Neurosci.* 20, 9071–9085 (2000).

Läuger, P. *Electrogenic ion pumps.* Sinauer: Sunderland, Mass. (1991).

Lauritzen, M. Cerebral blood flow in migraine and cortical spreading depression. *Acta Neurol. Scand.* 76(Suppl. 113), 9–40 (1987).

Lauritzen, M., Fabricius, M., and Jensen, L.H. On the role of glutamate receptor subtypes in spreading depression. In A. Lehmenkühler, K.-H. Grotemeyer, and F. Tegtmeier (eds.), *Migraine: basic mechanisms and treatment.* Urban & Schwarzenberg: München, 345–353 (1993).

Lauritzen, M. and Hansen, A.J. The effect of glutamate receptor blockade on anoxic depolarization and cortical spreading depression. *J. Cereb. Blood Flow Metab.* 12, 223–229 (1992).

Lauritzen, M., Jorgensen, M.B., Diemer, N.H., Gjedde, A., and Hansen, A.J. Persistent oligemia of rat cerebral cortex in the wake of spreading depression. *Ann. Neurol.* 12, 469–474 (1982).

Lauritzen, M., Rice, M.E., Okada, Y., and Nicholson, C. Quisqualate, kainate and NMDA can initiate spreading depression in the turtle cerebellum. *Brain Res.* 475, 317–327 (1988).

Lavoisier, A.-L. *Mémoires sur la respiration et la transpiration des animaux.* (*Collected reprints of papers originally published between 1777 and 1790*). Gauthier-Villars: Paris (1920).

Leão, A.A.P. Spreading depression of activity in the cerebral cortex. *J. Neurophysiol.* 7, 359–390 (1944).

Leão, A.A.P. Further observations on the spreading depression of activity in the cerebral cortex. *J. Neurophysiol.* 10, 409–414 (1947).

Leão, A.A.P. The slow voltage variation of cortical spreading depression of activity. *Electroencephalogr. Clin. Neurophysiol.* 3, 315–321 (1951).

Leão, A.A.P. On the spread of spreading depression. In M.A.B. Brazier (ed.), *Brain function: cortical excitability and steady potentials.* University of California Press, Berkeley, 73–85 (1963).

Leão, A.A.P. and Martins-Ferreira, H. Alteraçao de impedancia electrica no decurso de depressão alastrante da atividade do córtex cerebral. *An. Acad. Brasil. Ciênc.* 25, 259–266 (1953).

Leão, A.A.P. and Morison, R.S. Propagation of spreading cortical depression. *J. Neurophysiol.* 8, 33–45 (1945).

Leblond, J. and Krnjević, K. Hypoxic changes in hippocampal neurons. *J. Neurophysiol.* 62, 1–14 (1989).

Lee, A.C., Wong, R.K.S., Chuang, S.-C., Shin, H.-S., and Bianchi, R. Role of synaptic metabotropic glutamate receptors in epileptiform discharges in hippocampal slices. *J. Neurophysiol.* 88, 1625–1633 (2002).

Lee, J. and Wu, C.-F. Electroconvulsive seizure behavior in *Drosophila*: analysis of the physiological repertoire underlying stereotyped action pattern in bang-sensitive mutants. *J. Neurosci.* 22, 11065–11079 (2002).

Lee, K.S., Schubert, P., and Heinemann, U. The anticonvulsive action of adenosine: a postsynaptic, dendritic action by a possible endogenous anticonvulsant. *Brain Res.* 321, 160–164 (1984).

Lehmann, T.N., Gabriel, S., Kovacs, R., Eilers, A., Kivi, A., Schulze, K., Lanksch, W.R., Meencke, H.-J., and Heinemann, U. Alterations of neuronal connectivity in area CA1 of hippocampal slices from temporal lobe epilepsy patients and from pilocarpine-treated epileptic rats. *Epilepsia* 41(Suppl. 6), S190–S194 (2000).

Lehmenkühler, A. Änderungen des Mikromilieus van Nervenzellen in der Hirnrinde bei epileptischen Anfällen. Experimentelle Beobachtungen. *EEG-Labor.* 10, 145–161 (1988).

Lehmenkühler, A. Spreading depression—Reaktionen an der Hirnrinde: Störungen des extrazellulären Mikromilieus. *Z. EEG-EMG* 21, 1–6 (1990).

Lehmenkühler, A., Grotemeyer, K.-H., and Tegtmeier, F. (eds.). *Migraine: basic mechanisms and treatment.* Urban & Schwarzenberg: München (1993a).

Lehmenkühler, A., Syková, E., Svoboda, J., Zilles, K., and Nicholson, C. Extracellular space parameters in the rat neocortex and subcortical white matter during postnatal development determined by diffusion analysis. *Neuroscience* 55, 339–351 (1993b).

Lehmenkühler, A., Zidek, W., and Caspers, H. Changes of extracellular Na^+ and Cl^- activity in the brain cortex during seizure discharges. In M.R. Klee, H.D. Lux, and E.-J. Speckmann (eds.), *Physiology and pharmacology of epileptogenic phenomena.* Raven Press: New York, 37–45 (1982a).

Lehmenkühler, A., Zidek, W., Staschen, M., and Caspers, H. Cortical pH and pCa in relation to DC potential shifts during spreading depression and asphyxiation. In E. Syková, P. Hník, and L. Vyklicky (eds.), *Ion-selective microelectrodes and their use in excitable tissues.* Plenum Press: New York, 225–229 (1982b).

Leibowitz, D.H. The glial spike theory: I. On an active role of neuroglia in spreading depression and migraine. *Proc. R. Soc. B.* 250, 287–295 (1992).

Leite, J.P., Garcia-Cairasco, N., and Cavalheiro, E.A. New insights from the use of pilocarpine and kainate models. *Epilepsy Res.* 50, 95–105 (2002).

Leniger, T., Wiemann, M., Bingmann, D., Widman, G., Hufnagel, A., and Bonnet, U. Carbonic anhydrase inhibitor sulthiame reduces intracellular pH and epileptiform activity of hippocampal CA3 neurons. *Epilepsia* 43, 469–474 (2002).

Leniger-Follert, E. Mechanisms of regulation of cerebral microflow during bicuculline-induced seizures in anaesthetized cats. *J. Cereb. Blood Flow Metab.* 4, 150–165 (1984).

Lepik, I.E. Status epilepticus: the next decade. *Neurology* 40 (Suppl. 2), 4–9 (1990).

Lerche, H., Jurkat-Rott, K., and Lehman-Horn, F. Ion channels and epilepsy. *Am. J. Med. Genet.* 106, 146–159 (2001).

Leresche, N., Parri, H.R., Erdemli, G., Guyon, A., Turner, J.P., Williams, S.R., Asprodini, E.K., and Crunelli, V. On the action of the anti-absence drug ethosuximide in the rat and cat thalamus. *J. Neurosci.* 18, 4842–4853 (1998).

Lester, H.A. and Karschin, A. Gain of function mutants: ion channels and G protein-coupled receptors. *Annu. Rev. Neurosci.* 23, 89–125 (2000).

Leung, L.S., Ma, J.Y., and McLachlan, R.S. Behaviors induced or disrupted by complex partial seizures. *Neurosci. Biobehav. Rev.* 24, 763–775 (2000).

Lewandowsky, M. Zur Lehre der Cerebrospinal Flüssigkeit. *Z. Klin. Med.* 40, 480–494 (1900).

Lewis, D.V., O'Connor, M.J., and Schuette, W.H. Oxidative metabolism during recurrent seizures in the penicillin treated hippocampus. *Electroencephalogr. Clin. Neurophysiol.* 36, 347–356 (1974).

Lewis, D.V. and Schuette, W.H. NADH fluorescence and $[K^+]_o$ changes during hippocampal electrical stimulation. *J. Neurophysiol.* 38, 405–417 (1975).

Lewis, T.J. and Rinzel, J. Self-organized synchronous oscillations in a network of excitable cells coupled by gap junctions. *Network-Comput. Neural. Syst.* 11, 299–320 (2000).

Li, P.-A., Kristián, T., He, Q.-P., and Siesjö, B.K. Cyclosporin A enhances survival, ameliorates brain damage, and prevents secondary mitochondrial dysfunction after a 30-minute period of transient cerebral ischemia. *Exp. Neurol.* 165, 153–163 (2000a).

Li, P.-A., Rasquinha, I., He, Q.-P., Siesjö, B.K., Csiszár, K., Boyd, C.D., and MacManus, J.P. Hyperglycemia enhances DNA fragmentations after transient cerebral ischemia. *J. Cereb. Blood Flow Metab.* 21, 568–576 (2001).

Li, P.-A., Shuaib, A., Miyashita, H., He, Q.-P., and Siesjö, B.K. Hyperglycemia enhances extracellular glutamate accumulation in rats subjected to forebrain ischemia. *Stroke* 31, 183–191 (2000b).

Li, P.-A., Vogel, J., He, Q.-P., Smith, M.-L., Kuschinsky, W., and Siesjö, B.K. Preischemic hyperglycemia leads to rapidly developing brain damage with no change in capillary patency. *Brain Res.* 782, 175–183 (1998).

Lian, J., Bikson, M., Shuai, J., and Durand, D.M. Propagation of non-synaptic epileptiform activity across a lesion in rat hippocampal slices. *J. Physiol.* 537, 191–199 (2001).

Liberson, W.T. and Cadilhac, J. Les crises hippocampiques expérimentales. *Montpellier Med.* 45, 515–542 (1954).

Lieberman, D.N. and Mody, I. Properties of single NMDA receptor channels in human dentate gyrus granule cells. *J. Physiol.* 518, 55–70 (1999).

Lin, D.D., Cohen, A.S., and Coulter, D.A. Zinc-induced augmentation of excitatory synaptic currents and glutamate receptor responses in hippocampal CA3 neurons. *J. Neurophysiol.* 85, 1185–1196 (2001).

Lindvall, O., Kokaia, Z., Elmér, E., Ferencz, I., Bengzon, J., and Kokaia, M. Neurotrophins and kindling epileptogenesis. In M.E. Corcoran and S.L. Moshé (eds.), *Kindlking 5.* Plenum Press: New York, 299–310 (1998).

Link, M.J., Anderson, R.E., and Meyer, F.B. Effects of magnesium sulfate on pentylenetetrazole induced status epilepticus. *Epilepsia* 32, 543–549 (1991).

Lipton, P. Ischemic cell death in brain neurons. *Physiol. Rev.* 79, 1431–1568 (1999).

Lipton, P. and Whittingham, T.S. Reduced ATP concentration as a basis for synaptic transmission failure during hypoxia in the in vitro guinea pig hippocampus. *J. Physiol.* 325, 51–65 (1982).

Lisman, J.E. Bursts as a unit of neural information: making unreliable synapses reliable. *Trends Neurosci.* 20, 38–43 (1997).

Liu, S., Peterson, S.L., and Liu, K.J. Visualization of the early "no-reflow phenomenon" in rats subjected to focal cerebral ischemia and reperfusion. *Soc. Neurosci. Abstr.* 27, Prog. No. 434.16 (2001).

Llinas, R. and Sugimori, M. Electrophysiological properties of in vitro Purkinje cell dendrites in mammalian cerebellar slices. *J. Physiol.* 305, 197–213 (1980a).

Llinas, R. and Sugimori, M. Electrophysiological properties of in vitro Purkinje cell somata in mammalian cerebellar slices. *J. Physiol.* 305, 171–195 (1980b).

Lloyd, D.P.C. Post-tetanic potentiation of responses in monosynaptic reflex pathways of the spinal cord. *J. Gen. Physiol.* 33, 147–170 (1949).

Lockard, J.S. and Ward, A.A. (eds.) *Epilepsy. a window to brain mechanisms.* Raven Press: New York (1980).

Loewi, O. Über humorale Übertragbarkeit der Herznervenwirkung. *Pflügers Arch.* 189, 239–242 (1921).

Loiseau, P. Seizure precipitants. In J. Engel, Jr., and T.A. Pedley (eds.), *Epilepsy: a comprehensive textbook*, Vol. 1. Lippincott-Raven: Philadelphia, 93–97 (1998).

Lombardo, A.J., Kuzniecky, R., Powers, R.E., and Brown, G.B. Altered brain sodium channel transcript levels in human epilepsy. *Mol. Brain Res.* 35, 84–90 (1996).

Lømo, T. Potentiation of monosynaptic EPSPs in the perforant path granule cells synapse. *Exp. Brain Res.* 12, 46–63 (1971).

Lopantsev, V. and Avoli, M. Laminar organization of epileptiform discharges in the rat entorhinal cortex *in vitro*. *J. Physiol.* 509, 785–796 (1998).

Lopes da Silva, F.H. Neural mechanisms underlying brain waves: from neural membranes to networks. *Electroencephalogr. Clin. Neurophysiol.* 79, 81–93 (1991).

Lopes da Silva, F.H., Faas, G.C., Kamphuis, W., Titulaer, M., Vreugdenhil, M., and Wadman, W.J. Regional specific changes in glutamate and GABA$_A$ receptors, PKC isoenzymes and ionic channels in kindling epileptogenesis of the hippocampus of the rat. In M.E. Corcoran and S.L. Moshé (eds.), *Kindling 5*. Plenum Press: New York, 229–242 (1998).

Lopes da Silva, F.H. and Wadman, W.J. Pathophysiology of epilepsy. In H. Meinardi (ed.), *Handbook of clinical neurology*, Vol. 72 (28): *The Epilepsies*, Part I. Elsevier Science: Amsterdam, 39–81 (1999).

Lorente de Nó, R. Studies on the structure of the cerebral cortex. II. Continuation of the study of the ammonic system. *J. Psychol. Neurol.* 46, 113–177 (1934).

Löscher, W., Ebert, U., and Lehmann, H. Kindling induces a lasting, regionally selective increase in kynurenic acid in the nucleus accumbens. *Brain Res.* 725, 252–256 (1996).

Löscher, W. and Hönack, D. Anticonvulsant and behavioral effects of two novel competitive *N*-methyl-D-aspartic acid receptor antagonists, CGP 37849 and CGP 39551, in the kindling model of epilepsy. Comparison with MK-801 and carbamazepine. *J. Pharmacol. Exp. Ther.* 256, 432–440 (1991).

Lothman, E.W. Biological consequences of repeated seizures. In J. Engel, Jr., and T.A. Pedley (eds.), *Epilepsy: a comprehensive textbook*, Vol. 1. Lippincott-Raven: Philadelphia, 481–497 (1998).

Lothman, E.W., Bertram, E.H., Bekenstein, J.W., and Perlin, J.B. Self-sustaining limbic status epilepticus induced by "continuous" hippocampal stimulation: electrographic and behavioral characterstics. *Epilepsy Res.* 3, 107–119 (1989).

Lothman, E.W., Bertram, E.H., Kapur, J., and Stringer, J.L. Recurrent spontaneous hippocampal seizures in the rat as a chronic sequela to limbic status epilepticus. *Epilepsy Res.* 6, 110–118 (1990).

Lothman, E.W., Bertram, E.H.I., and Stringer, J.L. Functional anatomy of hippocampal seizures. *Prog. Neurobiol.* 37, 1–82 (1991).

Lothman, E.W., Collins, R.C., and Ferrendelli, J.A. Kainic acid-induced limbic seizures: electrophysiologic studies. *Neurology* 31, 806–812 (1981).

Lothman, E.W., Hatlelid, J.M., and Zorumski, C.F. Functional mapping of limbic seizures originating in hippocampus: a combined 2-deoxyglucose and electrophysiologic study. *Brain Res.* 360, 92–100 (1985a).

Lothman, E.W., Hatlelid, J.M., Zorumski, C.F., Conry, J.A., Moon, J.A., and Perlin, J.B. Kindling with rapidly recurring hippocampal seizures. *Brain Res.* 360, 83–91 (1985b).

Lothman, E., LaManna, J., Cordingley, G., Rosenthal, M., and Somjen, G. Responses of electrical potential, potassium levels and oxidative metabolism in cat cerebral cortex. *Brain Res.* 88, 15–36 (1975).

Lothman, E.W. and Somjen, G.G. Extracellular potassium activity, intracellular and extracellular potential responses in the spinal cord. *J. Physiol.* 252, 115–136 (1975).

Lothman, E.W. and Somjen, G.G. Functions of primary afferents and responses of extracellular K^+ during spinal epileptiform seizures. *Electroencephalogr. Clin. Neurophysiol.* 41, 253–267 (1976a).

Lothman, E.W. and Somjen, G.G. Motor and electrical signs of epileptiform activity induced by penicillin in the spinal cords of decapitate cats. *Electroencephalogr. Clin. Neurophysiol.* 41, 237–252 (1976b).

Lothman, E.W. and Somjen, G.G. Reflex effects and postsynaptic membrane potential changes during epileptiform activity induced by penicillin in decapitate spinal cords. *Electroencephalogr. Clin. Neurophysiol.* 41, 337–347 (1976c).

Lothman, E.W., Stringer, J.L., and Bertram, E.H. The dentate gyrus as control point for seizures in the hippocampus and beyond. *Epilepsy Res.* (Suppl. 7), 301–313 (1992).

Louis, N.C.A., Niquet, J., Ben-Ari, Y., and Represa, A. Cellular plasticity. In J. Engel, Jr., and T.A. Pedley (eds.), *Epilepsy: a comprehensive textbook*, Vol. 1. Lippincott-Raven: Philadelphia, 387–396 (1998).

Lucas, D.R. and Newhouse, J.P. The toxic effect of sodium L-glutamate on the inner layers of the retina. *Arch. Ophthalmol.* 58, 193–201 (1957).

Lucké, B. and Parpart, A.K. Osmotic properties and permeability of cancer cells. I. Relative permeability of Ehrlich mouse ascites tumor cells and of mouse erythrocytes to polyhydric alcohols and to sodium chloride. *Cancer Res.* 14, 75–80 (1954).

Lüders, H.O. (ed.). *Epilepsy: comprehensive review and case discussions.* Martin Dunitz: London (2001).

Lüders, H.O., Dinner, D.S., Morris, H.H., Wyllie, E., and Comair, Y.G. Electrical stimulation of negative motor areas. In H.O. Lüders and S. Noachtar (eds.), *Epileptic seizures: pathophysiology and clinical semiology.* Churchill Livingstone: New York, 199–210 (1998).

Luhmann, H.J. and Heinemann, U. Hypoxia-induced functional alterations in adult rat neocortex. *J. Neurophysiol.* 67, 798–811 (1992).

Luhmann, H.J. and Kral, T. Hypoxia-induced dysfunction in developing rat neocortex. *J. Neurophysiol.* 78, 1212–1221 (1997).

Lukyanetz, E.A., Shkryl, V.M., and Kostyuk, P.G. Selective blockade of N-type calcium channels by levetiracetam. *Epilepsia* 43, 9–18 (2002).

Lundbaek, J.A. and Hansen, A.J. Brain interstitial volume fraction and tortuosity in anoxia. Evaluation of the ion-selective micro-electrode method. *Acta Physiol. Scand.* 146, 473–484 (1992).

Lundbaek, J.A., Tonnesen, T., Laursen, H., and Hansen, A.J. Brain interstitial composition during acute hyponatremia. *Acta Neurochir.* (Suppl. 51), 17–18 (1990).

Lux, H.D. Kaliumaktivität im Hirngewebe. Untersuchungen zim Krampfproblem. *Mitteilungen Max Planck Gesellsch.* 1, 34–52 (1973).

Lux, H.D. The kinetics of extracellular potassium: relation to epileptogenesis. *Epilepsia* 15, 375–393 (1974).

Lux, H.D. An invertebrate model of paroxysmal depolarizing shifts. In P.A. Schwartzkroin and H.V. Wheal (eds.), *Electrophysiology of epilepsy*. Academic Press: London, 343–352 (1984).

Lux, H.-D. and Heinemann, U. Ionic changes during experimentally induced seizure activity. *Electroencephalogr. Clin. Neurophysiol.* (Suppl. 34), 289–297 (1978).

Lux, H.-D., Heinemann, U., and Dietzel, I. Ionic changes and alterations in the size of the extracellular space during epileptic activity. In A.V. Delgado-Escueta, A.A. Ward, D.M. Woodbury, and R.J. Porter (eds.), *Basic mechanisms of the epilepsies: molecular and cellular approaches*. Raven Press: New York, 619–639 (1986).

Lynch, M. and Sutula, T. Recurrent excitatory connectivity in the dentate gyrus of kindled and kainic acid-treated rats. *J. Neurophysiol.* 83, 693–704 (2000).

Lytton, W.W., Contreras, D., Destexhe, A., and Steriade, M. Dynamic interactions determine partial thalamic quiescence in a computer network model of spike-and-wave seizures. *J. Neurophysiol.* 77, 1679–1696 (1997).

Lytton, W.W., Hellman, K.M., and Sutula, T.P. Computer models of hippocampal circuit changes of the kindling model of epilepsy. *Artif. Intell. Med.* 13, 81–97 (1998).

MacDonald, R.L. Anticonvulsant drug actions on neurons in cell culture. *J. Neural Transmiss.* 72, 173–183 (1988).

MacDonald, R.L. Cellular effects of antiepileptic drugs. In J. Engel, Jr., and T.A. Pedley (eds.), *Epilepsy: a comprehensive textbook*, Vol. 2. Lippincott-Raven: Philadelphia, 1383–1391 (1998).

MacVicar, B.A. Voltage dependent calcium channels in glial cells. *Science* 226, 1345–1347 (1984).

MacVicar, B.A. and Dudek, F.E. Dye coupling between CA3 pyramidal cells in slices of rat hippocampus. *Brain Res.* 196, 494–499 (1980).

MacVicar, B.A. and Dudek, F.E. Electrotonic coupling between pyramidal cells: a direct demonstration in rat hippocampal slices. *Science* 213, 782–785 (1981).

Madeja, M. Extracellular surface charges in voltage-gated ion channels. *News Physiol. Sci.* 15, 15–19 (2000).

Madeja, M., Musshoff, U., Lorra, C., Pongs, O., and Speckmann, E.-J. Mechanism of action of the epileptogenic drug pentylenetetrazol on a cloned neuronal potassium channel. *Brain Res.* 722, 59–70 (1996).

Madsen, T.M., Treschow, A., Bengzon, J., Bolwig, T.G., Lindvall, O., and Tingstrom, A. Increased neurogenesis in a model of electroconvulsive therapy. *Biol. Psychiatry* 47, 1043–1049 (2000).

Maeno, E., Ishizaki, Y., Kanseki, T., Hazama, A., and Okada, Y. Normotonic cell shrinkage because of disordered volume regulation is an early prerequisite to apoptosis. *Proc. Natl. Acad. Sci. USA* 97, 9487–9492 (2000).

Magee, J.C. and Carruth, M. Dendritic voltage-gated ion channels regulate the action potential firing mode of hippocampal CA1 pyramidal neurons. *J. Neurophysiol.* 82, 1895–1901 (1999).

Magee, J.C., Hoffman, D.A., Colbert, C.M., and Johnston, D. Electrical and calcium signaling in dendrites of hippocampal pyramidal neurons. *Annu. Rev. Physiol.* 60, 327–346 (1998).

Maglóczky, Z., Halász, P., Vajda, J., Czirják, S., and Freund, T.F. Loss of calbindin-D28K immunoreactivity from dentate granule cells in human temporal lobe epilepsy. *Neuroscience* 76, 377–385 (1997).

Malafosse, A. and Moulard, B. Situation et perspectives de la génétique des épilepsies. *Rev. Neurol.* 158, 283–291 (2002).

Malenka, R.C. and Nicoll, R.A. Long term potentiation—a decade of progress? *Science* 285, 1870–1874 (1999).

Mamelak, A.N. and Lowenstein, D.H. Regulation of gene expression. In J. Engel, Jr., and T.A Pedley (eds.), *Epilepsy: a comprehensive textbook*, Vol. 1. Lippincott-Raven: Philadelphia, 291–306 (1998).

Marcoux, F.W., Probert, A.W., and Weber, M.L. Hypoxic neuronal injury in tissue culture is associated with delayed calcium accumulation. *Stroke* 21 (Suppl III), III-71–III-74 (1990).

Marrannes, R., De Prins, E., Fransen, J., and Clincke, G. Neuropharmacology of spreading depression. In A. Lehmenkühler, K.-H. Grotemeyer, and F. Tegtmeier (eds.), *Migraine: basic mechanisms and treatment*. Urban & Schwarzenberg: München, 431–443, (1993).

Marrannes, R., De Prins, E., Willems, R., and Wauquier, A. NMDA antagonists inhibit cortical spreading depression, but accelerate the onset of neuronal depolarization induced by asphyxia. In G. Somjen (ed.), *Mechanisms of cerebral hypoxia and stroke*. Plenum Press: New York, 303–304 (1988a).

Marrannes, R., Willems, R., De Prins, E., and Wauquier, A. Evidence for a role of the *N*-methyl-D-aspartate (NMDA) receptor in cortical spreading depression in the rat. *Brain Res.* 457, 226–240 (1988b).

Marrocos, M.A. and Martins-Ferreira, H. Effect of Na^+ and Cl^- on the velocity of propagation of the spreading depression in chick retina. *Braz. J. Med. Biol. Res.* 23, 473–476 (1990).

Marsh, D.J., Baraban, S.C., Hollopeter, G., and Palmiter, R.D. Role of the Y5 neuropeptide Y receptor in limbic seizures. *Proc. Natl. Acad. Sci. USA* 96, 13518–13523 (1999).

Marshall, W.H. Spreading cortical depression of Leão. *Physiol. Rev.* 39, 239–279 (1959).

Martin, D., McNamara, J.O., and Nadler, J.V. Kindling enhances sensitivity to CA3 hippocampal pyramidal cells to NMDA. *J. Neurosci.* 12, 1928–1935 (1992).

Martins-Ferreira, H. Variações Lentas De Voltagem Do Córtex Cerebral. Doctoral dissertation. Rio de Janeiro: Instituto de Biofisica (1954).

Martins-Ferreira, H. and de Oliveira Castro, G. Light-scattering changes accompanying spreading depression in isolated retina. *J. Neurophysiol.* 29, 715–726 (1966).

Martins-Ferreira, H., Nedergaard, M., and Nicholson, C. Perspectives on spreading depression. *Brain Res. Rev.* 32, 215–234 (2000).

Martins-Ferreira, H., Oliveira Castro, G.d., and Albuquerque, A. Effet des ions chlorures sur les variations d'intensité de la lumière diffusée par la rétine pendant la "spreading depression". *C.R. Acad. Sci. Ser. D* 273, 414–417 (1971).

Martins-Ferreira, H., Oliveira Castro, G.d., Struchiner, C.J., and Rodrigues, P.S. Circling spreading depression in isolated chick retina. *J. Neurophysiol.* 37, 773–784 (1974a).

Martins-Ferreira, H., Oliveira Castro, G.d., Struchiner, C.J., and Rodrigues, P.S. Liberation of chemical factors during spreading depression in isolated retina. *J. Neurophysiol.* 37, 785–791 (1974b).

Martins-Ferreira, H. and Ribeiro, L.J. Biphasic effects of gap junctional uncoupling agents on the propagation of retinal spreading depression. *Braz. J. Med. Biol. Res.* 28, 991–994 (1995).

Maru, E., Tatsuno, J., Okamoto, J., and Ashida, H. Development and reduction of synaptic potentiation induced by perforant path kindling. *Exp. Neurol.* 78, 409–424 (1982).

Massimini, M. and Amzica, F. Extracellular calcium fluctuations and intracellular potentials in the cortex during the slow sleep oscillation. *J. Neurophysiol.* 85, 1346–1350 (2001).

Masson, C. Anomalies des canaux ioniques ("channelopathies"). dans les maladies neurologiques. *Presse Med.* 31, 244–248 (2002).

Masukawa, L.M., Higashima, M., Kim, J.H., and Spencer, D.D. Epileptiform discharges evoked in hippocampal brain slices from epileptic patients. *Brain Res.* 493, 168–174 (1989).

Mathern, G.W., Babb, T.L., and Armstrong, D.L. Hippocampal sclerosis. In J. Engel, Jr., and T.A. Pedley (eds.), *Epilepsy: a comprehensive textbook*, Vol. 1. Lippincott-Raven: Philadelphia, 133–155 (1998).

Matsumoto, H., Ayala, G.F., and Gumnit, R.J. Neuronal behavior and triggering mechanism in cortical epileptic focus. *J. Neurophysiol.* 32, 688–703 (1969).

Matsumoto, S., Friberg, H., Ferrand-Drake, M., and Wieloch, T. Blockade of the mitochondrial permeability transition pore diminishes infarct size in the rat after transient middle cerebral artery occlusion. *J. Cereb. Blood Flow Metab.* 19, 736–741 (1999).

Matsuura, S. Effects of changes in extracellular K^+ concentration on resting and action potentials of the toad spinal motoneuron. *Osaka City Med. J.* 15, 29–45 (1969).

Mattson, M.P., Rychlik, B., Chu, C., and Christakos, S. Evidence for calcium-reducing and excito-protective roles for the calcium binding protein calbindin-D28k in cultured hippocampal neurons. *Neuron*, 6 41–51 (1991).

Matz, R. Hyperosmolar nonacidotic diabetes (HNAD). In D. Porte, Jr., and R.S. Sherwin (eds.), *Elleberg and Rifkin's diabetes mellitus*. Appleton & Lange: Stamford, Conn., 845–860 (1997).

Mayevsky, A. and Chance, B. Repetitive patterns of metabolic changes during cortical spreading depression of the awake rat. *Brain Res.* 65, 529–533 (1974).

Mayevsky, A. and Chance, B. Metabolic responses of the awake cerebral cortex to anoxia, hypoxia, spreading depression and epileptiform activity. *Brain Res.* 98, 149–165 (1975).

Mayevsky, A., Doron, A., Manor, T., Meilin, S., Zarchin, N., and Ouaknine, G.E. Cortical spreading depression recorded from the human brain using a multiparametric monitoring system. *Brain Res.* 740, 268–274 (1996).

Mayevsky, A., Zarchin, N., and Sonn, J. Brain redox state and O_2 balance in experimental spreading depression and ischemia. In A. Lehmenkühler, K.-H. Grotemeyer, and F. Tegtmeier (eds.), *Migraine: basic mechanisms and treatment*, Urban & Schwarzenberg: München, 379–393 (1993).

Maynard, K.I., Kawamata, T., Ogilvy, C.S., Perez, F., Arango, P., and Ames, A. Avoiding stroke during cerebral arterial occlusion by temporarily blocking neuronal function in the rabbit. *J. Stroke Cerebrovasc. Dis.* 7, 287–295 (1998).

Mazarati, A.M., Langel, U., and Bartfai, T. Galanin an endogenous anticonvulsant? *Neuroscientist* 7, 506–517 (2001).

Mazarati, A.M., Liu, H., Soomets, U., Sankar, R., Shin, D., Katsumori, H., Langel, Ü., and Wasterlain, C.G. Galanin modulation of seizures and seizure modulation of galanin in animal models of status epilepticus. *J. Neurosci.* 18, 10070–10077 (1998).

McBain, C.J. Hippocampal inhibitory neuron activity in the elevated potassium model of epilepsy. *J. Neurophysiol.* 72, 2853–2863 (1994).

McBain, C.J., Traynelis, S.F., and Dingledine, R. Regional variation of extracellular space in hippocampus under physiological and pathological conditions. *Science* 249, 674–677 (1990).

McCormick, D.A. and Contreras, D. On the cellular and network bases of epileptic seizures. *Annu. Rev. Physiol.* 63, 815–846 (2001).

McCormick, D.A. and Huguenard, J.R. A model of the electrophysiological properties of thalamocortical relay cells. *J. Neurophysiol.* 68, 1384–1400 (1992).

McDonald, J.W., Bhattacharyya, T., Sensi, S.L., Lobner, D., Ying, H.S., Canzoniero, L.M.T., and Choi, D.W. Extracellular acidity potentiates AMPA receptor-mediated cortical neuronal death. *J. Neurosci.* 18, 6290–6299 (1998).

McIntyre, D.C. and Poulter, M.O. Kindling and the mirror focus. *Int. Rev. Neurobiol.* 45, 387–407 (2001).

McIntyre, D.C., Poulter, M.O., and Gilby, K. Kindling: some old and some new. *Epilepsy Res.* 50, 79–92 (2002).

McIntyre, D.C. and Wong, R.K.S. Cellular and synaptic properties of amygdala-kindled pyriform cortex in vitro. *J. Neurophysiol.* 35, 1295–1307 (1986).

McLachlan, R.S., Avoli, M., and Gloor, P. Transition from spindles to generalized spike and wave discharges in the cat: simultaneous single-cell recordings in cortex and thalamus. *Exp. Neurol.* 85, 413–425 (1984).

McLachlan, R.S. and Girvin, J.P. Spreading depression of Leão in rodent and human cortex. *Brain Res.* 666, 133–136 (1994).

McLean, M.J. and MacDonald, R.L. Multiple actions of phenytoin on mouse spinal cord neurons in culture. *J. Pharmacol. Exp. Ther.* 227, 779–789 (1983).

McLean, M.J. and MacDonald, R.L. Sodium valproate, but not ethosuximide, produces use- and voltage-dependent limitation of high frequency repetitive firing of action potentials of mouse central neurons in cell culture. *J. Pharmacol. Exp. Ther.* 237, 1001–1011 (1986).

McNamara, J.O. Drugs effective in the therapy of epilepsies. In J.G. Hardman and L.E. Limbird (eds.), *Goodman and Gilman's The Pharmacological basis of therapeutics*, 10th edition. McGraw-Hill: New York, 521–547 (2001).

McNamara, J.O., Byrne, M.C., Dasheiff, R.M., and Fitz, J.G. The kindling model of epilepsy: a review. *Prog. Neurobiol.* 15, 139–159 (1980).

McNamara, J.O., Russell, R.D., Rigsbee, L., and Bonhaus, D.W. Anticonvulsant and antiepileptogenic actions of MK-801 in the kindling and electroshock models. *Neuropharmacology* 27, 563–568 (1988).

McNamara, J.O. and Wada, J.A. Kindling model. In J. Engel, Jr., and T.A. Pedley (eds.), *Epilepsy: a comprehensive textbook*, Vol. 1. Lippincott-Raven: Philadelphia, 419–425 (1998).

Meech, R.W. and Thomas, R.C. Effects of measured calcium chloride injection on the membrane potential and internal pH of snail neurones. *J. Physiol.* 298, 111–129 (1980).

Meeren, H.K.M., Pijn, J.P.M., van Luijtelaar, E.L.J.M., Coenen, A.M.L., and Lopes da Silva, F.H. Cortical focus drives widespread corticothalamic networks during spontaneous absence seizures in rats. *J. Neurosci.* 22, 1480–1495 (2002).

Meisler, M.H., Kearney, J.A., Sprunger, L.K., MacDonald, B.T., Buchner, D.A., and Escayg, A. Mutations of voltage-gated sodium channels in movement disorders and epilepsy. *Novartis Found. Symp.* 241, 72–81 (2002).

Melchers, B.P., Pennartz, C.M.A., Wadman, W.J., and Lopes da Silva, F.H. Quantitative correlation between tetanus-induced decreases in extracellular calcium and LTP. *Brain Res.* 454, 1–10 (1988).

Meldrum, B.S. Epileptic brain damage: a consequence and a cause of seizures. *Neuropathol. Appl. Neurobiol.* 23, 185–201 (1997).

Meldrum, B.S. Do preclinical seizure models preselect certain adverse effects of anti-epileptic drugs? *Epilepsy Res.* 50, 33–40 (2002a).

Meldrum, B.S. Concept of activity-induced cell death in epilepsy: historical and contemporary perspectives. In T. Sutula and A. Pitkänen (eds.), *Do Seizures Damage the Brain?* Elsevier: Amsterdam, 3–11 (2002b).

Meldrum, B.S., Akbar, M.T., and Chapman, A.G. Glutamate receptors and transporters in genetic and acquired models of epilepsy. *Epilepsy Res.* 36, 189–204 (1999).

Meldrum, B.S. and Brierley, J.B. Prolonged epileptic seizures in primates. Ischemic cell change and its relation to ictal physiological events. *Arch. Neurol.* 28, 10–17 (1973).

Meldrum, B.S. and Corsellis, J.A.N. Epilepsy. In J. Hume Adams, J.A.N. Corsellis, and L.W. Duchen (eds.), *Greenfield's neuropathology*. Wiley: New York, 921–950 (1984).

Mello, L.E., Cavalheiro, E.A., Tan, A.M., Kupfer, W.R., Pretorius, J.K., Babb, T.L., and Finch, D.M. Circuit mechanisms of seizures in the pilocarpine model of chronic epilepsy: cell loss and mossy fiber sprouting. *Epilepsia* 34, 985–995 (1993).

Menna, G., Tong, C.K., and Chesler, M. Interstitial shifts in pH, K^+ and Na^+ during spreading depression evoked in zero calcium media. *Soc. Neurosci. Abstr.* 25, 2104 (1999).

Menna, G., Tong, C.K., and Chesler, M. Extracellular pH changes and accompanying cation shifts during ouabain-induced spreading depression. *J. Neurophysiol.* 83, 1338–1345 (2000).

Mercuri, N.B., Bonci, A., Johnson, S.W., Stratta, F., Calabresi, P., and Bernardi, G. Effects of anoxia on rat midbrain dopamine neurons. *J. Neurophysiol.* 71, 1165–1173 (1994).

Merritt, H.H. and Putnam, T.J. A new series of anticonvulsant drugs tested by experiments on animals. *Arch. Neurol. Psychiatry* 39, 1003–1015 (1938).

Messeter, K. and Siesjö, B.K. Electrochemical gradients for H^+ and HCO_3^- during sustained acid-base changes. In B.K. Siesjö and S.C. Sørensen (eds.), *Ion homeostasis of the brain*, Munksgaard: Copenhagen, 190–200 (1971).

Mi, H., Haeberle, H., and Barres, B.A. Induction of astrocyte differentiation by endothelial cells. *J. Neurosci.* 21, 1538–1547 (2001).

Midzianovskaia, I.S., Kuznetsova, G.D., Coenen, A.M.L., Spiridonov, A.M., and van Luijtelaar, E.L.J.M. Electrophysiological and pharmacological characteristics of two types of spike-wave discharges in WAG/Rij rats. *Brain Res.* 911, 70 (2001).

Mies, G., Iijima, T., and Hossmann, K.-A. Correlation between peri-infarct DC shifts and ischaemic neuronal damage in rat. *NeuroReport* 4, 709–711 (1993).

Mies, G. and Paschen, W. Regional chnages of blood flow, glucose and ATP content determined on brain sections during a single passage of spreading depression in rat brain cortex. *Exp. Neurol.* 84, 249–258 (1984).

Mikuni, N., Babb, T.L., Wylie, C., and Ying, Z. NMDAR1 receptor proteins and mossy fibers in the fascia dentata during rat kainate hippocampal electrogenesis. *Exp. Neurol.* 163, 271–277 (2000).

Miles, R., Traub, R.D., and Wong, R.K.S. Spread of synchronous firing in longitudinal slices from the CA3 region of the hippocampus. *J. Neurophysiol.* 60, 1481–1496 (1988).

Milner, P.M. Note on the possible correspondence between the scotomas of migraine and spreading depression of Leão. *Electroencephalogr. Clin. Neurophysiol.* 10, 705 (1958).

Mintz, I.M., Sabatini, B.L., and Regehr, W.G. Calcium control of transmitter release at a cerebellar synapse. *Neuron* 15, 675–688 (1995).

Mitani, A., Andou, Y., and Kataoka, K. Selective vulnerability of hippocampal CA1 neurons cannot be explained in terms of an increase in glutamate concentration during ischemia in the gerbil: brain microdialysis study. *Neuroscience* 48, 307–313 (1992).

Mitani, A., Kadoya, F., and Kataoka, K. Temperature dependence of hypoxia-induced calcium accumulation in gerbil hippocampal slices. *Brain Res.* 562, 159–163 (1991).

Mitani, A., Takeyasu, S., Yanase, H., Nakamura, Y., and Kataoka, K. Changes in intracellular Ca^{2+} and energy levels during in vitro ischemia in the gerbil hippocampal slice. *J. Neurochem.* 62, 626–634 (1994).

Mitani, A., Yanase, H., and Kataoka, K. Postischemic functional changes of glutamate receptors in field CA1 of the gerbil hippocampus. *J. Neurochem.* 61 (Suppl.), S139 (1993).

Mittmann, T., Qü, M., Zilles, K., and Luhmann, H.J. Long-term cellular dysfunction after focal cerebral ischemia: in vitro analyses. *Neuroscience* 85, 15–27 (1998).

Mitzdorf, U. Current source density method and application in cat cerebral cortex: investigation of evoked potentials and EEG phenomena. *Physiol Rev* 65, 37–100 (1985).

Miyazaki, S., Katayama, Y., Furuichi, M., Kinoshita, K., Kawamata, T., and Tsubokawa, T. Post-ischemic potentiation of Schaffer collateral/CA1 pyramidal cell responses of the rat hippocampus in vivo: involvement of *N*-methyl-D-aspartate receptors. *Brain Res.* 611, 155–159 (1993).

Mody, I. Ion channels in epilepsy. *Int. Rev. Neurobiol.* 42, 199–226 (1998).

Mody, I. Synaptic plasticity in kindling. *Adv. Neurol.* 79, 631–643 (1999).

Mody, I. and Heinemann, U. NMDA receptors of dentate gyrus granule cells participate in synaptic transmission following kindling. *Nature* 326, 701–704 (1987).

Mody, I., Lambert, J.D.C., and Heinemann, U. Low extracellular magnesium induces epileptiform activity and spreading depression in rat hippocampal slices. *J. Neurophysiol.* 57, 869–888 (1987).

Mody, I. and Lieberman, D.N. Lasting prolongation of NMDA channel openings after kindling. In M.E. Corcoran and S.L. Moshé (eds.), *Kindling 5.* Plenum Press: New York, 65–72 (1998).

Mody, I., Stanton, P.K., and Heinemann, U. Activation of *N*-methyl-D-aspartate receptors parallels changes in cellular and synaptic properties of dentate gyrus granule cells after kindling. *J. Neurophysiol.* 59, 1033–1054 (1988).

Möhnle, P. and Goetz, A.E. Physiologische Effekte, Pharmakologie und Indikationen zur Gabe von Magnesium. *Anaesthesist* 50, 377–391 (2001).

Molnár, P. and Nadler, J.V. Mossy fiber-granule cell synapses in the normal and epileptic rat dentate gyrus studied with minimal laser photostimulation. *J. Neurophysiol.* 82, 1883–1894 (1999).

Molnár, P. and Nadler, J.V. Synaptically released zinc inhibits *N*-methyl-D-aspartate receptor activation at recurrent mossy fiber synapses. *Brain Res.* 910, 205–207 (2001).

Moody, W.J., Futamachi, K.J., and Prince, D.A. Extracellular potassium activity during epileptogenesis. *Exp. Neurol.* 42, 248–263 (1974).

Mori, S., Miller, W.H., and Tomita, T. Microelectrode study of spreading depression (SD). in frog retina. General observations of field potential associated with SD. *Jpn. J. Physiol.* 26, 203–217 (1976a).

Mori, S., Miller, W.H., and Tomita, T. Microelectrode study of spreading depression (SD). in frog retina. Müller cell activity and [K^+] during SD. *Jpn. J. Physiol.* 26, 219–233 (1976b).

Mori, S., Miller, W.H., and Tomita, T. Müller cell function during spreading depression in frog retina. *Proc. Natl. Acad. Sci. USA* 73, 1351–1354 (1976c).

Morison, R.S. and Dempsey, E.W. Mechanism of thalamocortical augmentation and repetition. *Am. J. Physiol.* 138, 297–308 (1942).

Morrell, F. Physiology and histochemistry of the mirror focus. In H.H. Jasper, A.A.Ward, and A. Pope (eds.), *Basic Mechanisms of the Epilepsies*. Little, Brown: Boston, 357–370 (1969).

Morris, M.E., Baimbridge, K.G., El-Beheiry, H., Obrocea, G.V., and Rosen, A.S. Correlation of anoxic neuronal responses and calbindin-D28K localization in stratum pyramidale of rat hippocampus. *Hippoccampus* 5, 25–39 (1995).

Moruzzi, M. and Magoun, H.W. Brain stem reticular formation and activation of the EEG. *Electroencephalogr. Clin. Neurophysiol.* 1, 455–473 (1949).

Muir, K.W. New experimental and clinical data on the efficacy of pharmacological magnesium infusions in cerebral infarcts. *Magnesium Res.* 11, 43–56 (1998).

Müller, M. Effects of chloride transport inhibition and chloride substitution on neuron function and on hypoxic spreading depression-like depolarization in rat hippocampal slices. *Neuroscience* 97, 33–45 (2000).

Müller, M., Brockhaus, J., and Ballanyi, K. ATP-independent anoxic activation of ATP-sensitive K^+ channels in dorsal vagal neurons of juvenile mice *in situ*. *Neuroscience* 109, 313–328 (2002).

Müller, M. and Somjen, G.G. Inhibition of major cationic inward currents prevents spreading depression-like hypoxic depolarization in rat hippocampal tissue slices. *Brain Res.* 812, 1–13 (1998).

Müller, M. and Somjen, G.G. Intrinsic optical signals in rat hippocampal slices during hypoxia-induced spreading depression-like depolarization. *J. Neurophysiol.* 82, 1818–1831 (1999).

Müller, M. and Somjen, G.G. Na^+ and K^+ concentrations, extra- and intracellular voltages and the effect of TTX in hypoxic rat hippocampal slices. *J. Neurophysiol.* 83, 735–745 (2000a).

Müller, M. and Somjen, G.G. Na^+ dependence and the role of glutamate receptors and Na^+ channels in ion fluxes during hypoxia of rat hippocampal slices. *J. Neurophysiol.* 84, 1869–1880 (2000b).

Murphy, K.P. and Greenfield, S.A. ATP-sensitive potassium channels counteract anoxia in neurons of the substantia nigra. *Exp. Brain Res.* 84, 355–358 (1991).

Mutsuga, N., Schuette, W.H., and Lewis, D.V. The contribution of local blood flow to the rapid clearance of potassium from the cortical extracellular space. *Brain Res.* 116, 431–436 (1976).

Nadler, J.V., Evenson, D.A., and Cuthbertson, G.J. Comparative toxicity of kainic acid and other acidic amino acids toward rat hippocampal neurons. *Neuroscience* 6, 2505–2517 (1981).

Nadler, J.V., Perry, B.W., and Cotman, C.W. Selective reinnervation of area CA1 and the fascia dentata after destruction of CA3-CA4 afferents with kainic acid. *Brain Res.* 182, 1–9 (1980).

Nadler, J.V., Thompson, M.A., and McNamara, J.O. Kindling reduces sensitivity of CA3 hippocampal pyramidal cells to competitive NMDA receptor antagonists. *Neuropharmacology* 33, 147–153 (1994).

Nagelhus, E.A., Nielsen, S., Agre, P., and Ottersen, O.P. High resolution immunogold localization of aquaporin-4, a water channel, in rat brain. *Soc. Neurosci. Abstr.* 22, 625 (1996).

Nägerl, U.V., Mody, I., Jeub, M., Lie, A.A., Elger, C.E., and Beck, H. Surviving granule cells of the sclerotic human hippocampus have reduced Ca^{2+} influx because of a loss of calbindin-D_{28k} in temporal lobe epilepsy. *J. Neurosci.* 20, 1831–1836 (2000).

Najm, I.M., Ying, Z., Babb, T.L., Mohamed, A., Hadam, J., LaPresto, E., Wyllie, E., Kotagal, P., Bingaman, W., Foldvary, N., Morris, H., and Luders, H.O. Epileptogenicity correlated with increased N-methyl-D-aspartate receptor subunit NR2A/B in human cortical dysplasis. *Epilepsia* 41, 971–976 (2000).

Naquet, H. and Fernandes-Guardiola, A. Effects of various types of anoxia on spontaneous and evoked cerebral activity in the cat. In H. Gastaut and J.S. Meyer (eds.), *Cerebral hypoxia and the electroencephalogram.* Charles C. Thomas: Springfield, Ill., 72–88 (1961).

Neckelmann, D., Amzica, F., and Steriade, M. Spike-wave complexes and fast components of cortically generated seizures. III. Synchronizing mechanisms. *J. Neurophysiol.* 80, 1480–1494 (1998).

Neckelmann, D., Amzica, F., and Steriade, M. Changes in neuronal conductance during different components of cortically generated spike-wave seizures. *Neuroscience* 96, 475–485 (2000).

Nedergaard, M. Direct signalling from astrocytes to neurons in cultures of mammalian brain cells. *Science* 263, 1768–1771 (1994).

Nedergaard, M. Spreading depression as a contributor to ischemic brain damage. *Adv. Neurol.* 71, 75–83 (1996).

Nedergaard, M., Cooper, A.J.L., and Goldman, S.A. Gap junctions are required for the propagation of spreading depression. *J. Neurobiol.* 28, 433–444 (1995).

Nedergaard, M., Goldman, S.A., Desai, S., and Pulsinelli, W.A. Acid-induced death in neurons and glia. *J. Neurosci.* 11, 2489–2497 (1991).

Nedergaard, M. and Hansen, A.J. Spreading depression is not associated with neuronal injury in the normal brain. *Brain Res.* 449, 395–398 (1988).

Nelken, I. and Yaari, Y. The role of interstitial potassium in the generation of low-calcium hippocampal seizures. *Isr. J. Med. Sci.* 23, 124–131 (1987).

Nellgard, B., Gustafson, I., and Wieloch, T. Lack of protection by the N-methyl-D-aspartate receptor blocker dizocilpine (MK-801) after transient severe cerebral ischemia in the rat. *Anesthesiology* 75, 279–287 (1991).

Nelson, W.L. and Makielski, J.C. Block of sodium current by heptanol in voltage-clamped canine cardiac Purkinje cells. *Circ. Res.* 68, 977–983 (1991).

Néverlée, H. de and Laget, P. Propagation de la "dépression envahissante" (spreading depression). et maturation corticale régionale chez le jeune Lapin. *C.R. Soc. Biol.* 159, 1332–1337 (1965).

Newman, E.A. Regional specialization of retinal glial cell membrane. *Nature* 309, 155–157 (1984).

Newman, E.A. High potassium conductance in astrocyte endfeet. *Science* 233, 453–454 (1986).

Newman, E.A. Glial cell regulation of extracellular potassium. In H. Kettenmann and B.R. Ransom (eds.), *Neuroglia.* Oxford University Press: New York, 717–731 (1995).

Nicholson, C. Comparative neurophysiology of spreading depression in the cerebellum. *An. Acad. Bras. Cienc.* 56, 481–494 (1984).

Nicholson, C. Volume transmission and the propagation of spreading depression. In A. Lehmenkühler, K.-H. Grotemeyer, and F. Tegtmeier (eds.), *Migraine: basic mechanisms and treatment.* Urban & Schwarzenberg: München, 293–308 (1993).

Nicholson, C. and Freeman, J.A. Theory of current source density analysis and determination of conductivity tensor for anuran cebellum.. *J. Neurophysiol.* 38, 356–368 (1975).

Nicholson, C. and Kraig, R.P. The behavior of extracellular ions during spreading depression. In T. Zeuthen (ed.), *The application of ion-selective microelectrodes.* Elsevier: Amsterdam, 217–238 (1981).

Nicholson, C., Phillips, J.M., and Gardner-Medwin, A.R. Diffusion from an iontophoretic point source in the braIn role of tortuosity and volume fraction. *Brain Res.* 169, 580–584 (1979).

Nicholson, C. and Rice, M.E. Use of ion selective microelectrodes and voltametric microsensors to study brain cell microenvironment. In A.A. Boulton, G.B. Baker, and W. Walz (eds.), *Neuromethods*, Vol. 9. Humana: Clifton, N.J., 247–361 (1988).

Nicholson, C. and Syková, E. Extracellular space structure revealed by diffusion analysis. *Trends Neurosci.* 21, 207–215 (1998).

Nicholson, C., Ten Bruggencate, G., Stöckle, H., and Steinberg, R. Calcium and potassium changes in extracellular microenvironment of cat cerebellar cortex. *J. Neurophysiol.* 41, 1026–1039 (1978).

Nico, B., Frigeri, A., Nicchia, G.P., Quondamatteo, F., Herken, R., Errede, M., Ribatti, D., Svelto, M., and Roncali, L. Role of aquaporin-4 water channel in the development and integrity of the blood-brain barrier. *J. Cell Sci.* 114, 1297–1307 (2001).

Nicotera, P., Leist, M., and Manzo, L. Neuronal cell death: a demise with different shapes. *Trends Pharmacol. Sci.* 20, 46–51 (1999).

Niedermeyer, E. Abnormal EEG patterns. In E. Niedermeyer and F.H. Lopes da Silva (eds.), *Electroencephalography.* Williams & Wilkins: Baltimore, 235–260 (1999a).

Niedermeyer, E. The normal EEG of the waking adult. In E. Niedermeyer and F.H. Lopes da Silva (eds.), *Electroencephalography.* Williams & Wilkins: Baltimore, 149–173 (1999b).

Niedermeyer, E. and Lopes da Silva, F.H. (eds.), *Electroencephalography.* Williams & Wilkins: Baltimore (1999).

Nielsen, S., Nagelhus, E.A., Amiry-Moghaddam, M., Bourque, C., Agre, P., and Ottersen, O.P. Specialized membrane domains for water transport in glial cells: high-resolution immunogold cytochemistry of aquaporin-4 in rat brain. *J. Neurosci.* 17, 171–180 (1997).

Nielsen, S., Smith, B.L., Christensen, E.I., and Agre, P. Distribution of the aquaporin CHIP in secretory and resorptive epithelia and capillary endothelia. *Proc. Natl. Acad. Sci. USA* 90, 7275–7279 (1993).

Nioka, S., Chance, B., Smith, D.S., Mayevsky, A., Reilly, M.P., Alter, C., and Asakura, T. Cerebral energy metabolism and oxygen state during hypoxia in neonate and adult dogs. *Pediatr. Res.* 28, 54–62 (1990).

Noebels, J.L. Single gene control of excitability in central neurones. In P.A. Schwartzkroin and H.V. Wheal (eds.), *Electrophysiology of epilepsy.* Academic Press: London, 201–217 (1984).

Noebels, J.L. Single-gene models of epilepsy. *Adv. Neurol.* 79, 227–238 (1999).

Noebels, J.L. Sodium channel gene expression and epilepsy. *Novartis Found. Symp.* 241, 109–120 (2002).

Noebels, J.L., Rees, M., and Gardiner, R.M. Molecular genetics and epilepsy genes. In J. Engel, Jr., and T.A. Pedley (eds.), *Epilepsy: a comprehensive textbook*, Vol. 1. Lippincott-Raven: Philadelphia, 211–216 (1998).

O'Connor, M.J., Herman, C.J., Rosenthal, M., and Jöbsis, F.F. Intracellular redox changes preceding onset of epileptiform activity in intact cat hippocampus. *J. Neurophysiol.* 35, 471–483 (1972).

O'Kelly, I., Stephens, R.H., Peers, C., and Kemp, P.J. Potential identification of the O_2-sensitive K^+ current in a human neuroepithelial body-derived cell line. *Am. J. Physiol.* 276, L96–L104 (1999).

O'Leary, J.L. and Goldring, S. D-C potentials of the brain. *Physiol. Rev.* 44, 91–125 (1964).

O'Reilly, J.P., Cummins, T.R., and Haddad, G.G. Oxygen deprivation inhibits Na^+ current in rat hippocampal neurones via protein kinase C. *J. Physiol.* 503, 479–488 (1997).

Obeidat, A.S. and Andrew, R.D. Spreading depression determines acute cellular damage in the hippocampal slice during oxygen/glucose deprivation. *J. Neurosci.* 10, 3451–3461 (1998).

Obeidat, A.S., Jarvis, C.R., and Andrew, R.D. Glutamate does not mediate acute neuronal damage after spreading depression induced by O_2/glucose deprivation in the hippocampal slice. *J. Cereb. Blood Flow Metab.* 20, 412–422 (2000).

Oberleithner, H., Greger, R., and Lang, F. The effect of respiratory and metabolic acid-base changes on ionized calcium concentration: in vivo and in vitro experiments in man and rat. *Eur. J. Clin. Invest.* 12, 451–455 (1982).

Obrenovitch, T.P. and Zilkha, E. High extracellular potassium and not extracellular glutamate is required for the propagation of spreading depression. *J. Neurophysiol.* 73, 2107–2114 (1995).

Obrenovitch, T.P. and Zilkha, E. Inhibition of cortical spreading depression by L-701,324, a novel antagonist at the glycine site of the *N*-methyl-D-aspartate receptor complex. *Br. J. Pharmacol.* 117, 931–937 (1996a).

Obrenovitch, T.P. and Zilkha, E. Intracerebral microdialysis markedly inhibits the propagation of cortical spreading depression. *Acta Neurochirurg.* (Suppl. 67), 21–23 (1996b).

Obrenovitch, T.P., Zilkha, E., and Urenjak, J. Evidence against high extracellular glutamate promoting the elicitation of spreading depression by potassium. *J. Cereb. Blood Flow Metab.* 160, 923–931 (1996).

Ochs, S. The nature of spreading depression in neural networks. *Int. Rev. Neurobiol.* 4, 1–70 (1962).

Ogata, N. Mechanisms of the stereotyped high-frequency burst in hippocampal pyramidal neurons in vitro. *Brain Res.* 103, 386–388 (1976).

Ojemann, G.A. Brain mechanisms for language: observations during neurosurgery. In J.S. Lockard and A.A. Ward (eds.), *Epilepsy: a window to brain mechanisms.* Raven Press: New York, 243–260 (1980).

Ojemann, G.A. Surgical therapy for medically intractable epilepsy. *J. Neurosurg.* 66, 489–499 (1987).

Oka, H., Kako, M., Matsushima, M., and Ando, K. Traumatic spreading depression syndrome. Review of a particular type of head injury in 37 patients. *Brain* 100, 287–298 (1977).

Okada, Y.C., Huang, J.-C., Rice, M.E., Tranchina, D., and Nicholson, C. Origin of the apparent tissue conductivity in the molecular and granular layers of the in vitro turtle cerebellum and the interpretation of current source density analysis. *J. Neurophysiol.* 72, 742–753 (1994).

Okazaki, M.M., Aitken, P.G., and Nadler, J.V. Mossy fiber lesion reduces the probability that kainic acid will provoke CA3 hippocampal pyramidal cell bursting. *Brain Res.* 440, 352–356 (1988).

Okazaki, M.M., Molnár, P., and Nadler, J.V. Recurrent mossy fiber pathway in rat dentate gyrus: synaptic currents evoked in presence and absence of seizure-induced growth. *J. Neurophysiol.* 81, 1645–1660 (1999).

Okazaki, M.M. and Nadler, J.V. Protective effect of mossy fiber lesions against kainic acid-induced seizures and neuronal degeneration. *Neuroscience* 26, 763–781 (1988).

Oldendorf, W.H., Cornford, M.E., and Brown, W.J. The large apparent work capability of the blood-brain barrier: a study of the mitochondrial content of capillary endothelial cells in brain and other tissues. *Ann. Neurol.* 1, 409–417 (1977).

Oliveira Castro, G.d., Martins-Ferreira, H., and Gardino, P.F. Dual nature of the peaks of light scattered during spreading depression in chick retina. *An. Acad. Brasil. Ciênc.* 57, 95–103 (1985).

Olney, J.W. Brain lesions, obesity and other disturbances in mice treated with monosodium glutamate. *Science* 164, 719–721 (1969).

Olney, J.W., deGubareff, T., and Sloviter, R.S. "Epileptic" brain damage in rats induced by sustained electrical stimulation of the perforant path. II. Ultrastructural analysis of acute hippocampal pathology. *Brain Res. Bull.* 10, 699–712 (1983).

Olsen, J.S. and Miller, R.F. Spontaneous slow potentials and spreading depression in amphibian retina. *J. Neurophysiol.* 40, 752–767 (1977).

Olsen, R.W. and Avoli, M. GABA and epileptogenesis. *Epilepsia* 38, 399–407 (1997).

Opie, L.H. Pathophysiology and biochemistry of ischemia, necrosis and reperfusion. In B.J. Gersh and S.H. Rahimtoola (eds.), *Acute myocardial infarction.* Chapman & Hall: New York, 51–67 (1997).

Opitz, E. and Schneider, M. Über die Sauerstoffversorgung des Gehirns und den Mechanismus von Mangelwirkung. *Erg. Physiol.* 46, 126–260 (1950).

Orkand, R.K., Nicholls, J.G., and Kuffler, S.W. Effect of nerve impulses on the membrane potential of glial cells in the central nervous system of amphibia. *J. Neurophysiol.* 29, 788–806 (1966).

Ørskov, S.L. Eine Methode zur fortlaufenden photographischen Aufzeichnung von Volumänderungen der roten Blutkörperchen. *Biochem. Z.* 279, 241–249 (1935).

Otoom, S.A. and Alkadhi, K.A. Epileptiform activity of veratridine model in rat brain slices: effects of antiepileptic drugs. *Brain Res.* 38, 161–170 (2000).

Otoom, S.A., Tian, L.M., and Alkadhi, K.A. Veratridine-treated brain slices: a cellular model for epileptiform activity. *Brain Res.* 789, 150–156 (1998).

Ou-Yang, Y.-B., Kristián, T., Mellergård, P., and Siesjö, B.K. The influence of pH on glutamate- and depolarization-induced increases of intracellular calcium concentration in cortical neurons in primary culture. *Brain Res.* 646, 65–72 (1994).

Ouyang, Y.-B., Tan, Y., Comb, M., Liu, C.-L., Martone, M.E., Siesjö, B.K., and Hu, B.-R. Survival- and death-promoting events after transient cerebral ischemia: phosphorylation of Akt, release of cytochrome C, and activation of caspase-like proteases. *J. Cereb. Blood Flow Metab.* 19, 1126–1135 (1999).

Pal, S., Sombati, S., Limbrick, D.D., Jr., and DeLorenzo, R.J. In vitro status epilepticus causes sustained elevation of intracellular calcium levels in hippocampal neurons. *Brain Res.* 851, 20–31 (1999).

Pan, E. and Stringer, J.L. Burst characteristics of dentate gyrus granule cells: evidence for endogenous and nonsynaptic properties. *J. Neurophysiol.* 75, 124–132 (1996).

Pan, E. and Stringer, J.L. Role of potassium and calcium in the generation of cellular bursts in the dentate gyrus. *J. Neurophysiol.* 77, 2293–2299 (1997).

Pang, Z.-P., Deng, P., Ruan, Y.-W., and Xu, Z.C. Depression of fast excitatory synaptic transmission in large aspiny neurons of the neostriatum after transient forebrain ischemia. *J. Neurosci.* 22, 10948–10957 (2002).

Parent, J.M. and Lowenstein, D.H. Seizure-induced neurogenesis: are more new neurons good for an adult brain? In T. Sutula and A. Pitkänen (eds.), *Do seizures damage the brain?* Elsevier: Amsterdam, 121–131 (2002).

Parent, J.M., Yu, T.W., Leibowitz, R.T., Geschwind, D.H., Sloviter, R.S., and Lowenstein, D.H. Dentate granule cell neurogenesis is increased by seizures and contributes to aberrant network reorganization in the adult rat hippocampus. *J. Neurosci.* 17, 3727–3738 (1997).

Parri, H.R., Gould, T.M., and Crunelli, V. Spontaneous astrocytic calcium oscillations in situ drive NMDAR-mediated neuronal excitation. *Nature Neurosci.* 4, 803–812 (2001).

Payne, R.S., Schurr, A., and Rigor, B.M. Cell swelling exacerbates hypoxic neuronal damage in rat hippocampal slices. *Brain Res.* 723, 210–213 (1996).

Peck, C. and Meltzer, S.J.K. Anesthesia of human beings by intravenous injection of magnesium sulfate. *JAMA* 67, 1131–1133 (1916).

Pedley, T.A., Fisher, R.S., Futamachi, K.J., and Prince, D.A. Regulation of extracellular potassium concentration in epileptogenesis. *Fed. Proc.* 35, 1254–1259 (1976).

Peeters, B.W., Kerbusch, J.M., Coenen, A.M.L., Vossen, J.M., and van Luijtelaar, E.L.J.M. Genetics of spike-wave discharges in the electroencephalogram (EEG) of the WAG/Rij inbred rat straIn a classical medelian crossbreeding study. *Behav. Genet.* 22, 361–368 (1992).

Pellegrini-Giampietro, D.E., Zukin, R.S., Bennett, M.V.L., Cho, S., and Pulsinelli, W.A. Switch of glutamate receptor subunit gene expression in CA1 subfield of hippocampus following global ischemia in rats. *Proc. Natl. Acad. Sci. USA* 89, 10499–10503 (1992).

Pellmar, T.C. and Wilson, W.A. Synaptic mechanism of pentylenetetrazole: selectivity for chloride conductance. *Science* 197, 912–914 (1977).

Penfield, W. and Jasper, H. *Epilepsy and the functional anatomy of the brain.* Little, Brown: Boston (1954).

Pérez-Pinzón, M.A., Born, J.G., and Centeno, J.M. Calcium and increased excitability promote tolerance against anoxia in hippocampal slices. *Brain Res.* 833, 20–26 (1999).

Perez-Pinzon, M.A., Mumford, P.L., Carranza, V., and Sick, T.J. Calcium influx from the extracellular space promotes NADH hyperoxidation and electrical dysfunction after anoxia in hippocampal slices. *J. Cereb. Blood Flow Metab.* 18, 215–221 (1998).

Pérez-Pinzón, M.A., Mumford, P.L., Rosenthal, M., and Sick, T.J. Anoxic preconditioning in hippocampal slices: role of adenosine. *Neuroscience* 75, 687–694 (1996).

Pérez-Pinzón, M.A., Mumford, P.L., Rosenthal, M., and Sick, T.J. Antioxidants, mitochondrial hyperoxidation and electrical recovery after anoxia in hippocampal slices. *Brain Res.* 754, 163–170 (1997a).

Pérez-Pinzón, M.A., Tao, L., and Nicholson, C. Extracellular potassium, volume fraction and tortuosity in rat hippocampal CA1, CA3 and cortical slices during ischemia. *J. Neurophysiol.* 74, 565–573 (1995).

Pérez-Pinzón, M.A., Xu, G.P., Dietrich, W.D., Rosenthal, M., and Sick, T.J. Rapid preconditioning protects rats against ischemic neuronal damage after 3 but not 7 days of reperfusion following global cerebral ischemia. *J. Cereb. Blood Flow Metab.* 17, 175–182 (1997b).

Perreault, P. and Avoli, M. Physiology and pharmacology of epileptiform activity induced by 4-aminopyridine in rat hippocampal slices. *J. Neurophysiol.* 65, 771–785 (1991).

Petito, C.K., Feldmann, E., Pulsinelli, W.A., and Plum, F. Delayed hippocampal damage in humans following cardiorespiratory arrest. *Neurology* 37, 1281–1286 (1987).

Petito, C.K., Torres-Munoz, J., Roberts, B., Olarte, J.-P., Nowak, T.S., and Pulsinelli, W.A. DNA fragmentation follows delayed neuronal death in CA1 neurons exposed to transient global ischemia in the rat. *J. Cereb. Blood Flow Metab.* 17, 967–976 (1997).

Petsche, H. Pathophysiologie und Klinik des Petit Mal. *Wiener Z. Nervenheilk. Grenzgeb.* 19, 345–441 (1962).

Phillips, J.M. and Nicholson, C. Anion permeability in spreading depression investigated with ion sensitive microelectrodes. *Brain Res.* 173, 567–571 (1979).

Phillis, J.W., Ren, J., and O'Regan, M.H. Studies on the effects of lactate transport inhibition, pyruvate, glucose and glutamine on amino acid, lactate and glucose release from the ischemic rat cerebral cortex. *J. Neurochem.* 76, 247–257 (2001).

Phillis, J.W., Song, D., and O'Regan, M.H. Effect of hyperglycemia on extracellular levels of amino acids and free fatty acids in the ischemic/reperfused rat cerebral cortex. *Brain Res.* 837, 177–183 (1999).

Picker, S., Pieper, C.F., and Goldring, S. Glial membrane potentials and their relationship to $[K^+]_o$ in man and guinea pig. *J. Neurosurg.* 55, 347–363 (1981).

Picone, C.M., Grotta, J.C., Earls, R., Strong, R., and Dedman, J. Immunohistochemical determination of calcium-calmodulin binding predicts neuronal damage after global ischemia. *J. Cereb. Blood Flow Metab.* 9, 805–811 (1989).

Piper, R.D. and Lambert, G.A. Inhalational anesthetics inhibit spreading depression: relevance to migraine. *Cephalalgia* 16, 87–92 (1996).

Piper, R.D., Lambert, G.A., and Duckworth, J.W. Cortical blood flow changes during spreading depression in cats. *Am. J. Physiol.* 261, H96–H102 (1991).

Pitkänen, A., Nissinen, J., Nairismägi, J., Lukasiuk, K., Gröhn, O.H.J., Miettinen, R., and Kauppinen, R. Progression of neuronal damage after status epilepticus and during spontaneous seizures in a rat model of temporal lobe epilepsy. In T. Sutula and A. Pitkänen (eds.), *Do seizures damage the brain?* Elsevier: Amsterdam, 67–83 (2002).

Plesnila, N., Zinkel, S., Le, D.A., Amin-Hanjani, S., Wu, Y., Qiu, J., Chiarugi, A., Thomas, S.S., Kohane, D.S., Korsmeyer, S.J., and Moskowitz, M.A. BID mediates neuronal cell death after oxygen/glucose deprivation and focal cerebral ischemia. *Proc. Natl. Acad. Sci. USA* 98, 15318–15323 (2001).

Pockberger, H., Rappelsberger, P., and Petsche, H. Penicillin-induced epileptic phenomena in the rabbit's neocortex. II. Laminar specific generation of interictal spikes after the application of penicillin to different cortical depths. *Brain Res.* 309, 261–269 (1984).

Polischuk, T.M., Jarvis, C.R., and Andrew, R.D. Instrinsic optical signaling denoting neuronal damage in response to acute excitotoxic insult by domoic acid in the hippocampal slice. *Neurobiol. Dis.* 4, 423–437 (1998).

Pollen, D.A. and Lux, H.D. Intrinsic triggering mechanisms in focal paroxysmal discharges. *Epilepsia* 7, 16–22 (1966).

Pollen, D.A. and Richardson, E.P. Intracellular studies at the border zone of glial scars developing after penetrating wounds and freezing lesions of the sensorimotor area of the cat. In J.-P. Cordeau and P. Gloor (eds.), *Recent contributions to neurophysiology*. Elsevier: Amsterdam, 29–41 (1972).

Pollen, D.A. and Trachtenberg, M.C. Neuroglia: gliosis and focal epilepsy. *Science* 167, 1252–1253 (1970).

Poolos, N.P. and Kocsis, J.D. Elevated extracellular potassium concentration enhances synaptic activation of *N*-methyl-D-aspartate receptors in hippocampus. *Brain Res.* 508, 7–12 (1990).

Posner, J.B. and Plum, F. Spinal-fluid pH and neurologic symptoms in systemic acidosis. *N. Engl. J. Med.* 277, 605–613 (1967).

Pott, L. and Mechmann, S. Large-conductance ion channel measured by whole-cell voltage clamp in single cardiac cells: modulation by β-adrenergic stimulation and inhibition by octanol. *J. Memb. Biol.* 117, 189–199 (1990).

Prince, D.A. Inhibition in "epileptic" neurons. *Exp. Neurol.* 21, 307–321 (1968a).

Prince, D.A. The depolarization shift in "epileptic" neurons. *Exp. Neurol.* 21, 467–485 (1968b).

Prince, D.A. and Connors, B.W. Mechanisms of epileptogenesis in cortical structures. *Ann. Neurol.* 16(Suppl.), S59–S64 (1984).

Prince, D.A., Connors, B.W., and Benardo, L.S. Mechanisms underlying interictal-ictal transitions. *Adv. Neurol.* 34, 177–187 (1983).

Prince, D.A. and Farrell, D. "Centrencephalic" spike-wave discharges following parenteral penicillin injection in the cat. *Neurology* 19, 309–310 (1969).

Prince, D.A. and Jacobs, K. Inhibitory function in two models of chronic epileptogenesis. *Epilepsy Res.* 32, 83–92 (1998).

Prince, D.A., Lux, H.-D., and Neher, E. Measurement of extracellular potassium activity in cat cortex. *Brain Res.* 50, 489–495 (1973).

Prince, D.A., Salin, P.A., Tseng, G.-F., Hoffman, S., and Parada, I. Axonal sprouting and epileptogenesis. *Adv. Neurol.* 72, 1–8 (1997).

Prince, D.A. and Schwartzkroin, P.A. Nonsynaptic mechanisms in epileptogenesis. In N. Chalazonitis and M. Boisson (eds.), *Abnormal neuronal discharges*. Raven Press: New York, 1–12 (1978).

Pritchard, J.A. The use of magnesium sulfate in preeclampsia-eclampsia. *J. Reprod. Med.* 23, 107–114 (1979).

Proctor, D.F. (ed.). *A history of breathing physiology*. Marcel Dekker: New York (1995).

Ptacek, L.J. and Fu, Y.-H. Channelopathies: episodic disorders of the nervous system. *Epilepsia* 42 (Suppl. 5), 35–43 (2001).

Pulsinelli, W.A. Selective neuronal vulnerability: morphological and molecular characteristics. *Prog. Brain Res.* 63, 29–37 (1985).

Pulsinelli, W.A. and Brierley, J.B. A new model of bilateral hemispheric ischemia in the unanesthetized rat. *Stroke* 10, 267–272 (1979).

Pulsinelli, W.A., Brierley, J.B., and Plum, F. Temporal profile of neuronal damage in a model of transient forebrain ischemia. *Ann. Neurol.* 11, 491–498 (1982a).

Pulsinelli, W.A., Levy, D.E., Sigsbee, B., Scherer, P., and Plum, F. Increased damage after ischemic stroke in patients with hyperglycemia with or without established diabetes mellitus. *Am. J. Med.* 74, 540–544 (1983).

Pulsinelli, W.A., Waldman, S., Rawlinson, D., and Plum, F. Moderate hyperglycemia augments ischemic brain damage: a neuropathologic study in the rat. *Neurology* 32, 1239–1246 (1982b).

Pulst, S.-M. *Neurogenetics*. Oxford University Press: New York (2000).

Pumain, R. and Heinemann, U. Stimulus- and amino acid-induced calcium and potassium changes in rat neocortex. *J. Neurophysiol.* 53, 1–16 (1985).

Pumain, R., Kurcewicz, I., and Louvel, J. Fast extracellular calcium transients: involvement in epileptic processes. *Science* 222, 167–188 (1983).

Pumain, R., Menini, C., Heinemann, U., Louvel, J., and Silva-Barrat, C. Chemical transmission is not necessary for epileptic seziures to persist in the baboon *Papio papio*. *Exp. Neurol.* 89, 250–258 (1985).

Puranam, R.S. and McNamara, J.O. Epilepsy and all that jazz. *Nature Med.* 7, 1103–1105 (2001).

Purpura, D.P. Mechanisms of propagation. Intracellular studies. In H.H. Jasper, A. Pope, and A.A. Ward (eds.), *Basic mechanisms of the epilepsies*. Little, Brown: Boston, 441–451 (1969).

Purpura, D.P., McMurtry, J.G., Leonard, C.F., and Malliani, A. Evidence for dendritic origin of spikes without depolarizing prepotentials in hippocampal neurons during and after seizures. *J. Neurophysiol.* 29, 954–979 (1966).

Racine, R., Newberry, F., and Burnham, W.M. Post-activation potentiation and the kindling phenomenon. *Electroencephalogr. Clin. Neurophysiol.* 39, 261–271 (1975).

Racine, R.J. Modification of seizure activity by electrical stimulation. II. Motor seizure. *Electroencephalogr. Clin. Neurophysiol.* 32, 281–294 (1972).

Racine, R.J., Adams, B., Osehobo, P., Milgram, N.W., and Fahnestock, M. Neuronal growth and neuronal loss in kindling epileptogenesis. In M.E. Corcoran and S.L. Moshé (eds.), *Kindling 5*. Plenum Press: New York, 193–207 (1998).

Racine, R.J., Milgram, N.W., and Hafner, S. Long-term potentiation phenomena in the rat limbic forebrain. *Brain Res.* 260, 217–231 (1983).

Rader, R.K. and Lanthorn, T.H. Experimental ischemia induces a persistent depolarization blocked by decreased calcium and NMDA antagonists. *Neurosci. Lett.* 99, 125–130 (1989).

Raffin, C.N., Harrison, M., Sick, T.J., and Rosenthal, M. EEG suppression and anoxic depolarization: influences on cerebral oxygenation during ischemia. *J. Cereb. Blood Flow Metab.* 11, 407–415 (1991).

Rafiq, A., Zhang, Y.-F., DeLorenzo, R.J., and Coulter, D.A. Long-duration self-sustained epileptiform activity in the hippocampal-parahippocampal slice: a model of status epilepticus. *J. Neurophysiol.* 74, 2028–2042 (1995).

Raichle, M.E. A central neuroendocrine system regulating brain volume. *Adv. Neurol.* 28, 341–343 (1980).

Rakic, P. Adult neurogenesis in mammals: an identity crisis. *J. Neurosci.* 22, 614–618 (2002).

Rall, D.P., Oppelt, W.W., and Patlak, C.S. Extracellular space of brain as determined by diffusion of inulin from the ventricular system. *Life Sci.* 2, 43–48 (1962).

Ramón y Cajal, S. Contribución al conocimiento de la neuroglia del cerebro humano. *Trab. Lab. Invest. Biol. Madrid* 18, 255–315 (1913).

Ramsay, R.E. and DeToledo, J. Acetazolamide. In J. Engel, Jr., and T.A. Pedley (eds.), *Epilepsy: a comprehensive textbook.* Lippincott-Raven: Philadelphia, 1455–1461 (1997).

Ranck, J.B. Analysis of specific impedance of rabbit cerebral cortex. *Exp. Neurol.* 7, 153–174 (1963).

Ranck, J.B. Specific impedance of cerebral cortex during spreading depression, and an analysis of neuronal, neuroglial and interstitial contributions. *Exp. Neurol.* 9, 1–16 (1964).

Ransom, B.R. The behavior of presumed glial cells during seizure discharge in cat cerebral cortex. *Brain Res.* 69, 83–99 (1974).

Ransom, B.R. and Goldring, S. Ionic determinants of membrane potential of cells presumed to be glia in cerebral cortex of cat. *J. Neurophysiol.* 36, 855–868 (1973a).

Ransom, B.R. and Goldring, S. Slow depolarization in cells presumed to be glia in cerebral cortex of cat. *J. Neurophysiol.* 36, 869–878 (1973b).

Ransom, B.R. and Sontheimer, H. The neurophysiology of glial cells. *J. Clin. Neurophysiol.* 9, 224–251 (1992).

Ransom, C.B., Ransom, B.R., and Sontheimer, H. Activity-dependent K^+-accumulation in the rat optic nerve is cleared by temperature-sensitive and temperature insensitive mechanisms. *Soc. Neurosci. Abstr.* 21, 583 (1995).

Ransom, C.B., Ransom, B.R., and Sontheimer, H. Activity-dependent extracellular K^+ accumulation in rat optic nerve: the role of glial and axonal Na^+ pumps. *J. Physiol.* 522, 427–442 (2000).

Rash, J.E., Yasumura, T., Dudek, F.E., and Nagy, J.I. Cell-specific expression of connexins and evidence of restricted gap junctional coupling between glial cells and between neurons. *J. Neurosci.* 21, 1983–2000 (2001).

Rausche, G., Igelmund, P., and Heinemann, U. Effects of changes in extracellular potassium, magnesium and calcium concentration on synaptic transmission in area CA1 and the dentate gyrus of rat hippocampal slices. *Pflügers Archiv—European Journal of Physiology* 415, 588–593 (1990).

Ravagnan, L., Roumier, T., and Kroemer, G. Mitochondria, the killer organelles and their weapons. *J. Cell. Physiol.* 192, 131–137 (2002).

Rayport, M. Single neurone studies in human epilepsy. In G.G. Somjen (ed.), *Neurophysiology studied in man.* Excerpta Medica: Amsterdam, 100–109 (1972).

Read, S.J., Smith, M.I., Benham, C.D., Hunter, A.J., and Parsons, A.A. Furosemide inhibits regenerative cortical spreading depression in anaesthetized cats. *Cephalalgia* 17, 826–832 (1997).

Regehr, W.G., Connor, J.A., and Tank, D.W. Optical imaging of calcium accumulation in hippocampal pyramidal cells during synaptic activation. *Nature* 341, 533–536 (1989).

Reggia, J.A. and Montgomery, D. A computational model of visual hallucinations in migraine. *Comput. Biol. Med.* 26, 133–141 (1996).

Reibel, S., Larmet, Y., Carnahan, J., Lè, B.-T., Marescaux, C., and Depaulis, A. Protective effects of brain-derived neurotrophic factor in hippocampal kindling. In M.E. Corcoran and S.L. Moshé (eds.), *Kindling 5.* Plenum Press: New York, 409–419 (1998).

Reid, K.H., Marrannes, R., and Wauquier, A. Spreading depression and central nervous system pharmacology. *J. Pharmacol. Meth.* 19, 1–21 (1988).

Revett, J.A., Ruppin, E., Godall, S., and Reggia, J.A. Spreading depression in focal ischemia: a computational study. *J. Cereb. Blood Flow Metab.* 18, 998–1007 (1998).

Rex, A., Pfeifer, L., Fink, F., and Fink, H. Cortical NADH during pharmacological manipulation of the respiratory chain and spreading depression. *J. Neurosci. Res.* 57, 359–370 (1999).

Ringer, S. A further contribution regarding the influence of the different constituents of the blood on the contraction of the heart. *J. Physiol.* 4, 29–42 (1883).

Ringer, S. Further experiments regarding the influence of small quantities of lime, potassium and other salts on muscular tissue. *J. Physiol.* 7, 291–308 (1886).

Risinger, M.W. Noninvasive ictal electrophysiology in humans. In H.O. Lüders and S. Noachtar (eds.), *Epileptic seizures: pathophysiology and clinical semiology.* Churchill Livingstone: New York, 32–48 (2000).

Rizzuto, R. Intracellular Ca^{2+} pools in neuronal signalling. *Curr. Opin. Neurobiol.* 11, 306–311 (2001).

Roberts, E.L., He, J., and Chih, C.-P. The influence of glucose on intracellular and extracellular pH in rat hippocampal slices during and after anoxia. *Brain Res.* 783, 44–50 (1998).

Roberts, E.L. and Sick, T.J. Calcium-sensitive recovery of extracellular potassium and synaptic transmission in rat hippocampal slices exposed to anoxia. *Brain Res.* 456, 113–119 (1988).

Roberts, E.L. and Sick, T.J. Glucose enhances recovery of potassium ion homeostasis and synaptic excitability after anoxia in hippocampal slices. *Brain Res.* 570, 225–230 (1992).

Robertson, G.A. LQT2: amplitude reduction and loss of selectivity in the tail that webs the HERG channel. *Circ. Res.* 86, 492–496 (2000).

Robinson, J.R. Metabolism of intracellular water. *Physiol. Rev.* 40, 112–149 (1960).

Rock, D.M., MacDonald, R.L., and Taylor, C.P. Blockade of sustained repetitive action potentials in cultured spinal cord neurons by zonisamide. *Epilepsy Res.* 3, 138–143 (2002).

Rodrigues, P.S., Guimaraes, A.P.O., Azeredo, F.A.M.D., and Martins-Ferreira, H. Involvement of GABA and ACh in retinal spreading depression: effects of "low calcium–high magnesium" solutions. *Exp. Brain Res.* 73, 659–664 (1988).

Rodrigues, P.S. and Martins-Ferreira, H. Cholinergic transmission in retinal spreading depression. *Exp. Brain Res.* 38, 229–236 (1980).

Rogawski, M.A., Kurzman, P.S., Yamaguchi, S., and Li, H. Role of AMPA and GluR5 kainate receptors in the development and expression of amygdala kindling in the mouse. *Neuropharmacology* 40, 28–35 (2001).

Roitbak, A.I. and Bobrov, A.V. Spreading depression resulting from cortical punctures. *Acta Neurobiol. Exp.* 35, 761–768 (1975).

Rose, C.R. and Konnerth, A. Exciting glial oscillations. *Nature Neurosci.* 4, 773–774 (2001a).

Rose, C.R. and Konnerth, A. Stores not just for storage. Intracellular calcium release and synaptic plasticity. *Neuron* 31, 519–522 (2001b).

Rose, C.R. and Ransom, B.R. pH regulation in mammalian glia. In K. Kaila and B.R. Ransom (eds.), *pH and Brain Function.* Wiley-Liss: New York, 253–275 (1998).

Rosen, A.S. and Andrew, R.D. Osmotic effects upon excitability in rat neocortical slices. *Neuroscience* 38, 579–590 (1990).

Rosen, A.S. and Morris, M.E. Depolarizing effects of anoxia on pyramidal cells of rat neocortex. *Neurosci. Lett.* 124, 169–173 (1991).

Rosen, A.S. and Morris, M.E. Anoxic depression of excitatory and inhibitory postsynaptic potentials in rat neocortical slices. *J. Neurophysiol.* 69, 109–117 (1993).

Rosenblueth, A. and Garcia Ramos, J. Some phenomena usually associated with spreading depression. *Acta Physiol. Lat.* 16, 141–179 (1966).

Rosene, D.L. and van Hoesen, G.W. The hippocampal formation of the primate brain. In E.G. Jones and A. Peters (eds.), *Cerebral cortex*, Vol. 6. Plenum Press: New York, 345–456 (1987).

Rosenthal, M. and Jöbsis, F.F. Intracellular redox changes in functioning cerebral cortex. II. Effects of direct cortical stimulation. *J. Neurophysiol.* 36, 750–761 (1971).

Rosenthal, M., LaManna, J.C., Jöbsis, F.F., Levasseur, J.E., Kontos, H.A., and Patterson, J.L. Effects of respiratory gases on cytochrome a in intact cerebral cortex: is there a critical P_{O_2}? *Brain Res.* 108, 143–154 (1976).

Rosenthal, M. and Somjen, G. Spreading depression, sustained potential shifts and metabolic activity of cerebral cortex of cats. *J. Neurophysiol.* 36, 739–749 (1973).

Ross, W.N., Miyakawa, H., Lev-Ram, V., Lasser-Ross, N., Lisman, J., Jaffe, D., and Johnston, D. Dendritic excitability in CNS neurons: insight from dynamic calcium and sodium imaging in single cells. *Jpn. J. Physiol.* 43 (Suppl. 1), S83–S89 (1993).

Rossen, R., Kabat, H., and Anderson, J.P. Acute arrest of cerebral circulation in man. *Arch. Neurol. Psychiatry* 50, 510–528 (1943).

Rossi, D.J., Oshima, T., and Attwell, D. Glutamate release in severe brain ischaemia is mainly by reversed uptake. *Nature* 403, 316–321 (2000).

Rothman, S.M. Synaptic activity mediates death of hypoxic neurons. *Science* 220, 536–537 (1983).

Rothman, S.M. The neurotoxicity of excitatory amino acids is produced by passive chloride influx. *J. Neurosci.* 5, 1483–1489 (1985).

Rothman, S.M. and Olney, J.W. Excitotoxicity and the NMDA receptor. *Trends Neurosci.* 10, 299–302 (1987).

Rothman, S.M., Thurston, J.H., Hauhart, R.E., Clark, G.D., and Solomon, J.S. Ketamine protects hippocampal neurons from anoxia *in vitro*. *Neuroscience* 21, 673–678 (1987).

Rudolphi, K.A., Schubert, P., Parkinson, F.E., and Fredholm, B.B. Adenosine and brain ischemia. *Cerebrovasc. Brain Metab. Rev.* 4, 346–369 (1992).

Rundfeldt, C. Charecterization of the K^+ channel opening effect of the anticonvulsant retigabine in PC12 cells. *Epilepsy Res.* 35, 99–107 (1999).

Rusakov, D.A. The role of perisynaptic glial sheath in glutamate spillover and extracellular Ca^{2+} depletion. *Biophys. J.* 81, 1947–1959 (2001).

Rusakov, D.A., Kullmann, D.M., and Stewart, M.G. Hippocampal synapses: do they talk to their neighbours? *Trends Neurosci.* 22, 382–388 (1999).

Rutecki, P.A., Lebeda, F.J., and Johnston, D. Epileptiform activity induced by changes in extracellular potassium in hippocampus. *J. Neurophysiol.* 54, 1363–1374 (1985).

Rutecki, P.A., Lebeda, F.J., and Johnston, D. 4-Aminopyridine produces epileptiform activity in hippocampus and enhances synaptic excitation and inhibition. *J. Neurophysiol.* 57, 1911–1924 (1987).

Rutecki, P.A., Lebeda, F.J., and Johnston, D. Epileptiform activity in the hippocampus produced by tetraethylammonium. *J. Neurophysiol.* 64, 1077–1088 (1990).

Rutter, G.A., Burnett, P., Robb-Gaspers, L.D., Thomas, A.P., Denton, R.M., Griffiths, E.J., and Rizzuto, R. Mitochondrial Ca^{2+} signalling. In A. Verkhratsky and C. Toescu (eds.), *Integrative aspects of calcium signalling*. Plenum Press: New York, 1998).

Sabbatani, L. Importanza del calcio che trovasi nella corteccia cerebrale. *Riv. Sper. Freniatria* 27, 946–956 (1901).

Sager, T.N., Lundbaek, J.A., and Hansen, A.J. Rat brain interstitial volume fraction and *N*-acetyl-aspartate (NAA) measured by microdialysis during acute hyponatremia. *Soc. Neurosci. Abstr.* 22, 627–1996).

Sanabria, E.R.G., Su, H., and Yaari, Y. Initiation of network bursts by Ca^{2+}-dependent intrinsic bursting in the rat pilocarpine model of temporal lobe epilepsy. *J. Physiol.* 532, 205–216 (2001).

Sankar, R., Shin, D., Mazarati, A.M., Liu, H., Katsumori, H., Lezama, R., and Wasterlain, C.G. Epileptogenesis after status epilepticus reflects age- and model-dependent plasticity. *Ann. Neurol.* 48, 580–589 (2000).

Saris, N.-E.L., Mervaala, E., Karppanen, H., Khawaja, J.A., and Lewenstam, A. Magnesium. An update on physiological, clinical and analytical aspects. *Clin. Chim. Acta* 294, 1–26 (2000).

Sarna, G.S., Obrenovitch, T.P., Matsumoto, T., Symon, L., and Curzoni, G. Effect of transient cerebral ischaemia and cardiac arrest on brain extracellular dopamine and serotonin as determined by in vivo dialysis in the rat. *J. Neurochem.* 55, 937–940 (1990).

Sawa, M., Maruyama, N., and Kaji, S. Intracellular potential during electrically induced seizures. *Electroencephalogr. Clin. Neurophysiol.* 15, 209–220 (1963).

Schachter, S.C. Current evidence indicates that antiepileptic drugs are anti-octal, not antiepileptic. *Epilepsy Res.* 50, 67–70 (2002).

Schanne, F.A.X., Kane, A.B., Young, E.E., and Farber, J.L. Calcium dependence of toxic cell death: a final common pathway. *Science* 206, 700–792 (1979).

Scharfman, H.E. Epileptogenesis in the parahippocampal region. Parallels with the dentate gyrus. *Ann. N.Y. Acad. Sci.* 911, 305–327 (2000).

Scharfman, H.E., Goodman, J.H., and Schwarcz, R. Electrophysiological effects of exogenous and endogenous kynurenic acid in the rat brain: studies *in vivo* and *in vitro*. *Amino Acids* 19, 283–297 (2000).

Scharfman, H.E., Goodman, J.H., Sollas, A.L., and Croll, S.D. Spontaneous limbic seizures after intrahippocampal infusion of brain-derived neurotrophic factor. *Exp. Neurol.* 174, 201–214 (2002).

Scheibel, A.B. Morphological correlates of epilepsy: cells in the hippocampus. In G.H. Glaser, J.K. Penry, and D.M. Woodbury (eds.), *Antiepileptic drugs: mechanism of action.* Raven Press: New York, 49–61 (1980).

Scheller, D., Heister, U., Kolb, J., and Tegtmeier, F. On the role of excitatory amino acids during generation and propagation of spreading depression. In A. Lehmenkühler, K.-H. Grotemeyer, and F. Tegtmeier (eds.), *Migraine: basic mechanisms and treatment.* Urban & Schwarzenberg: München, 355–366 (1993).

Scheller, D., Kolb, F., Tegtmeier, F., and Lehmenkühler, A. Extracellular changes of inorganic phosphate are different during spreading depression and global cerebral ischemia of rats. *Neurosci. Lett.* 141, 269–272 (1992a).

Scheller, D., Kolb, J., Peters, U., and Tegtmeier, F. The measurement of extracellular inorganic phosphate gives a more reliable indication for severe impairment of cerebral cell function and cell death than the measurement of extracellular lactate. *Acta Neurochirurg.* Suppl. 67, 28–30 (1996).

Scheller, D., Kolb, J., and Tegtmeier, F. Lactate and pH change in close correlation in the extracellular space of the rat brain during cortical spreading depression. *Neurosci. Lett.* 135, 83–86 (1992b).

Scheller, D., Tegtmeier, F., and Schlue, W.-R. Dose-dependent effects of tetraethylammonium on circling spreading depression in chicken retina. *J. Neurosci. Res.* 51, 85–89 (1998).

Schielke, G.P. and Betz, A.L. Electrolyte transport. In M.W.B. Bradbury (ed.), *Physiology and pharmacology of the blood-brain barrier.* Springer: Berlin, 221–243 (1992).

Schiff, S.J. and Somjen, G.G. Hyperexcitability following moderate hypoxia in hippocampal tissue slices. *Brain Res.* 337, 337–340 (1985).

Schiff, S.J. and Somjen, G.G. The effect of graded hypoxia on the hippocampal slice: an in vitro model of the ischemic penumbra. *Stroke* 18, 30–37 (1987).

Schiff, S.J., Szerb, J.C., and Somjen, G.G. Glutamine can enhance synaptic transmission in hippocampal slices. *Brain Res.* 343, 366–369 (1985).

Schmidt-Kastner, R. and Freund, T.F. Selective vulnerability of the hippocampus in brain ischemia. *Neuroscience* 40, 599–636 (1991).

Schmitz, D., Schuchmann, S., Fisahn, A., Draguhn, A., Buhl, E.H., Petrasch-Parwez, E., Dermietzel, R., Heinemann, U., and Traub, R.D. Axo-axonal coupling. A novel mechanism for ultrafast neuronal communication. *Neuron* 31, 831–840 (2001).

Schousboe, A. and Westergaard, N. Transport of neuroactive amino acids in astrocytes. In H. Kettenmann and B.R. Ransom (eds.), *Neuroglia.* Oxford University Press: New York, 246–258 (1995).

Schuchmann, S., Buchheim, K., Meierkord, H., and Heinemann, U. A relative energy failure is associated with low-Mg^{2+} but not with 4-aminopyridine induced seizure-like events in entorhinal cortex. *J. Neurophysiol.* 81, 399–403 (1999).

Schuchmann, S., Kovacs, R., Kann, O., Heinemann, U., and Buchheim, K. Monitoring NAD(P)H autofluorescence to assess mitochondrial metabolic functions in rat hippocampal entorhinal cortex slices. *Brain Res. Protocols* 7, 267–276 (2001).

Schurr, A., Payne, R.S., Miller, J.J., and Rigor, B.M. Brain lactate, not glucose, fuels the recovery of synaptic function from hypoxia upon reoxygenation: an in vitro study. *Brain Res.* 744, 105–111 (1997).

Schurr, A., Payne, R.S., Miller, J.J., and Tseng, M.T. Preischemic hyperglycemia-aggravated damage: evidence that lactate utilization is beneficial and glucose-induced corticosterone release is detrimental. *J. Neurosci. Res.* 66, 782–789 (2001a).

Schurr, A., Payne, R.S., Miller, J.J., Tseng, M.T., and Rigor, B.M. Blockade of lactate transport exacerbates delayed neuronal damage in a rat model of cerebral ischemia. *Brain Res.* 895, 268–272 (2001b).

Schurr, A., Payne, R.S., and Rigor, B.M. Protection by MK-801 against hypoxia-excitotoxin- and depolarization-induced neuronal damage in vitro. *Neurochem. Int.* 26, 519–525 (1995a).

Schurr, A., Payne, R.S., and Rigor, B.M. Synergism between diltiazem and MK-801 but not APV in protecting hippocampal slices against hypoxic damage. *Brain Res.* 684, 233–236 (1995b).

Schurr, A., Payne, R.S., Tseng, M.T., Gozal, E., and Gozal, D. Excitotoxic preconditioning elicited by both glutamate and hypoxia and abolished by lactate transport inhibition in rat hippocampal slices. *Neurosci. Lett.* 307, 151–154 (2001c).

Schurr, A., Payne, R.S., Tseng, M.T., Miller, J.J., and Rigor, B.M. The glucose paradox in cerebral ischemia. New insights. *Ann. N.Y. Acad. Sci.* 893, 386–390 (1999).

Schurr, A., Reid, K.H., Tseng, M.T., West, C., and Rigor, B.M. Adaptation of adult brain tissue to anoxia and hypoxia in vitro. *Brain Res.* 374, 244–248 (1986).

Schurr, A. and Rigor, B.M. The mechanism of neuronal resistance and adaptation to hypoxia. *FEBS Lett.* 224, 4–8 (1987).

Schurr, A., West, C.A., Reid, K.H., Tseng, M.T., Reiss, S.J., and Rigor, B.M. Increased glucose improves recovery of neuronal function after cerebral hypoxia in vitro. *Brain Res.* 421, 135–139 (1987).

Schwarcz, R., Eid, T., and Du, F. Neurons in layer III of the entorhinal cortex. A role in epileptogenesis and epilepsy? *Ann. N.Y. Acad. Sci.* 911, 328–342 (2000).

Schwartz-Bloom, R.D., Miller, K.A., Evenson, D.A., Crain, B.J., and Nadler, J.V. Benzodiazepines protect hippocampal neurons from degeneration after transient cerebral ischemia: an ultrastructural study. *Neuroscience* 98, 471–484 (2000).

Schwartz-Bloom, R.D. and Sah, R. γ-Aminobutyric acid$_A$ neurotransmission and cerebral ischemia. *J. Neurochem.* 77, 353–371 (2001).

Schwartzkroin, P.A. Mechanisms underlying the anti-epileptic efficacy of the ketogenic diet. *Epilepsy Res.* 37, 171–180 (1999).

Schwartzkroin, P.A., Baraban, S.C., and Hochman, D.W. Osmolarity, ionic flux, and changes in brain excitability [review]. *Epilepsy Res.* 32, 275–285 (1998).

Schweitzer, J.S. and Williamson, A. Relationship between synaptic activity and prolonged field bursts in the dentate gyrus of the rat hippocampal slice. *J. Neurophysiol.* 74, 1947–1952 (1995).

Schwindt, P.C. and Crill, W.E. The spinal cord model of experimental epilepsy. In P.A. Schwartzkroin and H.V. Wheal (eds.), *Electrophysiology of epilepsy*. Academic Press: London, 219–251 (1984).

Scobey, R.P. and Gabor, A.J. Ectopic action potential generation in epileptogenic cortex. *J. Neurophysiol.* 38, 383–394 (1975).

Sebastião, A.M. and Ribeiro, J.A. Fine-tuning neuromodulation by adenosine. *Trends Pharmacol. Sci.* 21, 341–346 (2000).

Segal, M.M. Epileptiform activity in microcultures containing one excitatory hippocampal neuron. *J. Neurophysiol.* 65, 761–770 (1991).

Segal, M.M. Endogenous bursts underlie seizurelike activity in solitary excitatory hippocampal neurons in microcultures. *J. Neurophysiol.* 72, 1874–1884 (1994).

Segal, M.M. Sodium channels and epilepsy electrophysiology. *Novartis Found. Symp.* 241, 173–180 (2002).

Segal, M.M. and Douglas, A.F. Late sodium channel openings underlying epileptiform activity are preferentially diminshed by the anticonvulsant phenytoin. *J. Neurophysiol.* 77, 3021–3034 (1997).

Shanes, A.M. Electrochemical aspects of physiological and pharmacological action in excitable cells. *Pharmacol. Rev.* 10, 59–273 (1958).

Shapiro, B.E. Osmotic forces and gap junctions in spreading depression: a computational model. *J. Comput. Neurosci.* 10, 99–120 (2001).

Sharpless, S.K. Isolated and deafferented neurons: disuse supersensitivity. In H.H. Jasper, A.A. Ward, and A. Pope (eds.), *Basic Mechanisms of the Epilepsies.* Little, Brown: Boston, 329–348 (1969).

Sheardown, M.J. The triggering of spreading depression in the chicken retina: a pharmacological study. *Brain Res.* 607, 189–194 (1993).

Shen, A.C. and Jennings, R.B. Myocardial calcium and magnesium in acute ischemic injury. *Am. J. Pathol.* 67, 417–440 (1972).

Shen, P.J. and Gundlach, A.L. Prolonged induction of neuronal NOS expression and activity following cortical spreading depression (SD): implications for SD- and NO-mediated neuroprotection. *Exper. Neurol.* 160, 317–332 (1999).

Shetty, A.K. and Turner, D.A. Neurite outgrowth from progeny of epidermal growth factor-responsive hippocampal stem cells is significantly less robust than from fetal hippocampal cells following grafting onto hippocampal slice cultures: effect of brain-derived neurotropic factor. *Neurobiol.* 38, 391–413 (1999).

Shibasaki, F., Hallin, U., and Uchino, H. Calcineurin as a multifunctional regulator. *J. Biochem.* 131, 1–15 (2002).

Shimazawa, M. and Hara, H. An experimental model of migraine with aura: cortical hypoperfusion following spreading depression in the awake and freely moving rat. *Clin. Exp. Pharmacol. Physiol.* 23, 890–892 (1996).

Sick, T.J. and Perez-Pinzon, M.A. Optical methods for probing mitochondrial function in brain slices. *Methods* 18, 104–108 (1999).

Sick, T.J., Solow, E.L., and Roberts, E.L. Extracellular potassium ion activity and electrophysiology in the hippocampal slice: paradoxical recovery of synaptic transmission during anoxia. *Brain Res.* 418, 227–234 (1987).

Sick, T.J. and Somjen, G.G. Tissue slice. Application to study of cerebral ischemia. In M.D. Ginsberg and J. Bogousslavsky (eds.), *Cerebrovascular disease: pathophysiology, diagnosis and management.* Blackwell Science: Malden, Mass., 137–156 (1998).

Siesjö, B.K. A new perspective on ischemic brain damage? *Prog. Brain Res.* 96, 1–9 (1993).

Siesjö, B.K., Ekhom, A., Katsura, K., and Theander, S. Acid-base changes during complete brain ischemia. *Stroke* 21(Suppl.), III-194–III-199 (1990).

Siesjö, B.K., Hu, B.-R., and Kristián, T. Is the cell death pathway triggered by the mitochondrion or the endoplasmic reticulum? [Commentary]. *J. Cereb. Blood Flow Metab.* 19, 19–26 (1999).

Siggaard-Andersen, O., Thode, J., and Wandrup, J. The concentration of free calcium ions in blood plasma. *5th Meeting Int. Fed. Clin. Chem.* 163–190 (1980).

Silva-Barrat, C., Champagnat, J., and Menini, C. The GABA-withdrawal syndrome: a model of local status epilepticus. *Neural Plasticity* 7, 9–18 (2000).

Silver, I.A. and Erecińska, M. Intracellular and extracellular changes of $[Ca^{2+}]$ in hypoxia and ischemia in rat brain in vivo. *J. Gen. Physiol.* 95, 837–866 (1990).

Simon, R.P., Swan, J.H., Griffiths, T., and Meldrum, B.S. Blockade of N-methyl-D-aspartate receptors may protect against ischemic damage in the brain. *Science* 226, 850–862 (1984).

Singer, W. and Lux, H.D. Extracellular potassium gradients and visual receptive fields in the cat striate cortex. *Brain Res.* 96, 378–383 (1975).

Singh, R., Gardner, R.J.M., Crossland, K.M., Scheffer, I.E., and Berkovic, S.F. Chromosomal abnormalities and epilepsy: a review for clinicians and gene hunters. *Epilepsia* 43, 127–140 (2002).

Skou, J.C. The (Na$^+$ + K$^+$) activated enzyme system and its relationship to the transport of sodium and potassium. *Q. Rev. Biophys.* 7, 401–434 (1975).

Slaght, S.J., Leresche, N., Deniau, J.-M., Crunelli, V., and Charpier, S. Activity of thalamic reticular neurons during spontaneous genetically determined spike and wave discharges. *J. Neurosci.* 22, 2323–2334 (2002).

Slotkin, T.A. and Seidler, F.J. Stress in the fetus and newborn. *Adv. Exp. Med. Biol.* 245, 283–294 (1988).

Sloviter, R.S. "Epileptic" brain damage in rats induced by sustained electrical stimulation of the perforant path. I. Acute electrophysiological and light microscopic studies. *Brain Res. Bull.* 10, 675–697 (1983).

Sloviter, R.S. Decreased hippocampal inhibition and a selective loss of interneurons in experimental epilepsy. *Science* 235, 73–76 (1987).

Sloviter, R.S. Calcium-binding protein (calbindin-D28k) and parvalbumin immunocytochemistry: localization in the rat hippocampus with specific reference to the selective vulnerability of hippocampal neurons to seizure activity. *J. Comp. Neurol.* 280, 183–196 (1989).

Sloviter, R.S. Permanently altered hippocampal structure, excitability and inhibition after experimental status epilepticus in the rat: the "dormant basket cell" hypothesis and its possible relevance to temporal lobe epilepsy. *Hippocampus* 1, 41–66 (1991).

Sloviter, R.S. Possible functional consequences of synaptic reorganization in the dentate gyrus of kainate-treated rats. *Neurosci. Lett.* 137, 91–96 (1992).

Sloviter, R.S. Status epilepticus-induced neuronal injury and network reorganization. *Epilepsia* 40(Suppl. 1), S34–S39 (1999).

Sloviter, R.S. Apoptosis: a guide for the perplexed. *Trends Pharmacol. Sci.* 23, 19–24 (2002).

Sloviter, R.S. and Damiano, B.P. Sustained electrical stimulation of the perforant path duplicates kainate-induced electrophysiological effects and hippocampal damage in rats. *Neurosci. Lett.* 24, 279–284 (1981).

Smith, M.-L. and Siesjö, B.K. Acidosis-related brain damage: immediate and delayed events. In G.G. Somjen (ed.), *Mechanisms of cerebral hypoxia and stroke*. Plenum Press: New York, 57–71 (1994).

Smith, S.E. and Chesler, M. Effect of divalent cations on AMPA-evoked extracellular alkaline shifts in rat hippocampal slices. *J. Neurophysiol.* 82, 1902–1908 (1999).

Smith, S.E., Gottfried, J.A., Chen, J.C.T., and Chesler, M. Calcium dependence of glutamate receptor-evoked alkaline shifts in hippocampus. *NeuroReport* 5, 2441–2445 (1994).

Snow, R.W. and Dudek, F.E. Electrical fields directly contribute to action potential synchronization during convulsant-induced epileptiform nursts. *Brain Res.* 323, 114–118 (1984a).

Snow, R.W. and Dudek, F.E. Synchronous epileptiform bursts without chemical transmission in CA2, CA3 and dentate areas of the hippocampus. *Brain Res.* 298, 382–385 (1984b).

Snow, R.W., Taylor, C.P., and Dudek, F.E. Electrophysiological and optical changes in slices of rat hippocampus during spreading depression. *J. Neurophysiol.* 50, 561–572 (1983).

Solà, C., Barrón, S., Tusell, J.M., and Serratosa, J. The Ca^{2+}/calmodulin system in neuronal hyperexcitability. *Int. J. Biochem. Cell Biol.* 33, 439–455 (2001).

Somjen, G.G. Effects of anesthetics on spinal cord of mammals. *Anesthesiology* 28, 135–143 (1967).

Somjen, G.G. Evoked sustained focal potentials and membrane potential of neurones and of unresponsive cells of the spinal cord. *J. Neurophysiol.* 33, 562–582 (1970).

Somjen, G.G. Electrogenesis of sustained potentials. *Prog. Neurobiol.* 1, 199–237 (1973).

Somjen, G.G. Electrophysiology of neuroglia. *Ann. Rev. Physiol.* 37, 163–190 (1975).

Somjen, G.G. Metabolic and electrical correlates of the clearing of excess potassium in the cortex and spinal cord. In R. Porter (ed.), *Studies in neurophysiology.* Cambridge University Press: Cambridge, 181–201 (1978).

Somjen, G.G. Extracellular potassium in the mammalian central nervous system. *Annu. Rev. Physiol.* 41, 159–177 (1979).

Somjen, G.G. Stimulus-evoked and seizure-related responses of extracellular calcium activity in spinal cord compared to those in cerebral cortex. *J. Neurophysiol.* 44, 617–632 (1980).

Somjen, G.G. *Neurophysiology—the essentials.* Williams and Wilkins: Baltimore, Md. (1983).

Somjen, G.G. Acidification of interstitial fluid in hippocampal formation caused by seizures and by spreading depression. *Brain Res.* 311, 186–188 (1984).

Somjen, G.G. Functions of glial cells in cerebral cortex. In E.G. Jones and A. Peters (eds.), *Cerebral cortex*, Vol. 6. Plenum Press: New York, 1–39 (1987).

Somjen, G.G. Nervenkitt: notes on the history of the concept of neuroglia. *Glia* 1, 2–9 (1988).

Somjen, G.G. Mechanism of the reversible arrest of function during transient cerebral hypoxia and ischemia. In A. Schurr and B.M. Rigor (eds.), *Cerebral ischemia and resuscitation.* CRC Press: Boca Raton, Fla.: 301–317 (1990).

Somjen, G.G. Glial and neuronal generators of sustained potential shifts associated with electrographic seizures. In St. Zschoke, and E.-J. Speckmann (eds.), *Basic mechanisms of the EEG.* Springer-Birkhäuser: Boston, 97–108 (1993).

Somjen, G.G. Electrophysiology of mammalian glial cells in situ. In H. Kettenmann and B.R. Ransom (eds.), *Neuroglial cells.* Oxford University Press: Oxford, 319–331 (1995).

Somjen, G.G. Low external NaCl concentration and low osmolarity enhance voltage gated Ca currents but depress K-currents in freshly isolated rat hippocampal neurons. *Brain Res.* 851, 25, 189–197 (1999).

Somjen, G.G. Mechanisms of spreading depression and hypoxic spreading depression-like depolarization. *Physiol. Rev.* 81, 1065–1096 (2001).

Somjen, G.G. and Aitken, P.G. The ionic and metabolic responses associated with neuronal depression of Leão's type in cerebral cortex and in hippocampal formation. *An. Acad. Bras. Ciên.* 56, 495–504 (1984).

Somjen, G.G., Aitken, P.G., Balestrino, M., Herreras, O., and Kawasaki, K. Spreading depression-like depolarization and selective vulnerability of neurons. A brief review. *Stroke* 21, III179–III183 (1990).

Somjen, G.G., Aitken, P.G., Czéh, G., Herreras, O., Jing, J., and Young, J.N. The mechanism of spreading depression: a review of recent findings, and a hypothesis. *Can. J. Physiol. Pharmacol.* 70(Suppl.), S248–S254 (1992).

Somjen, G.G., Aitken, P.G., Czéh, G., Herreras, O., Jing, J., and Young, J.N. Spreading depression in hippocampus: membrane currents and ion mechanisms. In A. Lehmenkühler, K.H. Grotemeyer, and F. Tegtmeier (eds.), *Migraine: basic mechanisms and treatment*. Urban & Schwarzenberg: München, 329–344 (1993a).

Somjen, G.G., Aitken, P.G., Czéh, G., Jing, J., and Young, J.N. Cellular physiology of hypoxia of the mammalian central nervous system. In S.G. Waxman (ed.), *Molecular and cellular approaches to the treatment of neurological disease. Research Publications*, ARNMD, Vol. 71. Raven Press: New York, 51–65 (1993b).

Somjen, G.G., Aitken, P.G., Giacchino, J.L., and McNamara, J.O. Sustained potential shifts and paroxysmal discharges in hippocampal formation. *J. Neurophysiol.* 53, 1079–1097 (1985).

Somjen, G.G., Aitken, P.G., Giacchino, J.L., and McNamara, J.O. Interstitial ion concentrations and paroxysmal discharges in hippocampal formation and spinal cord. In A.V. Delgado-Escueta, A.A. Ward, D.M. Woodbury, and R.J. Porter (eds.), *Basic mechanisms of the epilepsies*. Raven Press: New York, 663–680 (1986).

Somjen, G.G., Allen, B.W., Balestrino, M., and Aitken, P.G. Pathophysiology of pH and Ca^{2+} in bloodstream and brain. *Can. J. Physiol. Pharmacol.* 65, 1078–1085 (1987a).

Somjen, G., Dingledine, R., Connors, B., and Allen, B. Extracellular potassium and calcium activities in the mammalian spinal cord, and the effect of changing ion levels on mammalian neural tissues. In E. Syková, P. Hník, and L. Vyklicky (eds.), *Ion-selective microelectrodes and their use in excitable tissues*. Plenum Press: New York, 159–180 (1981).

Somjen, G.G., Faas, G.C., Vreugdenhil, M., and Wadman, W.J. Channel shutdown: a response of hippocampal neurons to adverse environments. *Brain Res.* 632, 180–194 (1993c).

Somjen, G.G. and Giacchino, J.L. Potassium and calcium concentrations in interstitial fluid of hippocampal formation during paroxysmal responses. *J. Neurophysiol.* 53, 1098–1108 (1985).

Somjen, G.G. and Gill, M.B. The mechanism of blockade of synaptic transmission in the mammalian spinal cord by diethyl ether and by thiopental. *J. Pharmacol. Exp. Ther.* 140, 19–30 (1963).

Somjen, G., Hilmy, M., and Stephen, C.R. Failure to anesthetize human subjects by intravenous administration of magnesium sulfate. *J. Pharmacol. Exp. Ther.* 154, 652–659 (1966).

Somjen, G.G. and Müller, M. Potassium-induced enhancement of persistent inward current in hippocampal neurons in isolation and in tissue slices. *Brain Res.* 885, 102–110 (2000).

Somjen, G.G., Rosenthal, M., Cordingley, G., LaManna, J., and Lothman, E. Potassium, neuroglia, and oxidative metabolism in central gray matter. *Fed. Proc.* 35, 1266–1271 (1976).

Somjen, G.G., Schiff, S.J., Aitken, P.G., and Balestrino, M. Forms of suppression of neuronal function. In N. Chalazonitis and M. Gola (eds.), *Inactivation of hypersensitive neurons*. Alan R.Liss: New York, 137–145 (1987b).

Somjen, G.G., Segal, M.B., and Herreras, O. Osmotic-hypertensive opening of the blood-brain barrier in rats does not necessarily provide access for potassium to cerebral interstitial fluid. *Exp. Physiol.* 76, 507–514 (1991).

Somjen, G.G. and Tombaugh, G.C. pH modulation of neuronal excitability and central nervous system functions. In K. Kaila and B.R. Ransom (eds.), *pH and Brain Function*. Wiley: New York, 373–393 (1998).

Sommer, W. Erkrankung des Ammonshorns als aetiologisches Moment der Epilepsie. *Arch. Psychiatr. Nervenkr.* 10, 631–675 (1880).

Sonnen, A.E.H. Alternative and folk remedies. In J. Engel, Jr., and T.A. Pedley (eds.), *Epilepsy: a comprehensive textbook*, Vol. 2. Lippincott-Raven: Philadelphia, 1365–1378 (1998).

Sontheimer, H. and Ritchie, M. Voltage gated sodium and calcium channels. In H. Kettenmann and B.R. Ransom (eds.), *Neuroglia*. Oxford University Press: New York, 202–220 (1995).

Sørensen, S.C. Factors regulating [H$^+$] and [HCO$_3^-$] in brain extracellular fluid. In B.K. Siesjö and S.C. Sørensen (eds.), *Ion homeostasis of the brain*. Munksgaard: Copenhagen, 206–217 (1971).

Spampanato, J., Escayg, A., Meisler, M.H., and Goldin, A.L. Functional effects of two voltage-gated sodium channel mutations that cause generalized epilepsy with febrile seizures plus type 2. *J. Neurosci.* 21, 7481–7490 (2001).

Speckmann, E.-J. and Caspers, H. Die sogenannte Terminaldepolarisation und ihre Beziehung zur Wiederbelebungszeit des Gehirns. *Pflügers Arch.* 289, R1-R2 (1966).

Speckmann, E.-J. and Caspers, H. Verschiebungen des corticalen Bestandspotentials bei veränderungen der Ventilationsgrösse. *Pflügers Arch.* 310, 235–250 (1969).

Speckmann, E.-J. and Caspers, H. The effect of O$_2^-$ and CO$_2$-tensions in the nervous tissue on neuronal activity and DC potentials. In A. Rémond (ed.), *Handbook of electroencephalography and clinical neurophysiology*. Elsevier, Amsterdam, 2C-71–2C-89 (1974).

Speckmann, E.-J. and Elger, C.E. Introduction to the neurophysiological basis of the EEG and DC potentials. In E. Niedermeyer and F.H. Lopes da Silva (eds.), *Electroencephalography*. Williams & Wilkins: Baltimore, 15–27 (1999).

Spielmeyer, W. Die Pathogenese des epileptischen Krampfes. Histopathologischer Teil. *Z. Neurol. Psychiatrie* 109, 501–520 (1927).

Spielmeyer, W. Über örtliche Vulnerabilität. *Z. Neurol. Psychiatrie* 118, 1–16 (1929).

Šramka, M., Brozek, G., Bureš, J., and Nádvorník, P. Functional ablation by spreading depression: possible use in human stereotactic surgery. *Appl. Neurophysiol.* 40, 48–61 (1977).

Stagliano, N.E., Perez-Pinzon, M.A., Moskowitz, M.A., and Huang, P.L. Focal ischemic preconditioning induces rapid tolerance to middle cerebral artery occlusion in mice. *J. Cereb. Blood Flow Metab.* 19, 757–761 (1999).

Starr, M.S. The role of dopamine in epilepsy. *Synapse* 22, 159–194 (1996).

Stasheff, S.F., Bragdon, A.C., and Wilson, W.A. Induction of epileptiform activity in hippocampal slices by trains of electrical stimuli. *Brain Res.* 344, 296–302 (1985).

Stasheff, S.F., Hines, M., and Wilson, W.A. Axon terminal hyperexcitability associated with epileptogenesis in vitro. I. Origin of ectopic spikes. *J. Neurophysiol.* 70, 961–975 (1993).

Steinhäuser, C., Berger, T., Jabs, R., Frotscher, M., and Kettenmann, H. Voltage- and ligand-gated membrane currents of identified glial cells in the hippocampal slice. In W. Haschke, A.I. Roitbak, and E.-J. Speckmann (eds.), *Slow potential changes in the brain*. Birkhäuser: Boston, 179–190 (1993).

Steinhäuser, C., Tennigkeit, M., Matthies, H., and Gündel, J. Properties of the fast sodium channels in pyramidal neurones isolated from the CA1 and CA3 areas of the hippocampus of postnatal rats. *Pflügers Arch.* 415, 756–761 (1990).

Steinlein, O.K. Genes and mutations in idiopathic epilepsy. *Am. J. Med. Genet.* 106, 139–145 (2001).

Steinlein, O.K. and Noebels, J.L. Ion channels and epilepsy in man and mouse. *Curr. Opin. Genet. Dev.* 10, 286–291 (2000).

Steriade, M. and Amzica, F. Intracortical and corticothalamic coherency of fast spontaneous oscillations. *Proc. Natl. Acad. Sci. USA* 93, 2533–2538 (1996).

Steriade, M. and Amzica, F. Slow sleep oscillation, athymic K-complexes and their paroxysmal developments. *J. Sleep Res.* 7(Suppl. 1), 30–35 (1998).

Steriade, M., Amzica, F., Neckelmann, D., and Timofeev, I. Spike-wave complexes and fast components of cortically generated seizures. II. Extra- and intracellular patterns. *J. Neurophysiol.* 80, 1456–1479 (1998).

Steriade, M. and Contreras, D. Relations between cortical and thalamic cellular events during transition from sleep patterns to paroxysmal activity. *J. Neurosci.* 15, 623–642 (1995).

Steriade, M., Contreras, D., and Amzica, F. Synchronized sleep oscillations and their paroxysmal developments. *Trends Neurosci.* 17, 100–208 (1994).

Steriade, M., Jones, E.G., and Llinas, R. *Thalamic oscillations and signaling.* Wiley: New York (1990).

Steriade, M., Timofeev, I., and Grenier, F. Natural waking and sleep states: a view from inside neocortical neurons. *J. Neurophysiol.* 85, 1969–1985 (2001).

Straub, V.A., Staras, K., Kemenes, G., and Benjamin, P.R. Endogenous and network properties of *Lymnaea* feeding central pattern generator interneurons. *J. Neurophysiol.* 88, 1569–1583 (2002).

Streit, D.S., Ferreira Fo, C.R., and Martins-Ferreira, H. Spreading depression in isolated spinal cord. *J. Neurophysiol.* 74, 888–890 (1995).

Stringer, J.L. and Lothman, E.W. Maximal dentate gyrus activation: characteristics and alterations after repeated seizures. *J. Neurophysiol.* 62, 136–143 (1989).

Stringer, J.L., Williamson, J.M., and Lothman, E.W. Induction of paroxysmal discharges in the dentate gyrus: frequency dependence and relationship to afterdischarge production. *J. Neurophysiol.* 62, 126–135 (1989).

Strong, A.J., Dardis, R. Depolarisation phenomena in traumatic and ischaemic brain injury. In J.D. Pickard, C. Di Rocco, V.V. Dolenc, R. Fahlbusch, J. Lobo Antunes, M. Sindou, N. De Tribolet, C.A.F. Tulleken, M. Vapalahti (eds), *Advances and Technical Standards in Neurosurgery*, Vol 29, Springer-Verlag: Wien, in press (2003).

Strong, A.J., Fabricius, M., Boutelle, M.G., Hibbins, S.J., Hopwood, S.E., Jones, R., Parkin, M.C., and Lauritzen, M. Spreading and synchronous depressions in cortical activity in acutely injured human brain. *Stroke* 33, 2738–2743 (2002).

Strong, A.J., Harland, S.P., Meldrum, B.S., and Whittington, D.J. The use of in vivo fluorescence image sequences to indicate the occurrence and propagation of transient focal depolarizations in cerebral ischemia. *J. Cereb. Blood Flow Metab.* 16, 367–377 (1996).

Strong, A.J., Smith, S.E., Whittington, D.J., Meldrum, B.S., Parsons, A.A., Krupinski, J., Hunter, A.J., Patel, S., and Robertson, C. Factors influencing the frequency of fluorescence transients as markers of peri-infarct depolarizations in focal cerebral ischemia. *Stroke* 31, 214–222 (2000).

Study, R.E. and Barker, J.L. Diazepam and (—)-pentobarbital: fluctuation analysis reveals different mechanisms for potentiation of gamma-aminobutyric acid responses in cultured central neurons. *Proc. Natl. Acad. Sci. USA* 78, 7180–7184 (1981).

Stys, P.K., Waxman, S.G., and Ransom, B.R. Effects of temperature on evoked electrical activity and anoxic injury in CNS white matter. *J. Cereb. Blood Flow Metab.* 12, 977–986 (1992a).

Stys, P.K., Waxman, S.G., and Ransom, B.R. Ionic mechanisms of anoxic injury in mammalian CNS white matter: role of Na^+ channels and Na^+-Ca^{2+} exchanger. *J. Neurosci.* 12, 430–439 (1992b).

Su, H., Alroy, G., Kirson, E.D., and Yaari, Y. Extracellular calcium modulates persistent sodium current-dependent burst-firing in hippocampal pyramidal neurons. *J. Neurosci.* 21, 4173–4182 (2001).

Sugar, O. and Gerard, R.W. Anoxia and brain potentials. *J. Neurophysiol.* 1, 558–572 (1938).

Sugawara, T., Fujimura, M., Morita-Fujimura, Y., Kawase, M., and Chan, P.H. Mitochondrial release of cytochrome c corresponds to the selective vulnerability of hippocampal CA1 neurons in rats after transient global cerebral ischemia. *J. Neurosci.* 19;RC39, 1–6 (1999).

Sugaya, E., Goldring, S., and O'Leary, J.L. Intracellular potentials associated with dircet cortical response and seizure discharge in cat. *Electroencephalogr. Clin. Neurophysiol.* 17, 661–669 (1964).

Sugaya, E. and Karahashi, Y. Intra- and extracellular potentials from "idle" cells in cerebral cortex of cat. *Jpn. J. Physiol.* 21, 149–157 (1971).

Sugaya, E., Takato, M., and Noda, Y. Neuronal and glial activity during spreading depression in cerebral cortex of cat. *J. Neurophysiol.* 38, 822–841 (1975).

Suter, K.J., Wuarin, J.P., Dudek, F.E., and Moenter, S.M. Whole-cell recording from preoptic/hypothalamic slices reveal burst firing in gonadotropin-releasing hormone neurons identified with green fluorescent protein in transgenic mice. *Endocrinology* 141, 3731–3736 (2000).

Sutula, T., He, X.X., Cavazos, J., and Scott, G. Synaptic reorganization in the hippocampus induced by abnormal functional activity. *Science* 239, 1147–1150 (1988).

Sutula, T.P. and Pitkänen, A. More evidence for seizure-induced neuron loss: is hippocampal sclerosis both cause and effect of epilepsy? *Neurology* 57, 169–170 (2001).

Sutula, T.P. and Pitkänen, A. (eds.). *Do seizures damage the brain?* Elsevier: Amsterdam (2002).

Suzuki, R., Yamaguchi, T., Kirino, T., Orzi, F., and Klatzo, I. The effect of 5-minute ischemia in Mongolian gerbils: I. Blood-brain barrier, cerebral blood flow, and local cerebral glucose utilization changes. *Acta Neuropathol.* 60, 216–1983a).

Suzuki, R., Yamaguchi, T., Li, C.-L., and Klatzo, I. The effect of 5-minute ischemia in Mongolian gerbils: II. Changes of spontaneous neuronal activity in cerebral cortex and CA1 sector of hippocampus. *Acta Neuropathol.* 60, 217–222 (1983b).

Svoboda, J., Motin, V., Hajek, I., and Syková, E. Increase in extracellular potassium level in rat spinal dorsal horn induced by noxious stimulation and peripheral injury. *Brain Res.* 458, 97–105 (1988).

Swartzwelder, H.S., Lewis, D.V., Anderson, W.W., and Wilson, W.A. Seizure-like events in brain slices: suppression by interictal activity. *Brain Res.* 410, 362–366 (1987).

Syková, E., Rothenberg, S., and Krekule, I. Changes in extracellular potassium concentration during spontaneous activity in the mesencephalic reticular formation of the rat. *Brain Res.* 79, 333–337 (1974).

Syková, E., Vargová, L., Kubinova, Š., Jendelová, P., and Chvátal, A. The relationship between changes in intrinsic optical signals and cell swelling in rat spinal cord slices. *NeuroImage* 18, 214–230 (2003).

Sypert, G.W. and Ward, A.A. Changes in extracellular potassium activity during neocortical propagated seizures. *Exp. Neurol.* 45, 19–41 (1974).

Szabó, C.A. and Lüders, H.O. Todd's paralysis and postictal aphasia. In H.O. Lüders and S. Noachtar (eds.), *Epileptic seizures*. Churchill Livingstone: New York, 652–657 (2000).

Szatkowski, M., Barbour, B., and Attwell, D. Non-vesicular release of glutamate from glial cells by reversed electrogenic glutamate uptake. *Nature* 348, 443–446 (1990).

Szerb, J.C. Glutamate release and spreading depression in the fascia dentata in response to microdialysis with high K$^+$: role of glia. *Brain Res.* 542, 259–265 (1991).

Takadera, T., Shimada, Y., and Mohri, T. Extracellular pH modulates *N*-methyl-D-aspartate receptor-mediated neurotoxicity and calcium accumulation in rat cortical cultures. *Brain Res.* 572, 126–131 (1992).

Takahashi, T. Activation methods. In E. Niedermeyer and F.H. Lopes da Silva (eds.), *Electroencephalography.* Wiliams & Wilkins: Baltimore, 261–284 (1999).

Takeda, A. Zinc homeostasis and functions of zinc in the brain. *BioMetals* 14, 343–351 (2001).

Tallon-Baudry, C., Bertrand, O., and Pernier, J. A ring-shaped distribution of dipoles as a source model of induced gamma-band activity. *Clin. Neurophysiol.* 110, 660–665 (1999).

Tallon-Baudry, C., Bertrand, O., Peronnet, F., and Pernier, J. Induced γ-band activity during the delay of a visual short-term memory task in humans. *J. Neurosci.* 18, 4244–4254 (1998).

Tanaka, E., Yamamoto, S., Kudo, Y., Mihara, S., and Higashi, H. Mechanisms underlying the rapid depolarization produced by deprivation of oxygen and glucose in rat hippocampal CA1 neurons in vitro. *J. Neurophysiol.* 78, 891–902 (1997).

Tancredi, V., D'Arcangelo, G., Zona, C., Siniscalchi, A., and Avoli, M. Induction of epileptiform activity by temperature elevation in hippocampal slices from young rats: an in vitro model for febrile seizures? *Epilepsia* 33, 228–234 (1992).

Tancredi, V., Hwa, G.G., Zona, C., Brancati, A., and Avoli, M. Low magnesium epileptogenesis in the rat hippocampal slice: electrophysiological and pharmacological features. *Brain Res.* 511, 280–290 (1990).

Tank, D.W., Sugimori, M., Connor, J.A., and Llinas, R.R. Spatially resolved calcium dynamics of mammalian Purkinje cells in cerebellar slice. *Science* 242, 773–777 (1988).

Tao, L. Light scattering in brain slices measured with a photon counting fiber optic system. *J. Neurosci. Meth.* 101, 19–29 (2000).

Tao, L., Masri, D., Hrabêtová, S., and Nicholson, C. Light scattering in rat neocortical slices differs during spreading depression and ischemia. *Brain Res.* 952, 290–300 (2002).

Tauck, D.L. and Nadler, J.V. Evidence of functional mossy fiber sprouting in hippocampal formation of kainic acid treated rats. *J. Neurosci.* 5, 1016–1022 (1985).

Taylor, C.P. and Dudek, F.E. Synchronous neural afterdischarges in rat hippocampal slices without active chemical synapses. *Science* 218, 810–812 (1982).

Taylor, C.P. and Dudek, F.E. Excitation of hippocampal pyramidal cells by an electrical field effect. *J. Neurophysiol.* 52, 126–142 (1984).

Taylor, C.P. and Weber, M.L. Effect of temperature on synaptic function after reduced oxygen and glucose in hippocampal slices. *Neuroscience* 52, 555–562 (1993).

Tegtmeier, F. Differences between spreading depression and ischemia. In A. Lehmenkühler, K.-H. Grotemeyer, and F. Tegtmeier (eds.), *Migraine: basic mechanisms and treatment.* Urban & Schwarzenberg: München, 511–532 (1993).

Tekkök, S., Medina, I., and Krnjević, K. Intraneuronal [Ca^{2+}] changes induced by 2-deoxy-D-glucose in rat hipocampal slices. *J. Neurophysiol.* 81, 174–183 (1999).

Telfeian, A.E. and Connors, B.W. Layer-specific pathways for the horizontal propagation of epileptiform discharges in neocortex. *Epilepsia* 39, 700–708 (1998).

Temkin, O. *The falling sickness.* Johns Hopkins University Press: Baltimore (1971).

Theis, M., Jauch, R., Zhuo, L., Speidel, D., Wallraff, A., Döring, B., Frisch, C., Söhl, G., Teubner, B., Euwens, C., Huston, J., Steinhäuser, C., Messing, A., Heinemann, U., and Willecke, K. Accelerated hippocampal spreading depression and enhanced locomotor activity in mice with astrocyte-directed inactivation of connexin43. *J. Neurosci.* 23, 766–776 (2003).

Theodore, W. and Wasterlain, C.G. Do early seizures beget epilepsy? *Neurology* 53, 898–899 (1999).

Thomas, E. and Grisar, T. Increased synchrony with increase of a low-threshold calcium conductance in a model thalamic network: a phase-shift mechanism. *Neural Comput.* 12, 1553–1571 (2000).

Thompson, S.M. and Gähwiler, B.H. Activity-dependent disinhibition. I. Repetitive stimulation reduces IPSP driving force and conductance in hippocampus in vitro. *J. Neurophysiol.* 61, 501–511 (1989a).

Thompson, S.M. and Gähwiler, B.H. Activity-dependent disinhibition. II. Effects of extracellular potassium, furosemide and membrane potential on E_{Cl^-} in hippocampal CA neurons. *J. Neurophysiol.* 61, 512–523 (1989b).

Thümmler, S. and Dunwiddie, T.V. Adenosine receptor antagonists induce persistent bursting in the hippocampal CA3 region vio and NMDA receptor-dependent mechanism. *J. Neurophysiol.* 83, 1787–1795 (2000).

Tobiasz, C. and Nicholson, C. Tetrodotoxin resistant propagation and extracellular sodium changes during spreading depression in rat cerebellum. *Brain Res.* 241, 329–333 (1982).

Tombaugh, G.C. Mild acidosis delays hypoxic spreading depression and improves neuronal recovery in rat hippocampal slices. *J. Neurosci.* 14, 5635–5643 (1994).

Tombaugh, G.C. Intracellular pH buffering shapes activity-dependent Ca^{2+} dynamics in dendrites of CA1 interneurons. *J. Neurophysiol.* 80, 1702–1712 (1998).

Tombaugh, G.C. and Sapolsky, R.M. Evolving concepts about the role of acidosis in ischemic neuropathology. *J. Neurochem.* 61, 793–803 (1993).

Tombaugh, G.C. and Somjen, G.G. Effects of extracellular pH on voltage-gated Na^+, K^+ and Ca^{2+} currents in isolated rat CA1 neurons. *J. Physiol.* 493, 719–732 (1996).

Tombaugh, G.C. and Somjen, G.G. pH modulation of voltage gated ion channels. In K. Kaila and B.R. Ransom (eds.), *pH and brain function.* Wiley: New York, 395–416 (1998).

Tomita, T. Spreading depression potential (SDP). in the frog retina. *An. Acad. Bras. Cienc.* 56, 505–518 (1984).

Tomkins, O., Kaufer, D., Korn, A., Shelef, I., Golan, H., Reichenthal, E., Soreq, H., and Friedman, A. Frequent blood-brain barrier disruption in the human cerebral cortex. *Cell. Mol. Neurobiol.* 21, 675–691 (2001).

Tong, C.K. and Chesler, M. Endogenous pH shifts facilitate spreading depression by effect on NMDA receptors. *J. Neurophysiol.* 81, 1988–1991 (1999).

Tong, C.K. and Chesler, M. Modulation of spreading depression by changes in extracellular pH. *J. Neurophysiol.* 84, 2449–2457 (2000).

Torp, R., Arvin, B., Le Peillet, E., Chapman, A.G., Ottersen, O.P., and Meldrum, B.S. Effect of ischaemia and reperfusion on the distribution of the extra- and intracellular distribution of glutamate, glutamine, aspartate and GABA in the rat hippocampus, with a note on the effect of the sodium channel blocker BW1003C87. *Exp. Brain Res.* 96, 365–376 (1993).

Towe, A.L., Mann, M.D., and Harding, G.W. On the currents that flow during the strychnine spike. *Electroencephalogr. Clin. Neurophysiol.* 51, 306–327 (1981).

Tower, D.B. Distribution of cerebral fluids and electrolytes *in vivo* and *in vitro.* In I. Klatzo and F. Seitelberg (eds.), *Brain Edema,* Springer, Wien, 303–332 (1967).

Tower, D.B. and Young, O.M. The activities of butyrylcholinesterase and carbonic anhydrase, the rate of anaerobic glycolysis, and the question of constant density of glial cells in cerebral cortices of various mammalian species from mouse to whale. *J. Neurochem.* 20, 269–278 (1973).

Trachtenberg, M.C. and Pollen, D.A. Neuroglia: biophysical properties and physiological function. *Science* 167, 1248–1252 (1970).

Trapp, S., Luckermann, M., Kaila, K., and Ballanyi, K. Acidosis of hippocampal neurones mediated by a plasmalemmal Ca^{2+}/H^+ pump. *NeuroReport* 7, 2000–2004 (1996).

Traub, R.D., Borck, C., Colling, S.B., and Jefferys, J.G.R. On the structure of ictal events in vitro. *Epilepsia* 37, 879–891 (1996a).

Traub, R.D. and Dingledine, R. Model of synchronized epileptiform bursts induced by high potassium in CA3 region of rat hippocampal slice. Role of spontaneous EPSPs in initiation. *J. Neurophysiol.* 64, 1009–1018 (1990).

Traub, R.D., Dudek, F.E., Taylor, C.P., and Knowles, W.D. Simulation of hippocampal afterdischarges synchronized by electrical interactions. *Neuroscience* 14, 1033–1038 (1985).

Traub, R.D. and Jefferys, J.G.R. Are there unifying principles underlying the generation of epileptic afterdischarges in vitro? *Prog. Brain Res.* 102, 383–394 (1994).

Traub, R.D. and Jefferys, J.G.R. Epilepsy in vitro: electrophysiology and computer modeling. In J. Engel, Jr., and T.A. Pedley (eds.), *Epilepsy: a comprehensive textbook*, Vol. 1. Lippincott-Raven: Philadelphia, 405–418 (1998).

Traub, R.D., Jefferys, J.G.R., and Whittington, M.A. Simulation of gamma rhythms in networks of interneurons and pyramidal cells. *J. Comput. Neurosci.* 4, 141–150 (1997).

Traub, R.D., Jefferys, J.G.R., and Whittington, M.A. Functionally relevant and functionally disruptive (epileptic). synchronized oscillations in brain slices. *Adv. Neurol.* 79, 709–724 (1999a).

Traub, R.D. and Llinas, R. Hippocampal pyramidal cells: significance of dendritic ionic conductances for neuronal function and epileptogenesis. *J. Neurophysiol.* 42, 476–496 (1979).

Traub, R.D., Miles, R., and Jefferys, J.G.R. Synaptic and intrinsic conductances shape picrotoxin-induced after-discharges in the guinea-pig hippocampal slice. *J. Physiol.* 461, 525–547 (1993).

Traub, R.D., Miles, R., and Wong, R.K.S. Models of synchronized hippocampal bursts in the presence of inhibition. I. Single population events. *J. Neurophysiol.* 58, 739–751 (1987).

Traub, R.D., Whittington, M.A., Buhl, E.H., Jefferys, J.G.R., and Faulkner, H.J. On the mechanism of the $\gamma \rightarrow \beta$ frequency shift in neuronal oscillations induced in rat hippocampal slices by tetanic stimulation. *J. Neurosci.* 19, 1088–1105 (1999b).

Traub, R.D., Whittington, M.A., Buhl, E.H., LeBeau, F.E., Bibbig, A., Boyd, S., Cross, H., and Baldeweg, T. A possible role for gap junctions in generation of very fast EEG oscillations preceding the onset of, and perhaps initiating, seizures. *Epilepsia* 42, 153–170 (2001).

Traub, R.D., Whittington, M.A., Colling, S.B., Buzsáki, G., and Jefferys, J.G.R. Analysis of gamma rhythms in the rat hippocampus in vitro and in vivo. *J. Physiol.* 493, 471–484 (1996b).

Traynelis, S.F. pH modulation of ligand-gated ion channels. In K. Kaila and B.R. Ransom (eds.), *pH and brain function.* Wiley-Liss: New York, 417–446 (1998).

Traynelis, S.F. and Dingledine, R. Potassium-induced spontaneous electrographic seizures in the rat hippocampal slice. *J. Neurophysiol.* 59, 259–276 (1988).

Traynelis, S.F. and Dingledine, R. Modification of potassium-induced interictal bursts and electrographic seizures by divalent cations. *Neurosci. Lett.* 98, 194–199 (1989).

Treiman, D.M. GABAergic mechanisms in epilepsy. *Epilepsia* 42 (Suppl. 3), 8–12 (2001).

Treiman, D.M. and Heinemann, U. Experimental models of status epilepticus. In J. Engel, Jr., and T.A. Pedley (eds.), *Epilepsy: a comprehensive textbook*, Vol. 1. Lippincott-Raven: Philadelphia, 443–455 (1998).

Truong-Tran, A.Q., Carter, J., Ruffin, R.E., and Zalewski, P.D. The role of zinc in caspase activation and apoptotic cell death. *BioMetals* 14, 315–330 (2001).

Tsakiridou, E., Bertolini, L., de Curtis, M., Avanzini, G., and Pape, H.C. Selective increase in T-type calcium conductance of reticular thalamic neurons in rat model of absence epilepsy. *J. Neurosci.* 15, 3110–3117 (1995).

Tschirgi, R.D. Blood-brain barrier: Fact or fancy? *Fed. Proc.* 21, 665–671 (1962).

Tsodyks, M.V. and Markram, H. The neural code between neocortical pyramidal neurons depends on neurotransmitter release probability. *Proc. Natl. Acad. Sci. USA* 94, 719–723 (1997).

Tsubokawa, H., Oguro, K., Masuzawa, T., and Kawai, N. Ca^{2+} dependent non-NMDA receptor mediated synaptic current in ischemic CA1 neurons. *J. Neurophysiol.* 71, 1190–1196 (1994).

Tuckwell, H.C. Simplified reaction-diffusion equations for potassium and calcium ion concentrations during spreading depression. *Int. J. Neurosci.* 12, 95–107 (1981).

Tuckwell, H.C. and Miura, R.M. A mathematical model for spreading cortical depression. *Biophys. J.* 23, 257–276 (1978).

Tuff, L.P., Racine, R.J., and Mishra, R.K. The effects of kindling on GABA-mediated inhibition in the dentate gyrus of the rat. II. Receptor binding. *Brain Res.* 277, 91–98 (1983).

Turner, D.A. and Fayuk, D.A. NADH/FAD imaging during hypoglycemia and ischemia in rat hippocampal slices. *Soc. Neurosci. Abstr.* Prog. No. 581.3 (2002).

Turner, D.A. and Schwartzkroin, P.A. Steady-state electrotonic analysis of intracellularly stained hippocampal neurons. *J. Neurophysiol.* 44, 184–199 (1980).

Turner, D.A. and Shetty, A.K. Clinical prospects for neural graft therapy for hippocampal lesions and epilepsy. *Neurosurgery* 52, 632–644 (2003).

Turski, L., Ikonomidou, C., Turski, W.A., Bortolotto, Z.A., and Cavalheiro, E.A. Review: cholinergic mechanisms and epileptogenesis. The seizures induced by pilocarpine: a novel experimental model of intractable epilepsy. *Synapse* 3, 154–171 (1989).

Twombly, D.A., Yoshii, M., and Narahashi, T. Mechanisms of calcium channel block by phenytoin. *J. Pharmacol. Exp. Ther.* 246, 189–195 (1988).

Urban, L., Aitken, P.G., Friedman, A., and Somjen, G.G. An NMDA-mediated component of excitatory synaptic input to dentate granule cells in "epileptic" human hippocampus studied in vitro. *Brain Res.* 515, 319–322 (1990a).

Urban, L., Neill, K.H., Crain, B.J., Nadler, J.V., and Somjen, G.G. Postischemic synaptic physiology in area CA1 of the gerbil hippocampus studied in vitro. *J. Neurosci.* 9, 3966–3975 (1989).

Urban, L., Neill, K.H., Crain, B.J., Nadler, J.V., and Somjen, G.G. Effects of transient forebrain ischemia in area CA1 of the gerbil hippocampus: an in vitro study. In Y. Ben-Ari (ed.), *Excitatory amino acids and neuronal plasticity*. Plenum Press: New York, 491–500 (1990b).

Urban, L., Neill, K.H., Crain, B.J., Nadler, J.V., and Somjen, G.G. Postischemic synaptic excitation and N-methyl-D-aspartate receptor activation in gerbils. *Stroke* 21, III23–III27 (1990c).

Urbán, L. and Somjen, G.G. Reversible effects of hypoxia on neurons in mouse dorsal root ganglia in vitro. *Brain Res.* 520, 36–42 (1990).

Urbanics, R., Leniger-Follert, E., and Lübbers, D.W. Time course of changes of extracellular H^+ and K^+ activities during and after direct electrical stimulation of the brain cortex. *Pflügers Arch.* 378, 47–53 (1978).

Uruno, K., O'Connor, M.J., and Masukawa, L.M. Alterations of inhibitory responses in the dentate gyrus of temporal lobe epileptic patients. *Hippocampus* 4, 583–593 (1994).

van Gelder, N.M. Calcium mobility and glutamic acid release associated with EEG abnormalities, migraine and epilepsy. In F. Andermann and E. Lugaresi (eds.), *Migraine and epilepsy.* Butterworth: Boston, 367–378 (1987).

Van Harreveld, A. Changes in the diameter of apical dendrites during spreading depression. *Am. J. Physiol.* 192, 457–463 (1958).

Van Harreveld, A. Compounds in brain extracts causing spreading depression of cerebral cortical activity and contraction of crustacean muscle. *J. Neurochem.* 3, 300–315 (1959).

Van Harreveld, A. Two mechanisms for spreading depression in the chicken retina. *J. Neurobiol.* 9, 419–431 (1978).

Van Harreveld, A., Crowell, J., and Malhotra, S.K. A study of extracellular space in central nervous tissue by freeze-substitution. *J. Cell Biol.* 25, 117–137 (1965).

Van Harreveld, A. and Fifková, E. Glutamate release from the retina during spreading depression. *J. Neurobiol.* 2, 13–29 (1970).

Van Harreveld, A. and Khattab, F.I. Changes in cortical extracellular space during spreading depression investigated with the electron microscope. *J. Neurophysiol.* 30, 911–929 (1967).

Van Harreveld, A. and Kooiman, M. Amino acid release from the cerebral cortex during spreading depression and asphyxiation. *J. Neurochem.* 12, 431–439 (1965).

Van Harreveld, A. and Ochs, S. Electrical and vascular concomitants of spreading depression. *Am. J. Physiol.* 189, 159–166 (1957).

Van Harreveld, A. and Schadé, J.P. Chloride movements in cerebral cortex after circulatory arrest and during spreading depression. *J. Cell. Comp. Physiol.* 54, 65–84 (1959).

Van Harreveld, A. and Schadé, J.P. On the distribution and movements of water and electrolytes in the cerebral cortex. In D.B. Tower and J.P. Schadé (eds.), *Structure and function of the cerebral cortex.* Elsevier: Amsterdam, 239–256 (1960).

Van Harreveld, A. and Stamm, J.S. Vascular concomitants of spreading cortical depression. *J. Neurophysiol.* 15, 487–496 (1952).

Van Harreveld, A. and Stamm, J.S. Cerebral asphyxiation and spreading cortical depression. *Am. J. Physiol.* 173, 171–175 (1953a).

Van Harreveld, A. and Stamm, J.S. Spreading cortical convulsions and depressions. *J. Neurophysiol.* 16, 352–366 (1953b).

Van Harreveld, A. and Stamm, J.S. Consequences of cortical convulsive activity in rabbit. *J. Neurophysiol.* 17, 505–520 (1955).

Van Harreveld, A., Stamm, J.S., and Christensen, E.I. Spreading depression in rabbit, cat and monkey. *Am. J. Physiol.* 184, 312–320 (1956).

Van Wylen, D.G.L., Park, T.S., Rubio, R., and Berne, R.M. Increase in cerebral interstitial fluid adenosine concentration during hypoxia, local potassium infusion and ischemia. *J. Cereb. Blood Flow Metab.* 6, 522–528 (1986).

Verkhratsky, A. and Kettenmann, H. Calcium signalling in glial cells. *Trends Neurosci.* 19, 346–352 (1996).

Vern, B.A., Schuette, W.H., Mutsuga, N., and Whitehouse, W.C. Effects of ischemia on the removal of extracellular potassium in cat cortex during pentylenetetrazol seizures. *Epilepsia* 20, 711–724 (1979).

Vezzani, A., Ravizza, T., Moneta, D., Conti, M., Borroni, A., Rizzi, M., Samanin, R., and Maj, R. Brain-derived neurotrophic factor immunoreactivity in the limbic system of rats after acute seizures and during spontaneous convulsions: temporal evolution of changes as compared to neuropeptide Y. *Neuroscience* 90, 1445–1461 (1999a).

Vezzani, A., Sperk, G., and Colmers, W.F. Neuropeptide Y: emerging evidence for a functional role in seizure modulation. *Trends Neurosci.* 22, 25–30 (1999b).

Világi, I., Klapka, N., and Luhmann, H.J. Optical recording of spreading depression in rat neocortical slices. *Brain Res.* 898, 288–296 (2001).

Vinogradova, L.V., Koroleva, V.I., and Bureš, J. Re-entry waves of Leão's spreading depression between neocortex and caudate nulceus. *Brain Res.* 538, 161–164 (1991).

Viveros, H. and Somjen, G.G. Magnesium-calcium antagonism in the contraction of arterioles. *Experientia* 24, 457–459 (1968).

Vogt, C. and Vogt, O. Erkrankungen der Grosshirnrinde im Lichte der Topistik, Pathoklise und Pathoarchitektonik. *J. Psychol. Neurol.* 28, 3–171 (1922).

Vogt, K., Mellor, J., Tong, G., and Nicoll, R. The actions of synaptically released zinc in hippocampal mossy fiber synapses. *Neuron* 26, 187–196 (2000).

Voipio, J. and Kaila, K. GABAergic excitation and K^+-mediated volume transmission in the hippocampus. *Prog. Brain Res.* 125, 329–338 (2000).

Voipio, J., Tallgren, P., Heinonen, E., Vanhatalo, S., and Kaila, K. Millivolt-scale DC shifts in the human scalp EEG: evidence for a non-neuronal generator. *J. Neurophysiol.* 89, 2208–2214 (2003).

Voskuyl, R.A. Basic mechanisms of antiepileptic drugs. In H. Meinardi (ed.), *Handbook of clinical neurology*, Vol. 73, *The epilepsies*, Part II. Elsevier: Amsterdam, 347–350 (2000).

Vreugdenhil, M., Faas, G.C., and Wadman, W.J. Sodium currents in isolated rat CA1 neurons after kindling epileptogenesis. *Neuroscience* 86, 99–107 (1998).

Vreugdenhil, M. and Wadman, W.J. Enhancement of calcium currents in rat hippocampal CA1 neurons induced by kindling epileptogenesis. *Neuroscience* 49, 373–381 (1992).

Vreugdenhil, M. and Wadman, W.J. Kindling-induced long-lasting enhancement of calcium current in hippocampal CA1 area of the rat: relation to calcium-dependent inactivation. *Neuroscience* 59, 105–114 (1994).

Vreugdenhil, M. and Wadman, W.J. Potassium currents in isolated CA1 neurons of the rat after kindling epileptogenesis. *Neuroscience* 66, 805–813 (1995).

Vreugdenhil, M. and Wadman, W.J. Modulation of sodium currents in rat CA1 neurons by carbamazepine and valproate after kindling epileptogenesis. *Epilepsia* 40, 1512–1522 (1999).

Vyskocil, F., Kriz, N., and Bureš, J. Potassium-selective microelectrodes used for measuring the extracellular brain potassium during spreading depression and anoxic depolarization in rats. *Brain Res.* 39, 255–259 (1972).

Wadman, W.J., Heinemann, U., Konnerth, A., and Neuhaus, S. Hippocampal slices of kindled rats reveal calcium involvement in epileptogenesis. *Brain Res.* 57, 404–407 (1985).

Wadman, W.J., Juta, A.J.A., Kamphuis, W., and Somjen, G.G. Current source density of sustained potential shifts associated with electrographic seizures and with spreading depression in rat hippocampus. *Brain Res.* 570, 85–91 (1992).

Walker, J.L. Ion specific liquid ion exchanger microelectrodes. *Anal. Chem.* 43, 89A–93A (1971).

Walton, J. *Brain's diseases of the nervous system.* Oxford University Press: Oxford (1985).

Walton, M., Connor, B., Lawlor, P., Young, D., Sirimanne, E., Gluckman, P., Cole, G., and Dragunow, M. Neuronal death and survival in two models of hypoxic-ischemic brain damage. *Brain Res. Rev.* 29, 137–168 (1999).

Walz, W. Swelling and potassium uptake in cultured astrocytes. *Can. J. Physiol. Pharmacol.* 65, 1051–1057 (1987).

Walz, W. Distribution and transport of chloride and bicarbonate ions across membranes. In H. Kettenmann and B.R. Ransom (eds.), *Neuroglia*. Oxford University Press: New York, 221–229 (1995).

Walz, W. Role of astrocytes in the spreading depression signal between ischemic core and penumbra. *Neurosci. Biobehav. Rev.* 21, 135–142 (1997).

Walz, W. Controversy surrounding the existence of discrete functional classes of astrocytes in adult gray matter. *Glia* 31, 95–103 (2000a).

Walz, W. Role of astrocytes in the clearance of excess extracellular potassium. *Neurochem. Int.* 36, 291–300 (2000b).

Walz, W. Chloride/anion channels in glial cell membranes. *Glia* 40, 1–10 (2002).

Walz, W. and Hertz, L. Intracellular ion changes of astrocytes in response to extracellular potassium. *J. Neurosci. Res.* 10, 411–423 (1983).

Walz, W. and MacVicar, B.A. Electrophysiological properties of glial cells: comparison of brain slices with primary cultures. *Brain Res.* 443, 321–324 (1988).

Walz, W. and Wuttke, W.A. Independent mechanisms of potassium clearance by astrocytes in gliotic tissue. *J. Neurosci. Res.* 56, 595–603 (1999).

Wang, J., Chambers, G., Cottrell, J.E., and Kass, I.S. Differential fall in ATP accounts for effects of temperature on hypoxic damage in rat hippocampal slices. *J. Neurophysiol.* 83, 3462–3472 (2000).

Ward, A.A. The epileptic neuron: Chronic foci in animals and man. In H.H. Jasper, A.A. Ward, and A. Pope (eds.), *Basic mechanisms of the epilepsies*. Little, Brown: Boston, 263–288 (1969).

Waxman, S.G. Transcriptional channelopathies: an emerging class of disorders. *Nature Rev.* 2, 652–659 (2001).

Waxman, S.G. Chair's introduction: sodium chanels and neuronal dysfunction—emerging concepts, converging themes. *Novartis Found. Symp.* 241, 1–4 (2002).

Weiss, J.H., Sensi, S.L., and Koh, J.-Y. Zn^{2+}: a novel ionic mediator of neural injury in brain disease. *Trends Pharmacol. Sci.* 21, 395–401 (2000).

Welsh, F.A. Role of vascular factors in regional ischemic injury. In K. Kogure, K.-A. Hossmann, B.K. Siesjö, and F.A. Welsh (eds.), *Molecular mechanisms of ischemic brain damage*. Elsevier: Amsterdam, 19–27 (1995).

Wenzel, H.J., Wooley, C.S., Robbins, C.A., and Schwartzkroin, P.A. Kainic acid-induced mossy fiber sprouting and synapse formation in the dentate gyrus of rats. *Hippocampus* 10, 244–260 (2000).

Westrum, L.E. and Blackstad, T.W. An electron microscopic study of stratum radiatum of the rat hippocampus (regio superior, CA1) with particular emphasis on synaptology. *J. Comp. Neurol.* 119, 281–309 (1962).

White, J.A., Alonso, A., and Kay, A.R. A heart-like Na^+ current in the medial entorhinal cortex. *Neuron* 11, 1037–1047 (1993).

Whitney, K.D. and McNamara, J.O. Autoimmunity and neurological disease. *Annu. Rev. Neurosci.* 22, 175–195 (1999).

Whittington, M.A., Traub, R.D., and Jefferys, J.G.R. Erosion of inhibition contributes to the progression of low magnesium bursts in rat hippocampal slices. *J. Physiol.* 486, 723–734 (1995).

Wieser, H.G. Historical review of cortical electrical stimulation. In H.O. Lüders and S. Noachtar (eds.), *Epileptic seizures: pathophysiology and clinical semiology*. Churchill Livingstone: New York, 141–152 (2000).

Wiley, J.W., Gross, R.A., Lu, Y., and MacDonald, R.L. Neuropeptide Y reduces calcium currents and inhibits acetylkcholine release in nodose neurons via a pertussis toxin-sensitive mechanism. *J. Neurophysiol.* 63, 1499–1507 (1990).

Williams, S.R., Toth, T.I., Turner, J.P., Hughes, S.W., and Crunelli, V. The "window" component of the low threshold Ca^{2+} current produces signal amplification and bistability in cat and rat thalamocortical neurones. *J. Physiol.* 505, 689–705 (1997).

Williamson, P.D. and Engel, J. Jr. Complex partial seizures. In J. Engel, Jr., and T.A. Pedley, (eds.), *Epilepsy: a comprehensive textbook*, Vol. 1. Lippincott-Raven: Philadelphia, 557–566 (1998).

Wilson, C.L., Maidment, N.T., Shomer, M.H., Behnke, E.J., Ackerson, L., Fried, I., and Engel, J., Jr. Comparison of seizure related amino acid release in human epileptic hippocampus versus a chronic, kainate rat model of hippocampal epilepsy. *Epilepsy Res.* 26, 245–254 (1996).

Wilson, W.A. and Wachtel, H. Negative resistance characteristics essential fo the maintenance of slow oscillations in bursting neurons. *Science* 186, 932–934 (1974).

Withrow, C.D. The ketoigenic diet: mechanism of anticonvulsant action. In G.H. Glaser, J.K. Penry, and D.M. Woodbury (eds.), *Antiepileptic drugs: mechanisms of action.* Raven Press: New York, 635–642 (1980).

Wolf, T., Lindauer, U., Obrig, H., Villringer, A., and Dirnagl, U. Extra- and intracellular oxygen supply during cortical spreading depression in the rat. *Adv. Exp. Med. Biol.* 388, 299–304 (1996).

Wong, R.K.S., Prince, D.A., and Basbaum, A.I. Intradendritic recordings from hippocampal neurons. *Proc. Natl. Acad. Sci. USA* 76, 986–990 (1979).

Wong, R.K.S. and Traub, R.D. Synchronized burst discharge in disinhibited hippocampal slice. I. Initiation in CA2-CA3 region. *J. Neurophysiol.* 49, 442–458 (1983).

Woodbury, D.M. Carbonic anhydrase inhibitors. In G.H. Glaser, J.K. Penry, and D.M. Woodbury (eds.), *Antiepileptic drugs: mechanisms of action.* Raven Press: New York, 617–633 (1980).

Wrogemann, K. and Pena, S.D.J. Mitochondrial calcium overload: a general mechanism for cell necrosis in muscle diseases. *Lancet* 1, 672–674 (1976).

Wuarin, J.-P. and Dudek, F.E. Excitatory synaptic input to granule cells increases with time after kainate treatment. *J. Neurophysiol.* 85, 1067–1077 (2001).

Wyler, A.R. and Ward, A.A. Epileptic neurons. In J.S. Lockard and A.A. Ward (eds.), *Epilepsy: window to brain mechanisms.* Raven Press: New York, 51–68 (1980).

Wynick, D., Thompson, S.W., and McMahon, S.B. The role of galanin as a multifunctional neuropeptide in the nervous system. *Curr. Opin. Pharmacol.* 1, 73–77 (2001).

Xie, X., Lancaster, B., Peakman, T., and Garthwaite, J. Interaction of the antiepileptic drug lamotrigine with recombinant rat brain type IIA Na^+ channels and with native Na^+ channels in rat hippocampal neurones. *Pflügers Arch.* 430, 437–446 (1995a).

Xie, Y., Dengler, K., Zacharias, E., Wilffert, B., and Tegtmeier, F. Effects of the sodium channel blocker tetrodotoxin (TTX) on cellular ion homeostasis in rat brain subjected to complete ischemia. *Brain Res.* 652, 216–224 (1994).

Xie, Y., Zacharias, E., Hoff, P., and Tegtmeier, F. Ion channel involvement in anoxic depolarization induced by cardiac arrest in rat brain. *J. Cereb. Blood Flow Metab.* 15, 587–594 (1995b).

Xiong, Z. and MacDonald, J.F. A novel non-selective cation channel which behaves as a calcium sensing receptor (CaSR) in hippocampal neurons. *Soc. Neurosci. Abstr.* 22, 2101–1996).

Xiong, Z.G. and MacDonald, J.F. Sensing of extracellular calcium by neurones. *Can. J. Physiol. Pharmacol.* 77, 715–721 (1999).

Xiong, Z.-G., Chu, X.-P., and MacDonald, J.F. Effect of lamotrigine on the Ca^{2+}-sensing cation current in cultured hippocampal neurons. *J. Neurophysiol.* 86, 2520–2526 (2001).

Xiong, Z.-G., Lu, W.-Y., and MacDonald, J.F. Extracellular calcium sensed by a novel cation channel in hippocampal neurons. *Proc. Natl. Acad. Sci. USA* 94, 7012–7017 (1997).

Xu, Z.C. and Pulsinelli, W.A. Electrophysiological changes of CA1 pyramidal neurons following transient forebrain ischemia: an in vivo intracellular recording and staining study. *J. Neurophysiol.* 76, 1689–1697 (1996).

Yaari, Y., Konnerth, A., and Heinemann, U. Spontaneous epileptiform activity of CA1 hippocampal neurons in low extracellular calcium solutions. *Exp. Brain Res.* 51, 153–156 (1983).

Yaari, Y., Konnerth, A., and Heinemann, U. Nonsynaptic epileptogenesis in the mammalian hippocampus in vitro. II. Role of extracellular potassium. *J. Neurophysiol.* 56, 424–438 (1986).

Yamamoto, C. and Kawai, N. Generation of the seizure discharge in thin sections from the guinea pig brain in chloride-free medium in vitro. *Jpn. J. Physiol.* 18, 620–631 (1968).

Yoon, R.S., Tsang, P.W., Lenz, F.A., and Kwan, H.C. Characterization of cortical spreading depression by imaging of intrinsic optical signals. *NeuroReport* 7, 2671–2674 (1996).

Young, J.N., Aitken, P.G., and Somjen, G.G. Calcium, magnesium, and long-term recovery from hypoxia in hippocampal tissue slices. *Brain Res.* 548, 343–345 (1991).

Young, J.N. and Somjen, G.G. Suppression of presynaptic calcium currents by hypoxia in hippocampal tissue slices. *Brain Res.* 573, 70–76 (1992).

Young, W. Spreading depression in elasmobranch cerebellum. *Brain Res.* 199, 113–126 (1980).

Yu, S.P., Canzoniero, L.M.T., and Choi, D.W. Ion homeostasis and apoptosis. *Curr. Opin. Cell Biol.* 13, 405–411 (2001).

Yu, S.P. and Choi, D.W. Ions, cell volume, and apoptosis. *Proc. Natl. Acad. Sci. USA* 97, 9360–9362 (2000).

Yuste, R. and Bonhoefer, T. Morphological changes in dendritic spines associated with long-term synaptic plasticity. *Annu. Rev. Neurosci.* 24, 1071–1089 (2001).

Yuste, R., Nelson, D.A., Rubin, W.W., and Katz, L.C. Neuronal domains in developing neocortex: mechanisms of coactivation. *Neuron* 14, 7–17 (1995).

Zhang, L. and Krnjević, K. Whole cell recording of anoxic effects on hippocampal neurons in slices. *J. Neurophysiol.* 69, 118–127 (1993).

Zhang, X., Cui, S.-S., Wallace, A.E., Hannesson, D.K., Schmued, L.C., Saucier, D.M., Honer, W.G., and Corcoran, M.E. Relations between brain pathology and temporal lobe epilepsy. *J. Neurosci.* 22, 6052–6061 (2002).

Zhang, Y. and Lipton, P. Cytosolic Ca^{2+} changes during in vitro ischemia in rat hippocampal slices: major roles for glutamate and Na^+-dependent Ca^{2+} release from mitochondria. *J. Neurosci.* 19, 3307–3315 (1999).

Zhang, Y.-F. and Coulter, D.A. Anticonvulsant drug effects on spontaneous thalamocortical rhythms in vitro: phenytoin, carbamazepine and phenobarbital. *Epilepsy Res.* 23, 55–70 (1996).

Zhang, Y.-F., Gibbs, J.W., and Coulter, D.A. Anticonvulsant drug effects on spontaneous thalamocortical rhythms in vitro: ethosuximide, trimethadione and dimethadione. *Epilepsy Res.* 23, 15–36 (1996a).

Zhang, Y.-F., Gibbs, J.W., and Coulter, D.A. Anticonvulsant drug effects on spontaneous thalamocortical rhythms in vitro: valproic acid, clonazepam and α-methyl-α-phenylsuccinimide. *Epilepsy Res.* 23, 37–53 (1996b).

Zhao, Y.-T. and Krnjević, K. 2-Deoxyglucose-induced long-term potentiation in CA1 is not prevented by intraneuronal chelator. *J. Neurophysiol.* 83, 177–180 (2000).

Zhou, M. and Kimelberg, H.K. Freshly isolated astrocytes from rat hippocampus show two distinct current patterns and different [K$^+$]$_o$ uptake capabilities. *J. Neurophysiol.* 84, 2746–2757 (2000).

Zhou, M. and Kimelberg, H.K. Freshly isolated hippocampal CA1 astrocytes comprise two populations differing in glutamate transporter and AMPA receptor expression. *J. Neurosci.* 21, 7901–7908 (2001).

Zhou, M., Schools, G.P., and Kimelberg, H.K. GFAP mRNA positive glia acutely isolated from rat hippocampus predominantly show complex current patterns. *Mol. Brain Res.* 76, 121–131 (2000).

Zhu, D.Y., Liu, S.H., Sun, H.S., and Lu, Y.M. Expression of inducible nitric oxide synthase after focal cerebral ischemia stimulates neurogenesis in the adult rodent dentate gyrus. *J. Neurosci.* 23, 223–229 (2003).

Zhu, P.J. and Krnjević, K. Anoxia selectively depresses excitatory synaptic transmission in hippocampal slices. *Neurosci. Lett.* 166, 27–30 (1994).

Zhu, P.J. and Krnjević, K. Persistent block of CA1 synaptic function by prolonged hypoxia. *Neuroscience* 90, 759–770 (1999).

Zini, S., Roisin, M.P., Langel, U., Bartfai, T., and Ben-Ari, Y. Galanin reduces release of endogenous excitatory amino acids in the rat hippocampus. *Eur. J. Pharmacol.* 245, 1–7 (1993).

Zoratti, M. and Szabó, I. The mitochondrial permeability transition. *Biochim. Biophys. Acta* 1241, 139–176 (1995).

Zuckermann, E.C. and Glaser, G.H. Hippocampal epileptic activity induced by localized ventricular perfusion with high-potassium cerebrospinal fluid. *Exp. Neurol.* 20, 87–110 (1968).

Zuckermann, E.C. and Glaser, G.H. Activation of experimental epileptogenic foci. Action of increased K$^+$ in extracellular spaces of brain. *Arch. Neurol.* 23, 358–364 (1970a).

Zuckermann, E.C. and Glaser, G.H. Slow potential shifts in dorsal hippocampus during "epileptogenic" perfusion of the inferior horn with high-potassium CSF. *Electroencephalogr. Clin. Neurophysiol.* 28, 236–246 (1970b).

Zweig, S. *Drei Meister*. Fischer: Frankfurt am Main (1958).

Index

Note: Page numbers followed by *f* and *t* indicate figures and tables, respectively.